Biological Approaches to Cancer Treatment

Biomodulation

NOTICE

Medicine is an ever-changing science. As new research and clinical experience broaden our knowledge, changes in treatment and drug therapy are required. The editors and publisher of this work have checked with sources believed to be reliable in their efforts to provide information that is complete and generally in accord with the standards accepted at the time of publication. However, in view of the possibility of human error or changes in medical sciences, neither the editors, the publisher, nor any other party who has been involved in the preparation or publication of this work warrants that the information contained herein is in every respect accurate or complete, and they are not responsible for any errors or omissions or for the results obtained from use of such information. Readers are encouraged to confirm the information contained herein with other sources. For example and in particular, readers are advised to check the product information sheet included in the package of each drug they plan to administer to be certain that the information contained in this book is accurate and that changes have not been made in the recommended dose or in the contraindications for administration. This recommendation is of particular importance in connection with new or infrequently used drugs.

Biological Approaches to Cancer Treatment

Biomodulation

EDITOR

Malcolm S. Mitchell, M.D.

Professor of Medicine and Microbiology
Kenneth J. Norris, Jr. Comprehensive Cancer Center
University of Southern California
Los Angeles, California

McGraw-Hill, Inc.
Health Professions Division

New York
St. Louis
San Francisco
Auckland
Bogotá
Caracas
Lisbon
London
Madrid
Mexico
Milan
Montreal
New Delhi
Paris
San Juan
Singapore
Sydney
Tokyo
Toronto

Biological Approaches to Cancer Treatment: Biomodulation

1234567890 DOCDOC 98765432

ISBN 0-07-105397-2

This book was set in Times Roman and Helvetica by Compset, Inc. The editors were Jane E. Pennington and Mariapaz Ramos Englis; the production supervisor was Richard Ruzycka. The project was supervised by Faye Zucker Editorial Service. The printer and binder was R.R. Donnelley & Sons Company.

Library of Congress Cataloging-in-Publication Data

Biological approaches to cancer treatment : biomodulation / edited by Malcolm S. Mitchell.
p. cm.
Includes bibliographical references and index.
ISBN 0-07-105397-2
1. Biological response modifiers—Therapeutic use. 2. Cancer—Immunotherapy. I. Mitchell, Malcolm S.
[DNLM: 1. Biological Response Modifiers—therapeutic use. 2. Immunity, Natural. 3. Immunotherapy. 4. Neoplasms—immunology. 5. Neoplasms—therapy. QW 541 B615]
RC271.B53B57 1992
616.99'406—dc20
DNLM/DLC
for Library of Congress 91-2570
CIP

CONTENTS

CONTRIBUTORS

Paul G. Abrams, M.D., University of Washington School of Medicine, Seattle, Washington 98195; NeoRx Corporation, 410 West Harrison, Seattle, Washington 98119 [12]

Darrell R. Anderson, Ph.D., IDEC Pharmaceuticals Corporation, 11099 North Torrey Pines Road, La Jolla, California 92037 [7]

Robert W. Baldwin, Ph.D., Cancer Research Campaign Laboratories, University of Nottingham, University Park, Nottingham NG7 2RD, England [11]

William C. Biddle, Ph.D., Life Technologies, Inc., 3175 Staley Road, Grand Island, New York 14072 [10]

Reinder L. H. Bolhuis, M.D., Ph.D., Department of Immunology, Dr. Daniel den Hoed Cancer Center, Groene Hilledijk 301, 3075 EA Rotterdam, The Netherlands [3]

Ernest C. Borden, M.D., Departments of Medicine, Microbiology, and Pediatrics, Medical College of Wisconsin Cancer Center, 8701 Watertown Plank Road, Milwaukee, Wisconsin 53226 [18]

Valerie I. Brown, University of Pennsylvania School of Medicine, 36th and Hamilton Walk, Philadelphia, Pennsylvania 19104 [1]

Numbers in brackets refer to chapter authored or co-authored by the contributor.

Vera S. Byers, M.D., Ph.D., XOMA Corporation, 2910 7th Street, Berkeley, California 94710 [11]

Isaiah J. Fidler, D.V.M., Ph.D., Department of Cell Biology, The University of Texas, M. D. Anderson Cancer Center, 1515 Holcombe Boulevard, Houston, Texas 77030 [15]

Kenneth A. Foon, M.D., Division of Hematology-Oncology, The Scripps Research Institute, 10666 North Torrey Pines Road, La Jolla, California 92037 [10]

Alan R. Fritzberg, Ph.D., University of Washington School of Medicine, Seattle, Washington 98195; NeoRx Corporation, 410 West Harrison, Seattle, Washington 98119 [12]

Janice Lynn Gabrilove, M.D., Department of Hematology, Memorial Sloan-Kettering Cancer Center, 1275 York Avenue, New York, New York 10021 [19]

Donald L. Granger, B.S., Division of Infectious Diseases, Department of Medicine, Duke University Medical Center, Durham, North Carolina 27710 [2]

Jan Willem Gratama, M.D., Ph.D., Department of Immunology, Dr. Daniel den Hoed Cancer Center, Groene Hilledijk 301, 3075 EA Rotterdam, The Netherlands [3]

Mark I. Greene, M.D., Ph.D., Division of Immunology, Department of Pathology and Laboratory Medicine, University of Pennsylvania School of Medicine, 36th and Hamilton Walk, Philadelphia, Pennsylvania 19104 [1]

Elizabeth A. Grimm, Ph.D., Department of Tumor Biology and General Surgery, M. D. Anderson Hospital and Tumor Institute, 1515 Holcombe Boulevard, Houston, Texas 77030 [8]

Sidney Grossberg, M.D., Department of Microbiology, Medical College of Wisconsin Cancer Center, 8701 Watertown Plank Road, Milwaukee, Wisconsin 53226 [18]

Peter Hersey, F.R.A.C.P., Oncology and Immunology Unit, 4th Floor, David Maddison Building, Royal Newcastle Hospital, Newcastle, N.S.W. 2300, Australia [13]

Jennifer E. Hetrick, Case Western Reserve University School of Medicine, Cleveland, Ohio 44106 [1]

John B. Hibbs, Jr., M.D., Veterans Affairs Medical Center, Division of Infectious Diseases, Department of Medicine, University of Utah School of Medicine, 50 North Medical Drive, Salt Lake City, Utah 84132 [2]

Robert E. Humphreys, M.D., Ph.D., Departments of Pharmacology and

Medicine, University of Massachusetts Medical School, 55 Lake Avenue North, Worcester, Massachusetts 01655 [5]

Ann Jakubowski, M.D., Ph.D., Memorial Sloan-Kettering Cancer Center, 1275 York Avenue, New York, New York 10021 [19]

Jerald J. Killion, Ph.D., Department of Cell Biology, The University of Texas, M. D. Anderson Cancer Center, 1515 Holcombe Boulevard, Houston, Texas 77030 [15]

Heinz Köhler, M.D., Ph.D., IDEC Pharmaceuticals Corporation, 11099 North Torrey Pines Road, La Jolla, California 92037 [7]

Michael T. Lotze, M.D., Department of Surgery, University of Pittsburgh School of Medicine, 497 Scaife Hall, 3550 Terrace Street, Pittsburgh, Pennsylvania 15261 [16]

Shan Lu, M.D., Ph.D., Department of Pharmacology, University of Massachusetts Medical School, 55 Lake Avenue North, Worcester, Massachusetts 01655 [5]

Otoniel Martínez-Maza, Ph.D., Departments of Obstetrics and Gynecology, and Microbiology and Immunology, UCLA School of Medicine, Center for the Health Sciences, 10833 Le Conte Avenue, Los Angeles, California 90024 [9]

Frank L. Meyskens, Jr., M.D., Head and Neck Oncology, UCI Cancer Center, 101 The City Drive, Building 44, Route 81, Orange, California 92668 [20]

Malcolm S. Mitchell, M.D., Division of Medical Oncology, Department of Medicine, Kenneth J. Norris, Jr. Comprehensive Cancer Center, University of Southern California, 2025 Zonal Avenue, Los Angeles, California 90033 [14]

Barbara M. Mueller, Ph.D., Department of Immunology, The Scripps Research Institute, 10666 North Torrey Pines Road, La Jolla, California 92037 [6]

Sybille Müller, Ph.D., IDEC Pharmaceuticals Corporation, 11099 North Torrey Pines Road, La Jolla, California 92037 [7]

Quoc V. Nguyen, M.D., Departments of Pharmacology and Pediatrics, University of Massachusetts Medical School, 55 Lake Avenue North, Worcester, Massachusetts 01655 [5]

Donna M. Paulnock, Ph.D., Department of Medical Microbiology, University of Wisconsin, Madison, Wisconsin 53792 [18]

James K. Pitcock, M.D., Head and Neck Oncology, UCI Cancer Center, 101 The City Drive, Building 44, Route 81, Orange, California 92668 [20]

Ralph A. Reisfeld, Ph.D., Department of Immunology, The Scripps Research Institute, 10666 North Torrey Pines Road, La Jolla, California 92037 [6]

Victor E. Reyes, Ph.D., Department of Pharmacology, University of Massachusetts Medical School, 55 Lake Avenue North, Worcester, Massachusetts 01655 [5]

Joshua T. Rubin, M.D., Department of Surgery, University of Pittsburgh School of Medicine, 497 Scaife Hall, 3550 Terrace Street, Pittsburgh, Pennsylvania 15261 [16]

Darrell J. Salk, M.D., University of Washington School of Medicine, Seattle, Washington 98195; NeoRx Corporation, 410 West Harrison, Seattle, Washington 98119 [12]

Hans Schreiber, M.D., Ph.D., Department of Pathology, The University of Chicago, 5841 South Maryland Avenue, Chicago, Illinois 60637 [4]

Paul M. Sondel, M.D., Ph.D., Departments of Pediatrics, Human Oncology, and Genetics, University of Wisconsin Medical School, Clinical Sciences Center, 600 Highland Avenue, Madison, Wisconsin 53792 [17]

Els Sturm, Ph.D., Department of Immunology, Dr. Daniel den Hoed Cancer Center, Groene Hilledijk 301, 3075 EA Rotterdam, The Netherlands [3]

Read R. Taintor, B.S., Veterans Affairs Medical Center, Division of Infectious Diseases, Department of Medicine, University of Utah School of Medicine, 50 North Medical Drive, Salt Lake City, Utah 84132 [2]

Zdenek Vavrin, B.S., Veterans Affairs Medical Center, Division of Infectious Diseases, Department of Medicine, University of Utah School of Medicine, 50 North Medical Drive, Salt Lake City, Utah 84132 [2]

Stephan D. Voss, M.D., Ph.D., Department of Human Oncology, University of Wisconsin Medical School, Clinical Sciences Center, 600 Highland Avenue, Madison, Wisconsin 53792 [17]

Patricia L. Ward, Ph.D., Department of Molecular Genetics and Cell Biology, The University of Chicago, 5841 South Maryland Avenue, Chicago, Illinois 60637 [4]

John R. Wingard, M.D., BMT Program, Emory University School of Medicine, Division of Hematology, The Emory Clinic, 1365 Clifton Road, NE, Atlanta, Georgia 30322 [21]

Patricia L. Witt, Ph.D., Department of Microbiology, Medical College of Wisconsin Cancer Center, 8701 Watertown Plank Road, Milwaukee, Wisconsin 53266 [18]

PREFACE

This book is intended to be both a logical successor to, yet fully independent of, an earlier volume entitled, *The Modulation of Immunity* (1985), published as a volume (Section 115) in the series *The International Encyclopedia of Pharmacology and Therapeutics*. That volume of extensive review articles dealt with specific types of immunological modulators set against a background of fundamental immunology. At the time, the use of biological approaches to the treatment of human cancers was in its infancy.

Since then, there has been a dramatic increase in the understanding and application of biological principles to cancer therapy, which has made it necessary to produce an entirely different sort of book. This volume is intended to summarize much of the body of knowledge concerning the principles and application of biological response modifiers, which we have abbreviated as "biomodulators," to the treatment of human cancers. In parallel, "biomodulation" is a term we have coined as an alternative to the lengthier phrase "biological response modification."

Although some of the treatments have been suggested for many years, knowledge and technology have now progressed sufficiently to allow us to test many of the concepts and specific biological agents alone or in combination against established tumors. This is particularly true of the cytokines such as interferons and interleukin-2, colony-stimulating factors, and monoclonal antibodies. Immunological adjuvants such as *Mycobacterium bovis* (strain bacillus Calmette-Guérin [BCG]) and *Corynebacterium parvum* (*Propionibacterium acnes*), which previously dominated our attention, are now being used as their names have always implied: as adjuncts to specific immunotherapy.

We view biomodulation as connoting a far broader field than immunotherapy, which it subsumes. Anything that modifies the host–tumor relationship, acting on either the host or the tumor (without simply killing the tumor cells), can legitimately be considered a biomodulator by our definition. That would include agents that permit the host to tolerate more chemotherapy, by supporting myeloid stem cells, or those that might cause maturation of the tumor cells such as retinoids and some colony-stimulating factors.

We have previously presented a set of definitions of biomodulators (Biological response modifiers: subcommittee report, 1983; Mitchell, 1985, 1988; Mitchell and Bertram, 1985) that might be repeated here to illustrate our point more clearly. By these criteria, a biomodulator is a substance that does one or more of the following:

1 augments the host's antitumor response directly, by stimulating an increase in the number or activity of effector cells or by stimulating an increased production of soluble mediators such as lymphokines or monokines;

2 decreases suppressor mechanisms and thus increases the host's immune response to the tumor indirectly;

3 increases the host's defenses by being itself a natural or synthetic effector or mediator;

4 increases the ability of the host to tolerate damage by cytotoxic modalities, such as by increasing bone marrow leukocyte precursors;

5 changes the characteristics of the cell membrane of tumor cells sufficiently to increase their immunogenicity, to alter their pattern of metastasis, or to make the tumor cells more susceptible to killing by immunological mechanisms or cytotoxic drugs;

6 prevents or reverses transformation, or promotes the maturation of the "primitive" tumor cell.

Categories 4 through 6 are clearly outside the usual limits of what has been considered "immunotherapy" in the past and indicate the expansion implied by "biomodulation." It is also important to recognize that therapy with biomodulators includes treatment by any agent, whether a chemical or a biological substance, that has these effects on the host or the tumor. Biological therapy does not mean solely therapy with a biologically derived material such as a lymphokine, but applies equally to the use of the chemical cyclophosphamide in inhibiting suppressor T cells or humoral suppressor factors.

The authors have presented a review of their respective fields, but have been invited to do so from their unique point of view. All have tried to provide critical reviews rather than summaries of information. The first section of the book is intended to provide the basis, mainly immunological, on which biological therapy is grounded. Tumor-associated antigens as we currently understand them, principally through work with monoclonal antibodies, are discussed, as are the types of leukocytes that are responsible for reacting against tumors. Interactions among elements of the immune response are stressed throughout, to indicate the complexities that might be involved in attempts to modify immunity against a tumor. Immunological "lessons" from AIDS are also discussed. The second section of the book is devoted to treatment, but again, the principles upon which future therapy will be built are emphasized rather than a summary of current results. The immunological aspects of bone marrow transplantation, which can be regarded as an immunological treatment as well as a repletion of myeloid stem cells, are discussed in that section.

While there have been solid clinical gains in the treatment of cancer through biomodulators, none of us would suggest that dosages and schedules have been perfected for any of them. Combinations of agents, in parallel to the strategy successful with chemotherapeutic drugs, are now beginning to be used and will undoubtedly improve response rates.

If this book serves as a scientific reference from which to plan future strategies, many of which have not yet been anticipated by its editor and its authors, then it will have fulfilled its intended purpose.

REFERENCES

Biological response modifiers: subcommittee report. National Cancer Institute monograph 63. Bethesda, MD: NIH publication no. 83-2606; 1983.

Mitchell MS. Biomodulation: a classification and overview, In: Reif AE, Mitchell MS, eds. Immunity to cancer. Orlando, Fl: Academic; 1985:401–411.

Mitchell MS. Combining chemotherapy with biological response modifiers in treatment of cancer. J Natl Cancer Inst. 1988;80:1445–1450.

Mitchell MS, Bertram JH. Immunology and biomodulation of cancer. In: Calabresi P, Schein PS, Rosenberg SA, eds. Medical oncology. New York: Macmillan; 1985:363–391.

PART ONE

FUNDAMENTAL IMMUNOLOGY AND TUMOR BIOLOGY

CHAPTER 1

ADAPTIVE AND NONADAPTIVE IMMUNITY TO TUMORS: AN INTRODUCTION TO TUMOR IMMUNOLOGY

Valerie I. Brown
Jennifer E. Hetrick
Mark I. Greene

Ehrlich (1957) hypothesized that tumors express structures that can be recognized as foreign by the host and elicit an immune response. This mechanism was thought to contribute to the relatively low frequency of tumors. However, his experiments proved to be irreproducible because the data regarding transplantation antigens were not known at the time, and so one could not rule out the possibility that tumors were rejected because of major histocompatibility (MHC) alloantigen disparity.

With the advent of inbred strains of mice, Gross (1943) demonstrated that mice immunized with a methylcholanthrene (MCA)–induced sarcoma derived from the same inbred line do not develop tumors from subsequent intradermal injections of the same sarcoma cells, whereas nonimmunized mice of the same inbred line develop tumors. These studies suggest that the immunity of these mice is specifically against the tumor used for inoculation. Foley (1953) found that most MCA-induced tumors possess a unique antigen not shared by spontaneous tumors tested nor by normal murine tissues. The MCA-induced tumor cells can induce immunity whereas spontaneous tumors cannot produce transferred immunity. Prehn and Main (1957) extended these studies using the MCA-induced sarcoma system. They showed that chemically induced and transplanted neoplasms evoke specific cellular-mediated (T cell) responses in the host. The antigens evoking such a response were termed tumor-specific transplantation antigens (TSTA).

Thomas (1959) suggested that the host has a normal homeostatic cellular mechanism active in eliminating "non-self" antigens such as those from parasites, mutated and neoplastic cells. Burnet (1971) observed that patients with genetic defects in the immune system are prone to develop neoplasms, particularly of the immune system. Also, transplantation patients who were immunosuppressed show higher incidence of cancer. Burnet theorized that one function of the immune system was to recognize and destroy nascent neoplastic cells, serving as a mechanism to control carcinogenesis.

The concept of tumor antigens and immune surveillance inspired many investigators to isolate novel tumor antigens and develop specific antibodies that could be passively administered to cancer patients for therapy and diagnostic imaging. However, these protocols proved unsuccessful because of two major obstacles. First, large quantities of homogeneous, well-defined specific antibodies were unavailable; and second, the evidence for widespread existence for tumor-specific antigens on spontaneous tumors was lacking. The development of hybridomas allowed for the production of large quantities of monoclonal antibodies (Köhler and Milstein, 1975). This discovery has contributed to the resurgence of interest in tumor antigens and the immune response. The use of monoclonal antibodies has led many investigators to attempt the isolation and characterization of tumor-associated molecules that appear to be the result of altered or aberrant expression of normal antigens. The development of monoclonal antibodies has provided investigators with tools to design novel protocols for tumor therapy and imaging.

In this chapter, we present the current findings regarding tumor-specific and tumor-associated antigens. Furthermore, we present the theories regarding the immune response to neoplasms, focusing primarily on the immune surveillance theory and how it has evolved over the past 30 years. Finally, we briefly discuss the ways in which learning more about tumor-host interactions may lead to the development of protocols to treat human neoplasia.

TUMOR ANTIGENS

A tumor antigen is defined as a unique antigen expressed by cells as a result of transformation (reviewed in Carroll and Greene, 1989). These novel antigens are expressed only on a particular tumor or tumor type, and not on normal cells, and elicit an immune response by the host unless the host's immune system is compromised. However, many tumor antigens are only associated with transformation in that they are an indirect consequence of the transformation effects, such as an alteration in protein expression and/or localization. The expression of these antigens may occur at the same time as the transformation event or it may result from genetic instability during tumor progression.

Oncogene-Encoded Tumor Antigens

Initially, oncogenes were found to be associated with retroviruses (Bishop, 1983; Stehelin et al., 1976). Further investigation showed that these oncogenes are mutated versions of normal cellular genes, termed proto-oncogenes (Bishop, 1983). The protein products of proto-oncogenes are somehow involved with the regulation of cell growth and differentiation (Bishop, 1983; Yarden and Schlessinger, 1987). In general, oncogenes have either a cellular or viral origin, many of which have been described previously (Bishop, 1983), but the specific role they play in human cancer is unclear (Duesberg, 1985). This type of transformation is important to study since the specific antigens expressed by these oncogenes essentially label these cells as neoplastic. Investigators can therefore target these cancerous cells for elimination with in vivo–administered antibody. One such oncogene that seems very promising for this therapy is the protein product of the *neu* oncogene, which appears to be a growth factor receptor with tyrosine kinase activity and structurally similar to the epidermal growth factor receptor (EGFr). Neu oncogene expression is associated with rat neuro- or glioblastomas arising in offspring after injection of ethylnitrosourea into pregnant BDIX rats on day 15 of gestation. Padhy et al. (1982) first identified the transforming ability of a high molecular weight DNA from these ethylnitrosourea-induced rat tumors. Subsequently, investigators showed that these tumors all contain one identical transforming gene, termed *neu,* and that, by immunofluorescence and immunoprecipitation, the *neu* oncogene encodes a 185-kDa cell-surface phosphoprotein, termed p185-*neu* (Drebin et al., 1984; Schechter et al., 1984). Hung et al. (1986) cloned both the *neu* oncogene and proto-oncogene (termed p185c-*neu*), and Bargmann et al. (1986a) sequenced the cDNA. Deletional analyses and site-directed mutagenesis revealed that p185-*neu* differs from p185c-*neu* by a single amino acid substitution at residue 664 located in the transmembrane region (Bargmann et al., 1986b; Bargmann and Weinberg, 1988). This mutation converts a valine to a glutamic acid. The exact nature and location of this mutation are critical for activating the transformed phenotype. Thus, it appears that the expression of this p185-*neu* antigen plays an integral role in conferring the transformed phenotype.

To further characterize the structure and function of p185, Drebin et al. (1984) raised monoclonal antibodies against this rat protein. The *neu*-transfected NIH3T3 cell line, B104-1-1, was used to immunize C3H/HeJ mice. The spleen cells from these immunized mice were fused with NS-1 myeloma cells to produce p185-specific monoclonal antibodies. Five of 3000 hybridomas screened showed specific reactivity with the extracellular domain, and one of these five, an IgG_{2a} termed 7.16.4, induces the rapid down-modulation of p185-*neu* from the cell surface of B104-1-1 cells (Drebin et al., 1985). This rapid down-modulation of p185-*neu* leads to the reversion of the transformed phenotype in a cytostatic manner (Drebin et al., 1985). In vivo treatment with the anti-p185 monoclonal antibody 7.16.4 was able to inhibit significantly the specific tumorigenic growth of both B104-1-1 cells and the original rat neuroblastomas from which the *neu* gene was isolated when implanted into nude mice. However, these mice eventually succumbed to death due to tumor progression (Drebin et al., 1986). Although none of the five monoclonal antibodies individually was able to fully eradicate these tumors, combinations of these antibodies reactive with different regions of p185's extracellular domain exerted synergistic antitumor effects and, in many cases, completely eradicated tumors (Drebin et al., 1988).

A human homologue of *neu,* termed c-*erb*B-2, or HER-2, has been shown to be amplified and/or overexpressed in a wide variety of human malignancies, including squamous carcinomas and glioblastomas. Many investigators have reported that an overexpression of c-*erb*B-2 in human breast carcinomas correlates with a poor prognosis and increased probability of relapse (Berger et al., 1988; King et al., 1985; Slamon et al., 1987; Van de Vijver et al., 1987; Venter et al., 1987). Although the overexpression of normal rat p185c-*neu* does not transform fibroblasts alone, the cotransfection of p185c-*neu* and the EGFr does lead to the transformed phenotype (Kokai et al., 1989). Furthermore, the treatment of these p185c-*neu*/EGFr cotransfected fibroblasts with either mAb7.16.4 or with the anti-EGFr monoclonal antibody, mAb425, which binds to the extracellular domain of EGFr, inhibits tumorigenic growth of these cells (Wada et al., 1990). These data indicate that the synergistic interactions of p185c-*neu* and EGFr appear to play an important role in cellular transformation. Thus, these studies show that p185 plays an important role in tumorigenicity and suggest that a cancer therapy utilizing monoclonal antibodies specific for the p185 antigen may prove to be feasible in treating cancers associated with the abnormal expression of p185.

Another oncogene that encodes a cell-surface protein is one of the protein products of the SM-FeSV *fms,* the McDonough strain of feline sarcoma virus. Expression of SM-FeSV proteins induces fibrosarcomas in cats and is capable of transforming a variety of mammalian cells in culture (Porzig et al., 1979). The v-*fms* oncogene, which resulted from a recombination event between normal feline c-*fms* sequences and the feline leukemia virus, encodes a set of related glycoproteins termed gp180, gp140, and gp120 (Frankel et al., 1979). Anderson et al. (1982) produced rat monoclonal antibodies to syngeneic FeSV–transformed rat cells and selected for antibodies that specifically immunoprecipitated v-*fms* proteins. The majority of the v-*fms* protein products were organelle- or membrane-associated, as determined by subcellular fractionization analysis and by immunofluorescence of permeabolized v-fms–transformed rat and mink cells (Anderson et al., 1984). By two-color immunofluorescence, the v-*fms* product was shown to be associated with the internal membrane-associated intermediate filament. Also, a small population of v-*fms* protein (gp140) is expressed on the cell surface (Anderson et al., 1984). Manger et al. (1984) confirmed this observation by surface labeling and immunoprecipitation. Immunofluorescence of unpermeabolized SM-FeSV transformed mink cells revealed that v-*fms* gp140 is expressed on the cell surface in a fine, punctuated pattern. Two-color immunofluorescence revealed that v-*fms* gp140 is associated with clathrin-coated pits, suggesting that this protein encodes a growth factor receptor. Further evidence supporting this notion came with the sequencing of gp140, which showed homology with other tyrosine kinase-encoding oncogenes and contained a membrane spanning region (Hampe et al., 1984). The cellular homologue of v-*fms,* c-*fms,* is a 170-kDa glycoprotein with tyrosine kinase activity. This proto-oncogene appears to be the mononuclear phagocyte receptor for macrophage growth factor colony-stimulating factor (CSF-1) (Sherr et al., 1985). Deletional mutation analysis and microsomal proteolytic digestion of v-*fms* have shown that the surface expression of v-*fms* correlates with transformation (Rettenmeir et al., 1985; Roussel et al., 1984). Rat antisera, which were obtained from (Wistar-

FurthXFischer) F1 rats that were injected with SM-FeSV–transformed rat embryo cells and formed tumors at sites of injection appear to cause tumor regression, since the rats whose tumors regressed had a higher titer of anti–v-*fms* activity. Thus, it appears that the specific cell-surface expression of v-*fms* confers the transformed phenotype and that removal of this protein from the cell surface promotes tumor regression, analogous to the case of the p185 antigen.

Viral Antigens

Viruses other than v-*fms* have been implicated in the genesis of certain human cancers. A causal relationship between chronic hepatitis B virus infection and hepatocellular carcinoma appears to exist (Robinson et al., 1984); herpes virus has been implicated in cervical cancer etiology; and human papilloma virus appears to play a role in the induction of some UV-associated skin cancers (Kirchner, 1984). Also, infection with the herpes virus, Epstein-Barr virus (EBV), seems to be associated with Burkitt's lymphoma and undifferentiated nasopharngeal cancers (Thorley-Lawson et al., 1982). It is very difficult to study these viruses because they only infect human (and sometimes primate) cells. However, monoclonal antibodies have contributed significantly in determining the existence of specific virus-associated antigens expressed in these cancers. Specific cytotoxic T cell reactivity patterns to EBV-infected cells suggest that EBV transformation results in expression of membrane-associated transformation antigens, termed lymphocyte-derived membrane antigens (LYDMA) (Thorley-Lawson et al., 1982). It is interesting to note that newly diagnosed patients with nasopharyngeal carcinoma demonstrate an impaired EBV-specific T cell–mediated immunity when compared to long-term survivors and those who are uninfected. It is possible that suppression of immunity is responsible for the impaired cellular response. Monoclonal antibodies have been used to help identify LYDMA. Hoffman et al. (1980) produced a monoclonal antibody to EBV B95-8 virions that detected a 250-kDa glycoprotein specifically expressed by human and marmaset virus-producing cells, and Thorley-Lawson et al., (1982) produced a monoclonal antibody, 17D6, against EBV-transformed cells and immunoprecipitated a 45-kDa antigen, but it is unclear if these antigens play some important role in tumorigenesis.

Tumor Antigens Associated with Human Organs

Many human tumor antigens expressed by different organs have been identified by screening with monoclonal antibodies produced by rodents immunized with human tumor cell lines or human biopsied tissue. One human malignancy that has been studied extensively is malignant melanoma. Many investigators have searched for tumor antigens expressed specifically on human melanomas. In learning more about melanoma-specific and associated antigens, investigators will be able to develop an effective immunotherapy, since these neoplasias characteristically do not respond to conventional protocols involving chemotherapy and radiation treatment. Monoclonal antibodies against human melanomas have been generated (Koprowski et al., 1978), although some of the monoclonal antibodies generated cross-reacted with normal tissues. However, these specific antimelanoma antibodies are able to suppress melanoma tumor growth in nude mice. Woodbury et al. (1980) generated monoclonal antibodies against a human melanoma cell line, SK-mel 28. The antibodies reacted with approximately 90% of the melanomas and 55% of other tumor cell types tested, but did not react with normal cells or tissues tested. They determined that some antibody bound a 97-kDa protein termed p97. The p97 protein was detected on both cultured melanoma cells and biopsied melanoma tissues and on other tumor tissues, but p97 was not detected in eight different samples of normal adult epithelial or mesenchymal tissues (Woodbury et al., 1980). Subsequently, many groups have identified many different melanoma tumor antigens using a panel of antimelanoma antibodies (Reisfield, 1982). In addition, antigen heterogenicity has been found within tissues removed from the same patient (Albino et al., 1981; Brocker et al., 1985; Natali et al., 1983). Based on reaction patterns of monoclonal antibodies against melanoma, Brocker et al. (1985) classified melanoma tumor antigens as either constitutive (antigens expressed on all local and systemic tumors), early (antigen expression decreases with disease progression), or late (antigens expressed on invasive primary tumor or metastases). The biochemical and functional natures of these antigens are unclear at the present time and are, therefore, considered tumor-associated only. Further investigation may show that these antigens play some causal role in tumorigenesis.

Several groups have generated monoclonal antibodies against human mammary carcinomas. A series of monoclonal antibodies derived from a metastatic human mammary carcinoma have been generated (Colcher et al., 1981). These antibodies reacted specifically with mammary tumor cells, but not with normal cell lines, sarcoma or melanoma cell lines, and tissue sections derived from normal human organs. One of these monoclonal antibodies, B72.3, immunoprecipitated a 220 to 400-kDa protein complex from human metastatic mammary carcinoma cells (Nuti et al., 1982). They found different levels of expression, but it is unclear what this antigen is. Other groups have identified antigens that are present on mammary neoplastic epithelial cells as well as on differentiated mammary breast ductal epithelia. Therefore, the role these mammary carcinoma-associated antigens play in tumorigenesis is unclear (Croghan et al., 1983; Menard et al., 1983).

Other investigators have identified antigens associated with prostatic cancer (Carroll and Greene, 1989; Carroll et al., 1984), but many of the monoclonal antibodies used in detecting these tumor antigens cross-react with either normal or benign prostate tissues (Frankel et al., 1982; Wang et al., 1979). A tumor antigen that was associated with human prostate, human prostate tumor tissue, and bladder cancer cell lines has been identified (Starling et al., 1982). Since the bladder and prostate originate from the urogenital sinus during embryological development, the antigen detected by this monoclonal antibody may be a urogenital differentiation antigen that may be re-expressed during tumorigenesis (Starling et al., 1982). In addition, a prostate-specific antigen has been identified (Bazinet et al., 1988), and tumor-specific antigens for human bladder cancer have been identified (Fradet et al., 1984).

Other tumor-associated antigens have been identified in conjunction with human pancreatic cancer (Schmiegal et al., 1985), ovarian carcinoma (Bast et al., 1981), gliomas (Schnegg et al., 1988), small-cell lung carcinoma (Bernal et al., 1985), and acute lymphoblastic leukemia (Ritz et al., 1980). However, it is unclear whether these antigens play some role in tumorigenesis or whether they only serve as a marker for tumor progression. The functions of these antigens should become clear following their characterization. Also, Udea et al. (1981) have identified tissue-specific antigens that are found only on cells of renal origin, both normal and malignant, and appear to be differentiation antigens expressed on the human kidney. Muraro et al., (1989) have produced a monoclonal antibody, D612, which selectively reacts with only malignant and normal gastrointestinal epithelium. It is likely that the antigen recognized by this monoclonal antibody is a differentiation antigen as well. Identification of these tumor-specific, tumor-associated, and differentiation antigens will help in the aid of tumor detection and perhaps tumor progression.

Tumor Antigens as a Result of Aberrant Glycosylation

Many carbohydrates have been defined by monoclonal antibodies as tumor-associated antigens. In 1985, Feizi found that many tumor antigens are actually carbohydrate structures (Feizi, 1985). These antigenic carbohydrates may be modifications of cell surface structures normally present at low levels during different stages of development or normally associated in a nonimmunogenic fashion. Recent data indicate that these tumor-associated antigens may be the product of aberrant synthesis and activity of glycosylation enzymes. Two processes, precursor accumulation and neosynthesis, appear to be responsible for producing tumor-associated carbohydrates (Hakamori, 1984). Precursor accumulation is associated with suppression of glycosyltransferase activities, resulting in the presentation of altered or even incomplete glycosylated products. Precursor structures have now been identified in several tumor systems. Studies of hamster, virus-transformed cultured fibroblasts demonstrated such incomplete construction of surface glycolipids (Den et al., 1974; Hakamori, 1984; Kijimoto and Hakamori, 1971; Robbins and McPherson, 1971). A G_{D3} disialoganglioside associated with human melanoma was shown to be the result of precursor accumulation. Attempts to target these G_{D3} structures were unsuccessful, due to their organization or steric interactions (Houghton et al., 1985; Nudelman et al., 1984; Pukel et al., 1982).

Neosynthesis results from the stimulation, derepression, or altered substrate specificity of glycosylation enzymes. The neosynthesis of fucose-containing glycolipids associated with very common and lethal cancers (gastrointestinal, pancreas, lung, and mammary glands) has been studied extensively. Holmes and Hakomori (1983) have shown that the induction of fucosyltransferase causes alterations in rat livers treated with a chemical carcinogen. Liepkalns et al. (1985) have studied the fucosolipid, gastrointestinal-associated cancer antigen (GICA), and have shown that the synthesis of GICA as well as other fucosolipids may be associated with rapid division of undifferentiated tumor cells.

Glycolipids containing monosaccharides are sources of potential antigenic determinants in that they can be separated and used to develop monoclonal antibodies and to stimulate antibody-mediated cytotoxicity. Antibody responses to the GM_2 ganglioside of melanoma patients were induced by purified glycolipid (Cahan et al., 1982), and Brodin et al. (1989) generated monoclonal antibodies to glycolipids of the isoglobo-series for recognition of tumor-associated antigens in rats. Further study and characterization of these molecules may reveal that such tumor markers correspond to stage-specific tumor progression, which would allow for imaging and diagnosis and for targeting tumor cells for destruction.

Oncofetal Antigens

The carcinoembryonic antigen (CEA) described by Gold and Freedman (1965) represents a new species of tumor antigen, termed oncofetal antigens. Oncofetal antigens are found on the cell surface during stages of embryonic and fetal development but are not normally present or are present at very low levels in adult cells. They are nonimmunogenic to the host cell and are detected through generation of antisera in allogenic or xenogenic animals. Since these antigens are often shed from the cell surface, serum levels of oncofetal antigens are used to monitor tumor growth and regression in the management of patients (Fletcher, 1986; Goldenberg, 1981; Neville, 1981). Carcinoembryonic antigen, a secreted 200-kDa glycoprotein, is primarily found in patients with gastrointestinal cancer, especially cancer of the colon, although CEA is present in lung, pancreas, and some breast and stomach cancers (Harmenberg et al., 1988; Zimmerman et al., 1987). Elevated levels of serum CEA are also found in a variety of noncancerous diseases such as pancreatitis, ulcerative colitis, and alcoholism. Carcinoembryonic antigen has been used, nevertheless, as a target in radiolabeled antibody imaging and antibody-mediated, neutron-capture therapy (Goldenberg et al., 1984; Sfakianakis and DeLand, 1982a).

Further classification has shown CEA to be structurally heterogeneous; it is not a single molecule, but rather a family of related glycoproteins (Beatty and Terz, 1982). There is some indication that a tumor-specific form exists that is associated only with malignancy (Jothy et al., 1986). The alphafeto protein, discovered by Abelev, is also associated with a wide variety of tumor types, most commonly hepatomas and testicular teratoblastomas (Benjamini and Leskowitz, 1988). Oncofetal antigens may also include some lipid and peptide-associated carbohydrate structures (Feizi, 1985).

It is unclear what roles oncofetal antigens play in transformation: if their expression is causal or a consequence of another transforming event. Currently, oncofetal antigens are associated with tumors and are used as markers for the existence, growth, and regression of tumors. However, the presence of oncofetal antigens on such a variety of tumor types indicates that they may be the result of derepression of a developmental gene (Carroll and Greene, 1989). Since these structures are present on normal embryonic and fetal cells, the proteins and the genes encoding them may help regulate differentiation and development. Expression of such cell surface structures is shown to be reduced or eliminated after organogenesis. The re-expression of these genes in the context of differentiated cells may lead to tumorigenesis.

IMMUNE SURVEILLANCE

Although Burnet is credited with formalizing the theory of immune surveillance, the concept of immune surveillance has been discussed since the turn of the century. In 1909, Ehrlich proposed that one of the functions of the immune system is to recognize and destroy nascent neoplastic cells (Ehrlich, 1957). Thomas (1959) proposed that the immune response to cancer cells is the same type as that responsible for allograft rejection, that is, a systemic, antigen-specific T-cell response. He further theorized that allograft rejection represents a by-product of a host-recognition mechanism designed to destroy autologous cancer cells. However, it seems more plausible that both allograft rejection and rejection of cancer cells are by-products of a host's defense against virally infected cells, parasites, and intracellular microbial pathogens, and so it is likely that T cell–mediated immunity against allografts and cancer cells evolved as a protective mechanism against infectious diseases (Kripke, 1988).

Because the main assumption of immune surveillance is that the immune response to cancer cells is strictly T cell–mediated, as is that for allograft rejection, tumor antigens were first defined on a basis of their ability to induce resistance to transplantation. Burnet postulated that "when aberrant cells with proliferative potential arise in the body, they will carry new antigenic determinants on their cell surface" (Burnet, 1970). It is conceivable that small accumulations of tumor cells may develop, but because of their expression of novel antigens, they provoke an immunological response, leading to a regression of tumor cells (Burnet, 1970, 1971). Three main predictions of the immune surveillance theory were formulated: (1) transformed cells are antigenic, (2) transformed cells can be recognized and destroyed by a T cell–mediated response, and (3) immunological suppression is associated with an increase in incidence of neoplasia (Gatti and Good, 1971; Lin et al., 1985). Neonatal thymectomy and other forms of immunological suppression have been found to lead to an increase in tumor incidence (Bolton, 1973; Carbone and Parmiani, 1971; Kripke and Borsos, 1974). Initially, there appeared to be a correlation between immunodeficiency disease and a higher incidence of lymphomas and leukemias (Gatti and Good, 1971). Allograft recipients receiving immunosuppressive agents have an increased incidence of cancer, and patients who received chemotherapy have been found to subsequently develop relatively high frequencies of novel primary malignancies, predominantly of lymphoid origin. Also, there is a higher incidence of Kaposi's sarcoma in patients with acquired immunodeficiency syndrome (Purtillo, 1984). Chemical carcinogens and viruses cause immunological suppression (Balk et al., 1966). (Stjernsward, 1969) showed that the carcinogenic hydrocarbons, methylcholanthrene (MCA), benz-α-pyrene (BaP) and dimethylbenzanthracene (DMBA) are all immunosuppressive (Burnet, 1970, 1971). All these data support the concept of immune surveillance.

However, studies of immunodeficient patients and organ transplant recipients failed to reveal a dramatic increase in common malignancies of internal organs (Hewitt et al., 1976); it appears that immunological suppression is associated only with an increase in lymphoma and leukemia and is not associated with a complete array of tumor types. Also, athymic nude mice do not have a higher incidence of spontaneous tumors nor are they any more susceptible to chemical carcinogens (Rygaard, 1974; Stutman, 1978). A likely explanation for these results is that a variety of effector mechanisms may be involved in eliminating tumors (Herberman, 1984). This possibility is discussed below.

Based on studies of transplantation immunity against tumors induced in inbred mice, tumors have been categorized into three broad groups: (1) virus-induced tumors, (2) chemically induced tumors, and (3) spontaneous tumors. Virus-induced tumors are highly antigenic, expressing the same tumor antigens for the same virus (Klein, 1966). Chemically induced tumors are generally antigenic, but they vary in their ability to produce protective immunity (Old et al., 1962). The antigens associated with chemically induced tumors are often specific for the immunizing tumor, so various antigens are produced by the same chemical. Spontaneous tumors are defined as those arising with no apparent cause in aged animals that lack the ability to induce protective immunity (Baldwin, 1966). It appears that the antigenicity of a tumor depends on its etiology (Baldwin, 1966). The immune surveillance theory as originally stated appears to hold for only highly antigenic tumors, that is, those that are oncogenic-induced, virus-induced, or UV-radiation-induced. Tumors induced by the Shope fibroma virus in rabbits and polyoma virus in mice are subject to immunological destruction.

The incidence of tumor development is greatly influenced by the immunological competence of the host (Allison, 1970; Klein and Klein, 1977; Strayer et al., 1984). It is likely that immune surveillance against these tumors resembles the surveillance against infectious agents. Hewitt et al. (1976) found no evidence of tumor immunogenicity against tumors arising spontaneously in mice strains with limited susceptibility to cancer. They tested 27 different tumors of different origins and found that none of the transplanted tumors failed and none regressed, despite using a small inocula. It is important to state that these tumors were not chemically or virally induced. Thus, they concluded that immunity against these "spontaneous" tumors could not be immunologically transferred.

Fischer and Kripke (1982) showed that skin cancers in mice induced by UV radiation responded to immune surveillance because these highly antigenic tumors were rejected upon transplantation into normal syngeneic hosts. However, these tumors are not "virus-like" in that the immunity against these tumors is specific only for the immunizing tumors. They develop initially in the host perhaps because of some suppression, attributed to the suppressor T cells in these UV-irradiated animals. Our laboratory has shown that UV-treated mice possess suppressor T cells specific for a panel of UV-induced tumor antigens (Drebin et al., 1982; Perry and Greene, 1981).

Furthermore, suppressor T cells are present in spleens of UV-irradiated mice prior to tumor challenge, and so irradiation alone generates suppressor T cells that can enhance the growth of UV-induced tumors.

Adaptive Immunity

Since T cells seem to play an important role in the immune response against tumors, investigators have attempted to determine the role different T-cell subsets play in the rejection of certain tumors. We examined in mice the ability of different T-cell subsets in vivo to confer protection against the methylcholanthrene-induced sarcoma, S1509a (Bhan et al., 1981), and found that $CD5^+CD8^-$ cells and unfractionated T cells are capable of inhibiting tumor growth in vivo, whereas $CD8^+$ cells do not. These findings indicate that the $CD5^+CD8^-$ and Thy 1^+ cells are capable of eradicating growth of this sarcoma, presumably by eliciting an inflammatory reaction; the histologic findings of mononuclear cells with only a few intact tumor cells at the site of tumor injection support the theory that delayed-type hypersensitivity reaction occurs at the tumor site. However, $CD8^+$ cells, which mediate cell-mediated cytotoxicity, do not play a role in eliminating this sarcoma.

In addition, Greene et al. (1982) determined the T-cell subpopulation responsible for the destruction of papova virus-induced transformed cells in vitro. The killing of these cells in vitro is mediated by a $CD8^+$ T-cell subset, indicating that cytolytic T lymphocytes (CTL) are responsible for the elimination of these virus-transformed cells. They further showed that these CTL lyse these papova virus-transformed cells in a specific and MHC-restricted manner.

These observations indicate that different T-cell subsets are responsible for eliminating specific tumor types, depending upon the tumor's origin. In these cases, it appears that $CD5^+CD8^-$ cells inhibit chemically induced tumors, and that CTL killing mediated by $CD8^+$ cells lyses virally induced tumor cells. Therefore, in the case of transformation by chemical carcinogens, specific antigens need not be expressed on the cell surface. Specific antigens released by rapidly proliferating or dying tumor cells appear to be endocytosed by antigen-presenting cells. These antigen-presenting cells bearing tumor products then evoke $CD5^+CD8^-CD4^+$ T cells, which mediate inflammatory responses to antigens. In the case of virus-transformed cells, viral antigens associate with MHC class I molecules on the tumor cell surface and are directly responsive to $CD4^-CD8^+$ T cells.

Hellstrom et al. (1971, 1977) initially showed that the ability to effectively destroy tumors could be adoptively transferred via sera from tumor-bearing animals. Specific blocking factors were thought to be the effectors of this response. However, our laboratory demonstrated that cells from the thymus or spleen conferred this inhibition. Further investigation implicated suppressor T cells and subsets of suppressor T cells as causative factors (Drebin et al., 1982; Perry and Greene, 1981).

Howie and McBride (1982) demonstrated that helper T cells are involved in various stages of tumor development, but that helper T-cell activity decreases, while suppressor T-cell activity increases, with the increasing of tumor size. Also, using the S1509a tumor system, Greene et al. (1979), found that certain T cells mediated immunity to S1509a tumors both in vivo and in vitro, but suppressor T cells existed that suppressed this activity. Suppressor T cells that appear in the thymus, spleen, and lymph nodes of tumor-bearing hosts, arose as a consequence of tumor antigen exposure in vivo within 48 hours after exposure to tumor antigens. However, suppressor T cells specific for S1509a tumor cells disappeared within 5 days of surgical removal of the tumor (Greene et al., 1979). This observation suggests that the presence of tumor antigens is required for the stimulation of suppressor T cells. Also, S1509a tumor-bearing mice expressed T cell–derived suppressor molecules (TsF) (Greene et al., 1979). In order to see if TsF was capable of stimulating the generation of effector suppressor cells in naive mice, S1509a-specific TsF was administered to naive mice over 5 days and resulted in the generation of S1509a-specific second-order suppressor T cells (Perry and Greene, 1981). Subsequently, these mice were unable to respond to an S1509a-specific tumor challenge. Thus, TsF abrogates the capacity of the host to respond to tumors.

The intravenous administration of S1509a membrane fragments to mice resulted in the induction of potent suppressor T cells (Greene et al., 1979; Perry and Greene, 1981). Splenic suppressor T cells taken from these mice were capable of markedly suppressing the immune response against S1509a tumor cells when transferred to an immunized host (Drebin et al., 1982). Splenectomy limited the inhibitory activity of mice since the spleen is the site of an active pool of mature suppressor T cells. The suppressor T cells harvested from these spleens were found to need constant antigen in order to stimulate suppressor T-cell function (Greene et al., 1979). When suppressor T precursors were eliminated with cyclophosphamide and the mice then challenged with S1509a tumor cells, suppressor T-cell generation was completely prevented. These mice were also capable of adoptively transferring augmented T-cell reactivity to normal mice (Greene et al., 1979). Mice given anti-I-A alloantiserum daily were no longer capable of rejecting tumor challenge or transferring immunity (Perry and Greene, 1981). This antibody, which is directed against the I-A subregion of the H-2 complex, impaired induction of T-cell responsiveness. Spleens of these antibody-treated mice contained suppressor T cells capable of inhibiting the development of S1509a-specific tumor rejection. These suppressor T cells may arise as a result of impaired antigen presentation which may lead to excess free antigen. These data suggest that suppressor T cells are stimulated preferentially by soluble tumor antigen shed into the circulation and bypassing normal antigen presentation. The continual presence of free antigen in tumor-bearing mice appears to lead to the activation of the T-cell suppressor system. Additionally, the role of suppressor T-cell immune regulation in response to peptides and haptens is thought to be analogous to that of tumors (Germain and Benacerraf, 1980; Gershon, 1974; Pierce and Kapp, 1976; Tada et al., 1975). Based on observations regarding the role of suppressor T cells, a comprehensive model regarding the inhibition of the immune response to tumors was proposed

(Nepom et al., 1983). This model involves the interaction of soluble tumor antigen, antigen-antibody complexes, anti-idiotypic antibodies, and T cell–derived suppressor factors.

Nonadaptive Immunity

It is thought that natural killer (NK) cells, a discrete subpopulation of lymphoid cells that are non-MHC–restricted, play a role in immune surveillance (Herberman, 1984; Kripke, 1988; Roder and Häliotis, 1980). Natural killer cells react against a variety of tumor cell lines, primary tumor cells, virally infected cells, and some normal cells. Evidence regarding the role of NK cells in immune surveillance has accumulated. Briefly, NK cells gather at sites of inflammation and in small primary and transplanted tumors (Herberman, 1984). They have a natural and rapidly activatable ability to lyse a variety of autochthonous tumors. There is an increase in tumor incidence in animals and individuals with depressed NK activity, such as beige mice and people with Chediak-Higashi syndrome, and in immunosuppressed transplant recipients (Herberman, 1984). Although they have a minimal ability to lyse solid tumors, NK cells appear to eliminate metastatic tumor cells (Hanna and Fidler, 1980). Hanna and Fidler (1980) have shown that animals treated with cyclophosphamide (Cy), which caused depletion or inactivation of various lymphoid cell populations, have enhanced survival of tumor cells injected by IV and, subsequently, a higher incidence of metastasis. Thus, they hypothesized that these NK cells play some role in the destruction of blood-borne tumor emboli. Also, NK activity was boosted with interferon, and inhibition of metastasis formation occurred. When animals with low NK activity were given NK cells with high activity before IV injection of tumor cells, there were fewer metastases. The cells killing these artificial metastases were non-T cells and Cy-sensitive cells that were nonadherent to nylon wool, and so they are most likely of NK origin. Brodt and Gordon (1982) have shown that mice deprived of B cells by chronic treatment with anti-IgM antibodies had heightened natural resistance to micro-organisms, parental bone marrow, and NK-sensitive tumors in vitro and in vivo. The latent period of primary tumors induced by injection of MCA was prolonged in these mice that had increased NK activity, and this increase in latency of tumor appearance may be due to some immune surveillance mechanism involving NK cells at work.

Other mechanisms appear to play a role in immune surveillance. Hibbs et al. (1971) found that macrophages can be activated to tumoricidal states. These activated macrophages can discriminate between neoplastic and normal cells (Hibbs, 1974), but this mechanism does not really appear to be a very good line of surveillance since there are very few activated macrophages in circulation or in tissues at any given time, and resting macrophages exhibit little cytotoxicity. However, if macrophages are depleted, the incidence of tumorigenicity increases (Norbury and Kripke, 1979). Thus, macrophages play a role in a natural mechanism of immune surveillance. Antibody-dependent, cell-mediated cytotoxicity (ADCC) may play a role in eliminating cancerous cells, too, but there is no direct evidence that this mechanism normally regulates the outgrowth of tumors during carcinogenesis (Den Otter, 1986).

Lymphokine-activated killer (LAK) cells, when incubated with interleukin-2 (IL-2) were capable of lysing fresh, noncultured NK-resistant tumor cells, but not normal cells. These cells were found in peripheral blood, lymph nodes, bone marrow, and thoracic duct (Rosenberg et al., 1985). It is thought that LAK cells may play some role in immune surveillance for tumor cells. Ting et al. (1987) determined that LAK cells are generated in tumor-bearing mice. After culturing murine spleen cells in vitro for 5 days, the LAK cells had greater cytotoxicity than cells generated from nontumor mice. The LAK cells were present in early or early advanced stage mice, but none were present at the terminal stage of tumor growth. In order to determine if tumor cells are somehow suppressing LAK-cell induction, X-irradiated tumor cells were incubated with LAK cells, resulting in a decrease in cytotoxicity of LAK cells (Rosenberg et al., 1987). Spiess et al. (1987) found that giving IL-2 to tumor-bearing mice could generate LAK cells that are capable of killing tumor cells in vitro, and furthermore, significant antitumor reactivity resulted when these LAK cells were adoptively transferred into other tumor-bearing hosts. This study showed the potential of such an LAK and IL-2 regimen in human cancer patients, and the results of such trials are discussed below.

Ellenhorn et al. (1988) found that the administration of low doses of monoclonal antibodies against the CD3 molecule of the T-cell receptor complex was able to prevent the outgrowth of tumors in mice. Furthermore, mice treated with anti-CD3 developed tumor immunity, since these animals failed to develop tumors following a second tumor challenge 60 days later with no additional antibody therapy. Yun et al. (1989) found that killer cells could be activated using anti-CD3 by activating endogenous lymphokine production. These activated killer cells, termed CD3-AK cells, when pre- and cocultured with anti-CD3 selectively killed tumor targets with a 10- to 50-fold higher cytotoxic activity than LAK cells. The CD3-AK cells were actively growing in vitro for 4 to 5 weeks, whereas LAK cells lasted for only 7 to 10 days in culture. In vivo, complete protection resulted against tumors with CD3-AK cells, but not against those with LAK cells. If CD3-AK cells are given 1 to 2 days after tumor challenge, tumor growth was slowed, and 20% of the mice remained tumor-free (Yun et al., 1989). Collectively, these data indicate that LAK and CD3-AK cells elicit nonspecific antitumor immunity.

The difficulty with non–T-cell immune surveillance is that there have not been enough studies done, particularly on spontaneous tumors. Currently, it appears that non–T-cell immunity against cancer is not as effective as T cell–mediated immune surveillance. Figure 1-1 summarizes the immune system's response to tumors arising from different origins. Recently, investigators have begun to investigate the host-tumor relationship in a local context, not a systemic one, as in the past. Bilik et al. (1989) characterized the lymphocytic infiltration present at or around the site of 56 primary mammary tumors. They found that these tumors were infiltrated with a disproportionately large number of suppressor T cells at these lesions as compared to the number in

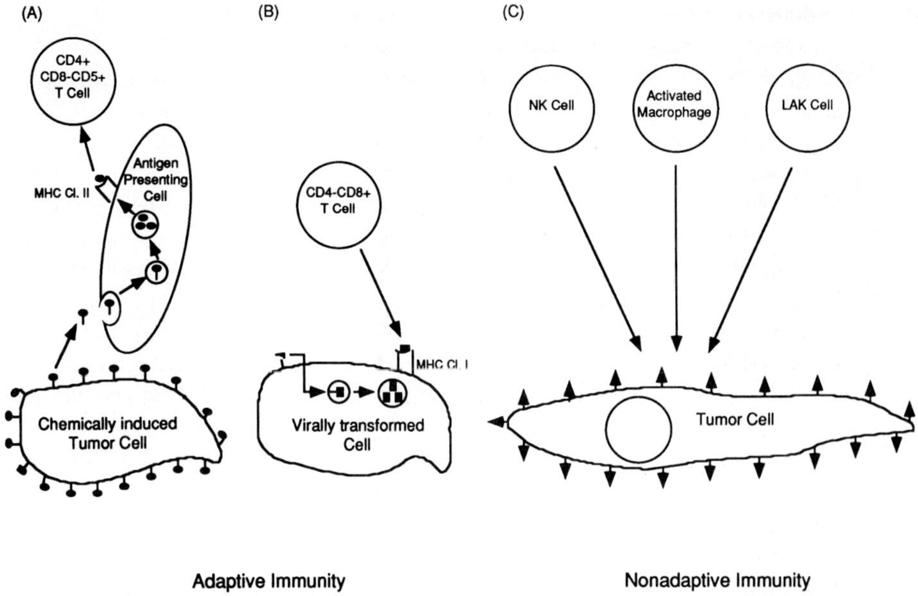

FIGURE 1-1
Mechanism of Adaptive and Nonadaptive Immunity Against Tumor Cells. The origin of the transforming factor(s) appears to play an important role in determining the way in which the immune system responds to a tumor cell. (A) Antigens expressed specifically by chemically induced tumor cells are processed by antigen-presenting cells (APC). These processed antigens are expressed on the cell surface of the APC in the context of MHC class II molecules and activate $CD4^+CD5^+CD8^-$ T cells. This immunity can be adoptively transferred. (B) Viral antigens of virally transformed cells are processed by the infected cells and are expressed on the cell surface in the context of MHC class I molecules. These complexes are recognized by specific $CD4^-CD8^+$ T cells and are activated. This immunity can be adoptively transferred. (C) Natural killer cells, activated macrophages, and LAK cells nonspecifically destroy tumor cells. This immunity is nonadaptive.

peripheral blood or normal tissues. Perhaps the presence of suppressor T cells at the tumor site is responsible for a depression of a T cell–mediated immune response.

IMMUNOLOGICAL APPROACHES TO ELIMINATING TUMORS

The crosslinking of monoclonal antibodies to radionuclides and toxins has been used successfully in targeting tumor cells for destruction (Baldwin, 1985; Bale et al., 1960; Persaud, 1988; Pressman, 1980; Sfakianakis and DeLand, 1982). Such labeling has been done using a variety of fluorescent chemicals for imaging and diagnosis of cancers (Koprowski, 1984; Tatsuta et al., 1989). This technology has been effectively utilized in intraoperative procedures, where localization of cancerous cells is accomplished through detection by a γ counter to radiolabeled monoclonal antibodies. This novel usage has resulted in a change in surgical course in 26% of patients with recurrent colorectal carcinoma. The use of monoclonal antibodies directed against tumor antigens allows for this specific and effective identification (Kaplan, 1989).

Since many tumor antigens are weakly immunogenic, attempts have been made at augmenting their immunogenicity. To date, many investigators have found that monoclonal antibodies directed against tumor antigens inhibit tumor growth, at least initially, and are effective in cancer therapy, both through direct interaction of monoclonal antibodies and through monoclonal antibodies' stimulation of an anti-idiotypic response (Drebin et al., 1986; Herlyn and Koprowski, 1982; Herlyn et al., 1980). Our laboratory has shown that mAb7.16.4 inhibits tumor growth in mice inoculated with *neu*-transformed cells. We showed the ability of mAb7.16.4, directed against extracellular p185-*neu,* to have cytostatic effects in vitro in the presence of spleen cells or complement. Also, we demonstrated that this monoclonal antibody inhibits tumor growth of both fresh inocula and already established tumors in nude mice. Although the tumors eventually progressed in the animals, mAb7.16.4 was shown to revert the transformed phenotype, mediate ADCC, trigger cell lysis in the presence of complement, and may crosslink p185, probably blocking its mode of activation or neutralizing it by steric changes. Administration of combinations of monoclonal antibodies also provided a more effective inhibition and, in some cases, elimination of tumor growth (Drebin et al., 1986, 1988).

Initially, monoclonal antibodies and anti-idiotypes were used in the treatment of lymphomas. Because T and B cells of lymphomas are thought to be derived from a single, original transformed lymphocyte, the population of lymphocytic cells expresses a single idiotype. Therefore, antibodies made against the specific receptors are highly specific and effective. Miller et al. (1982) and Meeker et al. (1985) reported that monoclonal antibody treatment achieved dramatic results.

Since many tumors seem to express either tumor-specific or tumor-associated antigens, many investigators have tried to increase antigen expression by treating cells with recombinant human interferon. Interferon has many different effects within the immune system. It appears to enhance the T cell–mediated response, but it also appears to decrease NK susceptibility, because interferon-γ appears to have the ability to increase MHC class I expression and de novo expression of MHC class II. In addition, interferon appears to enhance tumor antigen expression. Tran et al. (1988) studied eight different human breast carcinoma cell lines and clonally derived cell lines to determine the effects of interferon on these cells. These cell lines express a wide range of antigenic phenotypes. This group found that the cell lines that constitutively expressed low levels of mammary tumor–associated antigens were highly responsive to interferon-α and interferon-γ, whereas cell lines expressing high levels of tumor-associated antigens did not. Guadagni et al. (1989) showed that interferon-γ is the most potent in augmenting tumor-associated antigens in adenocarcinomas, malignant and benign nonepithelia. Interferon-γ also augmented CEA antigen expression (Guadagni et al., 1989). This same group determined the effects of interferon treatment in vivo.

They subcutaneously injected athymic mice with human mammary carcinoma and colorectal cancer cells. When these cells were given interferon in vitro, their tumor-antigen expression was augmented. Also, these tumor cells were responsive in vivo as long as interferon remained circulating within the animal via an osmotic pump. Thus, one can conclude that increasing antigen expression on tumor cells may render these cells more susceptible to T cell–mediated killing.

Because interferon can decrease NK activity, treatment with interferon may be detrimental to the tumor-bearing host since NK cells appear to play an important role in the regulation of metastatic spread. In order to compare the effects of interferon-γ on tumor management in mice, Zoller et al. (1988) used a cell line that is a weakly metastatic variant of B16 melanoma, termed B16-F1. After treatment with interferon in vitro, these cells had increased expression of MHC class I and class II, but these cells were not as susceptible to NK killing. Although in vivo treatment with interferon-γ resulted in a decrease in the efficiency of NK cells, this treatment resulted in increased antigenicity and immunogenicity resulting in tumor elimination. Thus, interferon-γ treatment appears to be a promising adjunct therapy for human tumors that are constitutively expressing low levels of tumor antigens and are weakly metastatic.

Based on the findings that murine tumors can be treated by administering LAK cells and IL-2 to tumor-bearing mice (Spiess et al., 1987), 25 patients with metastatic cancer that did not respond to conventional methods of therapy were given both autologous LAK cells and recombinant human IL-2. Eleven of these patients had marked tumor regression (Rosenberg et al., 1985). Based on these results, a more comprehensive study involving 157 patients treated with either LAK cells and IL-2 or IL-2 alone was performed (Rosenberg et al., 1987). Of the 106 patients receiving LAK and IL-2 treatment, 8 completely responded, and of the 46 patients receiving IL-2 alone, 1 completely responded. However, the effectiveness and optimization of this regimen need to be explored further, since there were four treatment-related deaths.

REFERENCES

Albino AP, Lloyd KO, Houghton AN, Oettgen HF, Old LJ. Heterogeneity in surface antigen and glycoprotein expression of cell lines derived from different melanoma metastases of the same patient: implications for the study of tumor antigens. J Exp Med. 1981;154:1764–1778.

Allison AC. Potentiation of viral carcinogenesis by immunosuppression. Br Med J. 1970;4:419–420.

Anderson SJ, Furth MW, Ruscetti SK, Sherr CJ. Monoclonal antibodies to the transformation-specific glycoprotein encoded by the feline retroviral oncogene v-fms. J Virol. 1982;44:696–702.

Anderson SJ, Gonda MA, Rettenmier CW, Sherr CJ. Subcellular localization of glycoproteins encoded by the viral oncogene v-fms. J Virol. 1984;51:730–741.

Baldwin RW. Tumor-specific immunity against spontaneous rat tumors. Int J Cancer. 1966;1:257–264.

Baldwin RW. Monoclonal antibody targeting of anti-cancer agents: Muhlbock Memorial Lecture. Eur J Clin Oncol. 1985;21:1281–1285.

Bale WF, Spar IL, Goodland RL. Experimental radiation therapy of tumors with I-131-carrying antibodies to fibrin. Cancer Res. 1960;20:1488–1494.

Balk JK, Sinclair NR, McCarter JA. Prolonged immunosuppression and tumor induction by a chemical carcinogen injected at birth. Science. 1966;152:650–651.

Bargmann CI, Hung M-C, Weinberg RA. The neu oncogene encodes an epidermal growth factor receptor–related protein. Nature. 1986a;319:226–230.

Bargmann CI, Hung M-C, Weinberg RA. Multiple independent activations of the neu oncogene by a point mutation altering the transmembrane domain of p185. Cell. 1986b;45:649–657.

Bargmann CI, Weinberg RA. Oncogenic activation of the neu-encoded receptor protein by point mutation and deletion. EMBO J. 1988;7:2043–2052.

Bast JRC, Feeney ME, Lazarus H, Nadler LM, Colvin RB, Knapp RC. Reactivity of a monoclonal antibody with human ovarian carcinoma. J Clin Invest. 1981;68:1331–1337.

Bazinet M, Cote RJ, Cordon-Cardo C, Myc A, Fair WR, Old LJ. Immunohistochemical characterization of two monoclonal antibodies, P25.48 and P25.91, which define a new prostate-specific antigen. Cancer Res. 1988;48:6938–6942.

Beatty JD, Terz JJ. Value of carcinoembryonic antigen in clinical medicine. Prog Clin Cancer. 1982;8:9–29.

Benjamini E, Leskowitz S. Immunology: a short course. New York: Alan R. Liss; 1988:313–330.

Berger MS, Locher GW, Saurer S, et al. Correlation of c-erbB-2 gene amplification and protein expression in human breast carcinoma with nodal status and nuclear grading. Cancer Res. 1988;48:1238–1243.

Bernal SD, Mabry M, Stahel RA, Griffen JD, Speak JA. Selective cytotoxicity of the SM1 monoclonal antibody towards small cell carcinoma of the lung. Cancer Res. 1985;45:1026–1032.

Bhan AK, Perry LL, Cantor H, Benacerraf MI, Mc Cluskey RT. Role of T cell sets in the rejection of a methylcholanthrene-induced sarcoma (S1509a) in syngeneic mice. Am J Pathol. 1981;102:20–27.

Bilik R, Mor C, Hazaz B, Moroz C. Characterization of T-lymphocyte subpopulations infiltrating primary breast cancer. Cancer Immunol Immunother. 1989;28:143–147.

Bishop J. Cellular oncogenes and retroviruses. Annu Rev Biochem. 1983;52:301–354.

Bolton PM. The effect of immune depression on chemical carcinogenesis in the rat. Oncology. 1973;27:525–532.

Brocker E-B, Suter L, Bruggen J, Ruiter DJ, Macher E, Sorg C. Phenotypic dynamics of tumor progression in human malignant melanoma. Int J Cancer. 1985;36:29–35.

Brodin NT, Thurin J, Karlsson K, Martensson S, Sjoegren HO. Monoclonal antibodies to glycolipids of the isoglobo series detect tumor-associated antigens in rats. Int J Cancer. 1989;43:317–326.

Brodt P, Gordon J. Natural resistance mechanisms may play a role in protection against chemical carcinogenesis. Cancer Immunol Immunother. 1982;13:125–127.

Burnet FM. The concept of immunological surveillance. Prog Exp Tumor Res. 1970;13:1–27.

Burnet FM. Immunological surveillance. Transplant Rev. 1971;7:3–25.

Cahan LD, Irie RF, Singh R, Cassidenti A, Paulson JC. Identification of a human neuroectodermal tumor antigen (OFA-I-2) as ganglioside GD2. Proc Natl Acad Sci USA. 1982; 79:7629–7633.

Carbone G, Parmiani G. Increased oncogenic effect of a low dose of methylcholanthrene in immunodepressed mice. Tumori. 1971;57:225–231.

Carroll AM, Greene MI. Tumor cell biology: tumor specific and associated antigen. In: Zalutsky MR, ed. Antibodies in radiodiagnosis and therapy. Boca Raton, FL: CRC Press; 1989:13–43.

Carroll AM, Zalutsky M, Schatten S, et al. Monoclonal antibodies to tissue-specific cell surface antigens. Characterization of an antibody to a prostate tissue antigen. Clin Immunol Immunopathol. 1984;132:268–274.

Colcher D, Hand PH, Nuti M, Schlom J. A spectrum of monoclonal antibodies reactive with mammary tumor cells. Proc Natl Acad Sci USA. 1981;5:3199–3203.

Croghan GA, Papsidero D, Valenzuela LA, Nemoto T, Penetrante R, Chu TM. Tissue distribution of an epithelial and tumor-associated antigen recognized by monoclonal antibody F36/22. Cancer Res. 1983;43:4980–4988.

Den H, Sela BA, Roseman S, Sachs L. Block in ganglioside synthesis in transformed hamster cells and their revertants. J Biol Chem. 1974;249:659–661.

Den Otter W. Immune surveillance and natural resistance: an evaluation. Cancer Immunol Immunother. 1986;21:85–92.

Drebin JA, Link VC, Greene MI. Monoclonal antibodies reactive with distinct domains of the neu oncogene-encoded p185 molecule exert synergistic anti-tumor effects in vivo. Oncogene. 1988;2:273–277.

Drebin JA, Link VC, Stern DF, Weinberg RA, Greene MI. Down-modulation of an oncogene protein product and reversion of the transformed phenotype by monoclonal antibodies. Cell. 1985;41:695–706.

Drebin JA, Link VC, Weinberg RA, Greene MI. Inhibition of tumor growth by a monoclonal antibody reactive with an oncogene-encoded tumor antigen. Proc Natl Acad Sci USA. 1986;83:9129–9133.

Drebin JA, Perry LL, Carter R, Greene MI. Regulation of the immune response to antigens on the malignant cell surface. Springer Semin Immunopathol. 1982;5:175–192.

Drebin JA, Stern DF, Link VC, Weinberg RA, Greene MI. Monoclonal antibodies identify a cell-surface antigen associated with an activated cellular oncogene. Nature. 1984;312:545–548.

Duesberg PH. Activated proto-oncogenic genes: sufficient or necessary for cancer? Science. 1985;228:669–677.

Ehrlich P. Uber den jetzigen Stand der Karzinomforschung. In: Himmelweit F, ed. The collected papers of Paul Ehrlich. Oxford: Pergamon Press; 1957:550.

Ellenhorn JDI, Hirsch R, Schreiber H, Bluestone JA. In vivo administration of anti-CD3 prevents malignant progressor tumor growth. Science. 1988;242:569–571.

Feizi T. Demonstration by monoclonal antibodies that carbohydrate structures of glycoproteins and glycolipids are onco-developmental antigens. Nature. 1985;314:53–57.

Fisher MS, Kripke ML. Suppressor T lymphocytes control the development of primary skin cancers in ultraviolet-irradiated mice. Science. 1982;216:1133–1134.

Fletcher RH. Carcinoembryonic antigen. Ann Intern Med. 1986;104:66–73.

Foley EJ. Antigenic properties of methylcholanthrene-induced tumors in mice of the same strain of origin. Cancer Res. 1953;13:835–837.

Fradet Y, Cordon-Cardo C, Thomson T, Daly ME, Whitmore JWF, Old LJ. Cell surface antigens of human bladder cancer defined by mouse monoclonal antibodies. Proc Natl Acad Sci USA. 1984;81:224–228.

Frankel AE, Gilbert JH, Porzig JH, Scolnick EM, Aaronson SA. Nature and distribution of feline sarcoma virus nucleotide sequences. J Virol. 1979;30:821–827.

Frankel AE, Rouse RV, Herzenberg LA. Human prostate specific and shared differentiation antigens defined by monoclonal antibodies. Proc Natl Acad Sci USA. 1982;79:903–907.

Gatti RA, Good RA. Occurrence of malignancy in immunodeficiency diseases. Cancer. 1971;28:89–98.

Germain R, Benacerraf B. Helper and suppressor T cell factors. Springer Semin Immunopathol. 1980;3:93–127.

Gershon RK. T cell control of antibody production. Contemp Topics Immunobiol. 1974;3: 1–40.

Gold P, Freedman SO. Demonstration of tumor-specific antigens in human colonic carcinomata by immunological tolerance and absorption techniques. J Exp Med. 1965;121:439–462.

Goldenberg DM. Carcinoembryonic antigen: its role as a marker in the management of cancer: A National Institutes of Health Consensus Development Conference. Ann Intern Med. 1981;94:407–409.

Goldenberg DM, Sharkey RM, Primus FJ, Mizusawa E, Hawthorne FM. Neutron-capture therapy of human cancer: in vivo results on tumor localization of boron-10-labeled antibodies to carcinoembryonic antigen in the GW-39 tumor model system. Proc Natl Acad Sci USA. 1984;81:560–563.

Greene MI, Perry L, Benacerraf B. Regulation of the immune response to tumor antigen. V. Modulation of suppressor T cell activity in vivo. Am J Pathol. 1979;95:159–169.

Greene MI, Perry LL, Kinney-Thomas E, Benjamin TL. Specific thymus-derived (T) cell recognition of papova virus-transformed cells. J Immunol. 1982;128:732–736.

Gross L. Intradermal immunization of C3H mice against a sarcoma that originated in an animal of the same line. Cancer Res. 1943;3:326–333.

Guadagni F, Schlom J, Johnston WW, et al. Selective interferon-induced enhancement of tumor-associated antigens on a spectrum of freshly isolated human adenocarcinoma cells. J Natl Cancer Inst. 1989;81:502–512.

Hakamori S. Tumor-associated carbohydrate antigens. Proc Natl Acad Sci USA. 1984;59:103.

Hampe A, Gobet M, Sherr C, Gailbert F. Nucleotide sequence of the feline retroviral oncogene v-*fms* shows unexpected homology with oncogenes encoding tyrosine-specific protein kinases. Proc Natl Acad Sci USA. 1984;81:85–89.

Hanna N, Fidler IJ. Role of natural killer cells in the destruction of circulating tumor emboli. J Natl Cancer Inst. 1980;85:801–809.

Harmenberg U, Wahren B, Wiechel KL. Tumor markers carbohydrate antigens CA19-9 and CA-50 and carcinoembryonic antigen in pancreatic cancer and benign diseases of the pancreatobiliary tract. Cancer Res. 1988;48:1985–1988.

Hellström KE, Hellström I. Immunological defences against cancer. In: Good RA, Fischer DW, eds. Immunobiology. Sunderland: Sinauer; 1971.

Hellström KE, Hellström I, Nepom JT. Specific blocking factors—are they important? Acta Biochem Biophys. 1977;473:121–143.

Herberman RB. Possible role of natural killer cells and other effector cells in immune surveillance against cancer. J Invest Dermatol. 1984;83:137s–140s.

Herlyn D, Koprowski H. IgG2a monoclonal antibodies inhibit human tumor growth through interaction with effector cells. Proc Natl Acad Sci USA. 1982;79:4761–4765.

Herlyn D, Steplewski Z, Herlyn MF, Koprowski H. Inhibition of growth of colorectal carcinoma in nude mice by monoclonal antibody. Cancer Res. 1980;40:717–721.

Hewitt HB, Blake ER, Walder AS. A critique of the evidence for active host defense against cancer, based on personal studies of 27 murine tumors of spontaneous origin. Br J Cancer. 1976;33:231–239.

Hibbs JJB. Discrimination between neoplastic and non-neoplastic cells in vitro by activated macrophages. J Natl Cancer Inst. 1974;53:1487–1492.

Hibbs JJB, Lambert JLH, Remington JS. Resistance to murine tumors conferred by chronic infection with intracellular protozoa. Toxoplasma gondii and Besnoitia jellisoni. J Infect Dis. 1971;124:587–592.

Hoffman G, Lazarowitz S, Hayward S. Monoclonal antibody against a 250,000 dalton glycoprotein of Epstein-Barr virus identifies a membrane antigen and a neutralizing antigen. Proc Natl Acad Sci USA. 1980;77:2979–2983.

Holmes EH, Hakomori S. Enzymatic basis for changes in fucoganglioside during chemical carcinogenesis. J Biol Chem. 1983;258:3706–3713.

Houghton AN, Mintzer D, Cordon-Cardo C, et al. Mouse monoclonal IgG3 antibody in detecting GD3 ganglioside: a phase I trial in patients with malignant melanoma. Proc Natl Acad Sci USA. 1985;82:1242–1246.

Howie S, McBride WH. Tumor-specific T helper activity can be abrogated by two distinct suppressor cell mechanisms. Eur J Immunol. 1982;12:671–675.

Hung M-C, Schechter AL, Chevray P-YM, Stern DF, Weinberg RA. Molecular cloning of the neu gene: absence of gross structural alteration on oncogenic alleles. Proc Natl Acad Sci USA. 1986;83:261–264.

Jothy S, Brazinsky SA, Chin-A-Loy M, et al. Characterization of monoclonal antibodies to carcinoembryonic antigen with increased tumor specificity. Lab Invest. 1986;54:108–117.

Kaplan EH. The diagnostic and therapeutic use of monoclonal antibodies in colorectal cancer. Hematol Oncol Clin N Am. 1989;3:125–134.

Kijimoto S, Hakamori S. Enhanced glycolipid: galactosyltransferase activity in contact-inhibited hamster cells, and loss of this response in polyoma transformants. Biochem Biophys Res Commun. 1971;44:557–570.

King CR, Kraus MH, Aaronson SA. Amplification of a novel v-*erb*B-related gene in a human mammary carcinoma. Science. 1985;29:974–976.

Kirchner H. Immunologic surveillance and human papilloma viruses. Immunol Today. 1984;5:272–275.

Klein G. Tumor antigens. Annu Rev Microbiol. 1966;20:223–253.

Klein G, Klein E. Immunosurveillance against virus-induced tumors and nonrejectability of spontaneous tumors: contrasting consequences of host versus tumor evolution. Proc Natl Acad Sci USA. 1977;74:2121–2125.

Köhler G, Milstein C. Continuous cultures of fused cells secreting antibody of predefined specificity. Nature (Lond). 1975;256:495–497.

Kokai Y, Myers JN, Wada T, et al. Synergistic interaction of p185c-neu and the EGF receptor leads to transformation of rodent fibroblasts. Cell. 1989;58:287–292.

Koprowski H. The Gordon Wilson lecture: monoclonal antibodies in human cancer. Transact Am Clin Clinatol Assoc. 1984;96:81–97.

Koprowski H, Steplewski Z, Herlyn D, Herlyn M. Study of antibodies against human melanoma produced by somatic cell hybrids. Proc Natl Acad Sci USA. 1978;7:3405–3409.

Kripke ML. Immunoregulation of carcinogenesis: past, present, and future. J Natl Cancer Inst. 1988;80:722–727.

Kripke ML, Borsos T. Immunosuppression and carcinogenesis: a review. Isr J Med Sci. 1974;10:888–903.

Liepkalns VA, Herrero-Zabaleta E, Fondaneche MC, Burtin P. Alterations in expression and synthesis of glycolipid antigens in human colonic tumor cell lines. Cancer Res. 1985;45:2255.

Lin Y, Patek PQ, Collins JL, Cohn M. Analysis of immune surveillance of sequentially derived cell lines that differ in their tumorigenic potential. J Natl Cancer Inst. 1985;74:1025–1030.

Manger R, Najita L, Nichols E, Hakomori S, Rohrshneider L. Cell surface expression of the McDonough strain of feline sarcoma virus *fms* gene product (gp140 fms). Cell. 1984;39:327–337.

Meeker TC, Lowder J, Maloney DG, et al. A clinical trial of anti-idiotype therapy for B cell malignancy. Blood. 1985;65:1349–1363.

Menard S, Tagliobue E, Canevari S, Fossati G, Colnagli MI. Generation of monoclonal antibodies reacting with normal and cancer cells of human breast. Cancer Res. 1983;43:1295–1300.

Miller RA, Maloney DG, Warnke R, Levy R. Treatment of B cell lymphoma with monoclonal anti-idiotype antibody. New Engl J Med. 1982;306:517–522.

Muraro R, Nuti M, Natali PG, et al. A monoclonal antibody (D612) with selective reactivity for malignant and normal gastro-intestinal epithelium. Int J Cancer. 1989;43:598–607.

Natali PG, Cavaliere R, Bigotti A, Nicotra MR, Russo C, Ng AK. Antigenic heterogeneity of surgically removed primary and autologous metastatic human melanoma lesions. J Immunol. 1983;130:1462–1466.

Nepom GT, Hellstrom I, Hellstrom KE. Suppressor mechanisms in tumor immunity. Experientia. 1983;39:235–242.

Neville AM. Carcinoembryonic antigen: its role as a marker in the management of cancer: summary of an NIH consensus statement. Br Med J [Clin Res]. 1981;282:373–375.

Norbury KC, Kripke ML. Ultraviolet-induced carcinogenesis in mice treated with silica, trypan blue or pyran copolymer. J Reticuloendothel Soc. 1979;26:827–837.

Nudelman E, Hakamori S, Kannagi R. Characterization of a human melanoma associated ganglioside antigen defined by a monoclonal antibody 4.2. J Biol Chem. 1984;257:12752–12756.

Nuti M, Teramoto YA, Mariani-Costantini R, Hand PH, Colcher D, Schlom J. A monoclonal antibody (B72.3) defines patterns of distribution of a novel tumor-associated antigen in human mammary carcinoma cell populations. Int J Cancer. 1982;29:539–545.

Old LJ, Boyse EA, Clarke DA. Antigenic properties of chemically induced tumors. Ann NY Acad Sci. 1962;101:80–106.

Padhy LC, Shih C, Cowing D, Finkelstein R, Weinberg RA. Identification of a phosphoprotein specifically induced by the transforming DNA of rat neuroblastomas. Cell. 1982;28:865–871.

Perry LL, Greene MI. T cell subset interaction in the regulation of syngeneic tumor immunity. Fed Proc. 1981;40:39–44.

Persaud RD. Biting the magic bullet. Radiolabelled monoclonal antibodies: the next great step forward in the diagnosis and treatment of cancer? Med Hyp. 1988;27:245–251.

Pierce C, Kapp J. Regulation of immune responses by suppressor T cells. Contemp Topics Immunobiol. 1976;5:91–143.

Porzig K, Barbacid M, Aaronson S. Biological properties and translational products of three independent isolates of feline sarcoma virus. Virology. 1979;92:91–107.

Prehn RT, Main JM. Immunity to methylcholanthrene-induced sarcomas. J Natl Cancer Inst. 1957;18:769–778.

Pressman D. The development and use of radiolabeled antitumor antibodies. Cancer Res. 1980;40:2960–2964.

Pukel CS, Lloyd KO, Travassos LR, Dippold WG, Oettgen HF, Old LJ. GD3, a prominent ganglioside of human melanoma: detection and characterization by mouse monoclonal antibody. J Exp Med. 1982;155:1133.

Purtillo DT. Biology of disease. Defective immune surveillance in viral carcinogenesis. Lab Invest. 1984;51:373–385.

Reisfield R. Monoclonal antibodies to human malignant melanoma. Nature. 1982;298:325–326.

Rettenmeir C, Roussel M, Quinn C, Kitchingman G, Look A, Sherr C. Transmembrane orientation of glycoproteins encoded by the v-*fms* oncogene. Cell. 1985;40:971–981.

Ritz J, Pesando JM, Notis-McConarty J, Lazarus H, Sclossman SF. A monoclonal antibody to human acute lymphoblastic leukemia antigen. Nature. 1980;283:583–585.

Robbins PW, McPherson I. Control of glycolipid synthesis in a cultured hamster cell line. Nature (Lond). 1971;229:569–570.

Robinson W, Miller R, Klote L, Marion P, Lee S. Hepatitis B virus and hepatocellular carcinoma. In: Vyas G, Dienstag J, Hoofnagle J, eds. Viral hepatitis and liver disease. Orlando, FL: Grune & Stratton; 1984:245.

Roder JC, Haliotis T. Do NK cells play a role in anti-tumor surveillance. Immunol Today. 1980;1:96–100.

Rosenberg SA, Lotze MT, Muul LM, et al. A progress report on the treatment of 157 patients with advanced cancer using lymphokine-activated killer cells and interleukin-2 alone. New Engl J Med. 1987;316:889–897.

Rosenberg SA, Lotze MT, Muul LM, et al. Observations on the systemic administration of autologous lymphokine-activated killer cells and recombinant interleukin-2 to patients with metastatic cancer. New Engl J Med. 1985;313:1485–1492.

Roussel M, Rettenmeir C, Look A, Sherr C. Cell surface expression of *v-fms* coded glycoproteins is required for transformation. Mol Cell Biol. 1984;4:1999–2009.

Rygaard JP. Is immunological surveillance not a cell-mediated immune function? Transplantation. 1974;17:135–136.

Schechter AL, Stern DF, Vaidyanathan L, et al. The neu oncogene: an *erb*B-related gene encoding a 185,000-Mr tumour antigen. Nature. 1984;312:513–516.

Schmiegal WH, Kalthoff H, Arndt R, et al. Monoclonal antibody-defined human pancreatic cancer-associated antigens. Cancer Res. 1985;45:1402–1407.

Schnegg JF, Discerens AC, Carrel S, Accolla RS, de Tribolet N. Human glioma-associated antigens detected by monoclonal antibodies. Cancer Res. 1988;41:1209–1213.

Sfakianakis GN, DeLand FH. Radioimmunodiagnosis and radioimmunotherapy. J Nucl Med. 1982;23:840–850.

Sherr CJ, Rettenmier CW, Sacca R, Roussel MF, Look AT, Stanley ER. The c-*fms* proto-oncogene product is related to the receptor for the mononuclear phagocyte growth factor, CSF-1. Cell. 1985;41:665–676.

Slamon DJ, Clark GM, Wong SG, Levin WJ, Ullrich A, McGuire WL. Human breast cancer: correlation of relapse and survival with amplification of the HER-2/*neu* oncogene. Science. 1987;235:177–182.

Spiess PI, Yang JC, Rosenberg SA. In vivo antitumor activity of tumor-infiltrating lymphocytes expanded in recombinant interleukin-2. JNCI. 1987;79:1067–1075.

Starling JJ, Sieg SM, Beckett ML, Schellhammer PF, Ladaga LE, Wright JGL. Monoclonal antibodies to human prostate and bladder tumor-associated antigens. Cancer Res. 1982; 42:3084–3089.

Stehelin D, Varmus H, Bishop J. DNA related to the transforming gene(s) of avian sarcoma viruses is present in normal avian DNA. Nature. 1976;260:170–173.

Stjernsward J. Immunosuppression by carcinogens. Antibiot Chemother. 1969;15:213–233.

Strayer DS, Skaletsky E, Sell S. Strain differences in Shope fibroma virus: an immunopathologic study. Am J Pathol. 1984;116:342–358.

Stutman O. Spontaneous, viral, and chemically induced tumors in the nude mouse. In: Fogh J, Giovanella B, eds. The nude mouse in experimental and clinical research. New York: Academic Press; 1978:411.

Tada T, Taniguichi M, Takemori T. Properties of primed suppressor T cells and their products. Transplant Rev. 1975;26:106–129.

Tatsuta M, Lishi H, Ichii M, et al. Diagnosis of gastric cancers with fluorescein-labeled monoclonal antibodies to carcinoembryonic antigen. Lasers Surg Med. 1989;9:422–426.

Thomas L. Reactions to homologous tissue antigens in relation to hypersensitivity. In: Lawrence HS, ed. Cellular and humoral aspects of the hypersensitive states. New York: Hoeber-Harper; 1959:529.

Thorley-Lawson D, Edson C, Geilinger K. Epstein-Barr virus antigens: a challenge to modern biochemistry. Adv Cancer Res. 1982;36:295–348.

Ting C-C, Hargrove ME, Stephany D. Generation of activated killer cells in tumor-bearing hosts. Int J Cancer. 1987;39.

Tran R, Greiner PH, Pestka JW, Schlom J. Enhancement of surface antigen expression on human breast carcinoma cells by recombinant human interferons. J Interferon Res. 1988;8:75–88.

Udea R, Ogata S-I, Morrissey DM, et al. Cell surface antigens of human renal cancer defined by mouse monoclonal antibodies: identification of tissue-specific kidney glycoproteins. Proc Natl Acad Sci USA. 1981;8:5122–5126.

Van de Vijver M, Van de Bersselaar R, Devilee P, Cornelisse C, Peterse J, Nusse R. Amplification of the neu (c-erbB-2) oncogene in human mammary tumors is relatively frequent and is often accompanied by amplification of the linked c-erbA oncogene. Mol Cell Biol. 1987;7:2019–2023.

Venter OJ, Kumar S, Tuzi NL, Gullick WJ. Overexpression of the c-erbB-2 oncoprotein in human breast carcinomas: immunohistological assessment correlates with gene amplification. Lancet. 1987;2:69–72.

Wada T, Myers JN, Kokai Y, et al. Anti-receptor antibodies reverse the phenotype of the cells transformed by two interacting proto-oncogene encoded receptor proteins. Oncogene. 1990;5:489–495.

Wang MC, Valenzuela LA, Murphy GP, Chu TM. Purification of a human prostate specific antigen. Invest Urol. 1979;17:159–163.

Woodbury RG, Brown JP, Yeh M-Y, Hellstrom I, Hellstrom KE. Identification of a cell surface protein, p97, in human melanomas and certain other neoplasms. Proc Natl Acad Sci USA. 1980;77:2183–2187.

Yarden Y, Schlessinger J. Self-phosphorylation of epidermal growth factor receptor: evidence for a model of intermolecular allosteric activation. Biochemistry. 1987;26:1434–1442.

Yun Y-S, Hargrove ME, Ting C-C. In vivo antitumor activity of anti-CD3-induced activated killer cells. Cancer Res. 1989;49:4770–4774.

Zimmerman W, Ortlieb B, Friedrich R, von Kleist S. Isolation and characterization of cDNA clones encoding the human carcinoembryonic antigen reveal a highly conserved repeating structure. Proc Natl Acad Sci USA. 1987;84:2960–2964.

Zoller M, Strubel A, Hammerling G, Andrighetto G, Raz A, Ben-Ze'ev A. Interferon-gamma treatment of B16 melanoma cells: opposing effects of non-adaptive and adaptive immune defense and its reflection by metastatic spread. Int J Cancer. 1988;41:256–266.

CHAPTER **2**

THE ROLE OF MACROPHAGES AS EFFECTOR CELLS AGAINST TUMORS

John B. Hibbs, Jr.
Read R. Taintor
Zdenek Vavrin
Donald L. Granger

Cancer and its complications remain one of the most common causes of death in the United States. At the cellular level the fundamental problem is the continuous and uncontrolled proliferation of tumor cells. Biochemical mechanisms that control cell proliferation are not understood. Tumor cells develop a profound and prolonged cytostasis when co-cultivated with cytotoxic-activated macrophages (CAM) (Keller, 1973; Krahenbuhl and Remington, 1974; Krahenbuhl, 1980; Granger et al., 1980; Hibbs and Granger, 1982; Hibbs et al., 1984; Drapier and Hibbs, 1986). Some tumor cell phenotypes undergo cytolysis after a period of CAM-induced cytostasis, while other tumor cell phenotypes eventually recover proliferative capability within 24 to 96 hours after being removed from CAM monolayers and cultured alone in fresh medium (Granger et al., 1980; Hibbs and Granger, 1982).

We have used the activated macrophage cytotoxic reaction as an in vitro model system for studying a cell-mediated mechanism that causes rapid and reproducible arrest of tumor cell proliferation. Our studies using this in vitro model show that the CAM effector mechanism causes inhibition of mitochondrial respiration and aconitase activity, in addition to DNA synthesis, and that these changes are caused by a perturbation of intracellular iron homeostasis (Granger et al., 1980; Hibbs and Granger, 1982; Hibbs et al., 1984; Drapier and Hibbs, 1986). A previously unrecognized biochemical pathway causes loss of intracellular iron from target cells as well as the pattern of CAM-induced selective metabolic inhibition (Hibbs et al., 1987a, 1987b, 1988; Drapier and Hibbs, 1988; Amber et al., 1988a, 1988b; Drapier et al., 1988). This pathway, unique in eukaryotic or prokaryotic biochemistry, synthesizes nitric oxide (NO) from a terminal guanidino nitrogen atom of L-arginine (Hibbs et al., 1988; Marletta et al., 1988; Stuehr et al., 1989a). This results in the formation of iron-nitrosyl complexes, particularly with nonheme iron, that can be readily detected by electron paramagnetic resonance spectroscopy (Lancaster and Hibbs, 1990). The other product of this pathway is L-citrulline, which is synthesized directly from L-arginine without loss of the guanidino carbon atom (Hibbs et al., 1987b; 1988; Amber et al., 1988b; Iyengar et al., 1987). It now becomes an important task to determine the biological significance of this recently discovered biochemical pathway. The best clues to its significance for cell-mediated immunity are found in studies that preceded and led to the discovery of the pathway. Our purpose here is to review this background information as well as to discuss current biochemical understanding of the L-arginine–dependent effector pathway.

PREVIOUS WORK SUGGESTS THAT A CLOSE RELATIONSHIP EXISTS BETWEEN CELL-MEDIATED RESISTANCE TO INTRACELLULAR MICROORGANISMS AND NEOPLASTIC CELLS

Since the early work of Metchikoff (1893), it was recognized that acquired resistance to intracellular microorganisms resulted from homeostatic mechanisms that rendered the intracellular habitat inhospitable for proliferation and/or survival of intracellular pathogens. Therefore, it is important conceptually to consider the intracellular environment as a unique compartment in terms of host defense (Hibbs, 1975b; Hibbs et al., 1980b). It is our view that the L-arginine–dependent effector mechanism has a central role in host resistance to intracellular microorganisms and that this same effector mechanism is involved in host resistance to neoplastic cells. Defense of the intracellular environment requires a biochemical effector mechanism that can inhibit the proliferation and/or kill intracellular microorganisms without causing irreversible damage to the host cell. In addition, it would be advantageous to the host if the biochemical defense against intracellular organisms altered the internal environment of the parasitized host cell so that factors (iron, high-energy phosphate molecules, etc.) required for the intracellular proliferation of intracellular pathogens were limited. It would not be surprising if the effector mechanism that targeted intracellular pathogens residing in the vacuolar system or in the cytoplasm of host cells also had the capability to inhibit the proliferation of normal and neoplastic mammalian cells. The pathway synthesizing NO from L-arginine is capable of causing these biological effects.

The first systematic investigation into mechanisms of host resistance to pathogens that reside in the intracellular environment began in the late 1950s and early 1960s by Mackaness (1962, 1964, 1969). He showed that a two-cell system (lymphocytes and macrophages) is required for expression of acquired cellular immunity to intracellular bacteria. Macrophages, the effector cells that express increased resistance to intracellular pathogens, are mobilized at sites of infection and are functionally modified by secreted products of sensitized lymphocytes responding to specific antigen. In vitro experiments demonstrated that sensitized lymphocytes, responding to specific antigen or conconavalin A, secrete a lymphokine(s) that delivers a signal to macrophages inducing physiological modification. These physiologically modified or "activated" macrophages are then able to inhibit the proliferation or kill the specific immunizing intracellular bacteria and also to nonspecifically inhibit the proliferation and/or kill unrelated intracellular bacteria. Remington and his colleagues demonstrated that increased nonspecific resistance generated during development of immunity to intracellular pathogens crossed phylogenetic lines (Ruskin and Remington, 1968; Remington and Merigan, 1969; Ruskin et al., 1969).

In 1970, Zbar, Rapp, and their colleagues showed that rejection of syngeneic tumor cell grafts in guinea pigs could be broken down into several steps (Zbar et al., 1970a, 1970b, 1972; Hanna et al., 1972). These workers noted a readily detectable component of nonspecificity in the host response that rejected neoplastic cells. This was an observation not explained by conventional concepts of tumor immunity of that time (host resistance to neoplastic cells was thought to be always highly specific). Recognition, the first step, was mediated by sensitized lymphocytes and was specific, but tumor cell destruction, the second step, was found to be nonspecific. They demonstrated that close contact between sensitized cells, sensitizing antigen, and the antigenically unrelated tumor cells or *Mycobacterium bovis* (strain bacillus Calmette-Guérin [BCG]) organisms was required to suppress the growth of antigenically unrelated tumor cells. These results showed a requirement for sensitized lymphocytes and specific antigen and, in addition, suggested the involvement of a nonspecific third factor.

In a series of studies, we provided evidence that the mechanisms of host resistance to intracellular pathogens are related to those for neoplasia and that the activated macrophage is a common effector arm for expression of this resistance (Hibbs et al., 1971, 1972a, 1972b, 1972c, 1972d; Hibbs, 1973, 1975a). In vivo experiments showed that mice infected with intracellular protozoa (*Toxoplasma gondii* or *Besnoitia jellsoni*) had increased resistance to autochthonous and transplanted tumors (Hibbs et al., 1971). In this experimental model, viable protozoa persist in multiple tissues for an extended period of time but the mice remain healthy. This provides the necessary context, coexistence of specific antigen and sensitized lymphocytes, for the expression of acquired as well as nonspecific resistance to intracellular pathogens and tumors. We observed an impressive delay in time to death due to spontaneous leukemia in AKR mice with chronic protozoan infection. In one group infected with *Besnoitia,* mice did not begin to die of leukemia until 10 months after chronic infection with the intracellular protozoan parasite was established (Hibbs et al., 1971). By that time 97% of control mice had died of leukemia. These mice were also more resistant than control mice to challenge with *Listeria,* a facultative intracellular bacterium; therefore, chronic infection with intracellular protozoa stimulates nonspecific resistance to a phylogenetically unrelated intracellular pathogen as well as to both autochthonous and transplanted tumor cell growth. Similar results were obtained with mice inoculated with killed *Mycobacterium butyricum* (present in complete Freund's adjuvant) (Hibbs et al., 1972c).

In the above and subsequent studies, we showed that the nonspecific effector component mediating resistance to neoplastic cell proliferation in mice infected with intracellular pathogens is a population of CAM (Hibbs et al., 1971, 1972a, 1972b, 1972c, 1972d; Hibbs, 1973, 1975a). Peritoneal macrophages from mice with chronic *Toxoplasma, Besnoitia,* or BCG infection, or from mice inoculated with killed *M. butyricum* were cytotoxic for syngeneic, allogeneic, and xenogeneic neoplastic cells in vitro. The results also showed that macrophages must undergo functional change in order to express nonspecific cytotoxicity for target cells in vitro. Normal resident peritoneal macrophages or normal macrophages elicited with sterile nonimmunogenic inflammatory stimulants, such as 10% peptone or thioglycolate broth, termed stimulated macrophages, were not cytotoxic for neoplastic cells (Hibbs et al., 1972a, 1972b, 1972d; Hibbs, 1973, 1975a). Therefore, from these studies, it was clear that signals generated during development of cellular immunity to intracellular pathogens in mice caused functional modification of host macrophages. This modification resulted in acquisition by peritoneal macrophages of the ability, when cultured in vitro, to express nonspecific cytotoxicity for tumor cells. In addition to being nonspecific at the effector cell level and an inducible function, the cytotoxic effect of activated macrophages was nonphagocytic and required close contact between the effector macrophages and target cells. Independently, Alexander and Evans (1971) showed that murine macrophages treated with lipopolysaccharide (LPS) in vitro were nonspecifically cytotoxic for syngeneic and allogeneic lymphoma cells by a nonphagocytic mechanism. At the same time, Keller and Jones (1971) demonstrated that macrophages infected with the nematode *Nippostrongylus brasiliensis* were also nonspecifically cytotoxic to neoplastic target cells in vitro. At the time, strict specificity was thought to form the foundation of all aspects of cell-mediated immunity. These experiments were generally viewed to be of little or only peripheral importance to host resistance to neoplastic cells because of the prominent component of nonspecificity observed. However, the original results were confirmed by subsequent experiments by others (Basic et al., 1974; Kaplan et al., 1974; Piessens et al., 1975; Meltzer et al., 1975a, 1975b; Fidler et al., 1976).

CYTOKINES INDUCED BY ANTIGEN-DEPENDENT AS WELL AS ANTIGEN-INDEPENDENT (MICROBIAL) SIGNALS ACTIVATE THE CELL-MEDIATED EFFECTOR MECHANISM THAT CONTAINS A COMPONENT OF NONSPECIFICITY

Once a nonspecific component of host resistance to intracellular pathogens and neoplastic cells mediated by CAM had been defined, it became important to identify the chemical signals that induced normal macrophages to undergo functional change and express nonspecific cytotoxicity for tumor cells. This functional change is caused by the local biochemical environment of a strong cell-mediated immune response often interacting with components of microorganisms (Hibbs et al., 1971, 1972a, 1972b, 1972c, 1972d; Hibbs, 1973, 1975a; Keller and Jones, 1971). When microorganisms invade the tissues, host-derived cytokine signals (particularly interferon-gamma [IFN-γ]) may also interact with signals of microbial origin (LPS, muramyl dipeptide [MDP], etc.). A number of years ago we reported that expression of nonspecific cytotoxicity by macrophages is the result of physiological changes induced by a sequence of differentiation signals (primary signals and second signals or cosignals) (Hibbs et al., 1977; Weinberg et al., 1978; Hibbs et al., 1980a). The experiments demonstrated that culture medium containing macrophage-activating factor (MAF) (activity of MAF later shown to be due to IFN-γ) (Schreiber et al., 1983; Svedersky et al., 1984) required picogram or nanogram quantities of LPS to induce normal or stimulated macrophages to express nonspecific cytotoxicity for tumor cells. These observations were confirmed by others (Russell et al., 1977; Ruco and Meltzer, 1978). The priming step was found to occur in vivo in an anatomical compartment undergoing a cell-mediated immune response or to be induced in vitro by MAF containing serum or supernatants, or by purified preparations of IFN-γ. Small amounts of LPS (nanogram or picogram quantities) or heat-killed *Listeria monocytogenes* were found to be second or cosignals. More recent experiments show that the bacterial cell wall component, MDP, can also function as a second signal (IFN-γ present as the priming signal) (Drapier et al., 1988). Induction of cytotoxicity by IFN-γ plus MDP was inhibited by antitumor necrosis factor-alpha (TNF-α) antibodies. This indicates that endogenously produced TNF-α is involved in the induction of the activated macrophage cytotoxic effector mechanism when MDP is the costimulant of microbial origin with IFN-γ. In contrast, anti-TNF-α antibodies did not fully suppress the effect of combined IFN-γ and LPS. In this case, induction of the cytotoxic effector mechanism may involve other factors in addition to TNF-α. Ding et al. (1988) independently showed that IFN-γ and TNF-α induce this cytotoxic effector mechanism in murine macrophages.

These experiments showed that expression of the activated macrophage cytotoxic effector mechanism required several signals for induction. The results suggested cooperation between signals generated by the cell-mediated immune response (particularly T lymphocyte–derived IFN-γ and macrophage-derived TNF-α) and signals of microbial origin (LPS, *Listeria* cell walls, and MDP). The cytotoxic effector mechanism remains poised but inactive (or only minimally active) in IFN-γ–primed macrophages (noncytotoxic activated macrophages) until contact is made with a microbial component or TNF-α. These results showed that microbial products can interact with MAF/IFN-γ causing activation of this effector mechanism. The response to microbial products could have been selected as a means to limit activation of this effector mechanism to IFN-γ–exposed macrophages that come in direct contact with certain microorganisms or their components. In this case, microbial molecules induce macrophages to secrete TNF-α (and perhaps other cytokines) that can have autocrine effects that cause expression of cytostatic or cytolytic activity for certain microorganisms or mammalian cells. These experiments show that microbial components such as LPS or MDP, in addition to cytokines, can participate in the complex network of regulation of the normal cell-mediated immune response.

Taken together, these studies provided evidence that infections with intracellular pathogens (or pathogens too large to be phagocytized) induced biochemical changes that cause increased nonspecific resistance to spontaneous and transplanted tumors in vivo. However, several questions had to be answered in order to fully understand the biological significance of these experimental observations demonstrating nonspecific elements to host resistance and to relate them in a meaningful way to other better defined host defense mechanisms. First, what are the biochemical changes induced in target cells (neoplastic cells or certain microorganisms) by the cell-mediated effector mechanism associated with expression of increased nonspecific resistance? And second, what is the effector mechanism that causes the biochemical changes?

THE ACTIVATED MACROPHAGE EFFECTOR MECHANISM CAUSES LOSS OF INTRACELLULAR IRON AND INHIBITION OF ENZYMES THAT HAVE CATALYTICALLY ACTIVE NONHEME IRON COORDINATED TO SULFUR

The results described above suggest that the cell-mediated response to intracellular microorganisms and neoplastic cells has similar elements. Experimental manipulation that enhanced resistance to intracellular pathogens in the tissues also enhanced resistance to the growth of neoplastic cells (Hibbs, 1975b; Hibbs et al., 1971, 1972c, 1980b). In vitro studies showed that macrophages from mice infected with intracellular bacteria or protozoans had potent cytotoxic effects for tumor target cells (Hibbs et al., 1971, 1972a, 1972b, 1972c, 1972d; Hibbs, 1973, 1975a). At this point it became important to attempt to understand this newly defined and nonspecific component of cell-mediated immunity at the biochemical level. Early studies demonstrated that CAM induce inhibition of DNA replication as determined by [^{3}H]-thymidine uptake by tumor target cells (Keller, 1973; Krahenbuhl and Remington, 1974; Krahenbuhl, 1980; Granger et al., 1980; Hibbs and Granger, 1982; Hibbs et al., 1984; Drapier and Hibbs, 1986). Ribonucleotide reductase, the rate-limiting enzyme in DNA synthesis, contains nonheme iron essential for its catalytic activity (Reichard and Ehrenberg, 1983). Figure 2-1 shows the kinetics of inhibition of [^{3}H]-thymidine incorporation in L10 cells cocultivated with CAM.

Approximately 10 years ago we observed that target cells cocultivated with CAM develop inhibition of mitochondrial respiration but remain viable and continue to synthesize adenosine triphosphate (ATP) via the glycolytic pathway (Granger et al., 1980). Glycolysis is a metabolic pathway that does not have catalytically active iron. Granger and Lehninger (1982) then demonstrated that this CAM-induced effect is due to inhibition of the proximal two oxidoreductases of the mitochondrial electron transport system; nicotinamide-adenine dinucleotide, reduced (NADH): ubiquinone oxidoreductase (complex I) and succinate:ubiquinone oxidoreductase (complex II). Other enzymes of the mitochondrial electron transport system of tumor target cells were not affected. Figure 2-2, a schematic representation of the citric acid cycle and the mitochondrial electron transport chain, is provided for reference. Complex I and complex II are iron-sulfur (Fe-S) flavoprotein dehydrogenases that contain most of the Fe-S complexes of the mitochondrial electron transport chain and that are essential for the catalytic function of these two oxidoreductases. We then performed experiments to

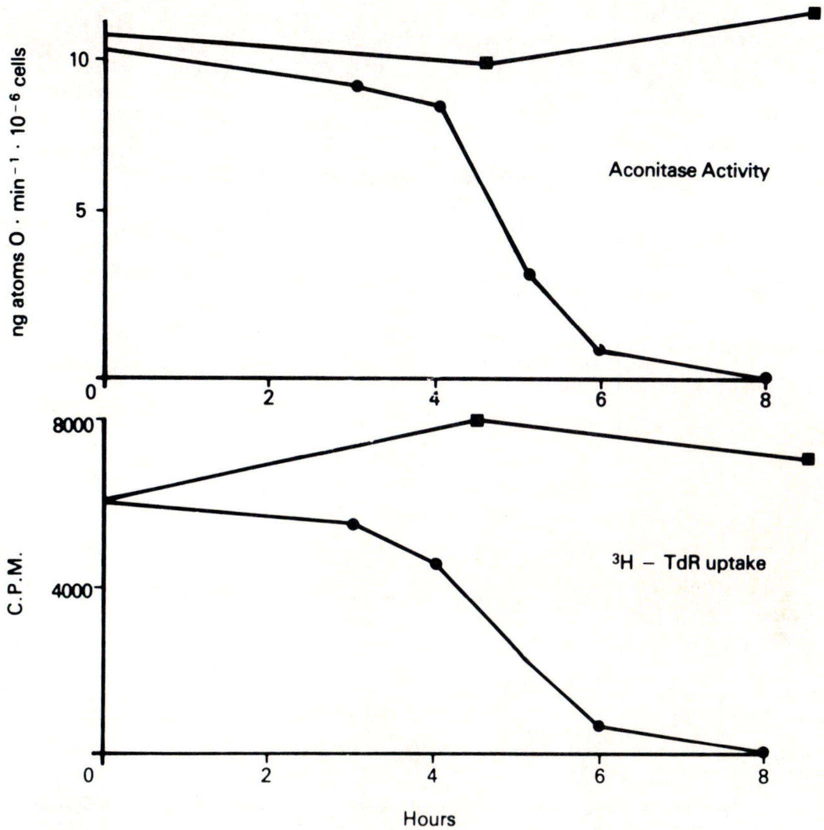

FIGURE 2-1
The kinetics of citrate-dependent respiration (aconitase activity and [^{3}H]-thymidine incorporation into DNA in L10 cells cultured alone or cocultivated with cytotoxic-activated macrophages. Measurement of aconitase activity and DNA synthesis were as described. (From Drapier and Hibbs, 1986, with permission.)

determine if the CAM effector mechanism causes perturbation of intracellular iron metabolism in target cells during cocultivation (Hibbs et al., 1984; Drapier and Hibbs, 1986). Results showed that tumor target cells cocultivated with CAM released a significant fraction of their intracellular iron content in parallel with development of inhibition of DNA synthesis and inhibition of mitochondrial respiration (Fig. 2-3). Kinetic studies showed that specific release of iron-59 from target cells began 4 to 6 hours after initiating cocultivation, which was the time point that inhibition of DNA synthesis was first detected (Fig. 2-1). Since both DNA replication and mitochondrial respiration are metabolic pathways with enzymatic activity vulnerable to inhibition by depletion of intracellular iron, this observation suggested a link between CAM-induced

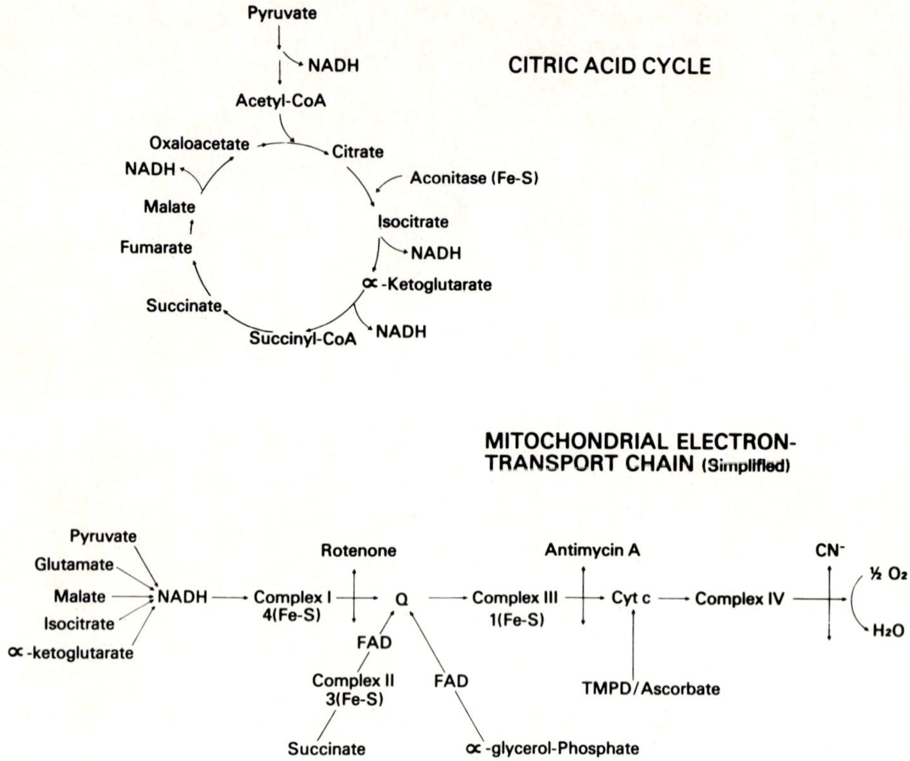

FIGURE 2-2
Schematic representation of the citric acid cycle and the mitochondrial electron transport chain. (From Drapier and Hibbs, 1986, with permission.)

iron mobilization in target cells and CAM-induced cytotoxicity. We next examined aconitase, a citric acid cycle enzyme with a catalytically active (4Fe-4S) cluster, to determine if Fe-S prosthetic groups are targets for CAM-induced iron removal (Drapier and Hibbs, 1986). Results showed that aconitase activity declined dramatically in target cells after 4 hours of cocultivation with CAM (Fig. 2-1). Aconitase inhibition occurred simultaneously with arrest of DNA synthesis, another CAM-induced metabolic change in target cells. Incubation of CAM-injured target cells in culture medium supplemented with ferrous ions plus a reducing agent caused near complete reconstitution of aconitase activity. These results showed that removal of a labile iron atom from the (4Fe-4S) cluster, by a CAM-mediated mechanism, is causally related to aconitase inhibition in tumor target cells.

We also observed that murine CAM developed the same pattern of metabolic inhibition that we had described earlier in their target cells (Drapier and Hibbs, 1988) (Fig. 2-4). Macrophages activated in vivo by infection with BCG or in vitro with IFN-γ or IFN-α/β (in the presence of the second or cosignal LPS in all cases) develop inhibition

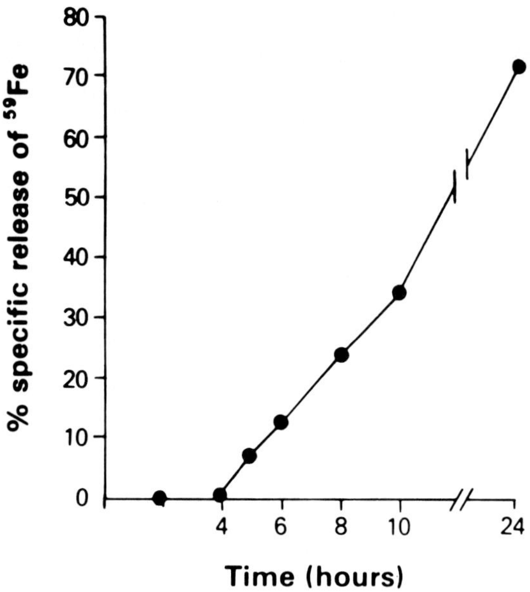

FIGURE 2-3
Kinetics of ^{59}Fe-specific release from viable murine L1210 leukemia cells cocultivated with CAM. (Adapted from Hibbs et al., 1984, with permission.)

of aconitase activity followed by inhibition of complex I and complex II of the mitochondrial electron transport chain. The pattern of inhibition of aconitase activity, complex I, and complex II in CAM is similar to that measured in earlier studies of the target cells of CAM (Drapier and Hibbs, 1986; Granger and Lehninger, 1982). However, the kinetics of inhibition of complex I and complex II are more rapid and residual enzymatic activity is less than we measure in target cells of CAM (Drapier and Hibbs, 1986). All enzymatic activities remained intact for at least 22 hours in stimulated macrophages cultured under the same conditions (Drapier and Hibbs, 1988). The same pattern of metabolic inhibition developed in parallel with loss of intracellular iron to the extracellular environment in the continuous murine macrophage cell line RAW 264.7 cells exposed to IFN-γ plus LPS (Drapier and Hibbs, 1988). These results strongly implicated the existence of an inducible activated macrophage cytotoxic effector mechanism that targeted intracellular iron. Interestingly, an earlier study had pointed to involvement of iron in expression of activated macrophage–induced cytotoxicity. We observed that endocytosis of erythrocytes or hemoglobin by activated macrophages inhibited their cytotoxic effect for tumor target cells (Weinberg and Hibbs, 1977). Erythrocytes that were added to the CAM tumor cell cocultures, but were not phagocytized, had no inhibitory effect. Hemoglobin as well as ferric and ferrous ions also inhibited the nonspecific cytotoxic effect of activated macrophages in this study.

The experimental evidence suggested that CAM cause inhibition of certain enzymatic activities by interfering with intracellular iron homeostasis. Certain enzymes with nonheme iron essential for catalytic activity (aconitase, complex I, and complex

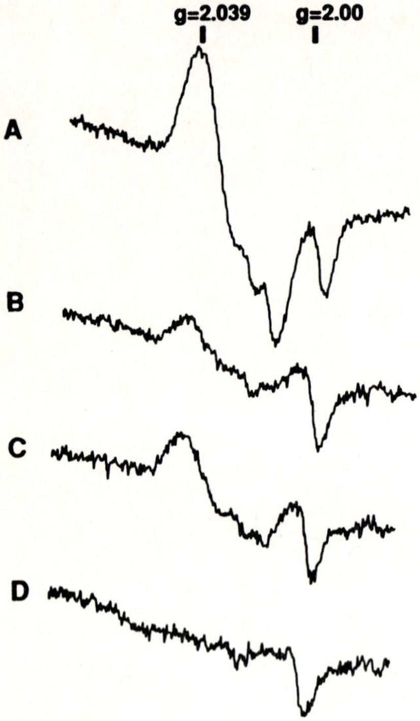

TREATMENT	NO_2^- (NMOL/10^7 CELLS)	NO_3^- (NMOL/10^7 CELLS)	CITRULLINE (NMOL/10^7 CELLS)
+L-ARGININE	425.5	569.4	650.0
+L-ARGININE + N^GMMA	66.7	68.1	142.2
NO ADDITION	108.3	81.5	221.3
+ N^GMMA	8.8	24.5	20.4

FIGURE 2-4
L-arginine-dependent simultaneous formation of nitrite, nitrate, citrulline, and the g = 2.039 signal by cytotoxic-activated macrophages. After a 20.5-hour incubation with the indicated additives, cells were treated and analyzed for nitrite, nitrate, and citrulline. Whole cell aliquots were examined by EPR spectroscopy as described with a modulation amplitude of 10 G (1 G = 0.1 mT) and a relative instrument gain of 1.6×10^3. N^GMMLA, N^G monomethyl-L-arginine. (From Lancaster and Hibbs, 1990, with permission.)

II) were strongly inhibited by the CAM effector mechanism. Enzymes containing heme prosthetic groups can also be inhibited by this effector mechanism. We have measured significant inhibition of cytochrome oxidase, a component of complex IV of the mitochondrial electron transport chain, in CAM and their target cells (Drapier and Hibbs, 1988). However, cytochrome oxidase is more resistant to inhibition mediated by the CAM effector mechanism than aconitase, complex I, and complex II. The experimental results suggest that the CAM effector mechanism causing cytostasis of tumor target cells removes or restricts intracellular iron that functions catalytically in certain enzymes and, in addition, restricts availability of the intracellular pool of iron available for recruitment into the catalytic iron compartment. This also could be a mechanism for controlling the proliferation of microorganisms that invade the intracellular environment of mammalian cells, as well as microorganisms that are too large to be phagocytized and, as a result, must be lysed or rendered static in the extracellular environment.

It has been recognized for many years that infection and inflammation cause a hypoferremic response in extracellular fluids (mediated at least in part by monocyte-macrophage derived IL-1α) that severely limits iron availability to extracellular pathogens (Weinberg, 1971, 1978; Lee, 1983). The results summarized above show that mouse peritoneal macrophages (when activated by a strong cell-mediated immune response) cause loss of intracellular iron from their own intracellular environment as well as the intracellular environment of target cells. This occurs in parallel with the development of inhibition of certain enzymes whose catalytic activity depends on iron containing-prosthetic groups. Therefore, these studies show that in addition to homeostatic controls that limit iron availability in the extracellular environment, there exists a component of cell-mediated immunity that targets intracellular iron and restricts iron availability in the intracellular environment. At this point the task turned to an attempt to identify an effector molecule(s) capable of causing these biochemical effects as well as an enzymatic pathway, induced by signals generated by the cell-mediated immune response, that synthesized the effector molecule.

THE BIOLOGICAL SYNTHESIS OF INORGANIC NITROGEN OXIDES FROM REDUCED ORGANIC NITROGEN

A brief summary of the biological synthesis of inorganic nitrogen oxides from reduced organic nitrogen will help place the recently observed synthesis of NO from L-arginine into a more general context. Until recently, the only known process for the biological synthesis of inorganic nitrogen oxides from reduced organic nitrogen was thought to be confined to chemoautotrophic soil bacteria (Lees, 1952; Suzuki, 1974; Hooper, 1984). Nitrogen in decomposing organic matter is largely converted to ammonia (NH_3). This volatile compound is then stabilized in the soil by oxidation through the action of nitrifying bacteria. *Nitrosomonas* oxidizes NH_3 to nitrite (NO_2^-) and *Nitrobacter* oxidizes the NO_2^- synthesized by *Nitrosomonas* to nitrate (NO_3^-). NO_3^- is absorbed by the root system of plants, reduced, and again incorporated into organic nitrogen–containing compounds. It was believed that the biological synthesis of inorganic nitrogen oxides was confined to nitrogen cycle activity described above and that mammals were not capable of synthesizing inorganic nitrogen oxides (although a metabolic balance study carried out in 1916 suggested humans were capable of NO_3^- synthesis [Mitchell et al., 1916], these results were either discounted or ignored).

In 1981 Tannenbaum and co-workers, as well as Witter et al., reported metabolic balance studies that showed that conventional and germ-free rats synthesize NO_3^- (Green et al., 1981b; Witter et al., 1981). This confirmed the earlier 1916 study and unequivocally demonstrated that NO_3^- synthesis is also a mammalian process. Equivalent results for germ-free and conventional rats eliminated the microflora as a significant contributor to NO_3^- production. Tannenbaum's group, with an interest in nitrosamine-induced carcinogenesis and working at the Massachusetts Institute of

Technology (MIT), then investigated NO_3^- metabolism in long-term metabolic balance studies in healthy humans. Under conditions of controlled low NO_3^- intake (less than 180 μmol/day/subject), the amount of NO_3^- excreted in the urine was fourfold greater than the amount ingested (Green et al., 1981a, 1981b). Balance studies with $^{15}NO_3^-$ showed that the source of excess NO_3^- in the urine was the endogenous synthesis of nitrate rather than emptying of a body storage pool. During one of these studies a human subject consuming a low and constant intake of dietary NO_3^- developed an unexpected increase of NO_3^- biosynthesis that occurred simultaneously with the onset of fever and diarrhea (Wagner and Tannenbaum, 1982). Compared to baseline levels, urinary NO_3^- excretion increased ninefold during the illness. Following this observation, Tannenbaum and co-workers examined the effect of LPS treatment on NO_3^- excretion in rats (Wagner et al., 1983). The results showed that LPS caused a marked (ninefold) increase in NO_3^- excretion. It was further demonstrated in these studies that the enhanced rate of NO_3^- excretion by LPS was not due to a reduction in NO_3^- metabolic loss but to an increased rate of synthesis.

Following these observations, Stuehr and Marletta (1985) (also working at MIT) examined the possibility that macrophages could be the source of NO_3^- synthesis. They administered LPS to mice and noted increased levels of NO_3^- in the blood and increased NO_3^- excretion in the urine, which confirmed the earlier studies in the rat. Then, using mouse peritoneal macrophages cultured in the presence of LPS, these workers showed that macrophages are capable of NO_2^- and NO_3^- biosynthesis from an unknown precursor(s). At this point our research program at the University of Utah intersected, from a very different point of experimental departure, with that of the MIT group. For many years we had been investigating the biology of the nonspecific cytotoxic reaction expressed by activated macrophages and the biochemical lesions induced in target cells of CAM (Hibbs et al., 1971, 1972a, 1972b, 1972c, 1972d; Hibbs, 1973, 1975a; Hibbs et al., 1977; Weinberg and Hibbs, 1977; Weinberg et al., 1978; Granger et al., 1980; Hibbs and Granger, 1982; Drapier and Hibbs, 1986). This is the work briefly discussed in the foregoing sections of this review. In the course of these studies we observed that L-arginine was required for development of activated macrophage–induced cytotoxicity (cytostasis) (Hibbs et al., 1987a). We also noted that, in parallel with the development of cytotoxicity, L-arginine was directly converted to L-citrulline without loss of the guanidino carbon atom (Hibbs et al., 1987b). The molecular mechanisms linking the direct synthesis of L-citrulline from L-arginine with expression of nonspecific cytotoxicity by activated macrophages were not immediately obvious. However, early in 1986 we became aware of the results published by Stuehr and Marletta (1985). Their findings provided the clue to the fate of the imino nitrogen atom lost from the guanidino group of L-arginine when CAM directly synthesize L-citrulline from L-arginine and express nonspecific cytotoxicity for tumor target cells. It seemed very likely that NO_2^- and NO_3^- were also products of the same pathway synthesizing L-citrulline from L-arginine and associated with expression of activated-macrophage cytotoxicity. We showed this to be the case in studies that will be described in detail later in this review (Hibbs et al., 1987a, 1987b, 1988; Drapier and Hibbs, 1988; Amber et al., 1988a, 1988b; Drapier et al., 1988). This work established a novel pathway synthesizing NO_2^-, NO_3^-, and L-citrulline (direct synthesis) from L-arginine by mammalian macrophages and that activation of this pathway resulted in the typical pattern of activated macrophage–induced cytotoxicity in tumor target cells.

The pathway synthesizing NO from L-arginine, which is the focus of this review, is an effector limb of the cell-mediated immune response that is induced in the tissues by cytokines. However, in addition to a role in macrophage effector functions, NO also has other bioregulatory activities. For example, before the biological synthesis of NO was discovered, it was known that organic nitrates and authentic NO can increase cyclic guanosine monophosphate (cGMP) levels by forming a nitrosyl heme moiety that associates with and activates soluble guanylate cyclase (Murad et al., 1978; Ignarro and Gruetter, 1980). Recently it has been found that NO synthesized from L-arginine by an enzymatic pathway similar to that existing in macrophages also functions as a signal, causing activation of soluble guanylate cyclase. Endothelial cell–dependent vascular smooth muscle relaxation and inhibition of platelet aggregation (in the presence of cyclooxygenase inhibition) (Palmer et al., 1987, 1988; Radomski et al., 1987) as well as N-methyl-D-aspartate–induced elevation of cGMP in neural tissue (Garthwaite et al., 1988; Knowles et al., 1989) are examples of modulation of cellular function via signal transduction by NO synthesized from L-arginine by a constitutive pathway. Ignarro and his colleagues (1987a, 1987b) independently demonstrated that endothelium-derived relaxing factor is NO. These findings show that NO synthesized from L-arginine functions in two ways. It is a cytotoxic effector molecular that causes enzymatic inhibition via iron–nitrosyl complex formation and, in addition, an intracellular messenger involved in cGMP-mediated functional linkage between cells. The quantity of NO synthesized, as well as other factors, may determine the type of biological activity observed.

DISCOVERY THAT L-ARGININE IS THE PRECURSOR MOLECULE, THAT L-CITRULLINE IS AN ADDITIONAL PRODUCT, AND THAT N^G-MONOMETHYL-L-ARGININE IS AN INHIBITOR OF THE MAMMALIAN PATHWAY SYNTHESIZING INORGANIC NITROGEN OXIDES

The L-arginine requirement for expression of activated-macrophage nonspecific cytotoxicity was identified while performing experiments asking an unrelated question. We noted that activated macrophages cultured in medium without amino acids, vitamins, or pyruvate were not cytotoxic for tumor target cells (Hibbs et al., 1987a). The cytotoxic activity of activated macrophages was not restored when the deficient culture medium was supplemented with vitamins or pyruvate. However, when modified Eagle's medium (MEM) amino acid mixture was added to the culture medium, activated macrophages were cytotoxic for tumor target cells. We then observed that the

TABLE 2-1A

Additives	Nitrite and L-citrulline concentrations in coculture medium: 7.5 hours coculture		10 hours coculture		24 hours coculture	
	Nitrite	Citrulline	Nitrite	Citrulline	Nitrite	Citrulline
None	7.5 ± 1.6	ND	10.1 ± 0.82	ND	21.0 ± 1.68	ND
L-arginine	33.1 ± 0.36	67.5 ± 7.5	44.8 ± 2.14	111.4 ± 0.09	106.0 ± 3.00	346.7 ± 46.5
L-NMMLA	3.1 ± 0.05	ND	3.1 ± 0.09	ND	4.3 ± 0.09	ND
L-arginine + L-NMMLA	11.4 ± 0.90	5.0 ± 3.0	15.8 ± 0.45	15.0 ± 9.0	24.2 ± 0.68	22.0 ± 18

TABLE 2-1B

Additives	L10 cell aconitase activity and DNA synthesis: Aconitase activity		[³H]-thymidine uptake	
	Nanomoles per minute per 10^6 cells	Percent of control L10 cells	Counts per minute	Percent of control L10 cells
None	3.54 ± 0.48	81.5	16,097 ± 637	93.7
L-arginine	0.30 ± 0.06	7.6	897 ± 90	6.0
N^GMMLA	4.06 ± 0.3	99.5	20,887 ± 739	138.2
L-arginine + N^GMMLA	3.16 ± 0.40	97.8	14,291 ± 1310	99.4

The CAM effector mechanism causing inhibition of aconitase and DNA synthesis in L10 cells requires L-arginine, converts L-arginine to L-citrulline plus nitrite, and is inhibited by N^GMMLA. Culture medium was supplemented with 1.2 mM L-arginine and/or 0.1 mM N^GMMLA where indicated. Data in Tables 2-1A and 2-1B were obtained by measuring the nitrite and L-citrulline levels in the culture medium and aconitase activity and [^{3}H]-thymidine uptake in L10 cells from the same experiment. Values are the mean ± SEM of three experiments (citrulline and DNA synthesis; aconitase activity) and five experiments (nitrite synthesis). ND, not detected by the method. See Hibbs et al., 1987b for experimental details.

cytotoxic effect of activated macrophages was expressed when L-arginine was added to the culture medium in the absence of all other amino acids (Hibbs et al., 1987a). The magnitude of inhibition of mitochondrial respiration in all target cells tested was directly proportional to the amount of L-arginine in the amino acid mixture. Activated macrophages were not cytotoxic for tumor cells when the cocultivation medium was supplemented with D-arginine rather than L-arginine. This demonstrated that the CAM effector mechanism had a stereospecific requirement for L-arginine. We also observed that L-citrulline was directly synthesized from L-arginine without loss of the guanidino carbon atom and the N^G-monomethyl-L-arginine (N^GMMLA) was a potent competitive inhibitor of the synthesis of L-citrulline from L-arginine as well as the nonspecific cytotoxic activity of activated macrophages (Hibbs et al., 1987a).

When we became aware of the findings of Stuehr and Marletta, it seemed very likely to us that, in addition to the precursor molecule L-arginine and the product L-citrulline identified in our studies (Hibbs et al., 1987b), NO_2^- and NO_3^- (identified by Stuehr and Marletta, 1985, 1987a, 1987b) were also products of this same pathway associated with expression of activated-macrophage cytotoxicity. This proved to be the case. We observed that CAM synthesized NO_2^- and L-citrulline in a coordinated manner from L-arginine and that N^GMMLA inhibited the synthesis of both products as well as the expression of cytotoxicity by activated macrophages (Tables 2-1A and 2-1B) (Hibbs et al., 1987b). These experiments demonstrated for the first time an enzymatic pathway synthesizing L-citrulline (direct synthesis) from L-arginine that was coupled to oxidation of the imino nitrogen derived from the guanidino group of L-arginine. In addition, N^GMMLA was identified as a specific inhibitor of this pathway. A cause-and-effect relationship was shown to exist between activity of this pathway and expression of nonspecific cytotoxicity by activated macrophages (Hibbs et al., 1987a, 1987b). Iyengar et al. (1987) confirmed that L-arginine is the precursor of NO_2^- and NO_3^- synthesized by activated macrophages and that L-citrulline is an additional product of the pathway.

NITRIC OXIDE IS THE PRECURSOR OF THE NITRITE/NITRATE SYNTHESIZED FROM L-ARGININE BY ACTIVATED MACROPHAGES AND, BY FORMING IRON-NITROSYL COMPLEXES WITH INTRACELLULAR IRON, IS AN EFFECTOR MOLECULE OF ACTIVATED MACROPHAGE–MEDIATED CYTOTOXICITY

Once the stable products of the L-arginine–dependent pathway (NO_2^-/NO_3^-/L-citrulline) had been identified, NO became the inorganic nitrogen oxide intermediate in the pathway of NO_2^-/NO_3^- synthesis most likely to cause iron loss and the pattern of CAM-induced metabolic inhibition observed in earlier studies. The possibility that NO could be the precursor of the NO_2^-/NO_3^- synthesized from L-arginine by CAM was supported by the findings of Palmer et al. (1987) and Ignarro et al. (1987a, 1987b).

These workers demonstrated that NO released by vascular endothelial cells accounted for the biological activity of endothelium-derived relaxing factor. This first demonstration of the synthesis of NO by mammalian cells was followed by a second report by Palmer et al. (1988) demonstrating that endothelial cell–derived NO is synthesized from a terminal guanidino nitrogen atom of L-arginine by the same or very similar pathway first identified in activated macrophages. Three laboratories then independently demonstrated that NO synthesized from a terminal guanidino nitrogen atom of L-arginine is the precursor of the NO_2^-/NO_3^- previously shown to be synthesized by activated macrophages (Hibbs et al., 1988; Marletta et al., 1988; Stuehr et al., 1989a). Furthermore, the pattern of activated macrophage–induced metabolic inhibition in tumor cells could be reproduced by treatment with authentic NO (Hibbs et al., 1988). Intracellular iron loss, inhibition of mitochondrial respiration, inhibition of aconitase activity, and inhibition of DNA synthesis was induced in guinea pig L10 hepatoma cells by treatment with authentic NO gas under anaerobic culture conditions. The NO effect for L10 hepatoma cells was cytostatic rather than cytolytic. Most of the NO-treated L10 hepatoma cells remained viable when cultured during a second incubation in medium containing glucose. However, more than 95% of the L10 hepatoma cells that had been treated with authentic NO underwent lysis during a second incubation in medium without glucose. This suggested that treatment of L10 hepatoma cells with authentic NO, similar to cocultivation with CAM, induced inhibition of complex I and complex II of the mitochondrial electron transport chain. This indeed is the case because Stuehr and Nathan (1989b) found that complex I and complex II were selectively inhibited in mitochondria of murine L1210 leukemia cells that had been treated with authentic NO.

These experiments demonstrated that NO is synthesized from L-arginine by CAM and that authentic NO causes iron loss, cytostasis, and the same pattern of biochemical inhibition in tumor cells as is induced by cocultivation with CAM (Hibbs et al., 1987a, 1987b, 1988; Drapier and Hibbs, 1988). The observations provided the information needed to elucidate a molecular explanation for the activated macrophage–mediated cytotoxicity that we had been studying. It was known that exposure of Fe-S groups to NO resulted in iron–nitrosyl complex formation (Salerno et al., 1976; Meyer, 1981; Reddy et al., 1983). Therefore, iron–nitrosyl complex formation could cause inactivation and/or degradation of Fe-S prosthetic groups and provide a molecular explanation for the pattern of biochemical inhibition induced by activated macrophages.

Since CAM develop the same pattern of L-arginine–dependent metabolic inhibition as is induced in their target cells (Drapier and Hibbs, 1988), we performed experiments to identify iron–nitrosyl complexes in the cytoplasm of CAM. The results demonstrated L-arginine–dependent nitrosyl–iron–sulfur complex formation in macrophages activated by a cell-mediated immune response in vivo but not in stimulated macrophages (Lancaster and Hibbs, 1990). Using electron paramagnetic resonance (EPR) spectroscopy, we observed that activated macrophages removed from the peritoneal cavity of mice with chronic BCG infection and subsequently exposed to small quantities of LPS in vitro had a strong axial signal at g = 2.039. This signal was similar to that previously recorded from nitrosyl–iron–sulfur complexes formed by the destruction of Fe-S centers by NO. The signal was dependent on the presence of L-arginine in the culture medium and was inhibited by N^{G}MMLA. We compared the hyperfine structure of the EPR signal from cells treated with L-arginine with terminal guanidino nitrogen atoms labeled with ^{14}N or ^{15}N. The results confirmed that the nitrosyl nitrogen in the paramagnetic complexes arises from one of the two terminal guanidino nitrogen atoms. Pellat et al. (1990) reported similar observations. They

FIGURE 2-5
Precursor and products of the biological synthesis of inorganic nitrogen oxides and L-citrulline from L-arginine. ^{15}N-containing products derived from L-[guanidino-$^{15}N_2$] arginine were identified by gas chromatography/mass spectrometry (Hibbs et al., 1988; Iyengar et al., 1987; Marletta et al., 1988; Palmer et al., 1988) or EPR spectroscopy (Lancaster and Hibbs, 1990) except for nitrogen dioxide (NO_2), which was detected by another method (Hibbs et al., 1988). The direct synthesis of L-citrulline from L-arginine has been identified with several techniques (Hibbs et al., 1987; Iyengar et al., 1987; Amber et al., 1988b; Hibbs et al., 1988; Palmer and Moncada, 1989; Knowles et al., 1989). The experiments utilizing L-[guanidino-^{14}C] arginine as precursor (Amber et al., 1988b; Hibbs et al., 1988) were performed as described. NO formed by reaction 1 can undergo oxidative degradation in aqueous solution (reactions 2 and 3) or react with nonheme iron associated with sulfur atoms to form sulfur–iron–nitrosyl complexes (reaction 4). Although not shown, certain other forms of intracellular iron, including ferritin iron, also probably complex with NO. (Hibbs JB Jr, unpublished data.)

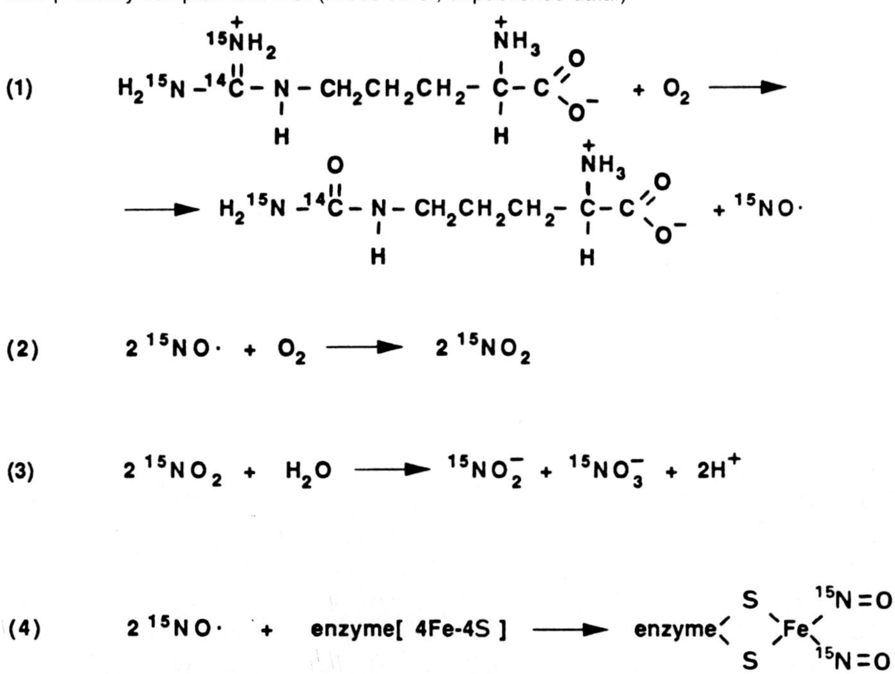

observed that stimulated macrophages treated with IFN-γ develop an EPR signal in the g = 2.04 region characteristic of paramagnetic nitrosyl–iron–sulfur complexes. Furthermore, exposure of control macrophages to excess $NaNO_2$ and ascorbate after helium deoxygenation (a treatment that generated NO in the culture medium) resulted in the appearance of the same g = 2.04 signal as was seen in the IFN-γ treated macrophages. The axial EPR signal that we and Pellat et al. observed in CAM was similar to that described earlier by Vanin (1967), who treated mitochondria and other biological materials containing Fe-S complexes with authentic NO.

This demonstrated that CAM synthesize NO and that this synthesis results in the formation of iron–nitrosyl complexes in the CAM effector cells (Lancaster and Hibbs, 1990; Pellat et al., 1990). The formation of iron–nitrosyl complexes with the Fe-S prosthetic groups of complex I and complex II of the CAM mitochondrial electron transport chain and with the Fe-S prosthetic group of aconitase in CAM explains the pattern of enzymatic inhibition caused by NO synthesis from L-arginine. In addition, in other experiments, we observed significant inhibition of cytochrome oxidase (>50%) following a 24-hour cultivation of RAW 264.7 macrophages with IFN-γ plus LPS (Drapier and Hibbs, 1988). It is of interest that cytochrome oxidase (a component of complex IV) is a heme protein sensitive to nitrosylation (Rousseau et al., 1988).

The identification of iron–nitrosyl complexes in these studies links iron, which is known to be lost from cells that develop activated-macrophage cytotoxicity (Hibbs et al., 1984; Drapier and Hibbs, 1986, 1988), the inhibition of enzymes with Fe-S prosthetic groups (Granger et al., 1980; Drapier and Hibbs, 1986; Hibbs et al., 1987a, 1987b, 1988; Drapier and Hibbs, 1988; Amber et al., 1988a, 1988b; Drapier et al., 1988; Kilbourn et al., 1984), and NO, which is synthesized by activated macrophages capable of expressing cytotoxicity (Hibbs et al., 1988; Marletta et al., 1988; Stuehr et al., 1989a). Although many details remain to be elucidated, with these observations, we have achieved an understanding at the biochemical and molecular level of the L-arginine–dependent effector pathway and the mechanism of expression of this pathway of activated macrophage–induced cytotoxicity. The sequence of reactions illustrated in Fig. 2-5 is compatible with the experimental results.

CYTOKINES INDUCE THE PATHWAY SYNTHESIZING INORGANIC NITROGEN OXIDES AND L-CITRULLINE FROM L-ARGININE IN NONMACROPHAGE CELLS

Induction of NO synthesis by CAM from L-arginine by an interacting network of cytokines or cytokines interacting with certain microbial products (e.g., LPS, MDP, *Listeria* cell walls) causes a reproducible pattern of biochemical effects including inhibition of DNA replication (Drapier and Hibbs, 1988; Drapier et al., 1988). However, in spite of developing profound cytostasis, many mammalian cells do not undergo cytolysis (Hibbs et al., 1987a, 1987b, 1988). If a network of cytokine signals, or cytokine signals plus signals of microbial origin, induces the synthesis of NO from

L-arginine in all or most somatic cells, this could markedly enhance the efficiency of cell-mediated immunity in controlling the proliferation of intracellular microorganisms or neoplastic cells in the tissues. In this manner, signals generated by a cell-mediated immune response could cause NO-induced biochemical changes locally in nonmacrophage cells of tissues invaded by certain microorganisms or within the cells comprising a tumor mass.

This may be a possibility because we observed that combinations of cytokines can induce the L-arginine–dependent effector system in nonmacrophage cells (Amber et al., 1988a, 1988b). This observation was confirmed by others (Lepoivre et al., 1989). Treatment of murine EMT-6 mammary adenocarcinoma cells with IFN-γ plus TNF-α and/or interleukin-1 (IL-1) caused release of ^{55}Fe label, inhibition of DNA replication, and inhibition of aconitase activity (Amber et al., 1988b) (Fig. 2-6). In addition, the same combination of cytokines induced EMT-6 cells to synthesize NO_2^-, NO_3^-, and L-citrulline directly from L-arginine (Amber et al., 1988b). These findings were identical to those obtained when macrophages were exposed to IFN-γ plus TNF-α or IFN-γ plus a microbial component (LPS or MDP) (Drapier and Hibbs, 1988; Drapier et al., 1988; Ding et al., 1988). We also observed that LPS can act as a cofactor in the induction of these metabolic effects when added to EMT-6 cells in the presence of IFN-γ (Amber et al., 1988b). These results demonstrated that increased levels of cytokines in the microenvironment can induce the L-arginine–dependent pathway in somatic cells not specialized for host defense, resulting in specific metabolic effects as well as the inhibition of cellular proliferation. (We have also found that murine fibroblasts synthesize NO, NO_2^-, NO_3^-, and L-citrulline from L-arginine [Hibbs JB Jr, Taintor RR, Vavrin Z, unpublished data]). These findings enlarge the frame of reference for the concept of cell-mediated immunity. The results suggest, at least in mice, that interleukin-2 (IL-2)–driven responses resulting in the synthesis of IFN-γ, IL-1, TNF-β, and/or TNF-α, as well as other cytokines, have the potential for inducing the pathway synthesizing NO from L-arginine in many types of nucleated somatic cells, including tumor cell phenotypes. In this more general context, macrophages can be viewed as highly mobile phagocytic cells that are recruited in large numbers to an anatomical compartment by cytokine signals generated by a cell-mediated immune response occurring in that anatomical area. As suggested by the experiments described above, it is possible that many or all fixed differentiated cells of that local anatomical area also actively participate biochemically in the cell-mediated immune response in a manner very similar to the macrophages recruited from the bone marrow. The local network of cytokines (molecules of microbial origin may contribute to the signaling when microorganisms invade the tissues) may induce the L-arginine–dependent effector pathway synthesizing NO from L-arginine in many or all cells of that local anatomical area. This could cause iron–nitrosyl complex formation in all cells within the local region affected by the cell-mediated immune response. In addition to producing the typical pattern of enzymatic inhibition, the local production of high levels of NO could limit iron availability for neoplastic cells or for invading microorganisms.

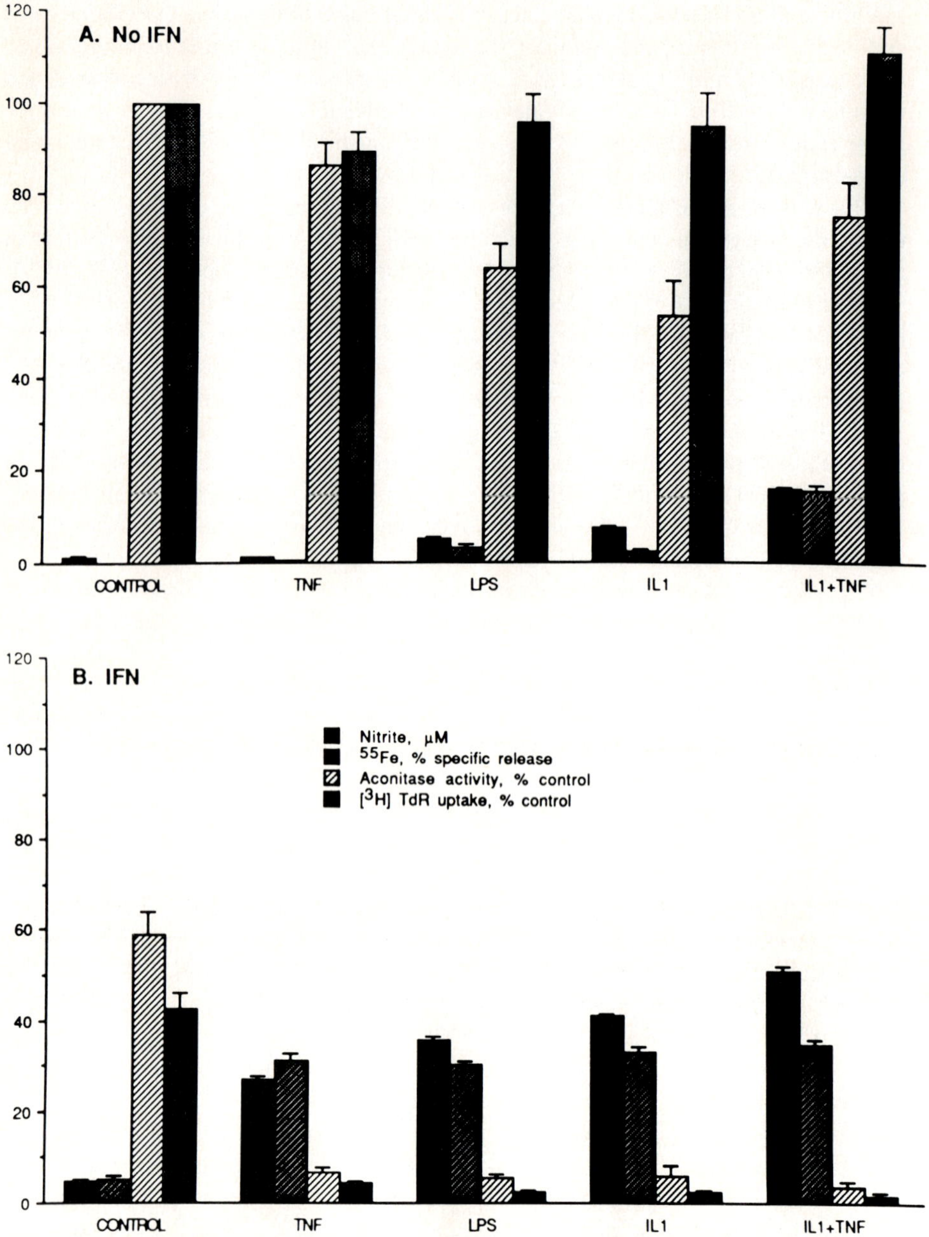

FIGURE 2-6
Cytokine treatment of EMT-6 cells results in development of biochemical changes characteristic of the L-arginine–dependent effector system. Cytokine and LPS concentrations were IFN-γ 10 U/ml, IL-1α, 10 U/ml, TNF-α 50 U/ml, and LPS 10 ng/ml. Control EMT-6 cells in panel A were cultured without added cytokines or LPS. Control EMT-6 cells in panel B were

EVIDENCE FOR THE EXISTENCE OF AN L-ARGININE INDEPENDENT ACTIVATED-MACROPHAGE CYTOTOXIC EFFECTOR MECHANISM THAT INDUCES CYTOLYSIS OF SOME TRANSFORMED CELL PHENOTYPES

In early studies we noted that transformed murine cells (L cells, KHT sarcoma cells, and EMT-6 mammary adenocarcinoma cells) responded differently to cocultivation with CAM than nontransformed murine cells (low-passage mouse embryo fibroblasts [MEF]). Mouse peritoneal macrophages activated in vivo by chronic infection with *Toxoplasma* or BCG, or by *M. butyricum* in complete Freund's adjuvant caused lysis of transformed target cells but had little or no cytolytic activity for the untransformed low-passage MEF (Hibbs et al., 1972a, 1972b, 1972d; Hibbs, 1973, 1974). Other groups reported similar results (Basic et al., 1974; Kaplan et al., 1974; Piessens et al., 1975; Meltzer et al., 1975a, 1975b; Fidler et al., 1976). We concluded from these results that a CAM-mediated surveillance mechanism exists that is not based on recognition of target cell antigen but that is apparently related to recognition of a cellular property associated with abnormal cellular proliferation (e.g., transformation) (Hibbs et al., 1972b, 1972d; Hibbs, 1973, 1974, 1975b, 1976). We then used MEF as target cells before and after spontaneous transformation in vitro. Newly established transformed lines of mouse fibroblasts reacted differently than untransformed mouse fibroblasts when cocultivated with monolayers of CAM (Hibbs et al., 1972d). Activated macrophages did not cause lysis of two allogeneic fibroblast cell lines differing from them at a strongly antigenic H-2 locus. In contrast, these macrophages were markedly cytolytic for the same allogeneic fibroblasts (and also for syngeneic fibroblasts) after the fibroblasts had spontaneously developed abnormal growth properties that included unlimited capacity to divide in vitro and loss of contact inhibition of cell division. Because H-2 antigens are more immunogenic than tumor-specific transplantation antigens or fetal antigens expressed on tumor cells, this study strongly suggested to us that changes associated with spontaneous in vitro transformation and the acquisition of abnormal growth properties by target cells, rather than a change in plasma membrane–associated antigens, are responsible for their susceptibility to destruction by activated macrophages. These experiments showed that cells at incipient stages of neoplast development were killed by contact with activated macrophages under conditions in which untransformed fibroblasts were not lysed.

---

cultured with IFN-γ as the only added cytokine. After 22 hours of culture, NO_2^- synthesis, iron-55 (^{55}Fe) release, mitochondrial aconitase, and [^3H]-thymidine uptake were measured. Culture medium NO_2^- concentration is expressed as micromoles per liter. ^{55}Fe release from prelabeled EMT-6 cells is expressed as percent specific release with spontaneous release taken as release of ^{55}Fe from control EMT-6 cells. Uptake of [^3H]-thymidine is expressed as percent control EMT-6 cells. EMT-6 cell mitochondrial aconitase activity is expressed as rate of *cis*-aconitase disappearance in nmol/min/mg protein. [^3H]-thymidine release from prelabeled EMT-6 cells was also measured as described and expressed as percent specific release. In no experimental group was the specific release of [^3H]-thymidine greater than 5.8% (data not shown). All assays were performed in parallel. The values are the mean ± for three to five separate experiments. (From Amber et al., 1988b, with permission.)

In subsequent studies it became clear that CAM did not cause cytolysis of all transformed target cells (Granger et al., 1980; Hibbs and Granger, 1982; Hibbs et al., 1984; Drapier and Hibbs, 1986; Hibbs et al., 1987a, 1987b; Cook et al., 1980, 1982). Based on response to cocultivation with CAM we identified two transformed cell phenotypes. The lytic transformed cell phenotype undergoes cytolysis following 18 to 48 hours of cocultivation with CAM. The nonlytic transformed cell phenotype does not undergo cytolysis but develops inhibition of DNA replication (cytostasis), inhibition of mitochondrial respiration, and inhibition of aconitase activity. The nonlytic transformed cell phenotype remains viable if glucose is available for glycolytic ATP formation.

Therefore, while some transformed cell phenotypes were susceptible to CAM-induced cytolysis, we showed that other transformed cells were resistant to CAM-induced cytolysis. However, the transformed cells with the nonlytic phenotype developed a reproducible pattern of metabolic inhibition that included inhibition of DNA replication, complex I, complex II, and aconitase activity (Granger et al., 1980; Hibbs and Granger, 1982; Hibbs et al., 1984; Drapier and Hibbs, 1986). Indeed, it was by using transformed cells with the nonlytic phenotype as target cells that we were able to identify the pattern of CAM-induced metabolic inhibition and subsequently the effector pathway synthesizing NO from L-arginine (Hibbs et al., 1987a, 1987b, 1988). The results showed that all transformed cells (lytic and nonlytic phenotypes) develop NO-induced metabolic inhibition when cocultivated with CAM and that NO-induced metabolic inhibition occurs in the absence of cytolysis in many transformed cells.

We also observed that normal low-passage MEF do not undergo cytolysis, but are induced to release intracellular iron and to develop inhibition of aconitase activity when cocultivated with CAM (Hibbs et al., manuscript in preparation). We also showed that CAM-induced cytolysis for several transformed cell phenotypes is L-arginine independent (Hibbs et al., manuscript in preparation). A recent preliminary report by others describes similar observations (Klostergaard and Leroux, 1989). These findings show that the selective cytotoxicity of activated macrophages for transformed target cells noted in our early in vitro studies was at the level of cytolysis. It is now apparent that NO-mediated enzymatic inhibition can be induced in most if not all transformed as well as normal untransformed cells. It is also clear that some transformed cells have the nonlytic phenotype and respond to cocultivation with CAM in a way that is similar to normal untransformed cells, for example, they are relatively resistant to cytolysis but develop L-arginine–dependent, NO-mediated metabolic inhibition. There is evidence to suggest that simian virus 40 transformed hamster cells with the nonlytic phenotype have increased virulence when transplanted into appropriate hosts (Cook et al., 1980, 1982).

In summary, these results demonstrate that CAM express two cytotoxic effector mechanisms. The first is L-arginine dependent and primarily cytostatic for mammalian cells. The second is L-arginine independent and primarily cytolytic for mammalian cells. It is possible that TNF-α is involved in activation of the L-arginine–independent cytolytic pathway in susceptible target cells. Identification of the biochemistry of the L-arginine–independent, activated-macrophage cytotoxic effector mechanism causing cytolysis is an important future goal.

CONCLUSION

The study of a nonspecific component of the cell-mediated immune response mediated by activated macrophages has resulted in the identification of a novel biochemical pathway that, when induced in the tissues, increases host resistance to intracellular pathogens and neoplastic cells. This newly discovered biochemical pathway may be the major biochemical defense of the intracellular environment invaded by microorganisms as well as an important defense against cells at incipient stages of neoplastic transformation. In vitro experiments showed that IFN-γ in cooperation with other cytokines (or IFN-γ interacting with certain microbial products) induces in macrophages and certain nonmacrophages cells an enzymatic pathway synthesizing NO and other inorganic nitrogen oxides from L-arginine (Hibbs et al., 1987b; Iyengar et al., 1987; Ding et al., 1988; Drapier and Hibbs, 1988; Amber et al., 1988a, 1988b; Drapier et al., 1988; Hibbs et al., 1988; Marletta et al., 1988; Stuehr et al., 1989a; Lancaster and Hibbs, 1990).

This work provided a biochemical explanation for the metabolic changes that occur in the tissues when cell-mediated defense mechanisms are activated (Granger et al., 1980; Hibbs and Granger, 1982; Hibbs et al., 1984; Drapier and Hibbs, 1986; Hibbs et al., 1987a, 1987b, 1988; Drapier and Hibbs, 1988; Amber et al., 1988a, 1988b; Drapier et al., 1988). In essence, this effector mechanism synthesizes high levels of NO, which limits the availability of iron in the intracellular environment and causes inhibition of certain enzymes with iron-dependent catalytic activity (Granger et al., 1980; Hibbs and Granger, 1982; Hibbs et al., 1984; Drapier and Hibbs, 1986; Hibbs et al., 1988; Lancaster and Hibbs, 1990; Pellat et al., 1990). The effector mechanism functions at the molecular level via NO-mediated nitrosylation of iron (Lancaster and Hibbs, 1990; Pellat et al., 1990). These biochemical insights, as well as those that will follow in the future, offer new opportunities for the therapeutic manipulation of the cell-mediated response to neoplastic cells and microorganisms.

ACKNOWLEDGMENT

This work was supported by the Department of Veterans Affairs, Washington, D.C.

REFERENCES

Alexander P, Evans R. Endotoxin and double stranded RNA render macrophages cytotoxic. Nature. 1971;232:76–78.

Amber IJ, Hibbs JB Jr, Taintor RR, Vavrin Z. The L-arginine dependent effector mechanism is induced in murine adenocarcinoma cells by culture supernatant from cytotoxic activated macrophages. J Leukoc Biol. 1988a;43:187–192.

Amber IJ, Hibbs JB Jr, Taintor RR, Vavrin Z. Cytokines induce an L-arginine-dependent effector system in nonmacrophage cells. J Leukoc Biol. 1988b;44:58–65.

Basic I, Milas L, Grdina DJ, Withers HR. Destruction of hamster ovarian cell cultures by peritoneal macrophages from mice treated with *Corynebacterium granulosum*. J Natl Cancer Inst. 1974;52:1839–1841.

Cook JL, Hibbs JB Jr, Lewis AM Jr. Resistance of simian virus 40-transformed hamster cells to the cytolytic effect of activated macrophages: a possible factor in species-specific viral oncogenicity. Proc Natl Acad Sci USA. 1980;77:6773–6777.

Cook JL, Hibbs JB Jr, Lewis AM Jr. DNA virus-transformed hamster cell-host effector cell interactions: level of resistance to cytolysis correlated with tumorigenicity. Int J Cancer. 1982;30:795–803.

Ding AH, Nathan CF, Stuehr DJ. Release of reactive nitrogen intermediates and reactive oxygen intermediates from mouse peritoneal macrophages. J Immunol. 1988;141:2407–2414.

Drapier J-C, Hibbs JB Jr. Murine cytotoxic activated macrophages inhibit aconitase in tumor cells. Inhibition involves the iron-sulfur prosthetic group and is reversible. J Clin Invest. 1986;78:790–797.

Drapier J-C, Wietzerbin J, Hibbs JB Jr. Interferon-γ and tumor necrosis factor induce the L-arginine-dependent cytotoxic effector mechanism in murine macrophages. Eur J Immunol. 1988;18:1587–1592.

Drapier J-C, Hibbs JB Jr. Differentiation of murine macrophages to express nonspecific cytotoxicity for tumor cells results in L-arginine-dependent inhibition of mitochondrial iron–sulfur enzymes in the macrophage effector cells. J Immunol. 1988;140:2829–2838.

Fidler IJ, Darnell JH, Budmen MB. Tumoricidal properties of mouse macrophages activated with mediator from rat lymphocytes stimulated with concanavalin A. Cancer Res. 1976; 36:3608–3615.

Garthwaite J, Charles SL, Chess-Williams R. Endothelium-derived relaxing factor release on activation of NMDA receptors suggests role as intercellular messenger in the brain. Nature. 1988;336:285–388.

Granger DL, Taintor RR, Cook JL, Hibbs JB Jr. Injury of neoplastic cells by murine macrophages leads to inhibition of mitochondrial respiration. J Clin Invest. 1980;65:357–370.

Granger DL, Lehninger AL. Sites of inhibition of mitochondrial electron transport in macrophage-injured neoplastic cells. J Cell Biol. 1982;95:527–535.

Green LC, Ruiz de Luzuriaga K, Wagner DA, et al. Nitrate biosynthesis in man. Proc Natl Acad Sci USA. 1981a;78:7764–7768.

Green LC, Tannenbaum SR, Goldman P. Nitrate synthesis in the germfree and conventional rat. Science. 1981b;212:56–58.

Hanna MG Jr, Zbar B, Rapp HJ. Histopathology of tumor regression after intralesional injection of *Mycobacterium bovis*. I. Tumor growth and metastasis. J Natl Cancer Inst. 1972;48:1441–1449.

Hibbs JB Jr, Lambert LJ Jr, Remington JS. Resistance to murine tumors conferred by chronic infection with intracellular protozoa, *Toxoplasma gondii* and *Besnoitia jellisoni*. J Infect Dis. 1971;124:587–592.

Hibbs JB Jr, Lambert LH Jr, Remington JS. Possible role of macrophage mediated nonspecific cytotoxicity in tumor resistance. Nature. 1972a;235:48–50.

Hibbs JB Jr, Lambert LH Jr, Remington JS. In vitro nonimmunologic destruction of cells with abnormal growth characteristics by adjuvant activated macrophages. Proc Soc Exp Biol Med. 1972b;139:1049–1052.

Hibbs JB Jr, Lambert LH Jr, Remington JS. Adjuvant induced resistance to tumor development in mice. Proc Soc Exp Biol Med. 1972c;139:1053–1056.

Hibbs JB Jr, Lambert LH Jr, Remington JS. Control of carcinogenesis: a possible role for the activated macrophage. Science. 1972d;177:998–1000.

Hibbs JB Jr. Macrophage nonimmunologic recognition: target cell factors related to contact inhibition. Science. 1973;180:868–870.

Hibbs JB Jr. Discrimination between neoplastic and nonneoplastic cells in vitro by activated macrophages. J Natl Cancer Inst. 1974;53:1487–1492.

Hibbs JB Jr. Activated macrophages as cytotoxic effector cells. II. Requirement for local persistence of inducing antigen. Transplantation. 1975a;19:81–87.

Hibbs JB Jr. Role of macrophages in resistance to cancer. In: Immunological aspects of neoplasia. Baltimore: Williams and Wilkins; 1975b;305–327.

Hibbs JB Jr. The macrophage as a tumoricidal effector cell: a review of in vivo and in vitro studies on the mechanism of the activated macrophage nonspecific cytotoxic reaction. In: Fink MA, ed. The macrophage in neoplasia. New York, NY: Academic Press; 1976:83–111.

Hibbs JB Jr, Taintor RR, Chapman HA Jr, Weinberg JB. Macrophage tumor killing: influence of the local environment. Science. 1977;197:279–282.

Hibbs JB Jr, Chapman HA Jr, Weinberg JB. Regulation of macrophage non-specific tumoricidal capability. In: van Furth R, ed. Mononuclear phagocytes. Functional aspects. Part II. Amsterdam: Martinus Nijhoff; 1980a:1681–1720.

Hibbs JB Jr, Remington JS, Stewart CC. Modulation of immunity and host resistance by microorganisms. Pharmacol Ther. 1980b;8:37–69.

Hibbs JB Jr, Granger DL. Activated macrophage-induced cytostasis and inhibition of aerobic energy metabolism in transformed cells: evaluation of lytic and nonlytic target cell responses. In: Mizuno D, Cohn ZA, Takeya K, Ishida N, eds. Self-defense mechanisms, role of macrophages. Tokyo: University of Tokyo Press; 1982:319–333.

Hibbs JB Jr, Taintor RR, Vavrin Z. Iron depletion: possible cause of tumor cell cytotoxicity induced by activated macrophages. Biochem Biophys Res Commun. 1984;123:716–723.

Hibbs JB Jr, Vavrin Z, Taintor RR. L-arginine is required for expression of the activated macrophage effector mechanism causing selective metabolic inhibition in target cells. J Immunol. 1987a;138:550–565.

Hibbs JB Jr, Taintor RR, Vavrin Z. Macrophage cytotoxicity: role for L-arginine deiminase activity and imino nitrogen oxidation to nitrite. Science. 1987b;235:473–476.

Hibbs JB Jr, Taintor RR, Vavrin Z, Rachlin EM. Nitric oxide: a cytotoxic activated macrophage effector molecule. Biochem Biophys Res Commun. 1988;157:87–94. (Erratum published Biochem Biophys Res Commun. 1989;158:624.)

Hooper AB. Ammonia oxidation and energy transduction in the nitrifying bacteria. In: Strohl WR, Tuovinan OH, eds. Microbial chemoautotrophy. Columbus, Ohio: Ohio State University Press; 1984:133–167.

Ignarro LJ, Gruetter CA. Requirement of thiols for activation of coronary arterial guanylate cyclase by glyceryl trinitrate and sodium nitrite. Biochim Biophys Acta. 1980;631:221–231.

Ignarro LJ, Byrns RE, Buga GM, Wood KS. Endothelium-derived relaxing factor from pulmonary artery and vein possesses pharmacological and chemical properties that are identical to those for nitric oxide radical. Circ Res. 1987a;61:866–879.

Ignarro LJ, Buga GM, Wood KS, Byrns RE, Chaudhuri G. Endothelium-derived relaxing factor produced and released from artery and vein is nitric oxide. Proc Natl Acad Sci USA. 1987b;84:9265–9269.

Iyengar R, Stuehr DJ, Marletta MA. Macrophage synthesis of nitrite, nitrate, and N-nitrosamines: precursors and role of the respiratory burst. Proc Natl Acad Sci USA. 1987;84:6369–6373.

Kaplan AM, Morahan PS, Regelson W. Induction of macrophage-mediated tumor-cell cytotoxicity by pyran copolymer. J Natl Cancer Inst. 1974;52:1919–1921.

Keller R. Cytostatic elimination of syngeneic rat tumor cells in vitro by nonspecifically activated macrophages. J Exp Med. 1973;138:625–644.

Keller R, Jones VE. Role of activated macrophages and antibody in inhibition and enhancement of tumor growth in rats. Lancet. 1971;1:847–849.

Kilbourn RG, Klostergaard J, Lopez-Berestein G. Activated macrophages secrete a soluble factor that inhibits mitochondrial respiration of tumor cells. J Immunol. 1984;133:2577–2581.

Klostergaard J, Leroux E. L-arginine independent macrophage tumor cytotoxicity. Biochem Biophys Res Commun. 1989;165:1262–1266.

Knowles RG, Palacios M, Palmer RMJ, Moncada S. Formation of nitric oxide from L-arginine in the central nervous system: a transduction mechanism for stimulation of the soluble guanylate cyclase. Proc Natl Acad Sci USA. 1989;86:5159–5162.

Krahenbuhl JE. Effects of activated macrophages on tumor target cells in discrete phases of the cell cycle. Cancer Res. 1980;40:4622–4627.

Krahenbuhl JL, Remington JS. The role of activated macrophages in specific and nonspecific cytostasis of tumor cells. J Immunol. 1974;113:507–516.

Lancaster JR Jr, Hibbs JB Jr. EPR demonstration of iron-nitrosyl complex formation by cytotoxic activated macrophages. Proc Natl Acad Sci USA. 1990;87:1223–1227.

Lee RG. The anemia of chronic disease. Semin Hematol. 1983;20:59–80.

Lees H. The biochemistry of the nitrifying organisms: the ammonia-oxidizing systems of nitrosomonas. Biochem J. 1952;52:134–139.

Lepoivre M, Boudbid H, Petit J-F. Antiproliferative activity of γ-interferon combined with lipopolysaccharide on murine adenocarcinoma: dependence on an L-arginine metabolism with production of nitrite and citrulline. Cancer Res. 1989;49:1970–1976.

Mackaness GB. Cellular resistance to infection. J Exp Med. 1962;116:381–417.

Mackaness GB. The immunological basis of acquired cellular resistance. J Exp Med. 1964; 120:105–120.

Mackaness GB. The influence of immunologically committed lymphoid cells on macrophage activity in vivo. J Exp Med. 1969;129:973–992.

Marletta MA, Yoon PS, Iyengar R, Leaf CD, Wishnok JS. Macrophage oxidation of L-arginine to nitrite and nitrate: nitric oxide is an intermediate. Biochemistry. 1988;27:8706–8711.

Meltzer MS, Tucker RW, Breuer AC. Interaction of BCG-activated macrophages with neoplastic and nonneoplastic cell lines in vitro: cinemicrographic analysis. Cell Immunol. 1975a;17:30–36.

Meltzer MS, Tucker RW, Sanford KK, Leonard EJ. Interaction of BCG-activated macrophages with neoplastic and nonneoplastic cell lines in vitro: quantitation of the cytotoxic reaction by release of tritiated thymidine from prelabeled target cells. J Natl Cancer Inst. 1975b;54:1177–1184.

Metchikoff E. Lectures in the comparative pathology of inflammation. London: Kegan, Paul, Trench and Co.; 1893.

Meyer J. Comparison of carbon monoxide, nitric oxide, and nitrate as inhibitors of the nitrogenase from *Clostridium pasteurianum*. Arch Biochem Biophys. 1981;210:246–256.

Mitchell HH, Shonle HA, Grindley HS. The origin of the nitrates in the urine. J Biol Chem. 1916;24:461–490.

Murad F, Mittal CK, Arnold WP, Katsuki S, Kimura H. Guanylate cyclase: activation by azide, nitro compounds, nitric oxide, and hydroxyl radical and inhibition by hemoglobin and myoglobin. Adv Cyclic Nucleotide Res. 1978;9:145–158.

Palmer RMJ, Ferrige AG, Moncada S. Nitric oxide release accounts for the biological activity of endothelium-derived relaxing factor. Nature. 1987;327:524–526.

Palmer RMJ, Ashton DS, Moncada S. Vascular endothelial cells synthesize nitric oxide from L-arginine. Nature. 1987;333:664–666.

Palmer RMJ, Moncada S. A novel citrulline-forming enzyme implicated in the formation of nitric oxide by vascular endothelial cells. Biochem Biophys Res Commun. 1989;158:348–352.

Pellat C, Henry Y, Drapier J-C. IFN-γ activated macrophages: detected by EPR of complexes between L-arginine derived nitric oxide and nonheme-iron proteins. Biochem Biophys Res Commun. 1990; in press.

Piessens WF, Churchill WH Jr, David JR. Macrophages activated in vitro with lymphocyte mediators kill neoplastic but not normal cells. J Immunol. 1975;114:293–299.

Radomski MW, Palmer RMJ, Moncada S. Comparative pharmacology endothelium-derived relaxing factor, nitric oxide and prostacyclin in platelets. Br J Pharmacol. 1987;92:181–187.

Reddy D, Lancaster JR Jr, Cornforth DP. Nitrite inhibition of *Clostridium botulinum*: electron spin resonance detection of iron-nitric oxide complexes. Science. 1983;221:769–770.

Remington JS, Merigan TC. Resistance to virus challenge in mice infected with protozoa or bacteria. Proc Soc Exp Biol Med. 1969;131:1184–1188.

Reichard P, Ehrenberg A. Ribonucleotide reductase—a radical enzyme. Science. 1983;221:514–519.

Rousseau DL, Singh S, Ching Y-C, Sassaroli M. Nitrosyl cytochrome c oxidase. Formation and properties of mixed valence enzyme. J Biol Chem. 1988;263:5681–5685.

Ruco LP, Meltzer MS. Macrophage activation for tumor cytotoxicity: development of macrophage cytotoxic activity requires completion of a sequence of short-lived intermediary reactions. J Immunol. 1978;121:2035–2042.

Ruskin J, Remington JS. Immunity and intracellular infection: resistance to bacteria in mice infected with a protozoan. Science. 1968;160:72–74.

Ruskin J, McIntosh J, Remington JS. Studies on the mechanisms of resistance to phylogenetically diverse intracellular organisms. J Immunol. 1969;103:252–259.

Russell SW, Doe WF, McIntosh AT. Functional characterization of a stable, noncytolytic stage of macrophage activation in tumors. J Exp Med. 1977;146:1511–1520.

Salerno JC, Ohnishi T, Lim J, King TE. Tetranuclear and binuclear iron-sulfur clusters in succinate dehydrogenase: a method of iron quantitation by formation of paramagnetic complexes. Biochem Biophys Res Commun. 1976;73:833–840.

Schreiber RD, Pace JL, Russell SW, Altman A, Katz DH. Macrophage-activating factor produced by a T cell hybridoma: physiochemical and biosynthetic resemblance to γ-interferon. J Immunol. 1983;131:826–832.

Stuehr DJ, Marletta MA. Mammalian nitrate biosynthesis: mouse macrophages produce nitrite and nitrate in response to *Escherichia coli* lipopolysaccharide. Proc Natl Acad Sci USA. 1985;82:7738–7742.

Stuehr DJ, Marletta MA. Synthesis of nitrite and nitrate in murine macrophage cell lines. Cancer Res. 1987a;47:5590–5594.

Stuehr DJ, Marletta MA. Induction of nitrite/nitrate synthesis in murine macrophages by BCG infection, lymphokines, or interferon-γ. J Immunol. 1987b;139:518–525.

Stuehr DJ, Gross SS, Sakuma I, Levi R, Nathan CF. Activated murine macrophages secrete a metabolite of arginine with the bioactivity of endothelium-derived relaxing factor and the chemical reactivity of nitric oxide. J Exp Med. 1989a;169:1011–1020.

Stuehr DJ, Nathan CF. Nitric oxide. A macrophage product responsible for cytostasis and respiratory inhibition in tumor target cells. J Exp Med. 1989b;169:1543–1555.

Suzuki I. Mechanisms of inorganic oxidation and energy coupling. Annu Rev Microbiol. 1974;28:85–101.

Svedersky LP, Benton CV, Berger WH, Rinderknecht E, Harkins RN, Palladino MA. Biological and antigenic similarities of murine interferon-γ and macrophage-activating factor. J Exp Med. 1984;159:812–827.

Vanin AF. Identification of divalent iron complexes with cysteine in biologic systems by the EPR method. Biokhimiia. 1967;32:277–282.

Wagner DA, Tannenbaum SA. Enhancement of nitrate biosynthesis by *Escherichia coli* lipopolysaccharide. In: Magee PN, ed. Nitrosamines in human cancer (Banbury report no. 12). New York: Cold Spring Harbor Laboratory; 1982;437–443.

Wagner DA, Young VR, Tannenbaum SR. Mammalian nitrate biosynthesis: incorporation of $^{15}NH_3$ into nitrate is enhanced by endotoxin treatment. Proc Natl Acad Sci USA. 1983; 80:4518–4521.

Weinberg ED. Roles of iron in host–parasite interactions. J Infect Dis. 1971;124:401–410.

Weinberg ED. Iron and infection. Microbiol Rev. 1971;42:45–66.

Weinberg JB, Hibbs JB Jr. Endocytosis of red blood cells or hemoglobin by activated macrophages inhibits their tumoricidal effect. Nature. 1977;269:245–247.

Weinberg JB, Chapman HA Jr, Hibbs JB Jr. Characterization of the effects of endotoxin on macrophage tumor cell killing. J Immunol. 1978;121:72–80.

Witter JP, Gatley SJ, Balish E. Evaluation of nitrate synthesis by intestinal microorganism in vivo. Science. 1981;213:449–450.

Zbar B, Wepsic HT, Borsos T, Rapp HJ. Tumor–graft rejection in syngeneic guinea pigs: evidence for a two-step mechanism. J Natl Cancer Inst. 1970a;44:473–481.

Zbar B, Bernstein I, Tanaka T, Rapp HJ. Tumor immunity produced by the intradermal inoculation of living tumor cells and living *Mycobacterium bovis* (strain BCG). Science. 1970b; 170:1217–1218.

Zbar B, Bernstein ID, Bartlett GL, Hanna MG Jr, Rapp HJ. Immunotherapy of cancer: regression of intradermal tumors and prevention of growth of lymph node metastases after intralesional injection of living *Mycobacterium bovis*. J Natl Cancer Inst. 1972;49:119–130.

CHAPTER 3

NATURAL IMMUNITY INCLUDING NATURAL KILLER AND MHC-UNRESTRICTED T LYMPHOCYTES

Reinder L. H. Bolhuis
Jan Willem Gratama
Els Sturm

TUMOR ANTIGENICITY AND IMMUNE ACTIVITY

It has been known for many years that experimentally induced tumor cells express "new" antigens (Ag) on the surface of their membrane. These new antigens are specific for that particular tumor and are immunogenic. Therefore, immune-specific cytotoxic T lymphocytes (CTL) can be elicited against these tumor cells. The search for tumor-specific immune reactions was initiated by the formulation of the immune surveillance hypothesis (Ehrlich, 1909) and by its later updates (Burnet, 1970). The central issue of this hypothesis is that immune-specific T lymphocytes play a crucial role as effector cells responsible for immunological surveillance, resulting in the arrest or elimination of cancer cells from the host. Generally, immune-specific T cells recognize their antigen in the context of the major histocompatibility complex (MHC) of the Ag presenting cell (i.e., MHC restriction). This hypothesis has been substantiated by numerous reports of actual studies describing such immune-specific T lymphocytes with antitumor reactivity. These tumor-specific T-cell responses indeed appeared MHC restricted. Some investigators claimed the existence of human immune-specific CTL reactivity against tumor cells, even in the absence of MHC differences between tumor and effector cells (Bubenik et al., 1971; Vose and White, 1983). These reports have boosted extensive investigations on host immune defenses in preclinical and clinical settings.

Around 1970 it was found that lymphocytes derived from healthy individuals were also quite capable of directly killing cancer cells in vitro, at that time a rather unexpected finding, which was neglected by the majority of tumorimmunologists as "background" killing. The subsequent detailed analysis of T-cell functions of cancer patients, in particular their cytolytic activity, yielded conflicting data, resulting in polarized views on the issue of whether or not immune responses would play a biologically significant role in the protection or defense against neoplastic growth.

A Third Wave of Immunotherapy

The first wave of immunotherapy was initiated at the end of the 19th century by William Coley (around 1890), who used anticancer "vaccines" consisting of bacteria, an approach that was eclipsed by the advent of radiotherapy. The second wave occurred in the late 1960s and early 1970s at a time when it was well-known that certain bacteria, notably bacillus Calmette-Guérin (BCG) or *Corynebacterium parvum (C parvum)* acted as adjuvants by enhancing antibody production and cell-mediated immune responses. This nonspecific stimulation of the immune system was widely applied for the immunotherapy of cancer. Later, the call for highly purified biological response modifiers (BRM) with better defined modes of action became stronger.

Since then, our knowledge of the (mammalian) immune system has increased exponentially, in parallel with that of molecular biology, which has led to the identification, cloning, and production of numerous pivotal cytokines involved in immune regulation. The large-scale production of recombinant cytokines has allowed their in vivo application. The advent of large-scale immune cell culture techniques has improved the ex vivo activation and expansion of patients' lymphocytes for clinical application. Monoclonal antibodies (mAb) selective for tumor cells have enabled immunological diagnosis and, in some instances, therapeutic applications. Now, with all the necessary tools at our disposal, our deepened knowledge of the immune system and the regulatory mechanisms that govern immune responses has to be translated into clinical protocols for the immunotherapy of cancer. The third wave of biotherapy is rolling.

Lymphocyte Subsets with MHC-Unrestricted Lytic Capacity

Natural Killer Lymphocytes Initially, MHC-unrestricted "spontaneous" cytolysis of tumor cells by lymphocytes was described as "natural killer" (NK) activity exerted by lymphocytes that now have been characterized as $CD3^-$/T-cell receptor (TCR^-). Therefore, their lytic activity is, by definition, MHC-unrestricted, and this represents the fundamental difference to the antigen-specific cytolysis displayed by "classic" $CD3^+/TCR\alpha\beta$ lymphocytes (Bolhuis et al., 1986a; Davis and Bjorkman, 1988; Trinchieri, 1989).

MHC-unrestricted cytolysis has also been termed nonspecific, anomalous, promiscuous, activated killer, natural killer-like, lymphokine-activated killer (LAK) activity, or lymphocyte-activated killer. It is directed against a wide variety of target cells including (autologous) tumor cells (Seeley and Golub, 1978; Poros and Klein, 1979; Masucci et al., 1980; Hersey et al., 1981; Vose and Bonnard, 1982; Grimm et al., 1982).

TCR$^+$ Lymphocytes The fact that NK lymphocytes lack the expression of the TCR$^-$/CD3$^-$ complex automatically leads to the conclusion that non-TCR structures must be involved in MHC-unrestricted lysis and that different lymphocyte populations may express such recognition elements (Ortaldo et al., 1989). Consequently, for years the debate centered on the question of whether all lymphocytes exerting MHC-unrestricted cytolysis are derived from TCR$^-$ lymphocytes or also from distinct (sub)lineages of TCR$^+$ lymphocytes that then would acquire MHC-unrestricted lytic activity following their activation.

That distinct subsets of lymphocytes can, in fact, exert MHC-unrestricted lysis was already suggested by early studies demonstrating that lymphocytes generated in mixed leukocyte cultures were different from MHC-restricted CTL (Seeley and Golub, 1978; Bolhuis and Ronteltap, 1980; Bolhuis and Schellekens, 1981; Van de Griend et al., 1984). These differences included: (1) target cells for MHC-unrestricted cytolysis did not cross-compete with CTL specific target cells; (2) distinct adherence properties of specific CTL and lymphocytes with MHC-unrestricted lytic activity; (3) MHC-restricted specific CTL, but not MHC-unrestricted lytic activity, showed a memory response; (4) MHC-unrestricted lysis is induced long before specific CTL lytic activity (Masucci et al., 1980; Bolhuis and Ronteltap, 1980; Bolhuis and Schellekens, 1981; Van de Griend et al., 1984; Hersey and Bolhuis, 1987); and (5) lymphocyte cell surface analysis clearly demonstrated that lymphocytes with the CTL phenotype also exerted MHC-unrestricted lytic activity (Hersey and Bolhuis, 1987). Therefore, the above-described differences cannot simply be explained by stating that distinct lytic activities are confined to different lymphocyte populations. Indeed, it is well documented that TCR$^-$ NK lymphocytes without prior activation, but also TCR$^+$ lymphocytes upon appropriate activation, can exert such MHC-unrestricted cytolytic activity (Hersey and Bolhuis, 1987), which is defined as LAK activity.

The TCR$^-$ NK and TCR$^+$ T lymphocytes belong to distinct lymphocyte subsets on the basis of whether or not functional TCR gene rearrangements have taken place. Thus, the precursor lymphocytes for the total population of lymphocytes displaying MHC-unrestricted cytolysis are distinct from mature effector cells, because LAK activity can also be generated from lymphocyte populations or tissues lacking NK activity. This also shows that precursor cells of lymphocytes with LAK activity are heterogeneous (Hersey and Bolhuis, 1987).

Taken together, the data demonstrate that both TCR$^-$ NK lymphocytes, as well as TCR$^+$ lymphocytes, are involved in MHC-unrestricted NK or LAK activities. Within the TCR$^+$ lymphocyte population, two subsets able to exert cell-mediated cytotoxicity can be identified: (1) T lymphocytes that express an antigen receptor, that is, a disulfide-linked heterodimer composed of the α and β proteins that are noncovalently linked to the CD3 complex (TCRαβ) (Bolhuis et al., 1986a); and (2) T lymphocytes with an antigen-receptor composed of γ and δ proteins, which is also a heterodimer that is noncovalently linked to CD3. The γ and δ chains can be either disulfide or nondisulfide linked (Brenner et al., 1986; Borst et al., 1987).

ANTIGEN-SPECIFIC RECEPTORS AND RESTRICTION ELEMENTS

The TCR

The T-lymphocyte structures capable of specific antigen recognition are the membrane-expressed polymorphic TCR (Acuto et al., 1983; Staertz et al., 1984). These TCR are noncovalently associated with the nonpolymorphic CD3 complex that comprises five different proteins. The TCR contains gene segments homologous to the variable (V), diversity (D), joining (J), and constant (C) gene segments of the immunoglobulin (Ig) gene of B cells. Thus, antigen-specific cellular cytoxicity is exerted by lymphocytes that express a surface TCR capable of discriminating between "altered self" or "foreign," i.e., "non-self" cells and normal autologous cells (non-self versus self discrimination). These antigen-specific TCR recognize and bind to their target cell, which triggers the delivery of an activation signal resulting in a lethal hit to target cells. Thereafter, the conjugate dissociates, the target cell disintegrates, and the effector lymphocyte is ready for another attack.

The target cell antigens for MHC-restricted CTL are presented by class I or II MHC molecules. The vast majority of antigen-specific T lymphocytes express the TCRαβ. Mature TCRαβ/CD3 lymphocytes are either $CD4^+$ or 8^+. The $CD4^+$ lymphocyte subset functions as helper or cytotoxic cells for T- and B-lymphocyte functions, interacting with MHC class II molecules on the target cells. The $CD8^+$ lymphocyte subset represents cytotoxic T lymphocytes interacting with MHC class I (HLA-A,B,C) expressing target cells (reviewed in Bolhuis et al., 1986a). As already illustrated above, upon appropriate activation, these specific CTL can also exert MHC-unrestricted lysis.

A minor fraction of the TCR^+ lymphocytes expresses the γδ-receptor and lacks the expression of CD4 or CD8 antigens (Borst et al., 1987; Brenner et al., 1987; Van de Griend et al., 1987a; Sturm et al., 1989). The gene organization of the TCRγδ is homologous to that of the TCRαβ after appropriate activation. These TCRγδ lymphocytes can be easily triggered to exert MHC-unrestricted lysis.

LYMPHOCYTE SURFACE STRUCTURES INVOLVED IN MHC-UNRESTRICTED CYTOLYSIS

Equally important is the question of which lymphocyte surface structures are involved in MHC-unrestricted lysis and, specifically, whether the distinct lymphocyte subsets employ the same recognition and/or signal-transducing molecules to exert MHC-unrestricted cytolysis.

Can TCR Be Involved in MHC-Unrestricted Cytolysis?

Already in 1983, Hercend and co-workers described a series of monoclonal antibodies, recognizing a broadly distributed target cell structure, TNK tar (VieF2), which blocked cytotoxic reactions at the target cell level. These anti-TNK tar monoclonal antibodies had no inhibitory effects on the lysis of the same target cells by randomly selected $CD3^-/TCR^-$ lymphocyte clones or $CD3^+/TCR\alpha\beta^+$ lymphocyte clones with MHC-unrestricted lytic activity. In fact, these reagents only blocked lytic activity of T lymphocytes, expressing a unique and infrequent clonotypic TCR determinant exclusively (Hercend et al., 1983, 1984; Schmidt et al., 1986). These and the earlier described data suggest that multiple receptors are involved in MHC-unrestricted lysis, including TCR. Other evidence that TCR may be involved in MHC-unrestricted lysis comes from the analysis of cloned $TCR\gamma\delta^+$ lymphocytes.

As described, a small portion of T lymphocytes expresses the TCRγδ heterodimer instead of the TCRαβ (Borst et al., 1987; Brenner et al., 1987). The majority of these TCRγδ lymphocytes lack the expression of the CD4 and CD8 molecules (Lanier et al., 1986; Van de Griend et al., 1987a; Ferrini et al., 1987).

Recently, we and others showed that human TCRγδ lymphocytes in peripheral blood consist mainly of two nonoverlapping subsets, which are defined on the basis of reactivity with anti-TCRγδ monoclonal antibody and selectively recognize protein products of particular functional TCR gene rearrangements (Triebel et al., 1988; Sturm et al., 1989; Casorati et al., 1989). The major subset expresses the Vγ9-Vδ2 encoded TCRγδ heterodimer, whereas the minor uses the Vδ1 gene segment for its functional TCR rearrangement. TCRγδ lymphocytes freshly isolated from peripheral blood do not display substantial cytolytic activities against K562 target cells (Lanier et al., 1985). After activation and culture in vitro, however, these lymphocytes acquire MHC-unrestricted cytolytic activity against a wide variety of histologically distinct tumor cells (Borst et al., 1987; Van de Griend et al., 1987a; Moingeon et al., 1987; Jitsukawa et al., 1988; Christmas, 1989; Bosnes et al., 1989). It is not known whether the broad spectrum of MHC-unrestricted cytotoxicity mediated by in vitro–activated TCRγδ lymphocytes involves the TCR molecule (Phillips et al., 1987; Van de Griend et al., 1987a). Although reports on Ag-specific and/or MHC-restricted TCRγδ lymphocytes have recently appeared (Bluestone et al., 1988; Haregewoin et al., 1989; Paliard et al., 1989; Kozbor et al., 1989; Holoshitz et al., 1989; Sturm et al., 1990), it is still enigmatic whether Ag recognition by TCRγδ lymphocytes is always MHC restricted.

We investigated whether the use of a particular Vγ or Vδ gene rearrangement corresponds with specific proliferative and/or cytolytic capacities. Our results revealed: (1) All TCRγδ clones exhibit MHC-unrestricted lytic activity; (2) On average, the Vγ9-Vδ2 clones exert higher levels of MHC-unrestricted cytolysis than the Vδ1 clones; and (3) Remarkably, the use of a Vγ9-Vδ2 gene rearrangement correlates with Daudi target-cell specificity.

It has to be realized that in vitro–activated TCRγδ lymphocytes possess two mechanisms by which they can exert cell-mediated cytotoxicity. Activated TCRγδ lymphocytes display MHC-unrestricted cytolysis (Borst et al., 1987; Van de Griend et al., 1987a; Moingeon et al., 1987; Triebel et al., 1988; Jitsukawa et al., 1988; Casorati et al., 1989; Christmas, 1989; Bosnes et al., 1989), that supposedly does not involve the TCR as a recognition structure (Phillips et al., 1987). However, recognition of target cells by TCRγδ lymphocytes may also be directly mediated via the TCR (Brenner et al., 1987; Kozbor et al., 1989). Although Daudi cells are known to be susceptible to MHC-unrestricted cytolysis by TCR^- lymphocytes, the fact that the ability to lyse Daudi cells correlates with the expression of a particular Vγ9-Vδ2 encoded TCRγδ supports a role for this type of TCRγδ in Daudi cell recognition. Also, the finding that freshly isolated Vγ9-Vδ2 peripheral blood lymphocytes (PBL), which do not display MHC-unrestricted lysis (Lanier et al., 1989) and specifically proliferate to Daudi cells but not to other stimulator cells, supports the idea of a TCRγδ-mediated recognition of Daudi cells.

The data described above suggest that the Vγ9-Vδ2 encoded TCRγδ is involved in MHC-unrestricted, but specific, recognition of Daudi target cells.

It is possible that the MHC-unrestricted recognition of Daudi cells by $V\gamma 9^+$ $V\delta 2^+$ TCRγδ lymphocytes may represent a specific TCR-"superantigen"-like interaction and therefore may qualitatively be distinct from MHC-unrestricted lysis by TCR^- NK or TCR^+ lymphocytes (Sturm et al., 1990). A superantigen response is the activation of a defined subset of lymphocytes, that is, all responder lymphocytes express an identical TCR-Vβ encoded TCRβ chain (Marrack and Kappler, 1988).

Non-TCR Lymphocyte Surface Receptors Involved in MHC-Unrestricted Cytolysis

Abundant data demonstrate that lymphocyte proliferation and/or lytic activity can be inhibited or induced by monoclonal antibodies directed against an array of their cell surface structures (e.g., CD2, 3, 16, 45, etc.) that are not directly involved in immune-specific antigen recognition based on the diversity of the TCR (Bolhuis and Van de Griend, 1985; Bolhuis et al., 1986a). It can be stated that inhibition of lymphocyte functions occurs when soluble monoclonal antibodies are used against distinct structures, whereas the same monoclonal antibodies will induce proliferative and lytic functions when presented in a cross-linked form.

Monoclonal Antibodies and Lymphokine-Mediated Functions A number of nonpolymorphic glycoproteins, such as CD3, CD16, CD28, CD45, etc., are involved in the lymphocyte activation and triggering for lysis. Some of these structures are functionally interrelated or interplay with the TCR and each other. Therefore, activation via one can be blocked via another using the relevant monoclonal antibodies (Bolhuis et al., 1986b; Pantaleo et al., 1987; Van de Griend et al., 1987a; Braakman et al., 1990; Goedegebuure et al., 1990).

Using combinations of monoclonal antibodies against the distinct activation sites, we and others have shown that activation via one activation site (e.g., CD3) can be inhibited by adding soluble antibodies against another (e.g., CD2) (Bolhuis et al., 1986b). However, when these combinations of monoclonal antibodies are both added in cross-linked form, synergism in the activation of lymphocytes is observed (Van de Griend et al., 1987b). As we originally proposed (Bolhuis et al., 1986b), synergism between, for instance, CD2 and CD3 has also been observed in MHC-restricted antigen recognition (Moingeon et al., 1989).

This functional interplay between distinct activation sites suggests that their individual activation pathways must intracellularly converge (Bolhuis et al., 1986b; Van de Griend et al., 1987b; Pantaleo et al., 1987; Alcover et al., 1988). Inhibition of lymphocyte function following the binding of soluble monoclonal antibodies to these activation molecules may be due to the delivery of an overall negative signal to the lymphocytes, thereby blocking antigen-specific, as well as nonspecific, lytic functions (Bolhuis et al., 1986b; Van de Griend et al., 1987b; Hersey and Bolhuis, 1987; Bolhuis and Braakman, 1988).

Inhibition of lysis by monoclonal antibodies against the CD45-T200 mAb has also been observed, but at a different level (i.e., the target-cell level). Using a cloned effector lymphocyte, anti-CD45 mAb inhibited the lysis of one (K562), but not another (Daudi) target cell (Van de Griend et al., 1984). All the data strongly argue in favor of the hypothesis that a multireceptor recognition process is involved in MHC-unrestricted target-cell recognition and lysis. The combination of the lymphocyte receptors involved will also depend on the target-cell antigenic makeup with which the lymphocyte effector cells interact.

The CD2 Antigen Activation of lymphocytes via CD2 is detailed here as an example. The CD2 antigen, formerly designated T11, is a glycoprotein originally known as the sheep red blood cell (SRBC) receptor on human TCR$\alpha\beta^+$ or TCR$\gamma\delta^+$ lymphocytes (Van de Griend et al., 1987b) and TCR$^-$ lymphocytes (Ortaldo et al., 1981; Bolhuis et al., 1986b; Goedegebuure et al., 1989). The CD2 antigen mediates adhesion of the lymphocytes to the target or antigen-presenting cells via binding to its natural ligand LFA-3 (Springer et al., 1987). Proliferation of TCR$^+$ lymphocytes and cytolysis by TCR$^+$ and TCR$^-$ lymphocytes can be induced by CD2 mAb (Van de Griend et al., 1987b).

Interestingly, TCR$\alpha\beta^+$, TCR$\gamma\delta^+$, and TCR$^-$ lymphocytes differ in their requirements to become activated by anti-CD2–specific monoclonal antibodies. The TCR$\alpha\beta^+$ lymphocytes require a combination of two CD2-specific monoclonal antibodies (i.e., anti-T11.2 and anti-T11.3 mAb). In contrast, TCR$\gamma\delta$ and TCR$^-$ lymphocytes, although the latter to a lesser extent, can be triggered by a single anti-CD2 monoclonal antibody (T11.1.) (Bolhuis et al., 1986b; Goedegebuure et al., 1989).

The differential activation of subsets of lymphocytes by different CD2-specific monoclonal antibodies, which each bind to distinct sites on the CD2 molecule, is not only expressed at the level of proliferation or cytolysis, as described (Bierer et al., 1989), but also in terms of induction of expression of lymphokine receptors, for example, CD25 (the interleukin-2 [IL-2] receptor) and/or via the induction of lymphokine production (Van de Griend et al., 1986). The type of response dictates whether or not proliferation and/or triggering of the lytic machinery will follow. For example, when production of both IL-2 and interleukin-4 (IL-4) is induced by a particular combination of CD2-specific monoclonal antibodies, no cytolytic response will follow because IL-4 inhibits differentiation of precursors of lymphocytes with LAK activity. Eight different human interleukins have meanwhile been cloned and each of these have shown to be pleiotropic and their activities to often be overlapping and dose-dependent. Moreover, cytokine antagonists have meanwhile been reported that counteract cytokine action, identifying a further complexity in the immune network. For instance, antagonists for interleukin-1 (IL-1) and tumor necrosis factor (TNF) have been identified (Durum and Mealy, 1990). These findings reflect the complex nature of immune networks.

In short, without reviewing all the literature data, the basic principle is as follows. Depending on the type of stimulus to the lymphocyte(s) and the subsequent modulation of expression of (1) TCR or putative NK lymphocyte receptors, (2) lymphocyte cell-surface activation sites, and/or (3) adhesion/signal transducing molecules, (4) cytokine receptors, or (5) combinations thereof, it can be expected that the production of distinct lymphokine repertoires is triggered, which, in turn, in combination exert differential effects on (1) the induction or enhancement of each or combinations of these lymphocyte cell surface molecules listed above; (2) the proliferative capacity of the lymphocytes; (3) differentiation and maturation of lymphocyte subsets; (4) secondary production of lymphokines; (5) migratory capacity; and (6) type, level, and specificity of the cytolytic response.

It is therefore clear that the distinct subsets of lymphocytes, each of which is capable of MHC-unrestricted lysis, display distinct tumor target-cell repertoires, ranging from almost exclusive for the stimulating tumor cell to virtually any type of tumor cell (for review, Hersey and Bolhuis, 1987; Bolhuis et al., 1988).

In conclusion, recognition of target cells by subsets of lymphocytes, that is, TCR$\alpha\beta$ or $\gamma\delta$ or TCR$^-$ NK lymphocytes, MHC-restricted or not, clearly involves multiple receptors on the individual lymphocytes. Only in MHC-restricted antigen recognition is the specificity exclusively dictated by the unique quarternary structure of the TCR. In all other cases, the costimulatory and/or adhesion molecules (e.g., integrins, super immunoglobulin family molecules, etc.) contribute to the recognition selectively. The signal transduction resulting from these different forms of recognition may be mediated via the CD3 ζ chain (Anderson et al., 1989) that is expressed on all the different subsets of lymphocytes (Hersey and Bolhuis, 1987; Lanier et al., 1989; Hercend, unpublished results).

Lymphocyte Integrins and Tumor-Cell Antigenic Makeup

Integrins are a family of membrane glycoproteins consisting of two subunits, α and β. Both integrin subunits have a large extracellular domain, a transmembrane domain, and a short cytoplasmic domain. A large number of integrins have been identified and new ones are continually being detected. An individual α-subunit can associate with different (combinations of) β-subunits (Cheresh et al., 1989; Hemler et al., 1989). Lymphocytes express receptors that bind to ligands on tumor cells and vice versa. Interestingly, one particular ligand can bind to more than one integrin and vice versa.

So far, 11 α-subunits and 7 β-subunits have been identified to form 16 different heterodimers. Examples of target-cell ligands for lymphocytes that play a functional role in lymphocyte activation are intercellular adhesion molecules 1 and 2 (ICAM-1 and ICAM-2); fibronectin (FN) and the complement component 3bi (C3bi). The ICAM-1 and ICAM-2 have been identified as the counterparts for the lymphocyte function–associated antigen-1 (LFA-1) (CD11a/CD18) (Mortarini et al., 1990; Braakman et al., 1990; Goedegebuure et al., 1990; for review, Staunton et al., 1989).

We have recently demonstrated that tumor cells that lack ICAM-1 on their membrane are resistant to antibody-triggered cytolysis via the TCR as well as to MHC-unrestricted cytolysis exerted by $TCR\gamma\delta^+$ lymphocytes and TCR^- NK lymphocytes (Braakman et al., 1990; Fisch et al., 1990; Goedegebuure et al., 1990; for review Staunton et al., 1989).

These and other kinetic studies (Hogg, 1989; Blanchard et al., 1990) also revealed that soluble anti-CD18 monoclonal antibodies inhibited CD3-mediated, as well as MHC-unrestricted, cytolysis of both $ICAM^+$ and $ICAM^-$ target cells without affecting conjugate formation to $ICAM^-$ target cells. Our data and other (Hogg, 1989) suggest that LFA-1/ICAM-1 effector-cell/target-cell interaction coactivates both MHC-restricted and MHC-unrestricted lymphocyte target-cell interactions and that the CD11a/CD18 (LFA-1) lymphocyte surface molecule also plays a functional role after the effector-cell/target-cell conjugate formation. The same integrins, and others not described here, also play a role in tumor-cell dissemination (metastasis) by interacting with extracellular matrix of other tissues (Ruoslahti and Giancotti, 1989).

Costimulatory Signals Determine Lymphocyte Responsiveness

Many studies, for instance, have conclusively shown that IL-1 is a requisite costimulator for growth of selected T lymphocytes. We already illustrated that many of the lymphocyte surface molecules have costimulatory activity in both MHC-unrestricted, as well as MHC-restricted, immune functions. It also appeared that different lymphocyte populations require different costimulators (Weaver and Unanue, 1990), as we detailed earlier regarding the differential monoclonal antibody–mediated activation of distinct lymphocyte subsets and via CD2.

The most important notion is that, in order to complete the activation program of a particular lymphocyte, this costimulus is a requisite. Consequently, lack of the structure providing the costimulus may lead to unresponsiveness, either as a result of lack of lymphocyte proliferation, tolerance induction, or otherwise (Lamb et al., 1983; Lamb and Feldmann, 1984). In fact, the cell that provides a tolerogenic or "suppression" signal to CTL precursors has been referred to as a "veto" cell (Fink et al., 1988). The veto cell probably lacks the costimulatory cell-surface ligand or the production of cytokine costimulatory signals, which therefore results in tolerance induction or lymphocyte paralysis.

It can therefore be hypothesized that tumor cells that do not express the ligand for the costimulator lymphocyte structure (e.g., LFA-1/ICAM-1) (Braakman et al., 1990; Goedegebuure et al., 1990), which is necessary to functionally activate unprimed lymphocytes, may not activate or even induce in vivo peripheral tolerization of potentially reactive lymphocyte clones (Miescher et al., 1988). Therefore, the expression of such additional signals, that is, ligands for costimulator molecules, may be crucial to convert a state of nonactivation or nonresponsiveness into a state of immune activation as originally proposed (Lafferty et al., 1983). Bispecific monoclonal antibodies (bs-mAb) directed against such costimulatory molecules can be instrumental to artificially restore costimulatory signals (Braakman et al., 1990; Goedegebuure et al., 1990).

RETARGETING OF SPECIFIC CTL FOR TUMOR-SELECTIVE, MHC-UNRESTRICTED LYSIS

Most efforts to produce human CTL specific for human tumors have failed, with the possible exception of melanoma CTL. However, many monoclonal antibodies are available that if not exclusively, at least selectively bind to tumor cells. In contrast to T lymphocytes, B lymphocytes use cell-surface Ig to recognize the three-dimensional confirmation of antigens, independently of a cellular or MHC-associated context (Davies et al., 1988).

Chimeric Immunoglobulin-TCR Proteins

Chimeric immunoglobulin (Ig)-TCR genes have been engineered, in which the V-region genes of the TCR are replaced with those of the V-region of an Ig with known specificity (Gross et al., 1989). Transfection of these chimeric receptor genes into T lymphocytes converts the Ig specificity for antigen to the transfected T lymphocytes. Thus, T lymphocytes that express such a chimeric Ig-TCR gene on their surface also display Ig-dictated antigen specificity, which consequently is MHC-unrestricted, in addition to their endogenous TCR. Activation of T lymphocytes via their chimeric Ig-TCR receptor results in activation of lymphokine production by T lymphocytes and triggering of the lytic machinery (Gross et al., 1989).

Transfection of V-region genes of tumor-selective monoclonal antibodies to lymphocytes allows Ig-dictated tumor specificity to be imposed on any transfected CTL, which now will lyse tumor cells in an MHC-unrestricted fashion, irrespective of their original TCR specificity.

It will be of utmost importance to determine whether a subset of T lymphocytes expressing chimeric Ig-TCR receptors retains immune memory function. Indeed, memory T lymphocytes are a requisite to maintain immune protection against "foreign structures," including tumor cells. These novel approaches open exciting new avenues for the development of immunotherapy protocols (Gross et al., 1989; Goverman et al., 1990).

Bispecific Monoclonal Antibody Retargeting of Lymphocytes

Another interesting exploitation of the phenomenon that monoclonal antibody–triggered lymphocyte activation results in lymphokine production as well as triggering of the lytic machinery is the use of bs-mAb (Staertz et al., 1985; Perez et al., 1985). Bs-mAb can be produced by chemically coupling a monoclonal antibody that is specific for the TCR-complex, for example, to a second monoclonal antibody specific for a given tumor target-cell structure, for example. Such a monoclonal antibody heteroaggregate bridges the effector lymphocyte to the target cell (conjugate formation) and consequently triggers the lymphocyte lytic machinery.

The bs-mAb can also be produced by fusion of two hybridomas that produce TCR-specific monoclonal antibody or the target-cell–specific monoclonal antibody, respectively (Milstein and Cuello, 1983).

Meanwhile, many preparations of bs-mAb that recognize the CD3 complex lymphocytes on the one hand and a tumor-associated antigen on the other (e.g., melanoma; renal, ovarian, lung, mammary carcinoma) have been produced and have been shown to effectively lyse tumor cells (Lanzavecchia and Scheidegger, 1987; Titus et al., 1987; Canevari et al., 1988; Van Dijk et al., 1989a, 1989b).

Use of bs-mAb in combination with highly cytolytic T lymphocytes thus also endows originally MHC-restricted cytotoxic T cells with the monoclonal antibody–dictated tumor specificity, in an MHC-unrestricted fashion (as in the case of the Ig-TCR chimeric receptor-expressing lymphocytes). These bs-mAb–retargeted CTL can effectively be used for adoptive transfer of immunity (Segal and Snider, 1989). This "laboratory-engineered" immune lymphocyte mechanism will be used for clinical adoptive immunotherapy. We have started a phase I-II clinical trial employing bs-mAb–retargeted lymphocytes for the intraperitoneal treatment of ovarian carcinoma patients.

The use of combinations of monoclonal antibodies directed at distinct activation and/or adhesion sites on the lymphocytes and at tumor-associated structures, respectively, may further increase the effectiveness of bs-mAb–retargeted CTL lymphocytes as described earlier (i.e., LFA-1/TCR costimulation).

Moreover, use of bs-mAb directed against costimulatory molecules on the lymphocytes may provide the costimulatory signal that is not provided by tumor cells as described earlier in this chapter. Employing such a combination of bs-mAb we may possibly be able to break tolerance or abrogate lymphocyte unresponsiveness.

HYPOTHESIS AND CONCLUSION

The major difference between MHC-unrestricted and MHC-restricted lymphocyte functions is that MHC-restricted lymphocyte function involves TCR binding to an Ag, in which the Ag is restricted to and presented by the MHC of the stimulator or target cell.

MHC-unrestricted lymphocyte function can occur (1) via TCR$\alpha\beta$- or TCR$\gamma\delta$-mediated recognition of target structures (e.g., superantigens), presented by, but not restricted to, the MHC of the stimulator or target cell, or totally independently from

MHC; or (2) independently from lymphocyte TCR and MHC by the stimulator or target cells, respectively.

We previously proposed the hypothesis that multiple receptors are involved in MHC-unrestricted NK and LAK cytolysis (Hersey and Bolhuis, 1987; Bolhuis and Braakman, 1988; Bolhuis et al., 1988). The prediction is that the target-cell specificity range of MHC-unrestricted lytic lymphocytes is dictated by the combination of receptors functionally involved in the effector-cell/target-cell interactions. The induction of the functional involvement of particular types of receptors is then the cumulative result of the interactions of multiple-effector surface molecules with their target-cell ligands and complex. These trigger a cascade of immune (regulatory) functions. The molecular interactions together contribute to the activation program of the lymphocyte, resulting in modulation of its migration capacity; proliferation; and differentiation, maturation, and, in particular, target-cell specificity repertoire(s) of the lymphocyte.

Induction of selective tumor-cell lysis by either TCRαβ, TCRγδ, or TCR^- NK lymphocytes can be obtained using the new techniques involving cytokines, chimeric Ig-TCR–expressing CTL, and bs-mAb–retargeted CTL. The non-MHC–restricted lytic function, either naturally occurring or laboratory engineered, may play a key role in the destruction of tumor or virus-infected cells. The employment of bs-mAb, chimeric Ig-TCR receptors, and/or cytokines prove promising approaches to advance our understanding of immune recognition and regulatory mechanisms (including tolerance) and to refine immunotherapy protocols.

REFERENCES

Acuto O, Hussey RE, Fitzgerald KA, et al. The human T-cell receptor: appearance in ontogeny and biochemical relationship of α and β subunits on IL-2 dependent clones and T-cell tumors. Cell. 1983;34:717–726.

Alcover A, Albertini C, Acuto O, et al. Interdependence of CD3-Ti and CD2 activation pathways in human T lymphocytes. EMBO J. 1988;7:1973–1977.

Anderson P, Caligiuri M, Ritz J, Schlossman SF. CD3-negative natural killer cells express zeta TCR as part of a novel molecular complex. Nature. 1983;341:159–162.

Bierer BE, Sleckman BP, Ratnofsky SG, Burakoff SJ. The biologic roles of CD2, CD4 and CD8 in T-cell activation. Annu Rev Immunol. 1989;7:579–599.

Blanchard DK, Hall RE, Djeu JY. Role of CD18 in lymphokine activated killer (LAK) cell-mediated lysis of human monocytes: comparison with other LAK targets. Int J Cancer. 1990;45:312–319.

Bluestone JA, Crom RQ, Cotterman M, Houlden BA, Matis LA. Structure and specificity of T-cell receptor γδ on major histocompatibility complex antigen specific $CD3^+$, $CD4^-$, $CD8^-$ T lymphocytes. J Exp Med. 1988;168:1899–1916.

Bolhuis RLH, Ronteltap CPM. Generation of natural killer (NK) cell activity after mixed lymphocyte culture (MLC): activation of effector cells in NK cell-depleted cell populations. Immunol Lett. 1980;1:191–196.

Bolhuis RLH, Schellekens SH. Induction of natural killer cell activity and allocytotoxicity in human peripheral blood lymphocytes after mixed lymphocyte culture. Scand J Immunol. 1981;13:401–412.

Bolhuis RLH, Van de Griend RJ. PHA induced proliferation and cytolytic activity in T3$^+$ but not in T3$^-$ cloned lymphocytes, requires the involvement of the T3 antigen for signal transmission. Cell Immunol. 1985;93:46–57.

Bolhuis RLH, Gravekamp C, Van de Griend RJ. Cell-Cell interactions. Clin Immunol Allergy. 1986a;6:29–90.

Bolhuis RLH, Roozemond RC, Van de Griend RJ. Induction and blocking of cytolysis in CD2$^+$ CD3$^-$ NK and CD2$^+$ CD3$^+$ cytotoxic T lymphocytes via CD2 50-Kd sheep erythrocyte receptor. J Immunol. 1986b;136:3939–3944.

Bolhuis RLH, Braakman E. Lymphocyte-mediated responses: activation of, and lysis by, cytotoxic lymphocytes. Curr Opin Immunol. 1988;1:236–240.

Bolhuis RLH, Braakman E, Van de Griend RJ. Are cognitive receptors involved in "non specific" MHC-unrestricted lytic activity? 23rd Forum in Immunol. Annales Inst Pasteur/ Immunologie. 1988;139:460–465.

Borst J, Van de Griend RJ, Van Oostveen H, et al. A T-cell receptor γ/CD3 complex found on cloned functional lymphocytes. Nature. 1987;325:683–688.

Bosnes V, Halvorsen R, Skaftadottir I, Gaudernack G, Thorsby E. Specificity of γδ receptor cytotoxic lymphocytes isolated from human peripheral blood. Scand J Immunol. 1989;29:723–731.

Braakman E, Goedegebuure PS, Vreugdenhil RJ, Segal DM, Shaw S, Bolhuis RLH. ICAM$^-$-melanoma cells are relatively resistant to CD3-mediated T-cell lysis. Int J Cancer. 1990;46:475–480.

Brenner MB, McLean J, Dialynas DPB, et al. Identification of a putative second T-cell receptor. Nature. 1986;322:145–149.

Brenner MB, McLean J, Scheft H, et al. Two forms of the T-cell receptor gamma protein found on peripheral blood cytotoxic T lymphocytes. Nature. 1987;325:689–694.

Bubenik J, Jakoubkova J, Krakora P, et al. Cellular immunity to renal carcinomas in man. Int J Cancer. 1971;8:503–513.

Burnet FM. The concept of immunological surveillance. Prog Exper Tumor Res. 1970;13: 1–27.

Canevari S, Ménard S, Mezzanzanica D, et al. Anti-ovarian carcinoma anti-T3 heteroconjugates or hybrid antibodies induce tumor cell lysis by cytotoxic T-cells. Int J Cancer. 1988;2: 18–21.

Casorati G, De Libero G, Lanzaveccia A, Migone N. Molecular analysis of human γ/δ$^+$ clones from thymus and peripheral blood. J Exp Med. 1989;170:1521–1535.

Cheresh DA, Smith JW, Cooper HM, Quaranta V. A novel vitronectin receptor integrin ($\alpha_v\beta_x$) is responsible for distinct adhesive properties of carcinoma cells. Cell. 1989;57:59–69.

Christmas SE. Most CD3$^+$ WT31$^-$ clones with T-cell receptor Cγ1 rearrangements show strong non-MHC-restricted cytotoxic activity in contrast to those with Cγ2 rearrangements. Eur J Immunol. 1989;19:741–746.

Davies DR, Sheriff S, Padlan EA. Antibody-antigen complexes. J Biol Chem. 1988;263:10541–10544.

Davis MM, Bjorkman PJ. T-cell antigen receptor genes and T-cell recognition. Nature. 1988;334:395–402.

Durum SK, Mealy K. Hilton Head revisited—cytokine explosion of the 80s takes shape for the 90s. News and features. Immunol Today. 1990;11(no. 4):103–106.

Ehrlich P. Uber den Jetzigen Stand der Karzinomforschung. Ned T voor Geneeskunde. 1909;35:273–290.

Ferrini SG, Bottino C, Blassoni R, et al. Characterization of $CD3^+$, $CD4^-$, $CD8^-$ clones expressing the putative T-cell receptor gamma gene product. J Exp Med. 1987;166:277–282.

Fink PJ, Shimonkevitz RP, Bevan MJ. VETO cells. Annu Rev Immunol. 1988;6:115–137.

Fisch P, Malkovsky M, Braakman E, et al. Gamma/delta T cell clones and natural killer cell clones mediate distinct cytolysis. J Exp Med. 1990;171:1567–1579.

Goedegebuure SP, Segal DM, Braakman E, et al. Induction of lysis by TCR $\gamma\delta^+/CD3^+$ T lymphocytes via CD2 requires triggering via the T11,1 epitope only. J Immunol. 1989; 142:1797–1802.

Goedegebuure SP, Braakman E, Segal DM, Vreugdenhil RJ, Bolhuis RLH. Lymphocyte leukocyte function-associated antigen-1 interacting with target cell intercellular molecule 1 coactivates cytolysis triggered via CD16 on the receptor involved in major histocompatibility antigen-unrestricted lysis. Int Immunol. 1990;2(no. 12):1213–1220.

Goverman J, Gomez SM, Segesman KD, Himakapiler T, Lang WE, Hood L. Chimeric immunoglobulin-T cell receptor complex formation and activation. Cell. 1990;60:929–939.

Grimm EA, Mazumder A, Zhang HZ, Rosenberg SA. Lymphokine-activated killer cells phenomenon or lysis of natural killer-resistant fresh solid tumor cells by interleukin 2-activated autologous human peripheral blood lymphocytes. J Exp Med. 1982;155:1823–1841.

Gross G, Waks T, Eshhar Z. Expression of immunoglobulin-T-cell receptor chimeric molecules as functional receptors with antibody-type specificity. Proc Natl Acad Sci USA. 1989; 86:10024–10028.

Haregewoin A, Soman G, Hom RC, Finberg RW. Human $\gamma\delta^+$ T cells respond to mycobacterial heat-shock protein. Nature. 1989;340:309–312.

Hemler ME, Crane C, Sonnenberg A. Association of the VLA α^6 subunit with a novel protein. J Biol Chem. 1989;264:6529–6535.

Hercend T, Meuer S, Brennan A, et al. Identification of a clonally restricted 90 kd heterodimer on two human cloned natural killer cell lines. Its role in cytotoxic effector functions. J Exp Med. 1983;158:1547–1560.

Hercend T, Schmidt R, Brennan A, et al. Identification of a 140 KDa activation antigen as a target structure for a series of human cloned natural killer cell lines. Eur J Immunol. 1984;14:844–852.

Hersey P, Bindon C, Edwards A. Induction of cytotoxic activity in human lymphocytes against autologous and allogeneic melanoma cells in vitro by culture with interleukin 2. Int J Cancer. 1981;28:695–703.

Hersey P, Bolhuis RLH. Non-specific MHC-unrestricted killer cells and their receptors. Immunol Today. 1987;8:233–239.

Hogg N. The leukocyte integrins. Immunol Today. 1989;10:111–114.

Holoshitz J, Koning F, Coligan JE, DeBruyn J, Strober S. Isolation of $CD4^-$, $CD8^-$ mycobacteria-reactive T lymphocyte clones from rheumatoid arthrites synovial fluid. Nature. 1989;339:226–229.

Jitsukawa S, Triebel F, Faure F, Miosse C, Hercend T. Cloned $CD3^+$ $TCR\alpha\beta^-$ $Ti\gamma A^-$ peripheral blood lymphocytes compared to the $Ti\gamma a^+$ counterparts: structural differences of the $\gamma\delta$ receptor and functional heterogeneity. Eur J Immunol. 1988;18:1671–1679.

Kozbor D, Trinchieri G, Monos DS, et al. Human TCR-γ^+/δ^+, $CD8^+$ T lymphocytes recognize tetanus toxoid in a MHC restricted fashion. J Exp Med. 1989;169:1847–1851.

Lafferty KJ, Prowse SJ, Simeonovic CJ. Immunobiology of tissue transplantation: a return to the passenger leucocyte concept. Annu Rev Immunol. 1983;1:143–173.

Lamb JR, Skidmore BJ, Green N, Chiller JM, Felman M. Induction of tolerance in influenza virus-immune T-lymphocyte clones with synthetic peptides of influenza hemagglutinin. J Exp Med. 1983;157:1434–1437.

Lamb JR, Feldmann M. Essential requirement for major histocompatibility complex recognition in T-cell tolerance induction. Nature. 1984;308:72–74.

Lanier LL, Kipps TJ, Phillips JH. Functional properties of a unique subset of cytotoxic $CD3^+$ lymphocytes that express Fc receptors for IgG (CD16/Leu11 antigen). J Exp Med. 1985;162:2089–2106.

Lanier LL, Ruitenberg JJ, Phillips JH. Human $CD3^+$ T lymphocytes that express neither CD4 nor CD8. J Exp Med. 1986;164:339–344.

Lanier LL, Yu G, Phillips JH. Co-association of CD3ζ with a receptor (CD16) for IgG Fc on human natural killer cells. Nature. 1989;342:803–805.

Lanzavecchia A, Scheidegger D. The use of hybrid hybridomas to target human cytotoxic T lymphocytes. Eur J Immunol. 1987;17:105–111.

Marrack P, Kappler J. The T cell receptor for antigen and MHC. Immunol Today. 1988;9:3081.

Masucci MG, Klein E, Argrov S. Disappearance of the NK effect after explantation of lymphocytes and generation of similar nonspecific cytotoxicity correlated to the level of blastogenesis in activated cultures. J Immunol. 1980;124:2458–2463.

Miescher S, Stoeck M, Qiao L, Barras C, Barrelet L, von Fliedner V. Proliferative and cytolytic potentials of purified human tumor-infiltrating T lymphocytes. Impaired response to mitogen-driven stimulation despite T-cell receptor expression. Int J Cancer. 1988;42:659.

Milstein C, Cuello AC. Hybrid hybridomas and their use in immunohistochemistry. Nature. 1983;305:537–540.

Moingeon P, Jitsukawa S, Faure F, et al. A γ-chain complex forms a functional receptor on cloned human lymphocytes with natural killer-like activity. Nature. 1987;325:723–726.

Moingeon P, Chang HC, Wallner BP, Stebbins C, Frey AZ, Reinherz EL. CD2-mediated adhesion facilitates T-lymphocyte antigen recognition function. Nature. 1989;339:312–314.

Mortarini R, Belli F, Parmiani G, Anichini A. Cytokine-mediated modulation of HLA-class II, ICAM-1, LFA-3 and tumor-associated antigen profile of melanoma cells. Comparison with anti-proliferative activity by rIL1-β, rTNF-α, rIFN-γ, rIL4 and their combinations. Int J Cancer. 1990;45:334–341.

Ortaldo JR, Sharrow SO, Timonen T, Herberman RB. Determination of surface antigens on highly purified human NK cells by flow cytometry with monoclonal antibodies. J Immunol. 1981;127:2401–2410.

Ortaldo JR, Kantor R, Segal D, Bolhuis RLH, Bino T. Identification of a proposed NK receptor. Natural Killer Cells and Host Defense. 1989;37:221–226.

Paliard X, Yssel H, Blanchard D, Waitz JA, De Vries JE, Spits H. Antigen specific and MHC non-restricted cytotoxicity of T cell receptor $\alpha\beta^+$ and $\gamma\delta^+$ human T-cell clones isolated in IL-4. J Immunol. 1989;143:452–457.

Pantaleo G, Olive D, Poggi A, Pozzan T, Moretta L, Moretta A. Antibody-induced modulation of the CD3/T-cell receptor complex causes T-cell refractoriness by inhibiting the early metabolic steps involved in T-cell activation. J Exp Med. 1987;166:619–624.

Perez P, Hoffman RW, Shaw S, Bluestone JA, Segal DM. Specific targeting of cytotoxic T-cells by anti-T3 linked to anti-target cell antibody. Nature. 1985;316:354–356.

Phillips JH, Weiss A, Gemlo TB, Rayner AA, Lanier L. Evidence that the T-cell antigen receptor may not be involved in cytotoxicity mediated by γδ and αβ thymic cell lines. J Exp Med. 1987;166:1579–1584.

Poros A, Klein E. Distinction of anti-K562 and anti-allocytotoxicity in in vitro stimulated populations of human lymphocytes. Cell Immunol. 1979;46:57–68.

Ruoslahti E, Giancotti FG. Integrins and tumor cell dissemination. Cancer Cells. 1989;1:119–125.

Schmidt RE, Murray C, Daley JF, Schlossman SF, Ritz J. A subset of natural killer cells in peripheral blood displays a mature T-cell phenotype. J Exp Med. 1986;164:351–356.

Seeley JK, Golub SH. Studies on cytotoxicity generated in human mixed lymphocyte cultures: 1. Time course and target spectrum of several distinct concomitant cytotoxic activities. J Immunol. 1978;120:1415–1422.

Segal DM, Snider DP. Targeting and activation of cytotoxic lymphocytes. Chem Immunol. 1989;47:179–213.

Springer TA, Dustin ML, Kishimoto TK, Marlin SD. The lymphocyte function-associated LFA-1, CD2 and LFA-3 molecules: cell adhesion receptors of the immune system. Annu Rev Immunol. 1987;5:223–252.

Staertz UD, Pasternack MS, Klein JR, Benedetto JD, Bevan MJ. Monoclonal antibodies specific for a murine cytotoxic T-lymphocyte clone. Proc Natl Acad Sci USA. 1984;1799–1803.

Staertz UD, Kanagawa O, Bevan MJ. Hybrid antibodies can target sites for attack by T-cells. Nature. 1985;314:628–631.

Staunton DE, Dustin ML, Springer TA. Functional cloning of ICAM-2, a cell adhesion ligand for LFA-1 homologous to ICAM-1. Nature. 1989;339:61–64.

Sturm E, Braakman E, Bontrop RE, et al. Coordinated Vγ and Vδ gene-segment rearrangements in human T-cell receptor γ/δ^+ lymphocytes. Eur J Immunol. 1989;19:1261–1265.

Sturm E, Braakman E, Fisch P, Vreugdenhil RJ, Sondel P, Bolhuis RLH. Human Vγ9-Vδ2 TCRγδ lymphocytes show specificity to Daudi Burkitt's lymphoma cells. J Immunol. 1990;145,10:3202–3208.

Titus JA, Garrido MA, Hecht TT, Winkler DF, Wunderlich JR, Segal DM. Human T-cells targeted with anti-T3 cross-linked to antitumor antibody prevent tumor growth in nude mice. J Immunol. 1987;138,11:4018–4022.

Triebel F, Faure F, Mami-Chouiab F, et al. A novel Vδ gene expressed predominantly in the TiγA fraction of γ/δ^+ peripheral lymphocytes. Eur J Immunol. 1988;18:2021–2027.

Trinchieri G. Biology of natural killer cells. Advances in Immunology. New York, NY: Academic Press: 1989;47:187–376.

Van de Griend RJ, Giphart MJ, Van Krimpen BA, Bolhuis RLH. Human T-cell clones exerting multiple cytolytic activities show heterogeneity in susceptibility to inhibition by monoclonal antibodies. J Immunol. 1984;133,3:1222–1229.

Van de Griend RJ, Ronteltap CPM, Gravekamp C, Monnikendam D, Bolhuis RLH. Interferon-β and recombinant IL-2 can both enhance but by different pathways, the non-specific cytolytic potential of T3-natural-killer-cell-derived clones rather than that of $T3^+$ clones. J Immunol. 1986;136,5:1700–1707.

Van de Griend RJ, Tax WJM, Van Krimpen BA, Vreugdenhil RJ, Ronteltap CPM, Bolhuis RLH. Lysis of tumor cells by $CD3^+$, 4^-, 8^-, 16^+ T-cell receptor $\alpha\beta^-$ clones regulated via CD3 and CD16 activation sites, recombinant interleukin 2 and interferon β. J Immunol. 1987a;138:1627–1633.

Van de Griend RJ, Bolhuis RLH, Stoter G, Roozemond RC. Regulation of cytolytic activity in CD3 and CD3$^+$ killer cell clones by monoclonal antibodies (anti-CD16, anti-CD2, anti-CD3) depends on subclass specificity of target cell IgG-FcR. J Immunol. 1987b;138:3137–3144.

Van Dijk J, Tsuruo T, Segal DM, et al. Bispecific antibodies reactive with the multidrug-resistance related glycoprotein and CD3 induce lysis of multidrug-resistant tumor cells. Int J Cancer. 1989a;44:738–743.

Van Dijk J, Warnaar SO, Van Eedenburg JDH, et al. Induction of tumor-cell lysis by bi-specific monoclonal antibodies recognizing renal-cell carcinoma and CD3 antigen. Int J Cancer. 1989b;43:344–349.

Vose BM, Bonnard GD. Specific cytotoxicity against autologous tumour and proliferative responses of human lymphocytes grown in interleukin 2. Int J Cancer. 1982;29:33–39.

Vose BM, White W. Tumour-reactive lymphocytes stimulated in mixed lymphocyte and tumour culture. Cancer Immunol Immunother. 1983;15:227–236.

Weaver CT, Unanue ER. The costimulatory function of antigen presenting cells. Immunol Today. 1990;11(no. 2):49–55.

CHAPTER 4

TUMOR ANTIGENS RECOGNIZED BY T CELLS

Patricia L. Ward
Hans Schreiber

Demonstration of the existence of tumor-specific antigens and identification of the genetic origins of these antigens have been the most difficult and elusive goals of tumor immunologists for many decades. The ability to define changes in malignant cells that are truly cancer-specific would provide not only potentially powerful tools for diagnosis and therapy of cancer but perhaps also provide insight into the basic mechanisms of malignant transformation. Although it has been proposed since the beginning of this century that it may be possible to immunize against cancer, the first convincing evidence for the existence of tumor-specific antigens came about 30 years ago from studies of chemically induced tumors in mice. While these studies established a firm basis for the existence of tumor-specific antigens, they could only describe the phenomenon.

In the last decade, it has become, however, increasingly clear that common tumors of man and mouse express mutant proteins that are tumor-specific in that these proteins are encoded by mutant genes that are found in the tumor or premalignant lesions, but not found in the germline of such individuals. For a detailed discussion of the important topic of mutant tumor-specific proteins, the reader is referred to a recent review (Urban and Schreiber, 1992). At least some of the common mutant tumor-specific proteins such as mutant RAS can be recognized by helper T cells of man (Jung and Schluesener, 1991) and mouse (Peace et al., 1991). The critical question that still needs to be answered is whether any of these mutant tumor-specific proteins encode the type of antigens that can lead to tumor rejection. Nevertheless, the unequivocal demonstration of tumor-specific mutant proteins that can be recognized by T cells provides a very strong foundation for the future of tumor immunology. One of the major defense mechanisms of the host against a tumor are cytotoxic T lymphocytes (CTL), which can recognize tumor-specific antigens on cancer cells. The importance of these immune effector cells for tumor rejection has been shown for a variety of experimentally induced murine tumors.

Surprisingly, the T cell–recognized antigens that lead to strong rejection responses in mice have been individually distinct for each independently induced tumor (for review, see Schreiber, 1989). Apparently tumor-specific cytolytic T cells have also been demonstrated for human tumors, in particular, malignant melanomas. The antigens that are the targets for these human T cells are mostly unknown, but recently the genetic origin of a human T cell–recognized melanoma antigen has been described (van der Bruggen et al., 1991). This antigen was found to be encoded by a previously unknown normal cellular gene and was expressed by other independently induced tumors. Remarkably, no expression has so far been found on normal cells. This finding would be unique because no previous similar claim of a shared normal antigen that is exclusively expressed on cancer cells has been upheld. Furthermore, experimental evidence suggests that tumor-specific unique antigens rather than normal shared antigens are the important targets for immunological tumor rejection by T cells. Therefore, it is essential to further study, characterize, and ultimately identify the molecular nature and genetic origin(s) of unique tumor antigens; it is necessary to generate specific probes that can be used for molecular analysis. The lack of permanent, specific probes has been a major stumbling block in the past. This chapter will concentrate on tumor antigens that are recognized by T cells and will review the current evidence for T cell–recognized antigens and their importance in tumor immunity.

EARLY STUDIES OF TUMOR ANTIGENS

Initial experiments early in this century appeared to demonstrate immune resistance to experimental cancers in rodents, but were complicated by the use of outbred animal strains. While these studies eventually led to the discovery of the major histocompatibility complex (MHC) (Gorer et al., 1948, 1956), the idea of tumor-specific antigens fell into disrepute. Experiments using syngeneic mice conducted by Gross in the 1940s (Gross, 1943) and Foley in the 1950s (Foley, 1953) also demonstrated resistance to chemically induced tumors, in particular, to tumors induced by the chemical carcinogen, 3-methylcholanthrene (MCA). Later, more extensive studies (Prehn and Main, 1957) showed very clearly that it was possible to immunize mice against tumors and that this response was distinct from self-reactivity. These authors demonstrated that immunization with one tumor could induce protection against challenge with the same tumor but not other tumors induced by the same carcinogen in the same strain of mice. Thus, the transplantation antigens expressed on these tumors were individually distinct or "unique." In addition, these authors showed that it was unlikely that the tumor antigens were widely expressed on normal tissues because normal tissue of the host from which the tumor had been isolated did not immunize the recipient to reject the tumor challenge, and mice immunized against the tumor still accepted normal skin grafts from the mouse of tumor origin. Furthermore, Klein et al. (1960) showed that immunization with tumor tissue could lead to resistance to tumor challenge even in the autochthonous host, that is, the host of tumor origin. Together, these studies supported the notion that residual heterozygosity, if it existed in these mouse strains, did not account for the immunogenicity of the transplanted tumors. Since these studies demonstrated tumor-specific protective immunity against transplantation of a tumor, these antigens are generally referred to as tumor-specific transplantation antigens. However, other tumor-specific antigens may exist on these tumors, which do not lead to transplantation resistance, but nevertheless stimulate specific immune responses. Since transplantation assays would not detect such antigens, it is possible these types of studies may underestimate the presence of tumor-specific antigens on cancer cells. Although most studies of tumor-specific transplantation antigens have focused on tumors induced by physical or chemical carcinogens, such transplantation antigens have also been reported on spontaneous tumors (Vaage, 1968; Morton et al., 1969; Carswell et al., 1970), that is, those tumors that arise without any experimental intervention.

Despite years of extensive research, the unequivocal demonstration of tumor-specific antigens on experimental tumors and the identification of their molecular nature has been difficult. For example, many tumor antigens originally thought to be tumor-specific were later found to be normal differentiation antigens that were expressed at higher levels on malignant cells (Bates and Longo, 1987). Furthermore, it was noted even by early investigators that immunization with normal tissue could provide some protection against tumors (Medawar and Hunt, 1983). Although transplantation studies have provided a clear framework for the study of tumor immunology, they have unfortunately not been useful in defining the genetic basis of the antigens that are the targets for immunological resistance. One reason for the lack of progress is that transplantation assays are cumbersome, not quantitative, and do not easily lend themselves to molecular analyses. Therefore, it is critical to develop probes that can be used for in vitro analysis and genetic studies. Certainly the lack of reliable probes has been a major stumbling block in elucidating the genetic origin(s) of unique tumor antigens.

TUMOR ANTIGENS DEFINED BY T-CELL PROBES

Animal Models

Ultraviolet Light–Induced Tumors Tumors induced by the physical carcinogen ultraviolet light (UV) have proven to be highly useful in the study of antigens recognized by cytolytic T cells. These tumors are frequently so immunogenic that they are rejected by normal mice without prior immunization but will grow out in immunosuppressed or in T cell–deficient nude mice (Kripke, 1974). This strong immunogenicity can lead to active immunity in the immunized host and can be used to generate cloned cytolytic T cells that are specific for these tumors. For example, previous studies in our laboratory showed that the UV-induced tumor 1591 induced in a C3H mouse expresses three altered MHC class I antigens (Philipps et al., 1985; Stauss et al., 1986a), one of which was shown to be the target for rejection in the normal host (Stauss et al., 1986b). All three antigens are recognized by cloned cytolytic T-cell probes, and these probes appeared to be specific for the UV-1591 tumor since they did not lyse syngeneic nonmalignant control cells. However, nonmalignant cells from the animal in which the UV-1591 tumor was induced were not available for analysis with these CTL probes, and thus it was not possible to exclude with absolute certainty that the antigens were not the result of germline mutation or residual heterozygosity in the C3H mouse strain. Indeed, it was subsequently shown that two of the three antigens defined on this tumor were similar, or identical, in their coding sequences to class I genes of two other mouse strains (Lee et al., 1988), which raised the possibility that contamination occurred during breeding and made results obtained using UV-1591 difficult to interpret. It has been argued that residual heterozygosity in inbred strains may be a rather common problem (Bailey, 1982), and thus it is critical to compare tumor cells with autologous nonmalignant cells from each individual host when conducting studies of specificity. More recent studies in our laboratory used newly derived tumors that were each isolated with autologous control cells as well as with DNA from nonmalignant tissues. These tumors allowed us to show that antigens detected with CTL clones on UV-induced regressor tumors were indeed unique (i.e., individually tumor-specific) and not detected on autologous normal cells (Ward et al., 1989).

One of the goals of studies of tumor antigens was to search for antigens that were unique to malignant cells but shared among different tumors. Such antigens would potentially be of great value in the diagnosis and therapy of cancer. However, transplantation studies suggested that the diversity of antigens expressed by experimentally induced tumors may be extremely large. An extensive search for cross-reactivity among different chemically induced tumors revealed no reproducible cross-reactivity between different tumors (Basombrío, 1970; Basombrío and Prehn, 1972a, 1972b) and thus demonstrated that the antigens were individually specific, or unique, for each tumor, although each was induced by the same carcinogen in the same organ system and in the same strain of mice (Table 4-1).

Ultraviolet light–induced tumors also appear to express unique antigens as evidenced by transplantation studies (12) and later by analysis in vitro using CTL clones (Ward et al., 1989), which represented the first permanent specific and transferable probe for unique tumor antigens. Figure 4-1 shows that a CTL clone raised against the UV-induced regressor tumor, UV-6138, kills cells of this tumor but not cells of 25 other tumors tested. Furthermore, when several tumors arose in the same animal following exposure to UV they displayed individually distinct CTL-recognized tumor antigens. An anti–UV-6132A CTL clone did not kill cells of a second tumor, UV-6132B, induced in the same animal, while in the reciprocal experiment, an anti–UV-6132B CTL clone did not kill UV-6132A tumor cells (Fig. 4-2). A CTL clone raised against an independently derived tumor, UV-6139B, also did not kill cells of two other tumors isolated from the same host (Fig. 4-2). All five tumors are differentiated spindle-cell tumors of very similar histologic appearance. These experiments, like earlier

TABLE 4-1
CHARACTERISTICS OF UNIQUE TUMOR ANTIGENS

1. Specific for an individual tumor when compared to other tumors
   — of the same histologic type
   — induced in the same organ system
   — by the same carcinogen
   — in the same mouse strain
2. Defined by tumor transplantation experiments using syngeneic hosts (not possible in humans)
3. Found in tumors induced by chemical and physical carcinogens as well as some spontaneous tumors
4. Very large antigenic diversity
5. Not detected on autologous normal cells using in vitro–derived probes
6. Origin(s) unknown; possibilities include
   — clonal amplification of preexistent antigens
   — activation of previously silent, normal genes
   — products of tumor-specific mutant genes

(Adapted from Schreiber, 1989.)

transplantation experiments in which no cross-protection was observed between multiple tumors arising in the same host (Globerson and Feldman, 1984), support the contention that the unique antigens expressed by the tumors are not due to genetic impurity in the mouse strain. However, because of the genetic instability of cancer cells (Nowell, 1976), genes encoding an alien antigenic specificity could be lost during continuous growth, particularly when tumors are transplanted in immunocompetent

FIGURE 4-1
Uniqueness of a CTL-defined antigen on the UV-induced tumor 6138. None of 25 other syngeneic C3H tumor cell lines are lysed by this CTL clone in a 4.5-hour ^{51}Cr-release assay. (Reprinted from Ward et al., 1989, with permission.)

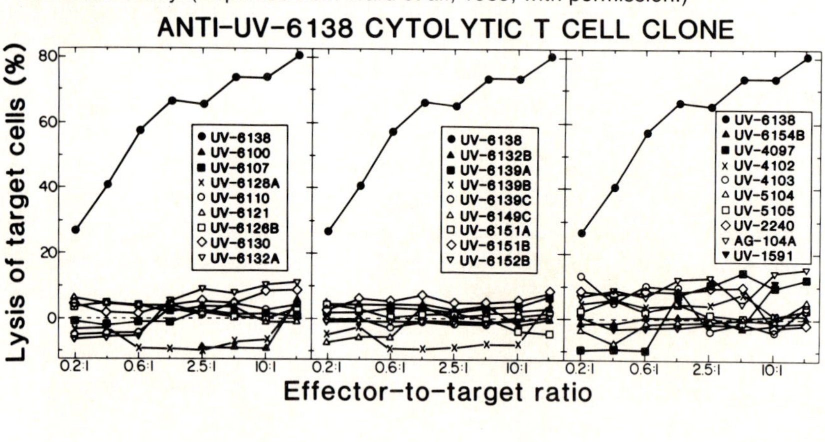

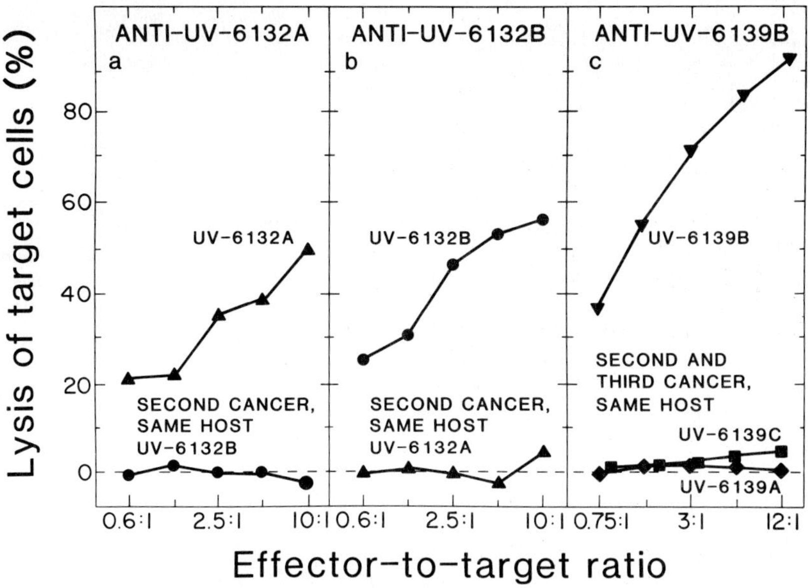

FIGURE 4-2
Multiple tumors isolated from a single host have individually distinct CTL-defined antigens. All five tumors are poorly differentiated spindle-cell tumors of very similar histologic appearance. (a,b) Tumors UV-6132A and UV-6132B were isolated from one individual mouse. (c) Tumors UV-6139A, UV-6139B, and UV-6139C were isolated from one individual mouse. Targets were tested in a 4.5-hour ^{51}Cr-release assay. (Reprinted from Ward et al., 1989, with permission.)

mice (Urban et al., 1986). Therefore, it is critical to test whether CTL clones that appear to display unique tumor specificity kill nonmalignant cells derived from the same mouse that gave rise to each tumor. Figure 4-3 shows that in the eight tumors tested, CTL clones that were raised against the tumors killed the appropriate tumor target and none of the autologous normal fibroblasts. Treatment of the nonmalignant cells with interferon-γ, a cytokine known to raise cell-surface expression of many proteins including, but not limited to, MHC class I antigens (Lindahl et al., 1973) did not reverse this resistance (Fig. 4-3, panel h). These normal fibroblasts could be lysed by an alloreactive CTL clone, indicating that the nonmalignant cells were not inherently resistant to lysis by CTL (Ward et al., 1989). It must be stated that these experiments do not prove that the antigens detected by these CTL clones are tumor-specific in the strictest sense, that is, that they are encoded by tumor-specific mutant genes. The possibility remains that the tumor antigens are comprised of a polymorphic family of molecules that are present on a small, undetectable number of normal cells (Lampson and Levy, 1979) and that malignant transformation simply fixes and selects for a certain antigenic phenotype (Srivastava and Old, 1988). However, the develop-

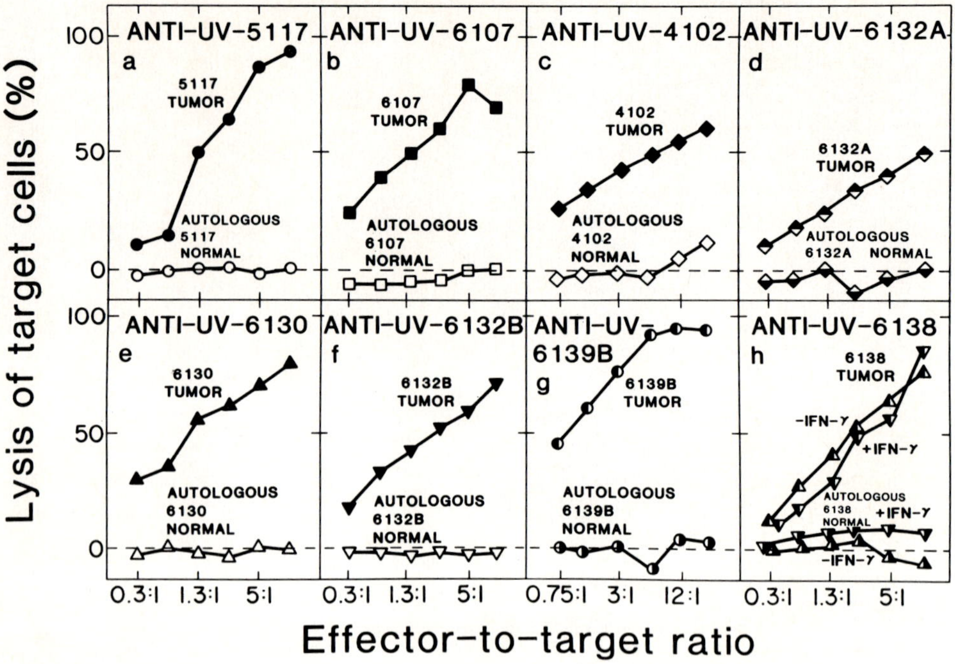

FIGURE 4-3
Absence of CTL-defined tumor antigens on autologous normal control cells. (a–g) Untreated targets. (h) Tumor and control cells were pretreated with 30 U/ml IFN-γ for 48 hours before testing in a 4.5-hour ^{51}Cr-release assay. (c, g) Effector cells are from bulk cultures generated in mixed lymphocyte tumor-cell cultures (MLTC). In all other panels, effector cells are from cloned CTL lines. (Reprinted from Ward et al., 1989, with permission.)

ment of a system that allows comparison of normal and malignant tissue of each host at the genetic level will allow a reliable search for the origins of these antigens.

Cytotoxic T-lymphocyte clones provide a sensitive means to dissect the complexity of tumor antigens. Coculture of tumor cells with a CTL clone that is specific for a particular antigen allows selection of resistant variants that can be used to generate new CTL clones with specificity for remaining antigens on the tumor cells. Using this approach, it was previously shown that the UV-1591 tumor expresses multiple, independent antigens recognized by CTL (Wortzel et al., 1983), at least one of which is responsible for rejection of the tumor by the unimmunized host (Stauss et al., 1986b) and which must be lost in order for the tumor to grow progressively (Wortzel et al., 1984). Therefore, we reexamined the question of multiple antigens using the tumors for which autologous nonmalignant cells were available. Following an approach similar to that used to dissect the antigenic specificity of UV-1591, we generated a CTL clone (called anti-A) against the UV-6139B regressor tumor. Using this anti-A CTL clone, variants were selected in vitro that were resistant to this CTL clone and were therefore A-negative. These variant tumor cells were then used as immunogen to generate an additional CTL clone (anti-B), which lysed not only the A-negative variant line, but also the parental UV-6139B tumor. The anti-B CTL clone was used to select a B-negative variant line. This B-negative variant still retained the A antigen (and, therefore, had an A^+B^- phenotype), while the A-negative variant was still killed by the anti-B CTL clone and, therefore, had an A^-B^+ phenotype (Fig. 4-4). Both the anti-A and anti-B CTL clones exhibited unique reactivity with the UV-6139B tumor and did not lyse autologous normal fibroblasts or other tumors (Ward et al., 1989), demonstrating that a single tumor can express multiple, independent, unique tumor antigens. Cross-reactivity among different UV-induced tumors has been detected using uncloned populations of CTL (Spellman and Daynes, 1978; Urban et al., 1982). However, analysis of this reactivity at the clonal level following limiting dilution (Urban et al., 1982a, 1982b) indicated that much of this reactivity was not due to activation of a single CTL clone directed against some common "UV" antigen, but rather due to polyclonal activation. The fact that CTL-resistant variants can be selected in vitro illustrates a problem faced by a tumor-bearing host, in which immunity directed against one antigen may allow variants to escape immune destruction. Multiple antigens could be ideal targets for combination therapy because the possibility that a cancer cell will lose several independent antigens simultaneously should be remote.

FIGURE 4-4
Demonstration of independence of two unique CTL-defined antigens expressed by a single tumor cell. The A and the B variants show a reciprocal sensitivity pattern to anti-A and anti-B CTL clones, indicating that the A variant had an A^-B^+ and the B variant an A^+B^- phenotype. Targets were tested in a 4.5-hour ^{51}Cr-release assay. (Reprinted from Ward et al., 1989, with permission.)

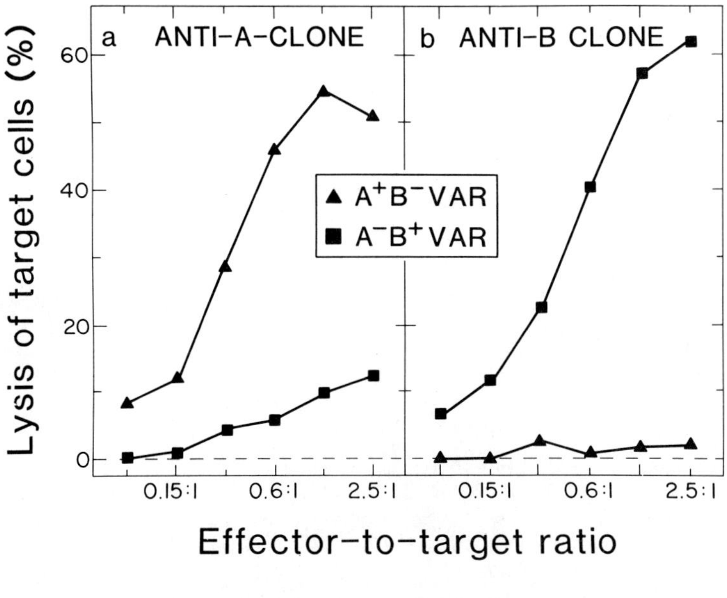

The Methylcholanthrene-Induced Tumor Meth A The MCA-induced tumor Meth A has been extensively studied for many years and is the prototype of chemically induced tumors that express individually distinct transplantation antigens. T cell–mediated immunity is clearly required for rejection of Meth A, but the contribution of the various T-cell subsets in the immune response is not fully understood. Isolation of permanent specific T-cell clones that recognize the Meth A tumor have been largely unsuccessful; however, antisera have repeatedly been generated. An antigen defined by these antisera was described whose encoding gene mapped close to the immunoglobulin locus (Pravtcheva et al., 1981), but it is not clear how this antigen relates to those that confer specific transplantation resistance. Despite the lack of T-cell probes, it has been possible to use transplantation studies for analysis of cell fractions to isolate and identify tumor antigens that appear to be targets for immune destruction in vivo. Antigens that were isolated from Meth A by this approach were cytosolic proteins of 75 to 86 kDa (Ullrich et al., 1986; Dubois et al., 1982). One of these proteins that conferred specific transplantation resistance was found to exist in two isoforms, and sequence analysis of the cloned gene indicated it was identical to that of a heat-shock protein. A 96-kDa glycoprotein capable of eliciting specific tumor immunity has been purified from plasma membranes of Meth A by lectin affinity and ion-exchange chromatography (Srivastava et al., 1986, 1987). Only fractions containing gp96 molecules were capable of eliciting a tumor-rejection response. Rabbit antisera derived after several immunizations with Meth A detected gp96 in CMS5 cells (another MCA-induced sarcoma antigenically distinct from Meth A), as well as other sarcomas, and in cells from a variety of normal tissues (Srivastava and Old, 1988). Despite the antigenic distinction evident from transplantation assays, biochemical analyses could not detect differences between the gp96 molecules among these different tissues. The gene-encoding gp96 has been mapped to mouse chromosome 10 (Srivastava et al., 1988) and contains a typical N-terminal signal sequence consistent with its apparent association with plasma membranes. Analysis of clones obtained from complementary DNA (cDNA) expression libraries defining the 5′ end of the gp96 gene indicate that gp96 antigens are encoded by a single gene specifying a single messenger RNA (mRNA) species without any discernable modifications (Srivastava et al., 1987). However, much of this gene remains to be investigated. It has been suggested from the available evidence that the specificity observed in transplantation assays is due to polymorphism in the gp96 molecule, which could arise from modifications in the amino acid sequence and which may be restricted to a particular region of the molecule. At present, it is not clear whether the gp96 and the 75- to 86-kDa proteins represent a family of unique tumor-specific antigens that are important for the rejection of methylcholanthrene-induced tumors.

P815 The P815 tumor is a mastocytoma induced with MCA in DBA/2 mice. This tumor displays relatively low immunogenicity, but chemical mutagenesis in vitro of the cancer cells led to the development of variants that exhibited lower tumorigenicity compared to the parental tumor and are therefore called tum$^-$ variants. These tum$^-$

variants form tumors in nude mice and express antigens not found on the parental (tum^+) tumor as evidenced by transplantation assays in vivo and CTL sensitivity in vitro (Uyttenhove et al., 1980; Maryanski et al., 1982). Like UV-induced tumors, the tum^- variants appear to express multiple antigens that can be independently lost and appear to be targets for rejection, since variants that escape immune destruction in vivo lose sensitivity to CTL clones in vitro (Uyttenhove et al., 1983; Urban et al., 1982a, 1982b). Expression of multiple antigens as demonstrated for UV-induced tumors may also occur on the mastocytoma P815 (Uyttenhove et al., 1983), suggesting this may be a common phenomenon among tumors. However, this tumor, like UV-1591, cannot be compared to autologous control cells, and allogenicity resulting from multiple, unlinked contaminating genes may mimic such multiple, unique tumor antigens. Recently, a CTL clone specific for the tum^- variant P91 was used in an in vitro system to clone the target antigen from a genomic library of the P815 tumor (De Plaen et al., 1988). This antigen, called P91A, is comprised of 12 exons and encodes a 60-kDa protein that contains no typical N-terminal signal sequence. Comparison of the gene encoding the CTL-recognized antigen with the normal allele in nonmalignant cells revealed a point mutation in exon 4 of this gene, which results in expression of the antigen. Tumorigenic variants that no longer express the P91A antigen carried deletions in this gene. Probes covering the various parts of the P91A gene hybridized to single bands on a Southern blot, indicating that this gene is probably not a member of a family of genes with closely related sequences. The function of the normal allele is unknown. The $H\text{-}2^k$ haplotype cells transfected with the P91A gene and the L^d gene were specifically lysed by CTL raised against P91A, while D^d transfected cells expressing the target gene were not lysed, demonstrating that recognition of the P91A antigen is class I restricted (Lurquin et al., 1989), as would be expected for an antigen recognized by $CD8^+$ CTL (Zinkernagel and Doherty, 1974, 1975). Furthermore, synthetic peptides corresponding to the region of the mutation in exon 4 were able to associate with the L^d molecule and were recognized as targets for CTL lysis, whereas peptides corresponding to the same region in the normal allele sequence failed to act as targets for CTL. This lack of recognition by CTL appeared to result from inability of the peptides generated from the normal allele to bind to the L^d restriction element, since these peptides could not compete with the P91A peptide for binding to L^d. Homology search revealed that the P91A gene is unrelated to genes of the MHC, immunoglobulin or T-cell receptor loci, retroviral genes, or to the gp96 molecule of Meth A. It is possible that the tum^- antigens are the result of chemical mutations in a large number of unrelated genes and it is unknown whether mutations in this gene or similar changes in other genes are found in any tumors as the origin of a natural, that is, not artificially introduced, tumor-specific antigen. In any event, the current evidence shows that carcinogen-induced mutations that are selected for during the clonal evolution of natural cancer development may be nonrandom and directed toward certain regions of a molecule. More recently, a gene encoding two of the antigens on the unmutagenized P815 mastocytoma has been identified (Van den Eynde et al., 1991). The antigen was found to be a normal protein also expressed by mast cells with little or no expression in other normal mouse cells and tissues of adult mice. It would be important to show that expression of this normal antigen can lead to tumor rejection in order to determine whether or not tissue or cell-type restricted differentiation antigens can provide useful target molecules for CTL-mediated therapy of human cancer.

Spontaneous Tumors Spontaneous cancers are generally much less immunogenic than experimentally induced tumors, thus analysis of these tumors presents additional experimental difficulties. Previous studies have demonstrated the presence of tumor-associated transplantation antigens on several spontaneous tumors of both rats and mice (Vaage, 1968; Morton et al., 1969; Carswell et al., 1970; Middle and Embleton, 1981). However, the use of serially transplanted tumors makes interpretation of these results difficult, since immunoselection can occur during a single passage through an immunocompetent animal (Urban et al., 1982b, 1986). Although spontaneous tumors may fail to elicit protective immunity, they may still possess antigens that could be useful for diagnosis and therapy (Koch et al., 1984) and are individually tumor-specific and not detected on autologous normal control cells (Ward et al., 1989). Furthermore, such antigens may reflect underlying changes in transformed cells, which could provide insight into the process of malignant transformation.

Since most experimentally induced tumors are the result of exposure to very high doses of physical or chemical carcinogens, it has been argued that the antigens detected on these tumors are merely laboratory artifacts of the induction process (Hewitt, 1978). For this reason, spontaneous cancers, which are presumably the result of continuous exposure to low doses of carcinogen(s), are considered by some scientists to be a more appropriate model of human cancer, also assumed to be caused by low doses of environmental carcinogens (Doll, 1980). While this issue has been subject to considerable debate (Rapp, 1979; Scott, 1984), it was of interest to test whether, as was true of UV-induced tumors, CTL probes could be generated that recognize antigens on these tumors that were not detectable on autologous normal cells. The C3H tumor AG-104A is a spontaneous tumor that was isolated in our laboratory. This tumor appeared particularly useful for analysis as two tumors arose independently in the same animal. The AG-104A tumor, like other spontaneous tumors, is poorly immunogenic and required multiple immunizations to generate CTL. Cytotoxic T lymphocytes generated in a 6-day, mixed-lymphocyte tumor culture were specific for the AG-104A tumor in that they did not kill cells of the second spontaneous skin tumor, AG-104B, isolated from the same host, nor autologous control fibroblasts (Fig. 4-5). We were consistently unsuccessful in deriving CTL clones for AG-104A. However, unlike the UV-induced tumors, we were able to generate a monoclonal antibody with the same degree of specificity as the CTL. The antibody did not react with any of 24 other tumors tested, which included other spontaneous cancers as well as experimentally induced cancers and various nonmalignant tissues (Ward et al., 1989), and thus appears to express a unique antigen. We do not know as yet whether these two probes recognize the same antigen on the AG-104A tumor. Based on the reported poor immunogenicity of spontaneous tumors in transplantation assays, it has been suggested that human cancers

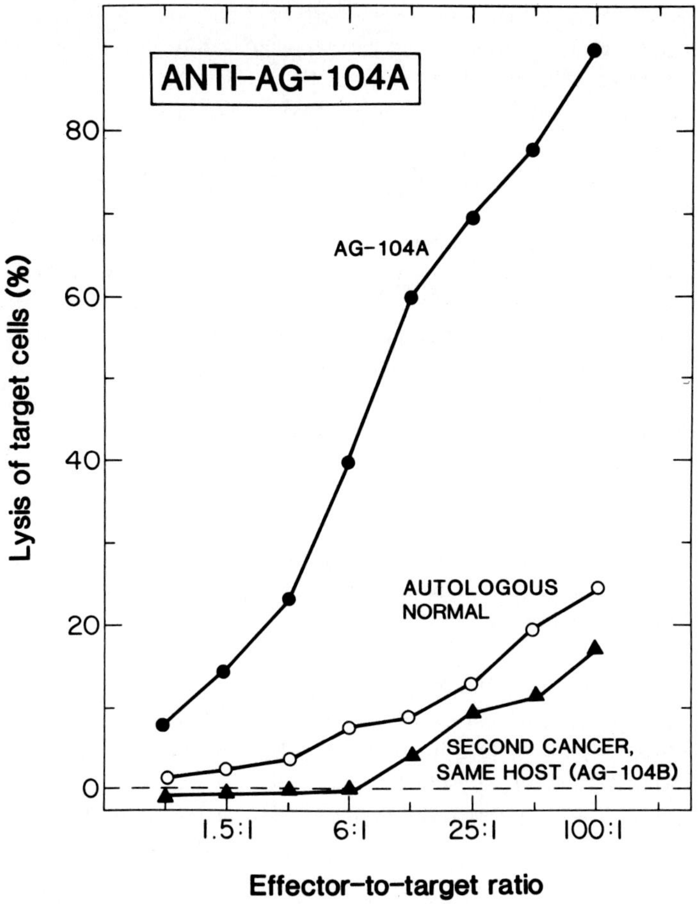

FIGURE 4-5
Unique tumor specificity of cytolytic T cells generated in an MLTC to the spontaneous tumor AG-104A. Neither a second tumor from the same host nor autologous fibroblasts are lysed in a 4.5-hour ^{51}Cr-release assay. (Reprinted from Ward et al., 1989, with permission.)

may also not express target antigens that could be useful for diagnosis and therapy. However, although AG-104A and other spontaneous cancers analyzed were much less immunogenic than those of our UV-induced tumor model, the results obtained with the AG-104A tumor clearly suggest that spontaneous cancers of mice can express unique tumor antigens.

Tumors Induced by DNA Viruses Oncogenic DNA viruses such as SV40, polyoma, and adenovirus encode functionally similar, but antigenically distinct, proteins that are required for induction and maintenance of the malignant phenotype. These proteins are primarily intracellular molecules and are located predominantly in the nucleus. However these antigens can be recognized at the cell surface by CTL and have been shown to be targets for rejection in vivo (Gooding and O'Connell, 1983; Tevethia, 1983; Tanaka and Tevethia, 1988). For example, resistance to SV40-induced tumors requires MHC class I restricted CTL that recognize the SV40 large T antigen. Conversely, purified large T antigen can induce protection against SV40 transformed cells and prevent development of SV40-induced tumors. Furthermore, cells transfected with SV40 large T antigen are specifically lysed by CTL that recognize SV40 transformed cells. Mouse embryo cells transformed in vitro by adenovirus also express proteins that are recognized by CTL. Tumors derived from such virus-transformed mouse embryo cells are apparently highly effective targets for adoptive immunotherapy in nude mice (Kast et al., 1989). These antigens, as well as those expressed by SV40 transformed cells, are tumor-specific in the sense that they are not present in nonmalignant cells, but are common to all tumors induced by the same virus regardless of tissue origin of the tumor or animal species (Schreiber, 1989).

It might be expected that tumor cells that express proteins that are not only recognized by the immune system, but are also essential for maintenance of malignancy, may evade host immunity by mechanisms other than loss of the virally encoded target antigen. However, mutations in these antigens might allow escape from CTL while still retaining the transforming properties of the protein. For example, SV40-induced tumors of C57BL/6 mice express four distinct predominant antigenic sites (I, II, III, IV) on SV40 large T antigen that are recognized by SV40 T antigen–specific CTL clones. Selection in vitro with CTL clones of an SV40 transformed mouse kidney cell line led to isolation of variants that lost expression of antigenic sites and consequently were resistant to lysis by CTL but retained expression of MHC class I antigens. Loss of these antigenic sites, however, did not preclude maintenance of the transformed phenotype (Tanaka and Tevethia, 1988).

Tumors Induced by RNA Viruses Tumors induced by oncogenic RNA viruses express virus-encoded antigens on the surface of the tumor cells. These antigens are encoded by the *env* gene (gp70 and p15E) and several viral core proteins encoded by the *gag* gene. As for tumors induced by DNA viruses, antigens expressed on tumors induced by oncogenic RNA viruses are shared by all tumors that carry the virus. The RNA tumor viral antigens such as the *env* gene product are also commonly expressed on normal cells since inbred mice carry normal murine leukemia proviral sequences in their genomic DNA without production of infectious particles (Old and Stockert, 1977). The *env* gene product gp70 molecules are also commonly expressed on chemically or physically induced tumors and it has been suggested that polymorphic gp70 proteins may represent the unique transplantation antigens observed on these tumors (Lennox et al., 1981; Roman et al., 1981). However, current evidence does not support this concept; no unique tumor-specific envelope sequence molecules have been isolated from chemically or UV-induced tumors, and there does not seem to be extensive polymorphism among these molecules, although recombinational events between different proviral sequences could conceivably generate considerable diversity. Furthermore, antibodies with unique tumor specificity have not reacted with gp70 molecules except in the case of one virally induced leukemia (Nakayama et al., 1984, 1986), but since normal autologous cells from the particular mouse of tumor origin were not available, such antigen could be a normal gene encoded in the germline of that mouse. Antibody reactivity to gp70 antigens on chemically induced tumors does not correlate with strong transplantation resistance (Brown et al., 1978), although weak cross-reactive resistance has been observed (Lennox et al., 1981).

The immunogenicity of murine leukemia viruses (MuLV) is illustrated by the ability of the immune system to reject these retrovirally infected cells, thereby controlling viremia and blocking growth of MuLV-induced leukemia and sarcomas. While some antibodies to viral proteins can neutralize the virus, rejection of RNA virus–induced tumors depends on MHC-restricted T cells that are specific for viral antigens and may include both helper and cytotoxic T-cell subsets (LeClerc and Cantor, 1980; Greenberg et al., 1981). Several studies have addressed the nature of the target antigen on MuLV-induced tumor cells (Flyer et al., 1983; Matis et al., 1985; van der Hoorn et al., 1985; Holt et al., 1986; Plata et al., 1987; Klarnet et al., 1988; Vasmel et al., 1989). Both *gag* and *env* gene products have been implicated as targets for CTL in vitro by transfection of fibroblasts with cloned viral and MHC class I genes and analysis of sensitivity of these target cells to specific CTL. The strength of the response to either antigen was highly influenced by the MHC class I antigen restriction element, and the genotype of the responding mouse determines whether the majority of the CTL will be directed against *gag* or *env* proteins (Holt et al., 1986).

Human Tumors

As briefly discussed in the introduction and in a recent review (Urban and Schreiber, 1992), the existence of T cell–recognized tumor-specific mutant proteins in man provides a firm foundation for the future of tumor immunology. Furthermore, knowledge of which genes or gene families encode tumor-specific antigens in the mouse (Lampson and Levy, 1979; Schreiber et al., 1988) might enable scientists to develop genetic probes to search for similar changes in human cancer cells. Isolation of monoclonal antibodies or CTL as specific and permanent probes for antigens on human tumors, however, remains a problem. Studies of malignant melanomas of humans suggest that T cells may prove to be an important tool in eradication of these tumors, and this idea has been exploited in the search of immunological approaches to therapy of human cancers. Adoptive transfer of immune lymphocytes as a therapeutic tool has been extensively explored in animal models, but these cases rely on the use of syngeneic immunized populations of cells that are unavailable for human cancers (for review, see Schreiber, 1989). Thus, much attention has been given to the isolation and characterization of CTL that specifically react with autologous tumor cells taken from tumor-bearing patients. Inconsistent results and undesirable side effects made therapy with lymphokine-activated killer (LAK) cells problematic. The variable success obtained with interleukin-2 (IL-2) and LAK cell therapy of human cancers may reflect a lack of induction of host-derived T cells that can recognize a specific target antigen or may be related to the immunogenicity of different types of tumors (Parmiani, 1990). Tumor-infiltrating lymphocytes (TIL) isolated directly from the tumor mass have been shown to be effective in eradication of metastatic lesions in experimental animals (Rosenberg et al., 1986), as well as useful for defining antigens on certain tumors in vitro (Barth et al., 1990). The action of the TIL was enhanced with low doses of IL-2 and cyclophosphamide, which did not result in the high level of toxicity previously seen with LAK and IL-2 therapy. Studies that expanded on this finding showed that CTL obtained from peripheral blood or from the tumor (TIL) of cancer patients can lyse autologous cancer cells in vitro (Muul et al., 1987; Topalian et al., 1989). At early passage times in culture, TIL behave like LAK cells in that they nonspecifically lyse an array of fresh and cultured tumor targets and are heterogeneous in their surface phenotype. However, specificity increased over time in culture and the phenotype of the specific cells are nearly uniformly $CD3^+$ $CD8^+$ cells. Both highly specific (lysing only autologous melanoma cells and not autologous normal cells or allogeneic targets) and moderately specific (lysing autologous melanoma cells and some allogeneic targets) T cells from melanoma patients have been reported. Generating CTL to human melanoma has consistently been more successful in the past than generating T cells specific for other human cancers (for review, see Schreiber, 1989). It is also difficult to assess whether melanoma antigens recognized by TIL are unique for each melanoma or shared among different melanomas, because the appropriate HLA restriction molecule may not have been present for recognition by $CD8^+$ CTL. This has important implications for therapy using adoptively transferred cytolytic T cells, since CTL would have to be tailored for each tumor and each individual. However, some reports show that when HLA antigens were shared with the allogeneic targets, CTL still showed specificity for autologous tumor cells, suggesting that melanomas and perhaps other human cancers do express unique antigens that are recognized by CTL (Slovin et al., 1986; Muul et al., 1987).

A major problem in therapy of human tumors is that, at the time of diagnosis, the tumor may have already undergone extensive selection (Knuth et al., 1989). In fact, available data from melanoma studies suggest there is vast heterogeneity within a given tumor (Herín et al., 1987; Knuth et al., 1989). Isolation of TIL from various metastatic deposits within the same individual showed different lytic specificities that may reflect differential antigen expression (or loss of some antigens in different populations). Furthermore, CTL clones derived from TIL and PBL of human melanoma patients revealed different patterns of reactivity, not only among clones of the same metastasis, but also among cells from tumor lesions isolated at different times from the same patient (Anichini et al., 1986, 1989).

Another class of CTL-recognized antigens found on human cancers is the mucins (Barnd et al., 1989). Mucins are high-molecular weight complex glycoproteins, or glycolipids, that are expressed on the surface or secreted by a variety of normal epithelial cells. These molecules, when expressed on certain types of tumors of epithelial origin, appear to be highly immunogenic in that they readily stimulate the production of antibodies as well as cytolytic T cells. Cytotoxic T-lymphocyte lines established from lymph nodes of patients with pancreatic adenocarcinomas and propagated in culture in IL-2 with an allogeneic pancreatic tumor cell line as stimulator lysed a panel of pancreatic adenocarcinoma and breast carcinoma lines, but not tumor lines established from other tissues. An antibody directed against mucin could inhibit lysis by this CTL line. An unusual finding was that the CTL lysed the tumor cells in an antigen-specific, but MHC-unrestricted, manner. Furthermore, biochemical analyses showed that these CTL appeared to utilize the alpha/beta T-cell receptor (TCR$\alpha\beta$) normally thought to recognize nominal antigen only in connection with MHC class I molecules. To reconcile this apparent paradox, it has been proposed that the multivalent nature of these large mucin molecules (demonstrated with monoclonal antibodies and analysis of the sequence of breast mucin) may allow direct recognition of the target antigen by CTL (Barnd et al., 1989). The question remaining is whether the tumor-associated mucin target antigens on breast and pancreatic cancer are different from those normally expressed in nonmalignant epithelial cells. As previously mentioned, antigens with strong immunogenicity, which are shared by a variety of tumors, but restricted to malignant cells, represent potentially powerful diagnostic and therapeutic tools, but it is not clear whether such antigens exist.

MECHANISMS OF TUMOR ESCAPE

T cell–mediated immunity is critical for rejection of virally and chemically induced tumors in immunized mice and for rejection of UV-induced tumors or allogeneic tumors in normal mice (Old et al., 1962; Rouse et al., 1972; Kripke, 1974; Tevethia, 1974). The relative importance of the different subsets of T cells in tumor rejection has been the subject of much controversy (Doherty et al., 1984; Robbins and Baldwin, 1985), and it is likely that the mechanism of rejection is influenced by the subset of T cells involved. Possibly the molecular nature of the antigen also influences the subset required for antigen recognition and rejection. Assuming that antigens recognized by CTL clones in vivo are important for tumor rejection, loss of a CTL-recognized target antigen and loss or reduction of MHC class I restriction elements required for CTL recognition of its target are two possible mechanisms of tumor escape from T cell–mediated immunity, both of which have been intensely investigated. Since CD8$^+$ T cells recognize antigens in the context of MHC class I molecules (Zinkernagel and Doherty, 1974, 1975), changes in expression of MHC class I molecules may allow tumors to escape immune destruction by CTL (Tanaka et al., 1985). Loss and/or reduction in expression of class I molecules have been reported for several virally induced tumors (Meruelo and McDevitt, 1978; Meruelo et al., 1978; Schmidt and Festenstein, 1982; Gooding, 1983; Bernards et al., 1983; Hui et al., 1984; Flyer et al., 1985; Meruelo et al., 1986) and for a few tumors of nonviral etiologies (Wallich et al., 1985; Burnham et al., 1989). Whether a similar mechanism occurs in human cancer is unclear. Reports of loss or down regulation of MHC class I antigen expression in human cancers include small-cell lung carcinoma, choriocarcinoma, and neuroblastoma. However, with the possible exception of a percentage of colorectal cancers that either appear to have downregulated expression of all class I antigens or show selective loss of certain class I antigens, it is unclear whether this loss of class I expression results in immune escape (Doyle et al., 1985; Momburg et al., 1989; Travers et al., 1982). For example, down regulation of class I expression observed in human choriocarcinoma may be a function of the depressed state of class I expression on the trophoblast cells from which these cancers originate. Other factors such as association of loss of class I with increased expression of certain oncogenes may account for the down regulation of class I expression in neuroblastoma and small-cell lung carcinoma. Thus, results seem to indicate that in tumors of both experimental animals and humans, there are examples in which loss or reduction of MHC class I antigen expression appears to be involved in escape of the tumors from immune destruction. However, there is not a consistent loss of class I expression for all tumors of any etiology reported to date (Haywood and McKhann, 1971; Burnham et al., 1989; Ward et al., 1990), and other mechanisms may also contribute to tumor escape.

Whether induced by the same or different carcinogens, tumors will undoubtedly be dissimilar enough as to utilize different mechanisms of escape from immune destruction. For example, while loss of class I antigens can account for tumor escape of some virally induced tumors, resistance to CTL could also occur via mutations in the target antigen (Tanaka and Tevethia, 1988) that may not alter the malignant state of the cell. Furthermore, some tumors induced with MuLV were found to escape immune destruction through loss of class I antigens (Flyer et al., 1985), while others retained expression of class I molecules but acquired resistance to CTL through failure to express viral antigens (Vasmel et al., 1989). The UV-induced tumors grow in T cell–deficient nude (but not normal) mice, which illustrates the importance of T-cell immunity for rejection of these tumors (Kripke, 1974). For example, rare progressor variants of the UV-1591 tumor were all found to have lost a CTL-defined antigen, and similarly, selection in vitro for cells that were resistant to the CTL clone resulted in tumors that were able to escape immune destruction and grow progressively in vivo. The $CD8^+$ T-cell subset alone can mediate rejection of this tumor (Fan and Edgington, 1989), and recently, we have found that all of the UV-induced regressor tumors we have tested are rejected by animals depleted of $CD4^+$ but not $CD8^+$ T cells (Ward et al., 1989). The UV-induced tumors were an ideal model for approaching the question of tumor escape since, as mentioned above, $CD8^+$ T cells require expression of class I antigens for recognition of target antigen. Furthermore, we could select CTL-resistant variants in vitro and look at growth behavior in vivo. Analysis of a large number of UV-induced regressor tumors, UV-induced progressor tumors, and spontaneous tumors showed no consistent loss or reduction in class I expression, although these tumors varied greatly in their ability to grow progressively in the normal host. Variants selected from regressor parent tumors showed no consistent loss in expression of MHC class I antigens compared to their regressor parents. Only 1 of 24 progressor tumors analyzed showed a selective loss of K antigen expression following T-cell selection, indicating that this mechanism must be a rare event as a means of escape. In vitro selected CTL-resistant variants that grew progressively in vivo all retained expression of class I molecules and thus appeared to have lost expression of a unique antigen (Ward et al., 1990). However, while some progressor variants that grew out as rare variants of regressors lost expression of a unique antigen, as was previously shown for the UV-1591 tumor, others retained both CTL sensitivity and class I expression (Ward et al., 1990) (Fig. 4-6).

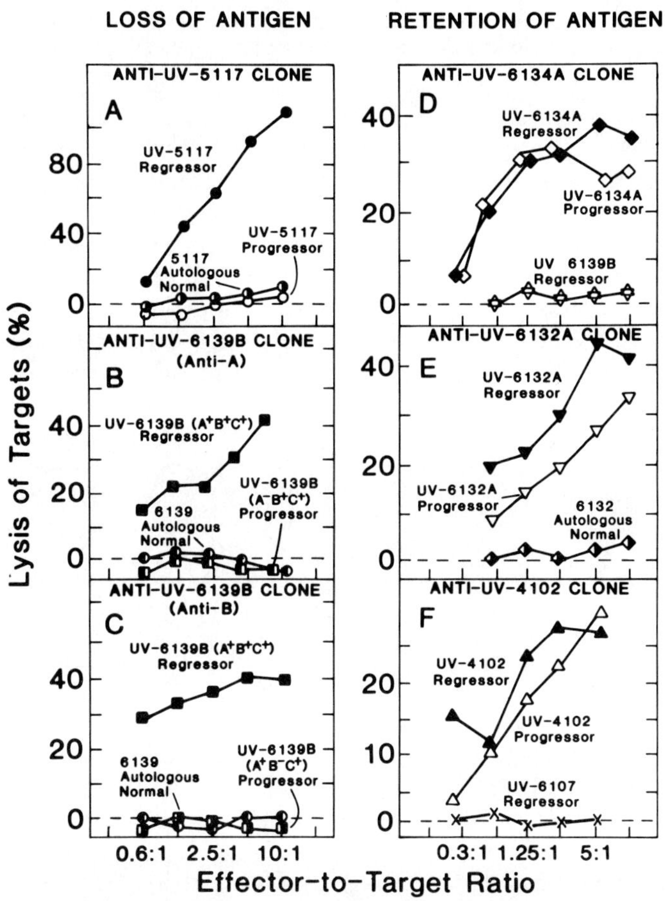

FIGURE 4-6
Analysis of progressor variants of UV-induced regressor tumors with CTL clones. Three variants, one derived in vivo and two derived in vitro, lose expression of a unique CTL-defined antigen (panels a, b, and c), but three other variants, all derived by host selection in vivo retain the antigen recognized by the CTL clones (panels d, e, and f). Variants were derived from highly immunogenic regressor tumors following selection in vivo (panels a, d, e, and f) or in vitro (panels b and c). Lysis of the targets was analyzed in a 4.5-hour ^{51}Cr-release assay. (Reprinted from Ward et al., 1990, with permission.)

It is possible that MCA tumors also do not frequently lose class I antigen expression as a means of tumor escape. One example is sarcoma T10, an MCA-induced tumor that lacks expression of Kk and Kb antigens and acquires increased immunogenicity after transfection and expression of these genes (Wallich et al., 1985). However, no consistent changes in class I expression that correlated with tumor immunity were found in a study of a number of MCA sarcomas (Haywood and McKhann, 1971). These tumors are, in general, much less immunogenic than UV-induced regressor tumors, and in contrast to the UV-induced tumors, variants that have lost transplantation antigens have not been isolated. Possibly, rejection of Meth A is mediated by helper T cells rather than cytolytic cells, and the immunity generated by helper cells may not be effective in selection of antigen loss variants (Van Waes et al., 1986). Like some UV-induced regressor tumors, escape variants of P815 that grew progressively have been attributed to loss of a CTL-recognized unique antigen (Maryanski and Boon, 1982), and to date, no evidence for loss of class I expression on these variants has been reported. While loss of class I antigen expression may be most frequently observed in virally induced tumors as a mechanism of escape from immune destruction, this may not be a common mechanism for tumors induced by chemical carcinogens or by UV. Furthermore, the mechanism(s) regulating expression of class I antigens in tumors are unknown (Burnham et al., 1989). Certainly, changes not directly related to loss of MHC class I expression or tumor antigen expression may also account for tumor escape, such as production of immunosuppressive substances that could prevent effective stimulation of $CD8^+$ immunity in vivo (Torre-Amione et al., 1990). Finally, effector mechanisms other than $CD8^+$ immunity may be adversely affected in tumor progression (Kärre et al., 1986).

NATURE OF TUMOR ANTIGENS RECOGNIZED BY T CELLS

The genetic origin(s) of unique tumor antigens has remained an enigma as has their relationship, if any, to malignant transformation. The diversity of the unique antigens has led some scientists to speculate that these molecules may originate from large polymorphic gene families such as the MHC or the immunoglobulin genes. Other theories include (1) genes that are expressed during fetal life and are derepressed during malignant transformation, (2) polymorphic gp70 envelope proteins of MuLV resulting from recombinational events, and (3) random carcinogen-induced mutations of many genes. Alternatively, these antigens may preexist on a small population of cells that may not be recognized until exposure to carcinogen leads to clonal amplification of cells expressing a particular antigen such as can occur in the idiotypes of B- or T-cell malignancies. This hypothesis, originally proposed by Burnet (1970), has been addressed experimentally. A nonmalignant fibroblast line was cloned and the progeny of the subclones were malignantly transformed. All of the transformants had distinct antigenic phenotypes based on immunological analyses even though they were all derived from the same precursor cell (Basombrío and Prehn, 1972a, 1972b; Embleton and Heidelberger, 1972). These experiments seemed to suggest that exposure to carcinogen resulted in mutations that led to appearance of neoantigens; however, the carcinogen could still have acted to activate previously nonexpressed random genes. Alternatively, since normal cells can acquire considerable diversity in surface phenotype following expansion in culture from a single precursor (Moscona, 1974; Hood et al., 1977), the action of the carcinogen may just have been to fix a particular antigenic phenotype already generated (Srivastava and Old, 1988). Both possibilities could lead to considerable antigenic diversity even if antigens were preexistent in normal cells. Finally, it is unclear whether these antigenic changes could lead to transplantation resistance since they were not tested in vivo.

So far, only a handful of examples exist in which genes encoding a unique transplantation antigen have been examined at the genetic level (Wortzel et al., 1984; Uyttenhove et al., 1983; Philipps et al., 1985; Stauss et al., 1986a; Srivastava et al., 1987). The gp96 antigen of MCA-induced tumors may represent an example of a preexistent cellular gene that is mutated by the carcinogen giving rise to polymorphic antigens that are recognized by the immune system and are targets for destruction of these tumors. A normal cellular counterpart to the CTL-recognized P91A antigen of P815 also has been identified and appears to be the result of mutagenization of the cancer cells by the chemical used to generate the tum$^-$ variant. Identification of the "novel" MHC class I rejection antigen of UV-1591 tumor was facilitated by use of an antibody that recognized the same antigen as the cloned CTL, but these antigens appear to be alloantigen present in the germline of the mouse of tumor origin (Lee et al., 1988). Results obtained with all of the other tumor models also suffer from the lack of appropriate autologous controls to determine conclusively the germline or somatic origin of the tumor-specific transplantation antigens.

Greater than 95% of known carcinogens are also mutagens (Ames, 1979), and there is considerable evidence that cancer is a result of multiple sequential mutations (Nigro et al., 1989). Very little is known, however, about the type of carcinogen-induced mutations that may be important for tumor formation in vivo or for the appearance of tumor antigens. Some of these mutations may lead to malignant transformation, while others may give rise to antigenic surface molecules that could serve as tumor-specific target antigens. Since the action of most mutagens are likely to be random events and may involve many different genes, mutations that lead to malignant transformation may not be completely independent of those that result in the appearance of unique cell-surface antigens. However, examples exist in which selected mutations are repeatedly found in certain types of tumors (Sukumar et al., 1986) and, if recognized by the immune system, would represent shared, but tumor-specific, antigens. Ideally, immune therapy could be directed against those mutant proteins that are responsible for maintaining malignant phenotype and that act as targets for CTL.

A clear example of a tumor-specific mutant protein is that produced by the chromosomal translocation that results in the generation of the *bcr-abl* fusion protein in chronic myelogenous leukemia. This is a result of a selective fusion between exons of the *bcr* and *abl* genes following a tumor-specific chromosomal translocation (Rowley, 1973; DeKlein et al., 1982; Shtivelman et al., 1985; Ben-Neriah, 1986). These mutant proteins represent changes that are tumor-specific, yet shared among tumors of the same type that are induced in different individuals, and may well encode shared tumor-specific antigens. This would represent an important difference between experimental tumors of nonviral etiology and human tumors, as common antigens have not as yet been described in experimental systems. Whether tumor-specific mutant proteins will frequently be found in human tumors, and whether these mutant proteins encode antigens that can be used for diagnostic or therapeutic purposes remains to be determined. If proteins such as *bcr-abl* are also essential for maintenance of the malignant phenotype, they would be ideal therapeutic targets, since variants that have lost the antigen could not retain the malignant phenotype and survive.

SUMMARY AND FUTURE GOALS

Studies of experimentally induced tumors and the discovery of T cell–recognized, tumor-specific mutant proteins in man and mouse clearly support the existence of tumor-specific antigens that can be recognized by T cells. While the nature of these antigens and their genetic origin(s) remain to be determined, the development of cloned T-cell probes and new methods to use these probes should pave the way towards this goal. Prospects for therapy based on expanding of specific cytolytic cells in vitro and reinfusing these cells into patients for treatment of cancer may be facilitated by the possibility of generation of large numbers of these T cells in vitro. Considerable problems and questions remain, however, especially with repeatedly generating these T cells with clear specificity from cancer patients, particularly those with cancer other than melanoma. The generation and selection of CTL-resistant variants that have lost expression of target antigens is a situation that may also be expected. Other treatment regimens such as treatment with certain T cell–stimulating antibodies that could result in generation of specific CTL and mediate tumor rejection in vivo remain to be explored further (Ellenhorn et al., 1990). The use of heteroconjugate antibody to attract T cells to the site of tumor growth also deserves careful study. Most human cancers are induced by environmental carcinogens, most of which are mutagenic. These human tumors, therefore, might express mutant proteins as antigenic targets for T cell–mediated therapeutic approaches. Furthermore, experimentally induced, as well as spontaneous, tumors of mice may well prove to be useful experimental models to search for the genetic origin of tumor-specific antigens on tumors. Finally, a major remaining problem is the rapid development of resistance to immunotherapy even by relatively minute solid cancers following establishment (e.g., Golumbek et al., 1991). This problem may be related to the as yet unknown large role of stroma surrounding malignant cells growing in vivo (Singh et al., 1992).

ACKNOWLEDGMENTS

This work was supported by a gift of the Passis family and by the National Institutes of Health grants R37 CA-22677, P01 CA-19266, R01-37156.

REFERENCES

Ames BN. Identifying environmental chemicals causing mutations and cancer. Science. 1979;204:587–593.

Anichini A, Fossati G, Parmiani G. Heterogeneity of clones from a human metastatic melanoma detected by autologous cytotoxic T lymphocyte clones. J Exp Med. 1986;163:215–220.

Anichini A, Fossati G, Parmiani G. Clonal analysis of the cytolytic T-cell response to human tumors. Immunol Today. 1987;8:385–389.

Anichini A, Mazzocchi A, Fossati G, Parmiani G. Cytotoxic T lymphocyte clones from peripheral blood and from tumor site detect intratumor heterogeneity of melanoma cells. Analysis of specificity and mechanisms of interaction. J Immunol. 1989;142:3692–3701.

Bahler DW, Frelinger JG, Harwell LW, Lord EM. Reduced tumorigenicity of a spontaneous mouse lung carcinoma following H-2 gene transfection. Proc Natl Acad Sci USA. 1987;84:4562–4566.

Bailey DW. How pure are inbred strains of mice? Immunol Today. 1982;3:210–214.

Barnd DL, Lan MS, Metzgar RS, Finn OJ. Specific major histocompatibility complex-unrestricted recognition of tumor-associated mucins by human cytotoxic T cells. Proc Natl Acad Sci USA. 1989;86:7159–7163.

Barth RJ Jr, Bock SN, Mule JJ, Rosenberg SA. Unique murine tumor-associated antigens identified by tumor infiltrating lymphocytes. J Immunol. 1990;144:1531–1537.

Basombrío MA. Search for common antigenicities among 25 sarcomas induced by methylcholanthrene. Cancer Res. 1970;30:2458–2462.

Basombrío MA, Prehn RT. Studies on the basis for diversity and time of appearance of antigens in chemically induced tumors. Natl Cancer Inst Monogr. 1972a;35:117–124.

Basombrío MA, Prehn RT. Antigenic diversity of tumors chemically induced within the progeny of a single cell. Int J Cancer. 1972b;10:1–8.

Bates SE, Longo DL. Use of serum tumor markers in cancer diagnosis and management. Sem Oncol. 1987;14:102–138.

Ben-Neriah Y, Daley G, Mes-Masson A, Witte O, Baltimore D. The chronic myelogenous leukemia-specific p210 protein is the product of the *bcr/abl* hybrid gene. Science. 1986; 233:212–214.

Bernards R, Schrier PI, Houweling A, et al. Tumorigenicity of cells transformed by adenovirus type 12 by evasion of T cell immunity. Nature (Lond). 1983;305:776–779.

Brown JP, Klitzman JM, Hellstrom I, Nowinski RC, Hellstrom KE. Antibody response of mice to chemically induced tumors. Proc Natl Acad Sci USA. 1978;75:955–958.

Burnet FM. The concept of immunological surveillance. Prog Exp Tumor Res. 1970;13:1–27.

Burnham DK, Mak CK, Webster RJ, Daynes RA. Relationship between inducible H-2 expression and the immunogenicity of murine skin neoplasms. I. Evidence that the immunogenicity of ultraviolet radiation–chemically induced tumors is associated with their susceptibility to γ-interferon–mediated enhancement of H-$2K^k$ expression. Transplantation. 1989;47:533–542.

Carswell EA, Wanebo HJ, Old LJ, Boyse EA. Immunogenic properties of reticulum cell sarcomas of SJL/J mice. J Natl Cancer Inst. 1970;44:1281–1288.

DeKlein A, Geurts van Kessel A, Grosveld G, et al. A cellular oncogene is translocated to the Philadelphia chromosome in chronic myelocytic leukemia. Nature. 1982;300:765–767.

DePlaen E, Lurquin C, Van Pel A, et al. Immunogenic (tum^-) variants of mouse tumor P815: cloning of the gene of tum^- antigen P91A and identification of the tum^- mutation. Proc Natl Acad Sci USA. 1988;85:2274–2278.

Doherty PC, Knowles BB, Wettstein PJ. Immunological surveillance of tumors in the context of major histocompatibility complex restriction of T cell function. Adv Cancer Res. 1984; 42:1–65.

Doll R. The epidemiology of cancer. Cancer. 1980;45:2475–2485.

Doyle A, Martin WJ, Funa K, et al. Markedly decreased expression of class I histocompatibility antigens, protein, and mRNA in human small-cell lung cancer. J Exp Med. 1985;161:1135–1151.

DuBois GC, Law LW, Appella E. Purification and biochemical properties of tumor-associated transplantation antigens from methylcholanthrene-induced murine sarcomas. Proc Natl Acad Sci USA. 1982;79:7669–7673.

Ellenhorn JDI, Schreiber H, Bluestone JA. Mechanism of tumor rejection in anti-CD3 monoclonal antibody-treated mice. J Immunol. 1990;144:2840–2846.

Embleton MJ, Heidelberger C. Antigenicity of clones of mouse prostate cells transformed in vitro. Int J Cancer. 1972;9:8–18.

Fan S-T, Edgington TS. Sufficiency of the CD8+ T cell lineage to mount an effective tumoricidal response to syngeneic tumor-bearing novel class I MHC antigens. J Immunol. 1989;143:4287–4291.

Flyer DC, Burakoff SJ, Faller DV. Retrovirus-induced changes in major histocompatibility complex antigen expression influence susceptibility to lysis by cytotoxic T lymphocytes. J Immunol. 1985;135:2287–2292.

Flyer DC, Burakoff SJ, Faller DV. Cytotoxic T lymphocyte recognition of transfected cells expressing a cloned retroviral gene. Nature (Lond). 1983;305:815–818.

Foley EJ. Antigenic properties of methylcholanthrene-induced tumors in mice of the strain of origin. Cancer Res. 1953;13:835–837.

Globerson A, Feldman M. Antigenic specificity of benzo[a]pyrene-induced sarcomas. J Natl Cancer Inst. 1984;32:1229–1243.

Golumbek PT, Lazenby AJ, Levitsky HI, et al. Treatment of established renal cancer by tumor cells engineered to secrete interleukin-4. Science. 1991;254:713–719.

Gooding LR, O'Connell KA. Recognition by cytotoxic T lymphocytes of cells expressing fragments of the SV40 tumor antigen. J Immunol. 1983;131:2580–2586.

Gorer PA. Some recent work on tumor immunity. Adv Cancer Res. 1956;4:149–186.

Gorer PA, Lyman S, Snell GD. Studies on the genetic and antigenic basis of tumour transplantation. Linkage between a histocompatibility gene and "fused" in mice. Proc R Soc Lond Ser B. 1948;135:499–505.

Greenberg PD, Cheever MA, Fefer A. Eradication of disseminated murine leukemia by chemoimmunotherapy with cyclophosphamide and adoptively transferred immune syngeneic Lyt-1+2-lymphocytes. J Exp Med. 1981;154:952–963.

Gross L. Intradermal immunization of C3H mice against a sarcoma that originated in an animal of the same line. Cancer Res. 1943;3:326–333.

Haywood GR, McKhann CF. Antigenic specificities on murine sarcoma cells. Reciprocal relationship between normal transplantation antigens (H-2) and tumor-specific immunogenicity. J Exp Med. 1971;133:1171–1187.

Herín M, Lemoine C, Weynants P, et al. Production of stable cytolytic T-cell clones directed against autologous human melanoma. Int J Cancer. 1987;39:390–396.

Hewitt HB. The choice of animal tumors for experimental studies on cancer therapy. Adv Cancer Res. 1978;27:149–200.

Holt CA, Osorio K, Lilly F. Friend virus-specific cytotoxic T lymphocytes recognize both gag and env gene-encoded specificities. J Exp Med. 1986;164:211–226.

Hood L, Huang HV, Dreyer WJ. The area code hypothesis: the immune system provides clues to understanding the genetic and molecular basis of cell recognition during development. J Supra Str. 1977;7:531–559.

Hui K, Grosveld F, Festenstein H. Rejection of transplantable AKR leukemia cells following MHC DNA-mediated cell transformation. Nature (Lond). 1984;311:750–752.

Jung S, Schluesener HJ. Human T lymphocytes recognize a peptide of single point-mutated, oncogenic ras protein. J Exp Med. 1991;173:273–276.

Kärre KHG, Ljunggren PG, Kiessling R. Selective rejection of H-2 deficient lymphoma variants suggests alternative immune defense strategy. Nature (Lond). 1986;319:675–678.

Kast WM, Offringa R, Peters PJ, et al. Eradication of adenovirus E1-induced tumors by E1A-specific cytotoxic T lymphocytes. Cell. 1989;59:603–614.

Klarnet JP, Kern DE, Okuno K, Holt C, Lilly F, Greenberg PD. FBL-reactive (Lyt-2 positive cytotoxic and L3T4-positive helper) T lymphocytes recognize distinct F-MuLV encoded antigens. J Exp Med. 1988;169:457–467.

Klein G, Sjögren HO, Klein E, Hellstrom KE. Demonstration of resistance against methylcholanthrene-induced sarcomas in the primary autochthonous host. Cancer Res. 1960;20:1561–1572.

Knuth A, Wölfel T, Klehmann E, Boon T, Meyer zum Buschenfelde KH. Cytolytic T-cell clones against an autologous human melanoma: specificity study and definition of three antigens by immunoselection. Proc Natl Acad Sci USA. 1989;86:2804–2808.

Koch S, Zaleberg JR, McKenzie IFC. Description of a murine B lymphoma tumor-specific antigen. J Immunol. 1984;133:1070–1077.

Kripke ML. Antigenicity of murine skin tumors induced by ultraviolet light. J Natl Cancer Inst. 1974;53:1333–1336.

Lampson LA, Levy R. A role for clonal antigens in cancer diagnosis and therapy. J Natl Cancer Inst. 1979;62:217–219.

LeClerc JC, Cantor H. T cell–mediated immunity to cornavirus-induced tumors. II. Ability of different T cell subsets to prevent tumor growth in vivo. J Immunol. 1980;124:851–854.

Lee DR, Rubocki RJ, Lie W, Hansen TH. The murine MHC class I genes, H-2D^q and H-2L^q are strikingly homologous to each other, H-2L^d and two genes reported to encode tumor-specific antigens. J Exp Med. 1988;168:1719–1739.

Lennox ES, Lowe AD, Cohn J, Evan G. Specific antigens on methylcholanthrene-induced tumors of mice. Transplant Proc. 1981;13:1759–1761.

Lindahl P, Leary P, Gresse I. Enhancement by interferon of the expression of surface antigens on murine leukemia L1210 cells. Proc Natl Acad Sci USA. 1973;70:2785–2788.

Lurquin C, Van Pel A, Mariame B, et al. Structure of the gene of tum$^-$ transplantation antigen P91A: the mutated exon encodes a peptide recognized with L^d by cytolytic T cells. Cell. 1989;58:293–303.

Maryanski JL, Boon T. Immunogenic variants obtained by mutagenesis of mouse mastocytoma P815. IV. Analysis of variant-specific antigens by selection of antigen-loss variants with cytolytic T cell clones. Eur J Immunol. 1982;12:406–412.

Matis LA, Ruscetti SK, Longo DL, et al. Distinct proliferative T cell clonotypes are generated in response to a murine retrovirus-induced syngeneic T cell leukemia: viral gp70 antigen-specific MT4$^+$ clones and Lyt-2$^+$ cytolytic clones which recognize a tumor-specific cell surface antigen. J Immunol. 1985;135:703–713.

Medawar PB, Hunt R. Can fetal antigens be used for prophylactic immunization? CIBA Found Symp. 1983;96:160–180.

Meruelo D, McDevitt HO. Recent studies on the role of the immune response to virus-induced leukemias and lymphomas. Semin Hematol. 1978;15:399–419.

Meruelo D, Nimelstein SH, Jones PP, Liebesman M, McDevitt HO. Increased synthesis and expression of H-2 antigens on thymocytes as a result of radiation leukemia virus infection: a possible mechanism for H-2 linked control of virus-induced neoplasia. J Exp Med. 1978;147:470–487.

Meruelo D, Kornreich R, Rossamondo A, et al. Lack of class I H-2 antigens in cells transformed by radiation leukemia virus is associated with methylation and rearrangement of H-2 DNA. Proc Acad Natl Sci USA. 1986;83:4504–4508.

Middle JG, Embleton MJ. Naturally arising tumors of the inbred WAB/not rat strain. II. Immunogenicity of transplanted tumors. J Natl Cancer Inst. 1981;67:637–643.

Momburg F, Ziegler A, Harpprecht J, Möller P, Moldenhauer G, Hämmerling GJ. Selective loss of HLA-A or HLA-B antigen expression in colon carcinoma. J Immunol. 1989;142:352–358.

Moscona AA. Surface specifications of embryonic cells: lectin receptors, cell recognition, and specific cell ligands. In: Moscona AA, ed. The cell surface in development. New York, NY: John Wiley and Sons; 1974:67–99.

Morton DL, Miller GF, Wood DA. Demonstration of tumor-specific immunity against antigens, unrelated to the mammary tumor virus in spontaneous mammary adenocarcinomas. J Natl Cancer Inst. 1969;42:289–301.

Muul LM, Spiess PJ, Director EP, Rosenberg SA. Identification of specific cytolytic immune responses against autologous tumor in humans bearing malignant melanoma. J Immunol. 1987;138:989–995.

Nakayama E, Uenaka A, Stockert E, Obata Y. Detection of a unique antigen on radiation leukemia virus-induced leukemia B6RV2. Cancer Res. 1984;44:5138–5144.

Nakayama E, Uenaka A, DeLeo AB, et al. Molecular basis of a unique tumor antigen of radiation leukemia virus–induced leukemia B6RV2: its relation to MuLV gp70 of xenotropic class. J Immunol. 1986;136:3502–3507.

Nigro JM, Baker SJ, Preisinger AC, et al. Mutations in the p53 gene occur in diverse human tumour types. Nature. 1989;342:705–708.

Nowell PC. The clonal evolution of tumor cell populations. Acquired genetic lability permits selection of variant sublines and underlies tumor progression. Science. 1976;194:23–28.

Old LJ, Stockert E. Immunogenetics of cell surface antigens of normal leukemia. Annu Rev Genet. 1977;17:127–160.

Old LJ, Boyse EA, Clarke DA, Carswell EA. Antigenic properties of chemically-induced tumors. Ann NY Acad Sci. 1962;101:80–106.

Parmiani G. An explanation of the variable clinical response to interleukin 2 and LAK cells. Immunol Today. 1990;11:113–115.

Peace DJ, Chen W, Nelson H, Cheever MA. T cell recognition of transforming proteins encoded by mutated ras proto-oncogenes. J Immunol. 1991;146:2059–2065.

Philipps C, McMillan M, Flood PM, et al. Identification of a unique tumor-specific antigen as a novel class I major histocompatibility molecule. Proc Natl Acad Sci USA. 1985;82:5140–5144.

Plata F, Langlade-Demoyen P, Abastado JP, Berbar T, Kourilsky P. Retrovirus antigens recognized by cytolytic T lymphocytes activate tumor rejection in vivo. Cell. 1987;48:231–240.

Pravtcheva DD, DeLeo AB, Ruddle FH, Old LJ. Chromosome assignment of the tumor-specific antigen of a 3-methylcholanthrene–induced mouse sarcoma. J Exp Med. 1981;154:964–977.

Prehn RT, Main JM. Immunity to methylcholanthrene-induced sarcomas. J Natl Cancer Inst. 1957;18:769–778.

Rapp HJ. Appropriateness of animal models for the immunology of human cancer. Cancer Res. 1979;39:4285–4286.

Robbins RS, Baldwin RW. T cell subsets in tumour rejection responses. Immunol Today. 1985;6:55–61.

Roman JM, Hirsch J, Readhead C, Levy D, DeOgny L, Dreyer WJ. Heritable differences among gp70-like molecules on C3H ultraviolet light–induced fibrosarcomas. Transplant Proc. 1981;13:1782–1786.

Rosenberg SA, Spiess P, Lafreniere R. A new approach to the adoptive immunotherapy of cancer with tumor-infiltrating lymphocytes. Science. 1986;233:1318–1321.

Rouse B, Roellinghoff TM, Warner NL. Anti-θ serum induced suppression of cellular transfer of tumor-specific immunity to a syngeneic plasma cell tumor. Nature New Biol. 1972;238: 116–117.

Rowley JD. A new consistent chromosomal abnormality in myelogenous leukemia identified by quinacrine fluorescence and Giemsa staining. Nature. 1973;243:290–293.

Schmidt W, Festenstein H. Resistance to cell-mediated cytotoxicity is correlated with reduction of H-2K gene products in AKR leukemia. Immunogenetics. 1982;16:257–264.

Schreiber H. Fundamental immunology, 2nd edition. New York, NY: Raven Press Ltd.; 1989;923–955.

Schreiber H, Ward PO, Rowley DA, Strauss HJ. Unique tumor-specific antigens. Ann Rev Immunol. 1988;6:465–483.

Scott O. Syngeneic tumor–host relationship. J Natl Cancer Inst. 1984;72:775.

Shtivelman E, Lifshitz B, Gale R, Canaani E. Fused transcripts of abl and bcr genes in chronic myelogenous leukemia. Nature. 1985;315:550–554.

Singh S, Ross SR, Acena M, Rowley DA, Schreiber H. Stroma is critical for preventing or permitting immunological destruction of antigenic cancer cells. J Exp Med. 1992;175:139–146.

Slovin SF, Lackman RD, Ferrone S, Kiely PE, Mastrangelo MJ. Cellular immune response to human sarcomas: cytotoxic T cell clones reactive with autologous sarcomas. I. Development, phenotype, and specificity. J Immunol. 1986;137:3042–3048.

Spellman CW, Daynes RA. Ultraviolet light–induced murine suppressor lymphocytes dictate specificity of anti-ultraviolet tumor immune responses. Cell Immunol. 1978;38:25–34.

Srivastava PK, Old LJ. Individually distinct transplantation antigens of chemically induced mouse tumors. Immunol Today. 1988;9:78–83.

Srivastava PK, DeLeo AB, Old LJ. Tumor rejection antigens of chemically induced sarcomas of inbred mice. Proc Natl Acad Sci USA. 1986;83:3407–3411.

Srivastava PK, Chen YT, Old LJ. 5′-Structural analysis of genes encoding polymorphic antigens of chemically induced tumors. Proc Natl Acad Sci USA. 1987;84:3807–3811.

Srivastava PK, Kozak CA, Old LJ. Chromosomal assignment of the gene encoding the mouse tumor rejection antigen gp96. Immunogenetics. 1988;28:205–207.

Stauss HJ, Linsk R, Fischer A, et al. Isolation of the MHC genes encoding the tumor-specific class I antigens expressed on an immune fibrosarcoma. J Immunogenet. 1986a;13:101–111.

Stauss HJ, Van Waes C, Fink MA, Starr B, Schreiber H. Identification of a unique tumor rejection antigen by molecular cloning and gene transfer. J Exp Med. 1986b;164:1516–1530.

Sukumar S, Notaria V, Marin-Zanca D, Barbacid M. Induction of mammary carcinoma in rats by nitroso-methylurea involves malignant activation of H-ras-1 locus by single point mutations. Nature (Lond). 1986;306:658–661.

Tanaka K, Isselbacher KJ, Khoury G, Jay G. Reversal of oncogenesis by the expression of a major histocompatibility complex class I gene. Science. 1985;228:26–30.

Tanaka Y, Tevethia SS. In vitro selection of SV40 T antigen epitope loss variants by site-specific cytotoxic T lymphocyte clones. J Immunol. 1988;140:4348–4354.

Tevethia SS, Blasecki JW, Waneck G, Goldstein AL. Requirement of thymus-derived θ positive lymphocytes for rejection of DNA virus (SV40) tumors in mice. J Immunol. 1974;113:1417–1423.

Tevethia SS, Tevethia MJ, Lewis AJ, Reddy VB, Weissman SM. Biology of simian virus 40 (SV40) transplantation antigen (TrAg) IX. Analysis of TrAg in mouse cells synthesizing truncated SV40 large T antigen. Virology. 1983;128:319–330.

Topalian SL, Solomon D, Rosenberg SA. Tumor-specific cytolysis by lymphocytes infiltrating human melanomas. J Immunol. 1989;142:3714–3725.

Torre-Amione G, Beauchamp DR, Koeppen H, et al. A highly immunogenic tumor transfected with a murine TGF-betal cDNA escapes immune surveillance. Proc Natl Acad Sci USA. 1990;87:1486–1490.

Travers PJ, Arklie JL, Trowsdale J, Patillo RA, Bodmer WF. Lack of expression of HLA-ABC antigens in choriocarcinoma and other human tumor cell lines. Natl Cancer Inst Monogr. 1982;60:175–180.

Ullrich SJ, Robinson EA, Law LW, Willingham M, Appela E. A mouse tumor–specific transplantation antigen is a heat shock–related protein. Proc Natl Acad Sci USA. 1986;83:3121–3125.

Urban JL, Schreiber H. Tumor antigens. Annu Rev Immunol. 1992;10:617–644.

Urban JL, Holland JM, Kripke M, Schreiber H. Immunoselection of tumor variants by mice suppressed with ultraviolet radiation. J Exp Med. 1982a;156:1025–1041.

Urban JL, Burton RC, Holland JM, Kripke ML, Schreiber H. Mechanisms of syngeneic tumor rejection. Susceptibility of host-selected progressor variants to various immunological effector cells. J Exp Med. 1982b;155:557–573.

Urban JL, Kripke ML, Schreiber H. Stepwise immunological selection of antigenic variants during tumor growth. J Immunol. 1986;137:3036–3041.

Uyttenhove C, Van Snick J, Boon T. Immunogenic variants obtained by mutagenesis of mouse mastocytoma P815. I. Rejection by syngeneic mice. J Exp Med. 1980;152:1175–1183.

Uyttenhove C, Maryanski J, Boon T. Escape of mouse mastocytoma P815 after nearly complete rejection is due to antigen loss variants rather than immunosuppression. J Exp Med. 1983;157:1040–1052.

Vaage J. Nonvirus-associated antigens in virus-induced mouse mammary tumors. Cancer Res. 1968;28:2477–2483.

Van den Eynde B, Leth B, Van Pel A, De Plaen E, Boon T. The gene coding for a major tumor rejection antigen of tumor P815 is identical to the normal gene of syngeneic DBA/2 mice. J Exp Med. 1991;173:1373–1384.

Van der Bruggen P, Traversari C, Chomez P, et al. A gene encoding an antigen recognized by cytolytic T lymphocytes on a human melanoma. Science. 1991;254:1643–1647.

Van der Hoorn FA, LaHaye T, Muller V, Ogle MA, Engers HD. Characterization of gP85^{gag} as an antigen recognized by Moloney leukemia virus-specific cytolytic T cell clones that function in vivo. J Exp Med. 1985;162:128–144.

Van Waes C, Urban JL, Rothstein JL, Ward PL, Schreiber H. Highly malignant tumor variants retain tumor-specific antigens recognized by T helper cells. J Exp Med. 1986;164:1547–1565.

Vasmel WLE, Sijts EJAM, Leupers CJM, Matthews EA, Melief CJM. Primary virus-induced lymphomas evade T cell immunity by failure to express viral antigens. J Exp Med. 1989;169:1233–1254.

Wallich RN, Bulbuc N, Hämmerling FJ, Katzav S, Segal S, Feldman M. Abrogation of metastatic properties of tumour cells by de novo expression of H-2K antigens following H-2 gene transfection. Nature (Lond). 1985;315:301–305.

Ward PL, Koeppen H, Hurteau T, Schreiber H. Tumor antigens defined by cloned immunological probes are highly polymorphic and are not detected on autologous normal cells. J Exp Med. 1989;170:217–232.

Ward PL, Koeppen HK, Hurteau T, Rowley DA, Schreiber H. MHC class I and unique antigen expression in tumor escape from $CD8^+$ T cell-dependent surveillance. Cancer Res. 1990;50:3851–3858.

Wortzel RD, Phillips C, Schreiber H. Multiplicity of unique tumor-specific antigens expressed on a malignant cell. Nature. 1983;304:165–167.

Wortzel RD, Urban JL, Schreiber H. Malignant growth in the normal host after variant selection in vitro with cytolytic T cell lines. Proc Natl Acad Sci USA. 1984;81:2186–2190.

Zinkernagel RM, Doherty PC. Restriction of in vitro T cell mediated cytotoxicity in lymphocytic choriomeningitis within a syngeneic or allogeneic system. Nature (Lond). 1974;248:701–702.

Zinkernagel RM, Doherty PC. H-2 compatibility requirement for T cell mediated lysis of target cells infected with lymphatic choriomeningitis virus. Different cytotoxic T cell specificities are associated with structures coded for in H-2K or H-2D. J Exp Med. 1975;141:1427–1441.

CHAPTER 5

PROCESSING AND PRESENTATION OF TUMOR-RELATED ANTIGENS

Victor E. Reyes
Shan Lu
Quoc V. Nguyen
Robert E. Humphreys

The purpose of this review is to summarize what is known about mechanisms for antigen processing and presentation to T cells and to project how this information might come to be exploited in immunological control of malignancies.

We are studying the mechanism of antigen processing, which is the digestion of proteins to peptides and the selection of some of them for presentation by major histocompatibility complex (MHC) proteins to antigen recognition receptors on T cells. We want to know why only some peptides are selected and the role of accessory molecules in charging and function of class II MHC proteins.

A principal question in this review is how the recurrent placement of hydrophobic amino acids in some antigenic peptide sequences might catalyze helical coiling of the peptide on a hydrophobic surface. Such coiling on the lipid bilayer of a vesicle or on a transfer molecule could lead either to protection of peptides of a foreign antigen from further proteolytic attack and/or to transfer to the desetopes of MHC molecules. These select peptides, when coiled as α-helices, have recurrent hydrophobic amino acids forming an axial strip with other axial quadrants having few or no competing hydrophobic residues. Understanding the biophysics of this process might lead to methods to engineer peptide vaccines in order to increase potency and widen the range of MHC restriction. Also, immunogenicity could be lessened for murine immunoglobulins used in therapy or diagnosis.

We also consider mechanisms that might regulate peptide charging of, and presentation by, class II MHC molecules, as reflected in structural changes, association and dissociation of accessory molecules that can be found with the MHC class II α and β chains.

PROCESSING AND PRESENTATION OF T CELL–PRESENTED ANTIGENS

Central to most immune responses to tumor and other antigens is a series of events termed antigen processing, in which antigenic proteins appear to be fragmented in a time- and energy-dependent process and only some peptides are selected for presentation to T lymphocytes (Ziegler and Unanue, 1982). That presentation of selected antigen fragments to antigen-specific T cells occurs through specific recognition by the T-cell antigen receptor (TCR) of determinants on both the presenting MHC molecules and on the antigenic peptides (Davis and Bjorkman, 1988). The specificity and magnitude of the immune response to a malignancy depend upon the pathways for processing and presentation of the tumor antigens. Toward an ultimate goal of exploiting knowledge about these mechanisms to modify the immune response to malignancies and to proteins used in the diagnosis and treatment of cancers, we have prepared this review following stepping stones of facts and hypotheses, which we try to distinguish clearly. First we consider the immunobiology and physical structure of T cell– and B cell (Ig)–recognized epitopes. Then, we contrast the processing pathway of class I and class II MHC-restricted, T cell–presented determinants. The role of physical structure in the selection of which sequences in a foreign protein will become T cell–presented is considered in detail. Finally, the associations, processing, cleavages, and dissociations of accessory proteins to class II MHC molecules are described. These changes might reflect mechanisms for catalysis of peptide charging of class II MHC desetopes. Facts are considered in light of theories about antigen processing and presenting mechanisms and about specific ways in which vaccines can be selected and engineered, or T-cell immunogenicity altered of therapeutic or diagnostic murine immunoglobulins.

T Cell–Presented, Tumor-Specific, and Tumor-Associated Antigens

The immune response to, and occasional control of, malignancies involves recognition of T cell–presented determinants that are expressed in malignant cells (Schreiber et al., 1988; Tanaka et al., 1988; Grey et al., 1989; Wölfel et al., 1989). To effect this control of malignancies, the immune system recognizes tumor-specific antigens (TSA) or tumor-associated antigens (TAA) (Carney, 1988). Such determinants can be created in a differentiation- or activation-specific molecule (TAA). Alternately, they arise as a result of expression of a cellular or viral oncogene (TSA). Aberrant forms of cellular proteins such as class I molecules have also been detected on various tumors (Festenstein and Hui, 1986; Schmidt and Festenstein, 1980; Wortzel et al., 1983). Tumor-specific antigens might be derived from the fragment of a proto-oncogene that has sustained a mutation leading to an altered growth-regulating function or might represent some protein that had been expressed during development but is no longer present in nonmalignant cells of the animal. Tumor-associated antigens might be expressed with increased abundance in malignancies, but if one looks closely, they are also on other, normal cells of the organism, at least in some stages of development. Aberrant or "novel" class I sequences present in tumor cells might arise from multiple recombination events among endogenous class I genes during tumorigenesis (Festenstein and Hui, 1986; Stauss et al., 1986; Tanaka et al., 1988). These tumor-specific or tumor-associated determinants can be recognized by either immunoglobulins or T-cell receptors.

T Cell– and B Cell–Recognized Epitopes of One Antigen

The immune system has evolved two types of receptors for specific recognition of two structurally distinct types of antigenic epitopes (Fig. 5-1). Immunoglobulins (Ig) recognize superficial, conformation-dependent determinants, for example, as hydrophilic, flexible segments on convex surfaces of native proteins or as externally placed, chemical modifications (haptens) (Geysen et al., 1987; Dyson et al., 1985). T-cell receptors recognize a second type of determinant that is still present in denatured or digested antigen and survives as peptides in such digests (Boyer et al., 1988; Allen et al., 1984; Shimonkevitz et al., 1983). Upon recognition of these "buried" or "carrier" determinants (peptides) by antigen- and MHC-specific receptors, $CD4^+$ helper T lymphocytes are activated to produce various lymphokines that have multiple immunoregulatory effects, such as the induction of proliferation and maturation of B lymphocytes to plasma cells (Balkwill and Burke, 1989). Until recent years, it was generally assumed that cytotoxic T lymphocytes (CTL) recognized intact proteins on the surfaces of tumor or virus-infected cells. That view changed with studies of Townsend and others, showing killing by CTL specific for proteins that are never expressed intact on virally infected cells (Townsend and Skehel, 1982, 1984; Townsend et al., 1984, 1986a). Influenza-specific CTL were observed to recognize proteins that were not present in the membrane of infected target cells. Studies using reassortant viruses led to the demonstration that genes encoding a viral polymerase (PB2) and nucleoprotein (NP) that are not cell surface–expressed were essential for the recognition by the influenza-specific CTL (Bennink et al., 1982; Kees and Krammer, 1984; Townsend and Skehel, 1982; Townsend et al., 1984). Furthermore, L cells transfected with NP were lysed by class I–restricted CTL, although NP-specific antibodies did not detect NP at the cell surface (Townsend and Skehel, 1984). In addition, cells transfected with a hemagglutinin (HA) gene, lacking the signal sequence needed for translocation into the ER and subsequent transport to the cell surface, were efficiently recognized by HA-specific, class I–restricted CTL (Townsend et al., 1986a). These observations led

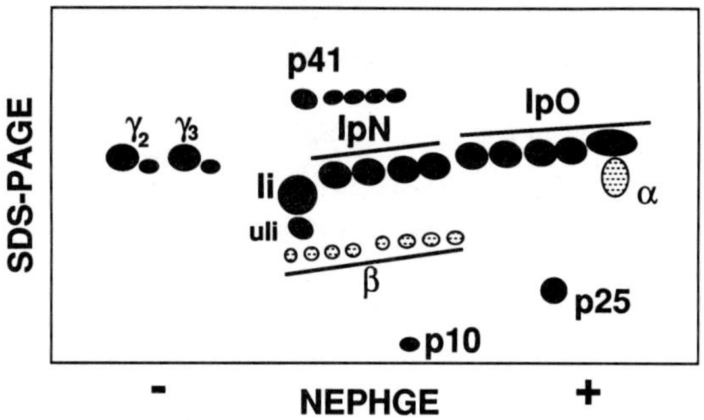

FIGURE 5-1
Multiple forms of I_i created by several transcriptional and posttranscriptional mechanisms. I_i itself is synthesized and glycosylated with two N-linked, high mannose chains. These can be modified to complex sugar chains with sialic acids (IpN) and O-linked chains can be added also with sialic acids (IpO). An alternate translational start site for the N-terminal, cytoplasmic tail of I_i yields γ2 and γ3 (p35) forms. An additional exon 6b and 64 amino acids can be inserted to form p41. I_i can be cleaved to p25, or in leupeptin- or antipain-treated cells, p21 and p10 can be found. Not shown is the chondroitin sulfate-derivatized form of I_i. The α and β chains of class II MHC molecules are illustrated.

to the view that CTL recognized degraded forms of NP and HA at the cell surface and, thus, such epitopes could be characterized with synthetic peptides in vitro, as initially shown for class II–restricted epitopes. A series of studies with influenza virus and other systems have shown that this is indeed the case (Rothbard et al., 1988; Townsend et al., 1986b; Morrison et al., 1986; Bastin et al., 1987; Pala et al., 1988; Sinigaglia et al., 1988; McMichael et al., 1986). Target cells coated with small, synthetic peptides representing sequences within the protein antigens are efficiently recognized by CTL (Bastin et al., 1987; Morrison et al., 1986; Kuwano et al., 1990; Ishioka et al., 1989; Nagy et al., 1989; Gotch et al., 1987).

In the case of antigen-presenting B lymphocytes, the linkage between Ig-recognized and helper T cell–recognized epitopes is defined by the presence of those B cell (Ig)– and T cell–recognized determinants in one molecule, complex, or virus that is internalized by the membrane Ig (mIg) of the B lymphocyte, which subsequently presents digested fragments to a helper T lymphocyte. Antibodies to all, or most, superficial B-cell epitopes can be generated with help from only those T cell–presented sequences that are bound to the particular MHC alleles expressed in the individual. Cytoxic T lymphocytes interact with specific fragments of TSA, TAA, or aberrant endogenous antigens presented by MHC class I (and in some instances by class II) molecules on the surfaces of tumors, initiating recognition that leads to lysis of the tumor cells (Wölfel et al., 1989; Grey et al., 1989; Martz and Howell, 1989). Likewise, helper T lymphocytes recognize fragments of tumor antigens to generate help to the structurally linked, Ig-recognized determinants. Some T cell–presented peptides can mediate suppression of all responses to the foreign protein (Krzych et al., 1988; Lakey et al., 1987a).

Intracellular Processing of Antigen by B Cells

Antigen uptake is the first event in the recognition of class II–restricted antigens. The uptake can be nonspecific through pinocytosis or specific through receptor-mediated endocytosis, that is, Ig on B cells or Fc receptors. The latter is a more efficient process. Antigen processing by B lymphocytes involves internalization of a foreign protein by surface immunoglobulin and digestion of the antigen into peptides, only some of which become T cell–presented (Shimonkevitz et al., 1983). Antigen processing by accessory cells is a time- and energy-dependent process (Ziegler and Unanue, 1982; Unanue and Cerottini, 1989). When a B lymphocyte processes a protein antigen, its mIg specifies the exact epitope for which help will be generated (Rock et al., 1984; Lanzavecchia, 1985; Tony and Parker, 1985). Foreign protein is digested into peptides, which become associated with class II MHC antigens for surface expression and presentation to TCR on $CD4^+$, helper T cells.

Recognition of the peptide-MHC molecule combination stimulates release from the helper T cell of interleukin-2 (IL-2) and other lymphokines, which promote differentiation and maturation of the B lymphocytes and other accessory cells. Although digested peptides from a foreign antigen can be presented by glutaraldehyde-fixed cells (Shimonkevitz et al., 1983) or by liposomal membranes (Walden et al., 1986), and although denatured protein (apparently without proteolytic digestion) can also be T cell–presented under some circumstances (Streicher et al., 1984), the main pathway in living B cells for processing of foreign antigen is by mIg-mediated endocytosis and endosomal or lysosomal digestion (Watts and Davidson, 1988). Agents that inhibit lysosomal function, such as chloroquine and NH_4Cl, inhibit the generation of immunogenic class II MHC-restricted peptides by antigen-presenting cells. Processing pathways of native foreign antigen are different for class II–restricted epitopes (exogenous, preformed antigen) and class I–restricted epitopes (endogenous, newly synthesized antigen) (Morrison et al., 1986; Moore et al., 1988; Whitton and Oldstone, 1989). The patterns of digestion of a foreign antigen by any given B cell depend upon the epitope to which its mIg is specific, at least in the case of Epstein-Barr virus (EBV)–transformed, B-cell clones with high-affinity mIgG receptors (Demotz et al., 1989b; Davidson and Watts, 1989). Davidson and Watts (1989) demonstrated that for human, EBV-transformed, anti-tetanus toxoid B clones, the patterns of digestion of [^{35}S]methionine-labeled tetanus toxoid by any given clone fit into one of several patterns. Addition of antibody secreted by one clone to antigen in a culture with a second clone with a different digestion pattern led to a hybrid pattern of digestion. These experiments were interpreted to mean that endosomal fragmentation of an antigen probably proceeded by attack on portions of the antigen not blocked by binding to mIg in the endosomal vesicle.

Assembly of Class I MHC/β_2-Microglobulin Complexes with Foreign Peptide

Different pathways exist for processing MHC class I– and class II–presented epitopes (Long and Jacobson, 1989; Morrison et al., 1986). In contrast to class II–restricted antigens, which are exogenous and whose digestion is sensitive to lysosomotropic agents, class I–presented epitopes depend upon de novo synthesis of antigen and/or receptors (Morrison et al., 1986; Whitton and Oldstone, 1989), and their generation is unaltered by agents that inhibit lysosomal proteases. In the case of endogenously synthesized and T cell–presented viral proteins, expression on the cell surface is not required (Townsend et al., 1986a; Townsend and Skehel, 1984). In fact, newly synthesized, class I–restricted antigens appear to be digested by cytoplasmic proteases prior to association with class I molecules and presentation at the cell surface. For instance, in experiments using a technique of pinosome lysis, it was shown that an exogenous antigen introduced into the cytoplasm of the target cell resulted in presentation of epitopes to class I–restricted CTL (Moore et al., 1988). In studies of a mutant cell line that had constitutively low levels of surface class I MHC molecules, Townsend et al. (1989) found that addition of a presented peptide to the culture enhanced surface expression of class I MHC molecules as well as the intracellular assembly of β_2-microglobulin class I chain complexes. Such assembly of class I chain with β_2-microglobulin might have been enhanced by folding of the desetope helices about the foreign peptide.

Possible Functions of Class II MHC Accessory Molecules

Our effort has been to characterize the accessory proteins that are associated with class II MHC molecules and the changing structures of such complexes as a function of time after synthesis and intracellular compartmentalization. From the time of their synthesis, class II MHC α and β chains are associated with an electrophoretically invariant chain (I_i), which might regulate antigen processing and presentation. Since I_i shows no allelic variation in electrophoretic mobility in two-dimensional (IEF or NEPHGE/SDS) gels, it was thought to have a regulatory role other than restriction of antigen presentation (Sung and Jones, 1981; Sant et al., 1983; Ploegh and Fuhrmann, 1985; Sivak et al., 1987; Sant et al., 1985; Giacoletto et al., 1986; Marks and Cresswell, 1986; Lipp and Dobberstein, 1986; Cresswell et al., 1987). Since L cells, which are transfected with genes for class II MHC α and β chains and I_i present foreign proteins as efficiently as peptides, and parallel transfectants with only α and β chains present only peptides efficiently, a role for I_i in processing and/or desetope charging of foreign proteins has been proposed (Stockinger et al., 1989).

There are many different products of I_i gene transcription and variably processed forms (Fig. 5-1). The I_i has alternate start sites leading to $\gamma2$ and $\gamma3$ (p35) forms of I_i. An exon 6b leads to a 41-kDa form incorporating a 64 amino acid insert, and I_i, itself, can be glycosylated with N- and O-linked sugars to which sialic acid can be variably added, as Ip (Quaranta et al., 1984; Machamer and Cresswell, 1982). The sialic acid additions to I_i do not occur in the P3HR-1 mutant or Jijoye lacking α and β chains (Spiro et al., 1984, 1985). Since α/β chain-freed Ip is not present in sequential immunoprecipitates with VIC-Y1 monoclonal antibodies (mAb) to I_i following preclearing with anti-MHC class II α and β serum (Nguyen and Humphreys, 1990b), the processing of I_i to Ip is thought to occur only in α/β/I_i trimers and Ip is not released intact from α/β chains but is degraded at or shortly after release.

We and others have studied the associations, processing and cleavages, and dissociations of class II MHC accessory molecules (Fig. 5-2). In studies of the time course for associations and dissociations of I_i forms and class II MHC molecules, Nguyen and Humphreys (1989) found that α/I_i dimers and α/β/I trimers were synthesized initially. The α/β/I_i were processed to O-glycosylated and sialic acid–derivatized forms, as described by others (Machamer and Cresswell, 1982, 1984; Kvist et al., 1982; Koch and Hämmerling, 1985; Kaufman et al., 1984). Only at 30 to 60 minutes did the γ2γ3 (p35) and p41 forms of I_i associate with α/β chains (Nguyen and Humphreys, 1989).

FIGURE 5-2
Accessory molecules might regulate class II MHC desetope charging with foreign peptides. The processing, associations, cleavages and dissociations of I_i and class II MHC molecules are illustrated. Upon synthesis, α/I_i dimers are formed to which β chain is added. Some α/I_i dimers persist and might be degraded. The α/β/I_i trimers are carbohydrate-processed through the Golgi apparatus. Presumably in the ER, a high mannose form of I_i is degraded to p25 from 20 to 60 minutes after synthesis. Later, from 2 to 6 hours after synthesis, a complex sugar form of I_i is degraded to p21 and p10, which are found in leupeptin- or antipain-treated cells. The time course of that cleavage parallels the time course of the appearance of I_i-freed α,β chains seen in sequential immunoprecipitations of pulse-chase radiolabeled cells. A chondroitin sulfate form of I_i is formed.

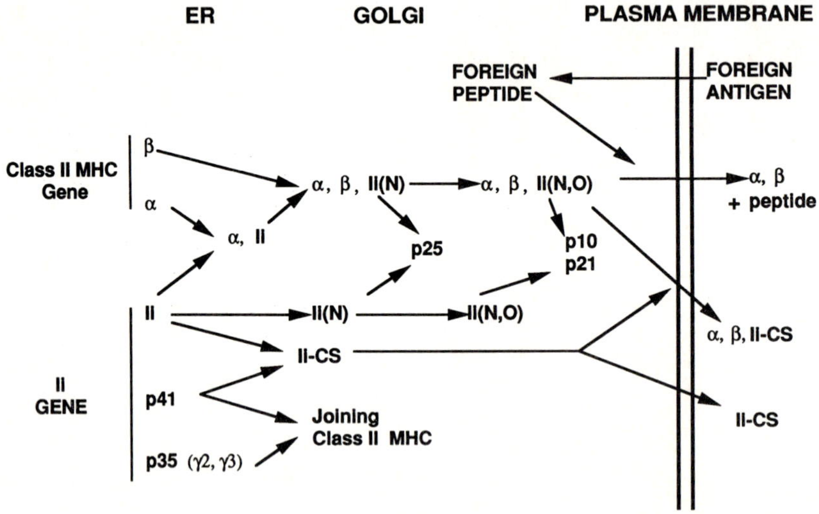

A p29 molecule associated with class II α/β chains transiently at 30-minute chase time. These associations and dissociations occurred during intracellular transport (Claesson and Peterson, 1983) within intracellular compartments of the density of endosomes in percoll gradients (Nguyen and Humphreys, 1989). Since I_i has been shown to have a role in the processing and presentation of foreign antigen (Stockinger et al., 1989), possibly through catalysis of desetope charging (Elliott et al., 1987; Stille et al., 1987), these endosomes might be related to a specific population that has been postulated to play a central role in antigen processing (Harding and Unanue, 1989).

We have identified two mechanisms of I_i proteolysis: (1) to yield C-terminal p25 from a high mannose form at 20 to 60 minutes after synthesis occurring in an ER or cis-Golgi compartment (Nguyen and Humphreys, 1989; Thomas et al., 1988, 1989); and (2) to yield N-terminal p21/p10 occurring in a mature sialic acid–derivatized form, at 2 to 4 hours after synthesis, in a post-Golgi (possibly endosomal) compartment (Blum and Cresswell, 1988; Nguyen and Humphreys, 1989a). Both cleavages can occur in class II–bound I_i molecules and could reflect removal of I_i associated with desetope charging, though other hypotheses have been considered. Leupeptin and antipain had been demonstrated to block a second stage of proteolytic cleavage of α/β-bound Ip (Blum and Cresswell, 1988; Nguyen and Humphreys, 1989a). Significant amounts of Ip were cleaved in the 3- to 5-hour interval of incubation with leupeptin as was significant additional release of I_i-freed α/β dimers from 4- to 6-hour chase times (Nguyen and Humphreys, 1990b). Cathepsin B and D were found to cleave I_i from class II MHC α and β chains without apparent damage to the α and β chains (Reyes et al., 1991). In sequential immunoprecipitates with four clearings with VIC-Y1 mAb to I_i to remove all I_i forms including α/β/I_i trimers, followed by a fifth set of immunoprecipitations with anti-class II α and β serum, no free α and β dimers were found at zero chase time, but free α and β dimers increased up to 6 hours of chase time. The time course for release of I_i-freed α/β dimers paralleled the appearance of I_i-derived p21 and p10 in leupeptin-blocked cells (Nguyen and Humphreys, 1990b). The time course of these two events also paralleled the finding of [^{35}S]methionine-labeled p70 and p80 molecules in crosslinked immunoprecipitates of class II α and β chains at 3, 6, and 9 hours of pulse chase–labeled cells (Sorli et al., 1990).

We have also found T cell–presented, amphipathic helices that are [^{125}I] labeled and crosslinked to bind principally (90%+) to a p70 in microsomal membranes, and to 32,000- and 44,000-dalton proteins to much lesser extents (Reyes VE, unpublished observation). This p70 might scavenge such peptides by recognizing hydrophobic surfaces of helices and transferring them to MHC molecules or to other disposals. It might be related to the p70, which is associated to class II MHC (Sorli et al., 1990). A p72/74 has been shown to bind and present an antigenic peptide from pigeon cytochrome c (Lakey et al., 1987b). This p72/74 was shown to be a member of the heat-shock protein family (Vanbuskirk et al., 1989). The cleavage of Ip to p21 and p10, the progressive release of I_i-freed α and β molecules, and the association of p70 and p80 with class II MHC complexes might all reflect stages in the process of charging the class II MHC desetope with foreign peptides.

While the above processes could reflect the mechanisms for charging of desetopes with T cell–presented sequences, we have pursued additional pathways to look for mechanisms for selection of T cell–presented sequences. Understanding the biophysical properties of such T cell–presented epitopes could lead to engineering of such determinants to alter potency or affect range of MHC restriction.

SELECTION OF T CELL–PRESENTED PEPTIDES

T cell–presented peptides were first found to be amphipathic structures (DeLisi and Berzofsky, 1985) and then proposed to resemble a "prototypic antigen," I_i (146-164), an α helix with an axial strip of aliphatic amino acids and otherwise variably hydrophilic amino acids (Elliott et al., 1987; Stille et al., 1987). While a superficial epitope (or hapten) determines mIg recognition of the foreign antigen, another buried determinant within the protein (or carrier) regulates the magnitude of T-cell response (Fig. 5-3). In some cases, only unfolding of the protein appears to be sufficient for T cells to recognize a determinant without a further cleavage being required (Streicher et al., 1984). However, most protein antigens require their digestion into small peptide fragments. Only one, or a few, of the peptides purified from proteolytic digests of foreign antigens have been found to substitute (at relatively higher concentrations) for intact foreign antigen in the generation of T-cell help when presented by antigen-presenting cells to helper T cells of the strain of mice that responds to the foreign protein (Allen et al., 1984). In most cases, synthetic peptides have been successfully used to elucidate the immunodominant epitopes within protein antigens. Furthermore, acid elutions from MHC class II molecules present in the preparations derived from a hen egg lysozyme (HEL)–pulsed, B-cell line were used to isolate physiologically processed antigenic peptides from 10% to 40% of the class II preparations. The naturally processed peptides corresponded to the HEL 107-116 determinant mapped previously with synthetic peptides (Demotz et al., 1989a). In most of these T cell–presented peptides, hydrophobic amino acids recurred at an average periodicity of 3.6 amino acids, consistent with coiling of the peptide in an α helix with axially opposing hydrophobic and hydrophilic surfaces (Elliott et al., 1987; Stille et al., 1987; DeLisi and Berzofsky, 1985). Similar amphipathic (or amphiphilic) peptide hormones have been analyzed in detail by Kaiser and his colleagues and are well documented to bind to hormone receptors and/or lipophilic surfaces (Kaiser and Kézdy, 1984). In this section of our review, we will summarize what is known about the structural nature of T cell–presented segments of antigenic proteins and how that structure might lead to selection and desetope charging of those peptides. Finally, we will speculate how this information might be used to increase potency or widen the range of MHC restriction of vaccines and to decrease immunogenicity of immunoglobulins or other proteins used in therapy or diagnosis of cancers and other diseases. Specifically, we will consider the structure of T cell–recognized and Ig-recognized epitopes, the presentation to T cells of amphipathic helical peptides by antigen-binding sites (desetopes) in MHC molecules, and the generic structure of such peptides. Biophysical principles governing

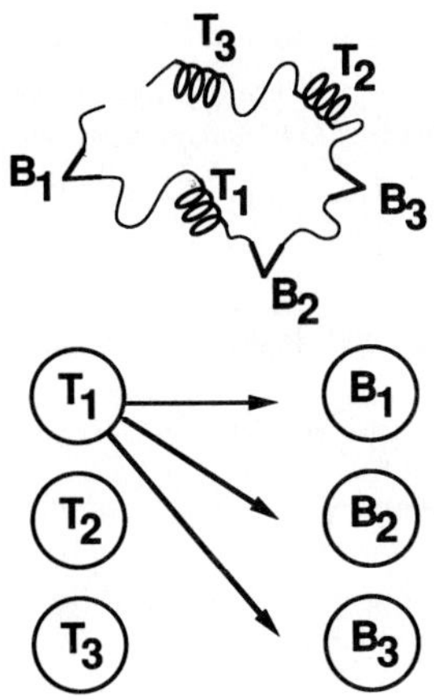

FIGURE 5-3
T and B epitopes of an antigen and MHC restriction on T-cell help. T-cell receptor– and B-cell immunoglobulin–recognized epitopes of one antigen are illustrated. The sequences that can form amphipathic helices and be T cell–presented are represented as helices T1, T2, T3. The external, flexible hydrophilic sequences that are recognized by immunoglobulins are indicated as B1, B2, B3. Only some MHC desetopes are capable of binding any given T cell–presented segment of a foreign antigen. Because the T-cell epitopes are variably restricted according to MHC alleles present in each responding person, help to B cells (or cytotoxicity) will be determined in any one individual usually by only some of several T-cell epitopes. In this example, only T1 regulates help to all three B-cell determinants.

selection of T cell–presented peptides might be exploited to alter potency and range of MHC restrictions of peptide vaccines for viral and tumor determinants. Finally, we will consider how these T cell–presented sequences come to be bound in the desetopes and presented to TCR. While we discuss our current understanding of antigen processing and presentation, and peptide vaccine design, we hope to summarize a foundation of knowledge needed to address continuing questions and future developments in this field.

We focus on biophysical principles in peptide selection for T-cell presentation and roles of accessory proteins in charging of MHC molecules with foreign peptides. By knowing what biophysical properties in a primary sequence of a foreign antigen lead to selection for T-cell presentation, we can better predict such selections for vaccine development and perhaps engineer those peptides to alter potency and range of MHC restriction. By understanding the mechanisms of antigen processing and peptide charging onto MHC molecules, we might better design vaccine(s) tailored for class I or class II MHC presentation, help, or suppression, and perhaps develop inhibitors.

In addition, patterns of digestion of a B-cell, Ig-recognized tetanus toxoid vary according to the antigen-specific, EBV-transformed clonal lines used (Davidson and Watts, 1989), suggesting that T-cell epitopes that survive digestion longest might be proximate to the B-cell epitope bound by the mIg of the B-cell line.

MHC Desetopes

Digested fragments of tumor antigens are thought to be presented to CTL or helper T lymphocytes after binding to antigen-presenting sites (desetopes) in class I and class II MHC molecules, respectively. The crystallographic structure of class I MHC molecules has been determined (Bjorkman et al., 1987b; Garrett et al., 1989), and the structure of the class II molecules' desetope has been deduced from sequence homologies to class I molecules and other information (Brown et al., 1986, 1988). These MHC molecules are composed of a β-pleated sheet on which two antiparallel, α helices sit, separated by 10 angstroms. Foreign peptides are bound in the space between the two helices (Bjorkman et al., 1987a), and the TCR recognizes residues on both the foreign peptide and the adjacent helices of the MHC molecules (Bjorkman et al., 1987a; Davis and Bjorkman, 1988). Binding of any peptide to MHC molecules for presentation to TCR depends upon fitting of the peptide into the desetope, that is, molding to the configuration of amino acids forming the walls and floor of the desetope. Since a given peptide will fit only some desetopes, or a given desetope will bind only a limited set of peptides, there is MHC restriction on presentation of any given epitope. While it has been proposed that class I MHC molecules are bound around a foreign peptide fragment thus charging themselves for presentation of the peptide, class II molecules appear to receive peptides into their desetopes differently. The class II MHC-associated I_i might initially play the role of the foreign peptide in the MHC class I case, allowing the class II molecules to assemble around it, and later, as I_i is excised or cleaved, it allows the class II molecules to bind the foreign peptides that are to be presented to T cells (Elliott et al., 1987; Stille et al., 1987). These catalytic mechanisms lead to the formation of stable peptide and class I or class II MHC complexes, which make it difficult to replace the associated peptides by exogenously added peptides.

Allele Specificity in Binding of T Cell–Presented Peptides

The genetic control of immune responsiveness can be explained, at least in part, by the differential ability of a T cell–presented peptide to bind in the antigen-binding site (desetope) of MHC molecules with various allelic structures (Babbitt et al., 1985, 1986; Buus et al., 1986a, 1986b, 1986c, 1988; Sette et al., 1989a, 1989b; Ceppellini et al., 1989; Chen and Parham, 1989; Bouillot et al., 1989; Reyes et al., unpublished observations). Since presentation of foreign peptides is governed by their binding to MHC desetopes, one might ask how the many antigenic foreign peptides form unique complexes with a limited number of MHC molecules. The MHC molecules are highly permissive in the sense that they function as restriction elements for a large number of antigens (Schaeffer et al., 1989). Furthermore, since various antigenic peptides known to be restricted by class I and class II MHC alleles were found to be structurally homologous, it was hypothesized that individual peptides might be restricted by both class I and class II alleles (Reyes et al., 1988). Peptides from influenza virus, originally described as restricted by human class I alleles, were shown to be restricted by murine class II alleles (Perkins et al., 1989). Sequence motifs in some antigenic peptides were related to binding to the Ia^d isotype (Sette et al., 1989a).

The interactions that take place between antigenic peptides and the desetope can be hypothesized in chemical terms. Two classes of interactions can be described for the binding of T cell–presented peptides with the MHC class II desetope: (1) allele-nonspecific binding, largely due to hydrophobic interactions of the axial, hydrophobic strip-of-helix (SOH) with the floor of the desetope; and (2) allele-specific interactions of the amino acids in the two axial quadrants of the foreign peptide helix with the lateral walls of the desetope. Such van der Waals, hydrophobic, and charge interactions are stereospecific with respect to the structures of both the foreign peptide and the helices forming the walls of the desetope. In anticipation of our later hypotheses on engineering T-cell determinants, we suggest there is a balance between these forces in that mild, competitive charge or steric interactions between groups of the peptide and walls of desetope could be overcome by increased binding of the hydrophobic SOH to the floor of the desetope.

Linkage of Presentation of T-Cell and B-Cell Epitopes Within Different Individuals

For a population of immunized individuals, all T cell–presented and B cell (Ig)–recognized determinants within one antigen are represented abstractly in Fig. 5-3. While all T cell–presented epitopes are recognized by different individuals within the population, any one epitope will be recognized only by an individual with a MHC desetope that accepts the peptide. The peptide within the desetope might be either coiled as an α helix or bound as an extended chain. In either case, amino acid side chains of the antiparallel helices that form the walls and β-pleated sheet floor of the desetope must accept the antigenic peptide. Since only some T cell–recognized peptides can bind to the MHC alleles of any given individual, the selections of T-cell epitopes generating help for the complete series of B cell (Ig)–recognized epitopes are restricted. As illustrated, only T1 provides help for the series of B cell (Ig)–recognized determinants. This restriction gives rise to a practical dilemma in vaccine development. That is, cocktails of multiple T cell–presented sequences need be devised for immunization of the population, for it is not practical to histotype all patients to immunize them with just the determinants that are T cell–presented by the MHC alleles they have. Perhaps this obstacle might be overcome using a prototypic foreign peptide or the putative desetope-binding helix in I_i, as described below, as a backbone onto which the critical residues for TCR recognition are transferred in analogy to the method of Lorenz et al. (1989). This maneuver would permit presentation of the antigen-specific residues in the context of most, if not all, MHC alleles.

Amphipathic Helical Structure of T Cell–Presented Antigens

DeLisi and Berzofsky (1985) proposed that a common structural characteristic of class II MHC-restricted, T cell–presented epitopes in antigenic proteins was amphipathic helicity. That is, peptides that when coiled as α or 3_{10} helices had axially opposing, hydrophilic and hydrophobic surfaces would be desetope-bound and presented to T cells. This hypothesis was based, in part, on the demonstrations of Emil Kaiser and colleagues that many polypeptide hormones bound to either receptors or a lipid surface through amphiphilic, helical structures, sometimes with peptidyl tails conferring biological function (Kaiser and Kézdy, 1984). The hydrophobic, axial side of such peptides was generic, that is, hydrophobic residues could be substituted with other hydrophobic residues. Berzofsky and colleagues developed and refined algorithms to identify such T cell–presented sequences by analysis of the periodicity of variations in hydrophilicity and hydrophobicity of amino acids in primary sequences of antigenic proteins (DeLisi and Berzofsky, 1985; Margalit et al., 1987; Cornette et al., 1987; Spouge et al., 1986).

Our past studies on the function of accessory molecules that associate with class II MHC molecules led to hypotheses that I_i could retain class II molecules from transport to the cell surface until complexed with a foreign peptide or act in an allosteric or directly competitive fashion to regulate peptide binding in the desetope. A striking amphipathic helix in I_i(Phe^{146}-Val^{164}) (Fig. 5-4) led to the specific hypothesis that I_i filled the desetope until its release to catalyze charging of the desetope with an antigenic peptide. Hypothesizing I_i(146-164) to be a prototypic foreign antigen, we developed an algorithm to search for other structurally similar sequences, that is, ones with axial, hydrophobic strips when coiled as α or 3_{10} helices (Fig. 5-5). That algorithm predicted MHC class II–presented and class I–presented peptides, and a derivative of it identified structural helices (Elliott et al., 1987; Stille et al., 1987; Reyes et al., 1988, 1989, 1990). Graphical displays with that algorithm can help one to judge secondary structure in proteins (Fig. 5-6).

Other Methods for T Cell–Presented Sequences

Three principal algorithms have been developed to predict T cell–presented sequences. DeLisi and Berzofsky (1985) proposed that similar amphipathic structures from anti-

FIGURE 5-4
Sheet projection of I_i(146-164). When the linear sequence is displayed in the pattern of an α helix, following the orientation of the arrow as the stripe around a barber's pole, we see clearly the axial hydrophobic strip Phe^{146}, Leu^{150}, Met^{153}, Ile^{157}, Val^{164}. Salt bridges are identified between Glu^{148} and Arg^{151} and between Lys^{154} and Glu^{158}. Glu^{148} can interact with the N-terminal, helical macrodipole and Lys^{163} with the C-terminal macrodipole. This projection is easier to read than the Edmundson wheel projection for four or more cycles of a helix and interactions among the loops of the helix are more easily identified.

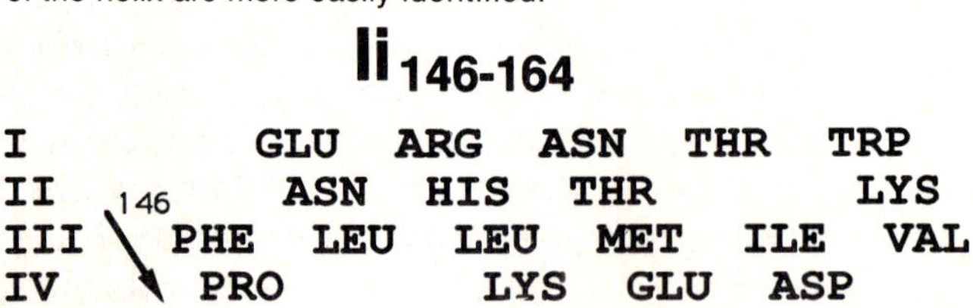

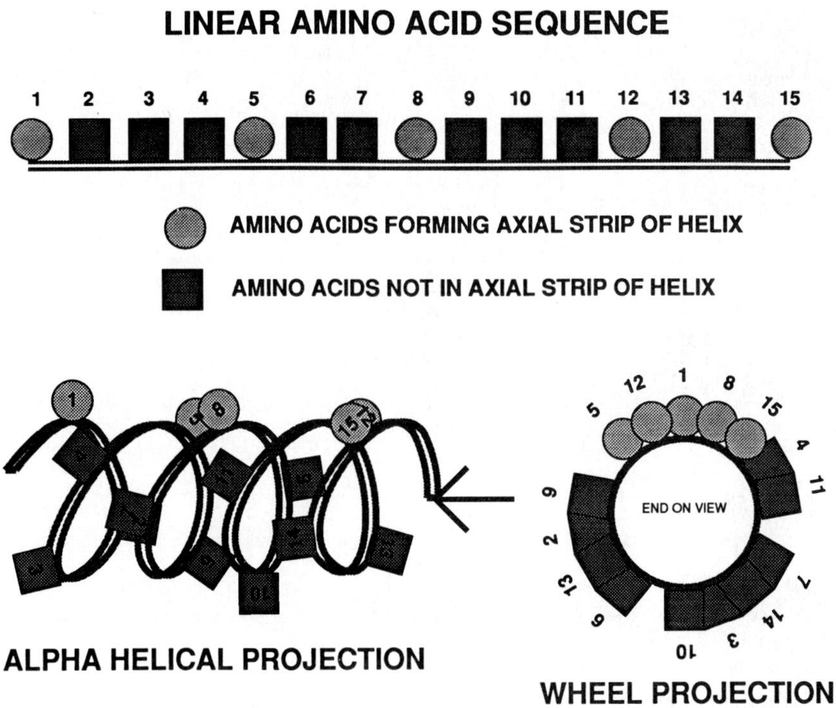

FIGURE 5-5
Strip-of-helix hydrophobicity algorithm (SOHHA). When hydrophobic residues (squares) recur among variably hydrophilic residues in a pattern of +4, +3, +4, +3, etc., then an axial hydrophobic strip will be formed when the sequence is coiled as an α helix. That helix will be amphipathic as seen in both lateral (sheet) and axial (Edmundson wheel) projections.

genic proteins were presented to TCR in association with class II MHC molecules. A second approach, the strip-of-helix hydrophobicity algorithm (SOHHA), was derived from the hypothesis that a "perfect" amphipathic helix I_i(146-164) bound at the desetope of class II MHC molecules until its release at the time of peptide charging (Elliott et al., 1987; Stille et al., 1987). This algorithm scored for periodic hydrophobicity of amino acids that would fall in an axial, hydrophobic strip when coiled as an α or 3_{10} helix. A third approach (Rothbard and Taylor, 1988b) identified generally the same sequences found with the algorithms of DeLisi and Berzofsky (1985) and of Stille et al. (1987) on the basis of amino acid sequence motifs: (charged or glycine)-(hydrophobic)-(hydrophobic)-(polar or glycine) or (charged or glycine)-(hydrophobic)-(hydrophobic or proline)-(proline or glycine). However, it did not rank selections within a protein or specify the extent of peptides to synthesize (Reyes et al., 1989, 1990).

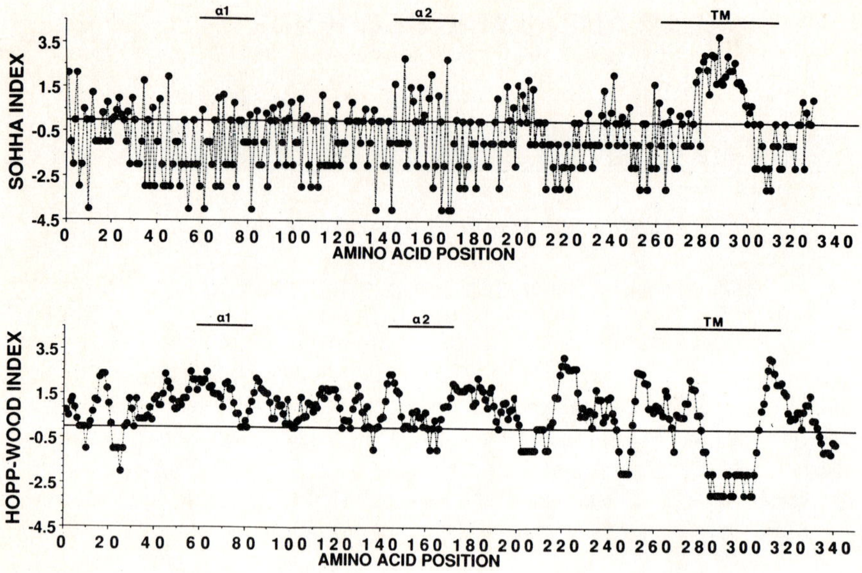

FIGURE 5-6
Hopp-Woods versus SOHHI plots of HLA-A2. A Hopp-Woods hydrophilicity plot and a four-cycle, α-helical SOHHA plot for the primary sequence of HLA-A2 is presented. Transmembranal regions are identified by both plots, though the beginning and ending are more sharply defined by the SOHHA. Regions that could coil as amphiphilic α helices are identified by rows of hydrophobic index points, for example, positions 149 to 166. That region is, in fact, the α_2 domain helix bordering the desetope. Such images of amphipathicity are not seen in the Hopp-Woods plot.

Function of the Narrow, Axial, Hydrophobic Strip

In studying a Hopp-Woods hydrophobicity plot of I_i, the invariant chain that associates with class II α and β chains from the time of their synthesis, Elliott et al. (1987) found a segment with seven cycles of 3.5 amino acid oscillations in hydrophobicity. They speculated that such a strip constituted an amphipathic helix and might fill the desetope until its release during a peptide-charging event. The oscillating hydrophobicity was found in a sheet projection of the I_i sequence (Fig. 5-4) to reflect a narrow, axial strip of aliphatic amino acids. If that structure represented a prototypic antigen filling the MHC class II desetope, then an algorithm identifying such narrow, axial strips might predict T cell–presented sequences. Stille et al. (1987) created the SOHHA to calculate mean hydrophobicities of sequences i, i+4, i+7, i+11, i+14, etc., for any number of turns (cycles + 1 amino acid) in an α helix (Fig. 5-5). This algorithm predicted T cell–presented determinants with similar sensitivity and greater efficiency than did the DeLisi-Berzofsky-Margalit method, and with greater sensitivity and efficiency than did the method of Rothbard and Taylor (Reyes et al., 1990). The projection of the strip-of-helix hydrophobicity index (SOHHI) permitted easy visualization of regions of potential amphipathicity and transmembranal hydrophobicity in I_i (Elliott et al., 1987 [Fig. 1]) and in antigenic proteins. Here we illustrate that projection with HLA-A2 (Fig. 5-6). We can review the development and use of these algorithms in order to understand the remaining biophysical hypotheses that might come to be exploited in vaccine development and engineering T cell–presented epitopes.

Appropriately placed, recurrent hydrophobic amino acids were hypothesized to catalyze the coiling of a peptide against a hydrophobic surface when an axial, hydrophobic strip would be formed (Elliott et al., 1987; Lu et al., 1990). To catalyze coiling of a peptide as an α helix, such hydrophobic amino acids would have to recur in positions that would form an axial, hydrophobic strip if the sequence were coiled as an α helix (Fig. 5-7). Hydrophobic amino acids not falling in the axial hydrophobic strip might actually compete for helix formation (Fig. 5-8). A maximal hydrophobic strip along an α helix might also stabilize that structure during the progressive folding of a nascent protein and thus be more likely to be preserved as a helix in the mature structure (Reyes et al., 1989). Likewise, such helices nucleating on the lipid membrane of a vesicle or hydrophobic surface of a scavenging, or transfer, molecule could bring the excised peptide, in a helical form relatively protected from further proteolysis, to a MHC

FIGURE 5-7
Catalysis of helix formation. This schema illustrates how appropriately recurrent hydrophobic residues in an otherwise hydrophilic peptide can catalyze helix formation on a hydrophobic surface. (B) Coiling on a membrane or in a hydrophobic trough of either an MHC desetope or scavenging and transfer molecule is initiated by two hydrophobic residues and the looping of the intervening residues. (C) That loop stabilizes an adjacent loop of the helix anchored by another appropriately placed hydrophobic residue. (D,E) The helix can extend, being anchored by additional hydrophobic residues.

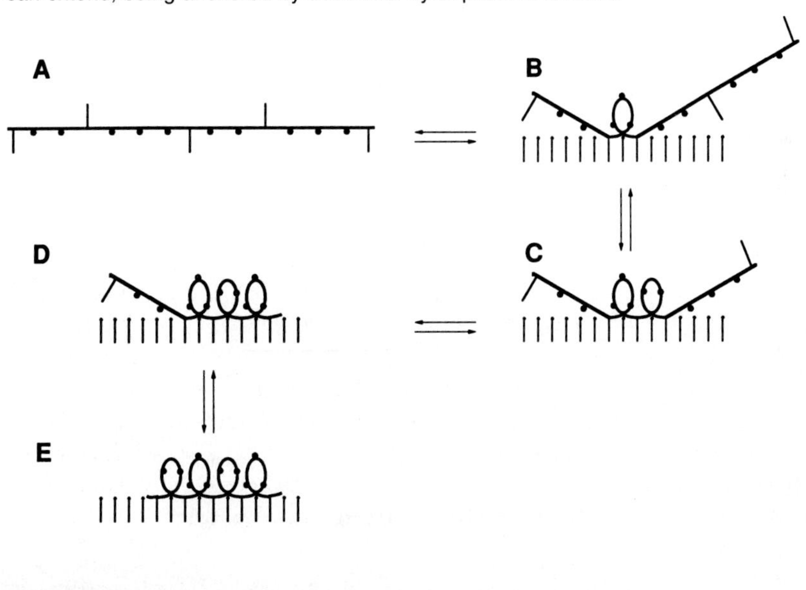

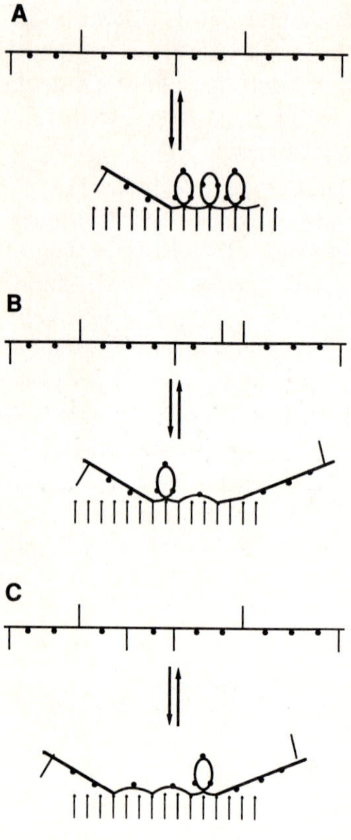

FIGURE 5-8
Competition for helix formation by hydrophobic residues not falling in an axial hydrophobic strip. (A) The coiling of a peptide with hydrophobic residues that only recur in positions falling in an axial hydrophobic strip is catalyzed or stabilized by insertion of the hydrophobic residues in the lipid membrane and by intercycle hydrogen bonds and ionic bridges among adjacent loops of the helix. When an additional aliphatic residue occurs, it can anchor the "tail" of the incipient helix to the membrane, competing for helix formation. Proteases might more readily digest sequences in (B) than in (A).

desetope (Reyes et al., 1989, 1990). Such a scavenging mechanism might have evolved to use a transport molecule derived from the heat-shock protein family (Lakey et al., 1987b; Vanbuskirk et al., 1989; Sorli et al., 1990) or might be so simple as to collect a subset of peptides that adhere to a vesicle wall while soluble components are extruded into a lysosome-directed compartment upon contraction of the endocytic vesicle prior to fusion with a class II MHC-containing compartment.

Strip-of-Helix Hydrophobicity Algorithm Derived from the "Prototypic T Cell–Presented Peptide": $I_i(Phe^{146}$-$Val^{164})$

The original hypothesis was that an amphipathic α helix of $I_i(Phe^{146}$-$Val^{164})$ binds to the foreign antigen-presenting site (desetope) of class II MHC molecules through hydrophobic amino acid residues (Phe^{146}, Leu^{150}, Leu^{153}, Met^{157}, Ile^{160}, Val^{164}) that are present in an axial strip along one side of the I_i helix. As an extension of this hypothesis, an algorithm was developed to search for T cell–presented peptides showing a similar hydrophobic SOH (Elliott et al., 1987; Stille et al., 1987; Reyes et al., 1988, 1990). Such peptides might bind to the class II MHC molecule site that was complementary to the I_i hydrophobic SOH. The SOHHI was the mean hydrophobicity (from Kyte-Doolittle values) of sets of amino acids in axial strips down sides of helices for three to six turns, at positions n, n+4, n+7, n+11, n+14, and n+18. Peptides correlating well with T-cell responsiveness had: (1) 12 to 19 amino acids (three to five turns of an α helix); (2) a strip with highly hydrophobic residues; (3) at least one adjacent, hydrophilic strip, scoring more hydrophilic than −1 in the SOHHA; (4) no prolines; and (5) no glycosylation sites. The degree of hydrophilicity of the remainder of a putative antigenic helix above a threshold value did not affect this index. That is, the magnitude of amphipathicity was not judged to be the principal selecting factor for T cell–presented peptides. This simple algorithm to quantitate SOH hydrophobicity in a putative amphipathic α helix, allowing otherwise generally hydrophilic residues, predicted 10 of 12 T cell–presented peptides in seven proteins for which T cell–presented peptides had been determined in some detail. It also predicted T cell–presented sequences in antigenic proteins that had not been analyzed in detail. The algorithm could also select the frequency of a 3_{10} helix (n, n+3, n+6, n+9, etc.) or a β-pleated sheet (n, n+2, n+4, n+6, etc.).

A SOHHA to predict class II MHC-restricted peptides, on the basis of their structural similarity to an amphipathic, α helix in I_i, also predicted peptides that were presented to cytotoxic T cells by class I MHC molecules (Reyes et al., 1988). This algorithm predicted the class I MHC-restricted, T cell–presented peptides in sequences of four proteins from which some class I MHC-restricted, T cell–presented sequences had been experimentally determined. Since the SOHHA predicted equally well peptides that were restricted by class I or class II MHC molecules, the antigenic peptide-binding sites were thought to be structurally related and receptive to amphipathic helices (Reyes et al., 1988). The crystallographic structures of the class I MHC HLA-A2 and HLA-Aw68 molecule (Bjorkman et al., 1987b; Garrett et al., 1989) and deduced model of class II MHC molecules (Brown et al., 1988) supported this proposal. Also, responses to several influenza viral peptides were found to be restricted, each by class I and class II MHC alleles (Perkins et al., 1989; Sweetser et al., 1989). For instance, a peptide corresponding to residues 252-271 of influenza virus hemagglutinin (HA) was found to be restricted for presentation to $CD8^+$ and $CD4^+$ T cells by $H\text{-}2^k$ and $I\text{-}A^d$, respectively (Sweetser et al., 1989).

Three methods to predict T cell–presented sequences within antigenic proteins were compared quantitatively, and possible biological principles underlying those approaches were considered in light of this comparison (Reyes et al., 1990). These methods were based on the amphipathicity algorithm of DeLisi and Berzofsky (1985) as modified by Margalit et al. (1987), SOHHA of Stille et al. (1987), and the motifs algorithm of Rothbard and Taylor (1988). Sensitivity (correct predictions/number of T cell–presented peptides) and efficiency (correct predictions/number of predictions) were quantitated in terms of overlapping predictions (intersection/union of predicted and experimentally determined sequences >0.5), touching predictions (0.5 >intersection/union >0.0), and neighboring predictions (predicted sequence and experimentally determined T cell–presented sequence being within six amino acids of each other). At the overlapping criterion, the SOHHA was more sensitive (0.43) than the amphipathicity (0.29) and motifs (0.0, 0.0) predictions, and more efficient (0.35) than the amphipathicity (0.14) and motifs (0.0, 0.0) predictions. At the less stringent criterion of overlapping + touching, the amphipathicity method (0.71) was as sensitive as Rothbard-4 (0.79) and more sensitive than SOHHA (0.57) and Rothbard-5 (0.43). At that criterion, the SOHHA was more efficient (0.47) than the Berzofsky (0.36) and Rothbard (0.25, 0.40) methods. Simple amalgamations of these approaches did not improve predictive scores, as would be anticipated from the view that the three methods reflected predominantly periodic hydrophobicity. Periodic hydrophobicity could promote helix formation that protected peptides from further proteolysis during antigen processing, or an axial, hydrophobic surface might actually promote binding to a desetope or to some peptidyl transferase for desetope charging.

While three methods to predict T cell–presented peptides (DeLisi-Berzofsky, Rothbard-Taylor, and SOHHA) are related, to the extent that they identify hydrophobic surfaces, only the SOHHA focuses explicitly on the magnitude of the mean strength of the hydrophobicity in the axial, hydrophobic strip. The DeLisi-Berzofsky algorithm scores the contribution of each amino acid to the periodicity of hydrophilic and hydrophobic moments along the axis of sometimes extended, possible helices. The magnitude of hydrophilicity in the T cell–presented surface of a peptide might not reflect on its binding to the desetope of a hydrophobic surface. And hydrophobic amino acids can be found among those thought to be recognized by TCR. The Rothbard-Taylor algorithm identifies motifs of four or five residues, respectively, centered on two or three hydrophobic ones. Functionally, it identifies one cycle of an amphipathic helix. Frequently, adjacent Rothbard-Taylor motifs occur, positioning the hydrophobic residues as if they were in an axial strip of a helix, but the algorithm does not weight such configurations and is less efficient than the DeLisi-Berzofsky and SOHHA methods.

Testing a Hypothesis on the Mechanism of Helical Nucleation

We hypothesized that mechanisms for folding of nascent proteins might depend on the same general principles of helical nucleation that control the selection of peptides for desetope binding and T-cell presentation. We found that a derivative of the SOHHA, the structural helices algorithm (SHA), predicted structural helices in crystallographically defined proteins (Reyes et al., 1989).

In the SHA, eight amino acid sequences, two cycles plus one amino acid in an α helix, with SOH hydrophobicity indices greater than 2.5, were selected with unions of overlapping segments. These selections were terminated according to simple "capping rules," which took into account the roles of N-terminal Asn or Pro and C-terminal Gly in stabilizing helices (Richardson and Richardson, 1988; Presta and Rose, 1988). In analyses of 35 crystallographically defined proteins with known α and 3_{10} helices, the predictions with this algorithm were coinciding (had intersection/union indices

≥0.5) with 32% of known helices, were overlapping (had intersection/union indices [0.5> × >0.0]) with 25% of structural helices, or were neighboring (came within six residues) for 12% of structural helices. This algorithm had a 68% sensitivity (percentage correct predictions/total number of known helices) and 63% efficiency (percentage correct predictions/total number of predictions). The sensitivity was not as great as that of the Chou-Fasman (Chou and Fasman, 1978) and Garnier-Robson methods (Garnier et al., 1978), but the efficiency was better (Reyes et al., 1989). The longitudinal hydrophobic strip was found to be relatively narrow. The distributions of amino acids in longitudinal quadrants of 255 helices in crystallographically studied proteins were determined on sequences that were fitted to sheet projections to maximize SOHHI (Torgerson et al., 1991). Leu, Ile, Val, and Phe were restricted to quadrant III (standardized deviations 5–7; p = 0.001) and Lys, Arg, Asp, and Glu were restricted from quadrant III. One might propose that the folding of a protein during its synthesis involves nucleation of progressively generated segments. For example, the formation of amphipathic helices can be catalyzed by association of hydrophobic axial strips with either unfoldases or with a hydrophobic strip of a previously synthesized and helically folded segment or with the hydrophobic surface of a β-pleated sheet. The nucleated, frequently helical segments might assemble progressively into structures defined principally by their order of synthesis and placement of hydrophobic strips in the growing aggregate.

Not all predicted helices with strong axial, hydrophobic strips were found as structural helices in the native protein. This observation was consistent with the failure of a helix to be stabilized in the mature structure or with migration of newly formed helices to adjacent regions. The identification of neighboring helices supported this view. In attempting to design a migration indicator based on analysis of axial, hydrophobic strips with SOH indices 2.5> × >2.0, we found that while some helices were improved in their index of prediction, for example, going from the overlapping to coincidental category, other helices were not improved, and some false-positives were also indicated. In general, we would not lessen the stringency of initial selections to include putative helices with SOH hydrophobicity indices less than 2.5. Nevertheless, since the SOH index is a continuum of values, an investigator focusing on a single protein, for example, in the context of determining a crystallographic structure, might wish to explore such additional calculations for clues that can be evaluated in the light of an evolving structural model.

We tested experimentally the hypothesis that the recurrence of hydrophobic amino acids in a polypeptide at positions falling in an axial, hydrophobic strip if the sequence were coiled as an α helix, can lead to helical nucleation on a hydrophobic surface (Lu et al., 1990). The hydrophobic surface could anchor such residues while the peptide sequence grows in a helical configuration that is stabilized by hydrogen bonds among carbonyl and amido NH groups along the peptidyl backbone of the helix, and by other intercycle interactions among amino acid side chains. Such a bound, helical structure might protect peptides from proteases and/or facilitate transport to a MHC-containing compartment and thus be reflected in the selection of T cell–presented segments. Helical structure in a series of high-pressure liquid chromatography (HPLC)–purified peptides was estimated from circular dichroism (CD) measurements in: (1) 0.01 M phosphate buffer, pH 7.0; (2) that buffer with 45% trifluoroethanol (TFE); and (3) that buffer with di-0-hexadecyl phosphatidylcholine vesicles. By decreasing the dielectric constant of the buffer, TFE enhances intrapeptide interactions generally, while the lipid vesicles only provide a surface for hydrophobic interactions. The peptides varied in their strip-of-helix hydrophobicity indices (SOHHI; the mean Kyte-Doolittle hydrophobicities of residues in an axial strip of an α helix) and in proline content. Structural order for peptides with helical CD spectra was estimated as percentage helicity from CD $\theta_{222\ \mathrm{nm}}$ values and peptide concentration. A prototypic α helical peptide with three cycles + two amino acids and an axial hydrophobic strip of four leucyl residues (SOHHI = 3.8) (Fig. 5-9) was disordered in phosphate buffer, 58% helical in that buffer with 45% TFE, and 36% helical in that buffer with vesicles. Percentage helicity in the presence of vesicles of the subset of peptides without proline followed their SOHHI values. Peptides with multiple prolyl residues had CD spectra with strong signals, but since they did not have altered spectra in the presence of vesicles relative to phosphate buffer alone, the hydrophobic surface of the vesicle did not appear to stabilize those structures. In a study of a series of structural analogs of the peptide Leu-Tyr-Gln-Glu-Leu-Gln-Lys-Leu-Thr-Gln-Thr-Leu-Lys in which one or two Leu were replaced with Thr, the number and placement of Leu residues were found to determine helix formation in the presence of lipid vesicles, while all peptides formed helices in trifluoroethanol (Lu et al., 1991).

Theories About Altering Potency and MHC Range of T Cell–Presented Peptides

Experiments can be proposed to test whether the strength of the axial hydrophobic strip, as measured with the SOHHI, correlates with catalysis of helix formation on lipid vesicles in phosphate buffer. We can test experimentally the helix stabilizing influences of the axial, hydrophobic strip and other intercycle bridging groups by analysis of helix formation in a series of homologs of the prototypic α-helical peptide shown in Figure 5-9. Percentage helicity will be measured by CD of the peptides in

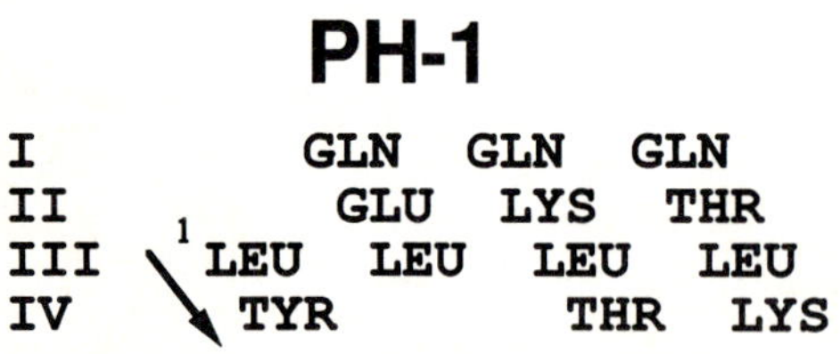

FIGURE 5-9
Sheet projection of prototypic helix (PH-1). This synthetic peptide with a narrow axial hydrophobic strip (Leu^{1}, Leu^{5}, Leu^{8}, Leu^{12}) and otherwise variably hydrophilic residues, forms an α helix in the presence of lipid vesicles. Analogs of it can be tested to ascertain the structural relationships between the hydrophobicity of the axial hydrophobic strip and the propensity to nucleate as a helix on a membrane surface.

phosphate buffer, 45% TFE, and lipid vesicles in phosphate buffer. Formation of helices in TFE may be due to multiple effects, but helices in the presence of lipid vesicles is hypothesized to be due primarily to interaction of aliphatic residues in an axial hydrophobic strip. Trifluoroethanol lessens hydrogen bonding of the peptide to water, enhancing intrapeptide hydrogen bonds and other interactions that stabilize helix formation. For example, amide-carboxyl hydrogen bonds between i and i + 4 (or i + 3, or i + 5) residues stabilize the core of the helix; salt bridges can form between the cycles of a helix; ionic side chains can interact (in a stabilizing manner) with the helix macrodipole; hydrophobic residues can interact between adjacent cycles. These secondary interactions can predominate in any given peptide. For example, some hydrophilic peptides with bulky side chains, but without potential axial hydrophobic strips, might form helices in TFE, but not in the presence of vesicles. To test the influence of the axial hydrophobic strip on helix stabilization in the presence of vesicles, we will synthesize a series of analogs of the prototypic helix-1, PH-1 (Fig. 5-9), replacing progressively the axial Leu residues with Thr. The influence of hydrophobic residues that "compete" for the dominance of the axial hydrophobic strip can be tested. With additional analogs, we can address the role of the salt bridge between the first and second cycles of the helix and the interactions of side chains with the helical macrodipole and charged groups at the termini.

With other peptides that are T cell–presented, we could also test whether a peptide's potency and range of presenting MHC alleles can be altered by engineering its axial hydrophobic strip (Lu et al., 1991b, 1992). Changing aliphatic residues (Leu, Ile, Val, Met) in such strips to Thr or altering Gly, Ser, or Ala in that strip to Leu will, respectively, decrease or increase the mean hydrophobicity of the strip and possibly dependent biological properties. The long-range applications of these engineerings would be in vaccine design and modifying immunogenicity of therapeutically or diagnostically administered proteins, for example, murine antibodies. For example, increasing potency of peptides could lead to priming of memory T cells in low-responder strains so that secondary challenges with the wild type virus elicits killing of virally infected cells when minimal amounts of wild type peptide is yet presented by the low-responder allele. This scenario assumes epitope presentation by high- and low-responder alleles is a dose-response, rather than an all-or-nothing, phenomenon. The second clinical goal would be in engineering proteins administered to patients, for example, murine antibodies, to decrease immunogenicity without a significant effect on either structural stability or recognition by the antibody combining site. Such murine mAb engineered to decrease the potencies of their helper T-cell epitopes could be used in diagnosis or therapy of cancers. By altering a few amino acids in the axial, hydrophobic strips of the T cell–presented, helper epitopes, the potencies of such peptides could fall below the thresholds needed to generate T-cell help.

ACKNOWLEDGMENTS

This work was supported by a grant from the American Cancer Society (R.E.H.), by the American Cancer Society, Massachusetts Division, Inc. (Q.V.N.), and by

NIH grant CA25783 and Diabetes-Endocrinology Research Center grant DK32520 (R.E.H.). V.E.R. and Q.V.N. were fellows of Immunovirology Training Grant T32-AI07272.

REFERENCES

Allen PM, Strydom DJ, Unanue ER. Processing of lysozyme by macrophages: identification of the determinant recognized by two T-cell hybridomas. Proc Natl Acad Sci USA. 1984; 81:2489–2493.

Babbitt BP, Allen PM, Matsueda G, Haber E, Unanue ER. Binding of immunogenic peptides to Ia histocompatibility molecules. Nature. 1985;317:359–361.

Babbitt BP, Matsueda G, Haber E, Unanue E, Allen PM. Antigenic competition at the level of peptide-Ia binding. Proc Natl Acad Sci USA. 1986;83:4509–4513.

Balkwill FR, Burke F. The cytokine network. Immunol Today. 1989;9:299–304.

Bastin J, Rothbard J, Davey J, Jones I, Townsend A. Use of synthetic peptides of influenza nucleoprotein to define epitopes recognized by class I–restricted cytotoxic T lymphocytes. J Exp Med. 1987;165:1508–1523.

Bennink JR, Yewdell JW, Gerhard W. A viral polymerase involved in recognition of influenza-infected cells by a cytotoxic T cell clone. Nature. 1982;296:75–76.

Bjorkman PJ, Saper MA, Samraoui B, Bennett WS, Strominger JL, Wiley DC. The foreign antigen binding site and T cell recognition regions of class I histocompatibility antigens. Nature. 1987a;329:512–518.

Bjorkman PJ, Saper MA, Samraoui B, Bennett WS, Strominger JL, Wiley DC. Structure of the human class I histocompatibility antigen, HLA-A2. Nature. 1987b;329:506–512.

Blum JS, Cresswell P. Role for intracellular proteases in the processing and transport of class II HLA antigens. Proc Natl Acad Sci USA. 1988;85:3975–3979.

Bouillot M, Choppin J, Cornille F, et al. Physical association between MHC class I molecules and immunogenic peptides. Nature. 1989;339:473–475.

Boyer M, Novak A, Fotear A, Singh B. Contribution of antigen processing to the recognition of a synthetic peptide antigen by specific T cell hybridomas. J Molec Recog. 1988;1:99–106.

Brown MA, Glimcher LA, Nielsen EA, Paul WE, Germain RN. T-cell recognition of Ia molecules selectively altered by a single amino acid substitution. Science. 1986;231:225–258.

Brown JH, Jardetzky T, Saper MA, Samraoui B, Bjorkman PJ, Wiley DC. A hypothetical model of the foreign antigen binding site of class II histocompatibility molecules. Nature. 1988;332:845–850.

Buus S, Colon S, Smith C, Freed RH, Miles C, Grey HM. Interactions between a "processed" ovalbumin peptide and Ia molecules. Proc Natl Acad Sci USA. 1986a;83:3968–3971.

Buus S, Sette A, Colon SM, Jenis DM, Grey HM. Isolation and characterization of antigen-Ia complexes involved in T cell recognition. Cell. 1986b;47:1071–1077.

Buus S, Sette A, Colon SM, Miles C, Grey HM. The relation between major histocompatibility complex (MHC) restriction and the capacity of Ia to bind immunogenic peptides. Science. 1986c;235:1353–1358.

Buus S, Sette A, Colon SM, Grey HM. Autologous peptides constitutively occupy the antigen binding site on Ia. Science. 1988;242:1045–1047.

Carney W. Human tumor antigens and specific-tumor therapy. Immunol Today. 1988;9:363–364.

Ceppellini R, Frumento G, Ferrara GB, Tosi R, Chersi A, Pernis B. Binding of labelled influenza matrix peptide to HLA DR in living B lymphoid cells. Nature. 1989;339:392–394.

Chen BP, Parham P. Direct binding of influenza peptides to class I HLA molecules. Nature. 1989;337:743–745.

Chou PY, Fasman GD. Prediction of the secondary structure of proteins from their amino acid sequence. Adv Enzymol. 1978;47:45–148.

Claesson L, Peterson PA. Association of human γ chain with class II transplantation antigens during intracellular transport. Biochemistry. 1983;22:3206–3213.

Cornette JL, Cease KB, Margalit H, Spouge JL, Berzofsky JA, DeLisi C. Hydrophobicity scales and computational techniques for detecting amphipathic structures in proteins. J Mol Biol. 1987;110:659–685.

Cresswell P, Blum JS, Kelner DN, Marks MS. Biosynthesis and processing of class II histocompatibility antigens. CRC Crit Rev Immunol. 1987;7:31–53.

Davidson HW, Watts C. Epitope-directed processing of specific antigen by B lymphocytes. J Cell Biol. 1989;109:85–92.

Davis MM, Bjorkman PJ. T-cell antigen receptor genes and T-cell recognition. Nature. 1988;334:395–402.

DeLisi C, Berzofsky JA. T-cell antigenic sites tend to be amphipathic structures. Proc Natl Acad Sci USA. 1985;82:7048–7052.

Demotz S, Grey HM, Appella E, Sette A. Characterization of a naturally processed MHC class II-restricted T-cell determinant of hen egg lysozyme. Nature. 1989a;342:682–684.

Demotz S, Lanzavecchia A, Eisel U, Niemann H, Widmann C, Corradin G. Delineation of several DR-restricted tetanus toxin T cell epitopes. J Immunol. 1989b;142:394–402.

Dyson HJ, Cross KJ, Houghten RA, Wilson IA, Wright PE, Lerner RA. The immunodominant site of a synthetic immunogen has a conformational preference in water for a type-II reverse turn. Nature. 1985;318:480–483.

Elliott WL, Stille CJ, Thomas LJ, Humphreys RE. An hypothesis on the binding of an amphipathic, alpha helical sequence in I_i to the desetope of class II antigens. J Immunol. 1987;138:2949–2952.

Festenstein H, Hui KM. Aberrant H-2-like allospecificities on K36.16 thymoma. Studies by radiobinding and immunoprecipitation with anti-H-2 monoclonal antibodies. J Immunogenet. 1986;13:113–116.

Garnier J, Osguthorpe D, Robson B. Analysis of the accuracy and implications of simple methods for predicting the secondary structure of globular proteins. J Mol Biol. 1978;120:97–120.

Garrett TPJ, Saper MA, Bjorkman PJ, Strominger JL, Wiley DC. Specificity pockets for the side chains of peptide antigens in HLA-Aw68. Nature. 1989;342:692–696.

Geysen HM, Tainer JA, Rodda SJ, et al. Chemistry of antibody binding to a protein. Science. 1987;235:1184–1190.

Giacoletto KS, Sant AJ, Bono C, et al. The human invariant chain is the core protein of the human class II-associated proteoglycan. J Exp Med. 1986;164:1422–1439.

Gotch F, Rothbard J, Howland K, Townsend A, McMichael A. Cytotoxic T lymphocytes recognize a fragment of influenza virus matrix protein in association with HLA-A2. Nature. 1987;326:881–882.

Grey HM, Sette A, Buus S. How T cells see antigen. Sci Am. 1989;261:56–64.

Harding CV, Unanue ER. Antigen processing and intracellular Ia: possible roles of endocytosis and protein synthesis in Ia function. J Immunol. 1989;142:12–19.

Ishioka GY, Colon S, Miles C, Grey HM, Chesnut RW. Induction of class I MHC-restricted, peptide-specific cytolytic T lymphocytes by peptide priming in vivo. J Immunol. 1989;143:1094–1100.

Kaiser ET, Kézdy FJ. Amphiphilic secondary structure: design of peptide hormones. Science. 1984;223:249–255.

Kaufman JF, Auffray C, Korman AJ, Shackelford DA, Strominger J. The class II molecules of the human and murine major histocompatibility complex. Cell. 1984;36:1–13.

Kees U, Krammer PH. Most influenza A-virus specific memory cytotoxic T lymphocytes react with antigenic epitopes associated with internal virus determinants. J Exp Med. 1984; 159:365–377.

Koch N, Hämmerling GJ. Ia-associated invariant chain is fatty acylated before addition of sialic acid. Biochemistry. 1985;24:6185–6190.

Krzych U, Fowler AV, Miller A, Sercarz EE. Induction of helper and suppressor T cells by nonoverlapping determinants on the large protein antigen, β-galactosidase. FASEB J. 1988;2:141–145.

Kuwano K, Reyes VE, Humphreys RE, Ennis F. Recognition of disparate HA and NSl peptides by an H-2k^{d}–restricted, influenza-specific CTL clone. Mol Immunol. 1990;28:1–7.

Kvist S, Wilman K, Claesson L, Peterson PA, Dobberstein B. Membrane insertion and oligomeric assembly of HLA-DR histocompatibility antigens. Cell. 1982;29:61–69.

Lakey EK, Casten LA, Anderson MS, Smolenski LA, Smith JA, Margoliash E, et al. T cell activation by processed antigen is equally blocked by I-E and I-A–restricted immunodominant peptides. Eur J Immunol. 1987a;17:1605–1609.

Lakey EK, Margoliash E, Pierce SK. Identification of a peptide binding protein that plays a role in antigen presentation. Proc Natl Acad Sci. 1987b;84:1659–1663.

Lanzavecchia A. Antigen-specific interaction between T and B cells. Nature. 1985;314:537–539.

Lipp J, Dobberstein B. The membrane-spanning segment of invariant chain (Iγ) contains a potentially cleavable signal sequence. Cell. 1986;46:1103–1112.

Long EO, Jacobson S. Pathway of viral antigen processing and presentation to CTL: defined by the mode of virus entry? Immunol Today. 1989;10:45–48.

Lorenz RG, Tyler AN, Allen PM. Reconstruction of the immunogenic peptide RNase(43-56) by identification and transfer of the critical residues into an unrelated peptide backbone. J Exp Med. 1989;170:203–215.

Lu S, Reyes VE, Lew RA, et al. Role of recurrent hydrophobic residues in catalysis of helix formation by T cell–presented peptides in the presence of lipid vesicles. J Immunol. 1990;145:899–904.

Lu S, Ciardelli T, Reyes VE, Humphreys RE. Number and placement of hydrophobic residues in a longitudinal strip governs helix formation of peptides in the presence of lipid vesicles. J Bio Chem. 1991a;266:10054–10057.

Lu S, Reyes VE, Torgerson RR, Lew RA, Humphreys RE. Common principles in protein folding and antigen presentation. Trends Biotechnol. 1991b;9:238–242.

Lu S, Reyes VE, Bositis CM, et al. Biophysical mechanisms of the scavenger site near T-cell presented epitopes. Vaccine. 1992;10:3–7.

Machamer CE, Cresswell P. Biosynthesis and glycosylation of the invariant chain associated with HLA-DR antigens. J Immunol. 1982;129:2564–2569.

Machamer CE, Cresswell P. Monensin prevents terminal glycosylation of the N- and O-linked oligosaccharides of the HLA-DR–associated invariant chain and inhibits its dissociation from the α-β chain complex. Proc Natl Acad Sci USA. 1984;81:1287–1291.

Margalit H, Spouge JL, Cornette JL, Cease KB, DeLisi C, Berzofsky JA. Prediction of immunodominant helper T cell antigenic sites from the primary sequence. J Immunol. 1987;138:2213–2229.

Marks MS, Cresswell P. Invariant chain associates with HLC class II antigens via its extracytoplasmic region. J Immunol. 1986;136:2519–2525.

Martz E, Howell DM. CTL: virus control cells first and cytolytic cells second? DNA fragmentation, apoptosis and the prelytic halt hypothesis. Immunol Today. 1989;10:79–86.

McMichael AJ, Gotch FM, Rothbard J. HLA-B37 determines an influenza A virus nucleoprotein epitope recognized by cytotoxic T lymphocytes. J Exp Med. 1986;164:1397–1406.

Moore MW, Carbone FR, Bevan MJ. Introduction of soluble protein into the class I pathway of antigen processing and presentation. Cell. 1988;54:777–785.

Morrison LA, Lukacher AE, Braciale VL, Fan DP, Braciale TJ. Differences in antigen presentation to MHC class I– and class II–restricted influenza virus-specific cytolytic T lymphocyte clones. J Exp Med. 1986;163:903–921.

Nagy ZA, Lehmann PV, Falcioni F, Muller S, Adorini L. Why peptides? Their possible role in the evolution of MHC-restricted T-cell recognition. Immunol Today. 1989;10:132–137.

Nguyen QV, Humphreys RE. Time course of intracellular associations, processing, and cleavage of I_i forms and class II MHC molecules. J Biol Chem. 1989;264:1631–1637.

Nguyen QV, Humphreys RE. Different processing pathways for I_i depending on association with class II MHC. 1991a; submitted for publication.

Nguyen QV, Humphreys RE. Time course for release of class II MHC α and β chains from I_i or Ip. 1991b; submitted for publication.

Nguyen QV, Knapp W, Humphreys RE. Inhibition by leupeptin and antipain of the intracellular proteolysis of I_i. Hum Immunol. 1989;24:153–163.

Pala P, Corridan G, Strachan T, et al. Mapping of HLA epitopes recognized by H-2-restricted cytotoxic T lymphocytes specific for HLA using recombinant genes and synthetic peptides. J Immunol. 1988;140:871–877.

Perkins DL, Lai M-Z, Smith JA, Gefter ML. Identical peptides recognized by MHC class I– and II–restricted T cells. J Exp Med. 1989;170:279–289.

Ploegh H, Fuhrmann U. Manipulation of glycans on antigens of the major histocompatibility complex. In Pernis B, Vogel HJ, eds. Cell biology of the major histocompatibility complex. New York, NY: Academic Press; 1985:133–151.

Presta LG, Rose GD. Helix signals in proteins. Science. 1988;240:1632–1641.

Quaranta V, Majdic O, Stingl G, Liszka K, Honigsmann H, Knapp W. A human Ia cytoplasmic determinant located on multiple forms of invariant chain (γ, γ2, γ3). J Immunol. 1984;132:1900–1905.

Reyes VE, Chin LT, Humphreys RE. Selection of class I MHC-restricted peptides with the strip-of-helix hydrophobicity algorithm. Mol Immunol. 1988;25:867–871.

Reyes VE, Phillips L, Humphreys RE, Lew RA. Prediction of protein helices with a derivative of the strip-of-helix hydrophobicity algorithm. J Biol Chem. 1989;264:12854-12858.

Reyes VE, Fowlie EJ, Lu S, et al. Comparison of three related methods to select T cell–presented sequences of antigenic proteins. Molec Immunol. 1990;27:1021–1027.

Reyes VE, Lu S, Humphreys RE. Cathespin B cleaves I_i from class II MHC molecules without apparent damage to the alpha and beta chains. J Immunol. 1991;146:3877–3880.

Richardson JS, Richardson DC. Amino acid preferences for specific locations at the ends of α helices. Science. 1988;240:1648–1652.

Rock KL, Benacerraf B, Abbas AK. Antigen presentation by hapten-specific B lymphocytes. I. Role of surface immunoglobulin receptors. J Exp Med. 1984;160:1102–1113.

Rothbard JB, Taylor WR. A sequence pattern common to T cell epitopes. EMBO J. 1988;7:93–100.

Rothbard JB, Lechler RI, Howland K, et al. Structural model of HLA-DR1 restricted T cell antigen recognition. Cell. 1988;52:515–523.

Sant A, Schwartz BD, Cullen SE. Identification of a new component in the murine Ia molecular complex. J Exp Med. 1983;158:1979–1992.

Sant AJ, Cullen SE, Schwartz BD. Biosynthetic relationships of the chondroitin sulfate proteoglycan with Ia and invariant chain glycoproteins. J Immunol. 1985;135:416–422.

Schaeffer EB, Sette A, Johnson DL, et al. Relative contribution of "determinant selection" and "holes in the T-cell repertoire" to T-cell responses. Proc Natl Acad Sci USA. 1989;86:4649–4653.

Schmidt W, Festenstein H. Serological and immunochemical studies of H-2 allospecificities on K36.16 syngeneic tumor of AKR. J Immunogenet. 1980;7:7–17.

Schreiber H, Ward PL, Rowley DA, Stauss HJ. Unique tumor-specific antigens. Ann Rev Immunol. 1988;6:465–483.

Sette A, Buus S, Appella E, Smith JA, Chesnut R, Miles C, et al. Prediction of major histocompatibility complex binding regions of protein antigens by sequence pattern analysis. Proc Natl Acad Sci USA. 1989a;86:3296–3300.

Sette A, Buus S, Colon S, Miles C, Grey HM. Structural analysis of peptides capable of binding to more than one Ia antigen. J Immunol. 1989b;142:35–40.

Shimonkevitz R, Kappler J, Marrack P, Grey H. Antigen recognition by H-2–restricted T cells. I. Cell-free antigen processing. J Exp Med. 1983;158:303–316.

Sinigaglia F, Guttinger M, Kilgus J, et al. A malaria T-cell epitope recognized in association with most mouse and human MHC class II molecules. Nature. 1988;336:778–780.

Sivak LE, Harris MR, Kindle C, Cullen SE. Inhibition of proteoglycan synthesis eliminates the proteoglycan form of Ia-associated invariant chain and depresses antigen presentation. J Immunol. 1987;138:1319–1321.

Sorli CH, Reisert PS, Welch WJ, Humphreys RE. Identification of p70 and p80 associations with class II MHC molecules and I_i. Am J Hematol. 1990;35:157–166.

Spiro RC, Sairenji T, Humphreys RE. Enhanced I_i expression after n-butyrate treatment of a P3HR-1 subline which does not express HLA-D. Hematol Oncol. 1984;2:239–247.

Spiro RC, Sairenji T, Humphreys RE. Kinetics of I_i synthesis, processing and turnover in n-butyrate-treated Burkitt's lymphoma cell lines which express or do not express class II antigens and in hairy leukemia cells. J Immunol. 1985;134:3539–3549.

Spouge JL, Guy HR, Cornette JL, et al. Strong conformational propensities enhance T cell antigenicity. J Immunol. 1986;138:204–212.

Stauss HJ, Linsk R, Fischer A, et al. Isolation of the MHC genes encoding the tumor-specific class I antigens expressed on a murine fibrosarcoma. J Immunogenet. 1986;13:101–111.

Stille CJ, Thomas LJ, Reyes VE, Humphreys RE. Hydrophobic strip-of-helix algorithm for selection of T cell–presented peptides. Mol Immunol. 1987;24:1021–1027.

Stockinger B, Pessara U, Lin RH, Habicht J, Grez M, Koch NA. A role of Ia-associated invariant chains in antigen processing and presentation. Cell. 1989;56:683–689.

Streicher HZ, Berkower IJ, Busch M, Gurd RFN, Berzofsky JA. Antigen conformation determines processing requirements for T-cell activation. Proc Natl Acad Sci USA. 1984; 81:6831–6835.

Sung E, Jones PP. The invariant chain of murine Ia antigens: its glycosylation, abundance and subcellular localization. Mol Immunol. 1981;18:899–913.

Sweetser MT, Morrison LA, Braciale VL, Braciale TJ. Recognition of pre-processed endogenous antigen by class I but not class II MHC-restricted T cells. Nature. 1989;342:180–182.

Tanaka K, Yoshioka T, Bieberich C, Jay G. Role of the major histocompatibility complex class I antigens in tumor growth and metastasis. Ann Rev Immunol. 1988;6:359–380.

Thomas LJ, Nguyen QV, Elliott WL, Humphreys RE. Proteolytic cleavage of I_i to p25. J Immunol. 1988;140:2670–2674.

Thomas LJ, Humphreys RE, Knapp W, Nguyen QV. Time-dependent cleavage of a high mannose form of I_i to p25 in an intracellular compartment. Am J Hematol. 1989;32:167–177.

Tony H-P, Parker DC. Major histocompatibility complex-restricted, polyclonal B cell responses resulting from helper T cell recognition of anti-immunoglobulin presented by small B lymphocytes. J Exp Med. 1985;161:223–241.

Torgerson RR, Leu RA, Reyes VE, Hardy L, Humphreys RE. Highly restricted distributions of hydrophobic and charged amino acids in longitudinal quadrants of alpha helices. J Biol Chem. 1991;266:5521–5524.

Townsend ARM, Skehel JJ. Influenza A-specific cytotoxic T-cell clones that do not recognize viral glycoproteins. Nature. 1982;300:655–657.

Townsend ARM, Skehel JJ. The influenza A virus nucleoprotein gene controls the induction of both subtype specific and crossreactive cytotoxic T cell. J Exp Med. 1984;160:552–563.

Townsend ARM, McMichael AJ, Carter NP, Huddleston JA, Brownlee GG. Cytotoxic T cell recognition of the influenza nucleoprotein and hemagglutinin expressed in transfected mouse L cells. Cell. 1984;39:13–25.

Townsend ARM, Bastin J, Gould K, Brownlee GG. Cytotoxic T lymphocytes recognize influenza haemagglutinin that lacks a signal sequence. Nature. 1986a;324:575–577.

Townsend ARM, Rothbard J, Gotch FM, Bahadur G, Wraith D, McMichael AJ. The epitopes of influenza nucleoprotein recognized by cytotoxic T lymphocytes can be defined with short synthetic peptides. Cell. 1986b;44:959–968.

Townsend A, Öhlén C, Bastin J, Ljunggren H-G, Foster L, Kärre K. Association of class I major histocompatibility heavy and light chains induced by viral peptides. Nature. 1989; 340:443–448.

Unanue ER, Cerottini J-C. Antigen presentation. FASEB. 1989;3:2496–2502.

Vanbuskirk A, Crump BL, Margoliash E, Pierce SK. A peptide binding protein having a role in antigen presentation is a member of the HSP70 heat shock family. J Exp Med. 1989;170:1799–1809.

Walden P, Nagy ZA, Klein J. Antigen presentation by liposomes: inhibition with antibodies. Eur J Immunol. 1986;16:717–720.

Watts C, Davidson HW. Endocytosis and recycling of specific antigen by human B cell lines. EMBO J. 1988;4:1937–1945.

Whitton JL, Oldstone MBA. Class I MHC can present an endogenous peptide to cytotoxic T lymphocytes. J Exp Med. 1989;170:1033–1038.

Wölfel T, Klehmann E, Müller C, Schütt K-H, Meyer Zum Büschenfelde K-H, Knuth A. Lysis of human melanoma cells by autologous cytolytic T cell clones: identification of human histocompatibility leukocyte antigen A2 as a restriction element for three different antigens. J Exp Med. 1989;170:797–810.

Wortzel RD, Philipps C, Schreiber H. Multiple tumor-specific antigens expressed on a single tumor cell. Nature. 1983;304:165–167.

Ziegler K, Unanue E. Decrease in macrophage antigen catabolism caused by ammonia and chloroquine is associated with inhibition of antigen presentation to T cells. Proc Natl Acad Sci USA. 1982;79:175–178.

CHAPTER **6**

HUMAN TUMOR–ASSOCIATED ANTIGENS IDENTIFIED BY MONOCLONAL ANTIBODIES

Ralph A. Reisfeld
Barbara M. Mueller

The progress of cancer research has been greatly influenced during the last 15 years by human tumor–associated antigens recognized by murine monoclonal antibodies (mAb). Developments, such as those of hybridomas secreting monoclonal antibodies together with the application of techniques of modern molecular biology, have stimulated considerable hope for improvements in the diagnosis and therapy of cancer. These technologies may also aid considerably in the experimental analysis of novel concepts that may ultimately lead to a better understanding of basic mechanisms involved in tumor invasion and metastasis. Although these new methods have led to some advances in cancer research, one has to realize that with the possible exception of oncogenes, few truly conceptual advances were made thus far that provide for a quantum jump in our basic knowledge of tumor invasion and metastasis. With these considerations and limitations in mind, the aim of this chapter is to focus on several monoclonal antibodies directed against antigens associated with human cutaneous melanoma and the impact made thus far by these molecular probes on the progress in cancer research.

Human cutaneous melanoma is selected as the topic of this chapter because of an increasing interest in its biology and pathophysiology, which developed during the last two decades, in part because of some unique biological characteristics and the rapidly mounting incidence of this disease. Although the 27,000 annual cases of malignant melanoma account for only about 2.5% of cancer in the United States and approximately 7% of all skin cancer, they cause approximately 65% of all skin cancer deaths. The fatal nature of this highly disseminated disease is caused by its poor response to conventional radiation and chemotherapy. Partly because of this rather dismal clinical outlook and possibly due to melanoma being among the tumors with the most rapidly mounting incidence, at 7% annually, an intense interest has developed in melanoma-associated antigens (MAA) as a potential means for diagnosis and therapy. This interest is also based, in part, on prior well-documented findings indicating that changes in cell-surface antigens were associated with neoplastic transformation. During the last 10 years, there has been considerable progress in the development of monoclonal antibodies to human MAA. These antibodies have some potential for adjuvant therapy of melanoma and offer themselves as effective molecular probes to define antigens that may prove useful in delineating some of the basic mechanisms involved in tumor invasion and metastasis.

It is the intent of this chapter to focus mainly on those MAA that were defined by murine monoclonal antibodies and that have the potential to serve as molecular probes to gain a better understanding of tumor invasion and metastasis. Particular emphasis has been placed on the biochemical and immunological characterization of these antigens and a delineation of their possible biological functions in normal and neoplastic cells. Finally, an effort has been made to provide some perspectives for future developments of monoclonal antibodies that identify human tumor–associated antigens.

STRUCTURAL AND FUNCTIONAL CHARACTERISTICS OF HUMAN MELANOMA–ASSOCIATED ANTIGENS

It should be recognized that few, if any, investigators initially set out to find a particular type of tumor antigen. Rather, the choice was made for them by the type of monoclonal antibodies that ultimately emerged as the result of immunizing mice with cells of a particular neoplasm. This approach, although eminently practical, created a certain amount of confusion at its inception. The field of antigens associated with human melanoma provides a particularly good example of this, since it has been investigated quite thoroughly by a critical mass of researchers who, within a few years after the development of the hybridoma technology (Köhler and Milstein, 1975) already made use of monoclonal antibodies. Among research investigators studying solid tumors of human origin, it was also this group of scientists who compared and critically evaluated over 30 MAA defined by numerous monoclonal antibodies in two workshops organized at the beginning of the last decade (Steplewski, 1982). From this relatively large number of antigens, only relatively few are still being investigated. However, monoclonal antibodies directed against MAA have provided molecular probes that led to the identification of several antigenic structures with distinct biochemical and immunological characteristics. Based on these characteristics and on their established, as well as putative, biological functions, these antigens and the monoclonal antibodies recognizing them are ordered here into several major categories and their biochemical, immunological, and biological characteristics are described. These categories can be extended to those antigens that are expressed on the cell surface and/or shed into the circulation during melanoma tumor progression. Thus, gangliosides and cell-substrate interacting proteins, such as the MAA-chondroitin sulfate proteoglycan are both expressed on the cell surface and shed. A number of cell-surface receptors for various growth factors, as well as several ion-transport and binding proteins, are concerned with the intracellular transport of biologically relevant material. The HLA antigens are involved in immune recognition and are both expressed and shed by melanoma cells. Finally, some pigmentation antigens are located in the cytoplasm and can be found in the spent medium of pigmented melanoma cells.

Cell-Substrate Interacting Glycoproteins

Several molecules of relatively high molecular weight belong to this class of MAA, which are uniformly expressed and show little heterogeneity within each tumor when analyzed either on cultured cells or tumor tissue sections.

Chondroitin Sulfate Proteoglycans

Biochemical and immunological characteristics. The gene-encoding, melanoma-associated chondroitin sulfate proteoglycan (CSP) was mapped to chromosome 15 (Rettig et al., 1986) and this major MAA has produced several murine monoclonal antibodies because of its high expression on human melanoma cells and its immunogenicity in mice. Thus, a unique glycoprotein-proteoglycan complex associated with human melanoma cells has been defined by mAb 9.2.27 (Morgan et al., 1981). Biosynthetic studies indicated that this molecule consists of an N-linked glycoprotein of 250 kDa and a proteoglycan component of >450 kDa. Pulse-chase analysis demonstrated that the 250-kDa glycoprotein has endo-β-N-acetylglucosaminidase–sensitive (Endo-A) precursors that are N-asparagine–linked, unprocessed, high mannose oligosaccharides. The selective digestion of the proteoglycan with chondroitin lyases and glycosaminoglycan analysis showed it to be a CSP (Bumol and Reisfeld, 1982) with a 250-kDa core glycoprotein. Biosynthetic analysis also showed that the catonic ionophore monensin blocks biosynthesis of the proteoglycan, and its appearance appeared to be linked kinetically to biosynthetic functions of the Golgi apparatus, the proposed site of glycosyltransferases involved in proteoglycan biosynthesis. Taken together, these data suggest that the chondroitin sulfate chains are added onto the 250-kDa core glycoprotein to form the >450-kDa proteoglycan. This conclusion was confirmed by pulse-chase analysis, which demonstrated that mAb 9.2.27 recognizes several N-linked, glycosylated precursors of 210 and 220 kDa, as judged by their sensitivity to Endo-H, as well as another precursor of 240-kDa and the 250-kDa core glycoprotein. Consequently, the addition of N-linked oligosaccharides appears to be an early biosynthetic event in CSP core protein biosynthesis (Bumol et al., 1984).

A number of other monoclonal antibodies have been reported that recognize antigens designated as melanoma-associated, high-molecular-weight antigens (MAA-HMW). There is considerable evidence from several laboratories indicating that these monoclonal antibodies also recognize epitopes on a melanoma-associated proteoglycan. The most intensely investigated among these reagents is mAb 225.28S (IgG1) (Imai et al., 1981; Kantor et al., 1982). Comparison of this antibody with mAb 9.2.27 in a competition antibody binding assay revealed a striking difference in reactivity. Also, by sodium dodecyl sulfate polyacrylamide gel electrophoresis (SDS-PAGE) analysis of appropriate immunoprecipitates of detergent lysate from the same melanoma cell line and by digestion with chondroitin lyases ABC and AB, it was established that although both these antibodies bind to the core glycoprotein of CSP, they clearly recognize different epitopes. Moreover, only mAb 225.28S reacts slightly with the fibrosarcoma cell line HT 1080, leading to the speculation that only the epitope recognized by 225.28S is on proteoglycans found on such cells (Harper et al., 1982). This would support the argument for structural heterogeneity of CSP. This certainly seems to be a possibility in view of the very complex structure of proteoglycan aggregates, which can include isomeric, sulfate-substituted carbohydrates and differential chain length of oligosaccharides, such as hyaluronic acid. This type of molecular complexity could easily explain why a whole variety of antigen epitopes are recognized by different monoclonal antibodies. Since additional data of several investigators obtained from antibody-binding inhibition and immunodepletion assays also confirmed the conclusion that mAb 225.28S indeed recognizes a different epitope on the same antigen structure recognized by mAb 9.2.27, that is, melanoma-associated CSP, it is most likely that the antigen designated as MAA-HMW is also a melanoma-associated proteoglycan (Harper et al., 1982).

Recently, an anti-idiotype (anti-id) antibody exhibited mimicry for the human high-molecular-weight, melanoma-associated antigen (HMW-MAA) recognized by mAb 225.28 (Chattopadhey et al., 1991). Thus, a mouse anti-id monoclonal antibody (IMEL-1) was able to be recognized by an idiotope in the antigen combining site of this antibody. Furthermore, mAb IMEL-1 induces an immune response against self-cross-reacting HMW-MAA in rabbits that express this antigen in normal tissues. The rabbit anti-id antibodies inhibited interactions of melanoma cells with elements of the extracellular matrix. Thus, it was postulated that this may be an additional mechanism by which anti–HMW-MAA immunity affects the biology of melanoma cells in melanoma patients immunized with anti-id mAb IMEL-1.

Functional properties. Proteoglycans have been implicated in growth control, involvement in adhesion in cell–substratum interactions, cell–cell contacts, and other functional properties of potential biological relevance. The potential of CSP as a functional molecule is brought in focus by its presence on >90% of melanoma cultures where 80% to 100% of cells express this molecule at densities ranging from 1×10^5 to 6×10^6 binding sites per cell. The CSP is expressed on the melanoma cell's surface on microspikes, that is, structures of 1 to 2 μ on the upper cell surface that range up to 20 μ at the cell periphery. These peripheral CSP microspikes are involved in cell–cell contacts and also form complex footpads that make contact with the substratum. The CSP antigen is also very well expressed on adhesion plaques that are deposited along cell membranes (Harper et al., 1985).

A possible functional role of CSP in human melanoma was demonstrated in their interaction with basement membrane components. Thus, mAb 9.2.27 can block the early events of melanoma cell spreading on endothelial basement membranes, while only slightly inhibiting cell adhesion, suggesting a possible role for CSP in stabilizing cell–substratum interactions in this in vivo model for metastatic invasion. Another potential functional role for CSP was indicated when mAb 9.2.27 specifically inhibited anchorage-independent growth of human melanoma cells in a soft agar clonogenic assay. The precise mechanism underlying this phenomena is not entirely clear, and it has been proposed that it relates to the physicochemical nature and location of CSP recognized by mAb 9.2.27 on the microspikes of the melanoma cell surface (Harper and Reisfeld, 1983).

Another functional property of melanoma-associated proteoglycans was suggested when mAb 9.2.27, employed as a molecular and functional probe, demonstrated that the core protein of the CSP recognized by this antibody is present in two forms on the cell surface, either free or modified by the addition of chondroitin sulfate chains. These findings suggest that the addition of glycosaminoglycan chains may not be a prerequisite for cell-surface expression of proteoglycan core protein (Harper et al., 1986; Spiro et al., 1986). Since the addition of these chains is not a prerequisite for cell-surface expression of the core protein, it is unlikely that such a modification serves as a marker to segregate molecules on the cell surface. Signals involved in targeting CSP or its core protein to the cell surface are more likely to reside in the N- and/or O-linked oligosaccharides that are added to the core protein prior to addition of glycosaminoglycan chains (Harper et al., 1985, 1986).

Melanoma-Associated Cell-Adhesion Molecules Several monoclonal antibodies have been reported that, under nonreducing conditions, immunoprecipitate from melanoma cells a series of molecules ranging from 130 to 150 kDa and from 90 to 105 kDa. Under reducing conditions, these molecular species are of 116 to 120, 95, 29, and 25 to 26 kDa. Among the monoclonal antibodies that identify these molecules are Nu4B, which binds to most cultured melanoma and glioma cells and to most melanomas in situ. Another mAb, DA3, was reported to have a similar binding pattern, but higher binding affinity. The mAb DA3 and AMF7 inhibit attachment of melanoma cells to different substrates, and the antigen recognized by mAb AMF7 has been designated melanoma-associated, cell-adhesion molecule-1 (MECAM-1), as it is reported to play a role in motility and migration of melanoma cells.

Among the various monoclonal antibodies recognizing melanoma-associated, cell-adhesion molecules, mAb LM609 is probably best defined by its recognition of the biochemically well-characterized vitronectin receptor $\alpha_v\beta_3$, expressed on human endothelial cells and on the cultured human melanoma cell line M21. The $\alpha_v\beta_3$ vitronectin receptor is promiscuous, since it is capable of recognizing the arginine-glycine-aspartic acid (RGD) sequence, not only in vitronectin, but also in such adhesive proteins as fibrinogen and von Willebrand factor (Cheresh, 1987). The heterodimeric adhesion receptor complex recognized by LM609 consists of noncovalently associated α and β subunits that, under reducing conditions, have molecular masses of 135 and 115 kDa, respectively. The α subunit also contains a disulfide bridge–linked 27-kDa light chain that can be detected under reducing conditions of SDS-PAGE (Cheresh and Spiro, 1987).

Additional monoclonal antibodies have been reported that recognize melanoma-associated, cellular-adhesion molecules. Among these is mAb CL203.4, which is secreted from hybridomas produced by immunizing BALB/c mice with human melanoma cells COLO 38 treated with interferon (IFN)-γ. This antibody recognizes a single-chain glycoprotein of 96 kDa with a polypeptide moiety of 50 kDa. This antigen is identical in biochemical and immunological properties to the well-characterized intercellular adhesion molecule (ICAM-1) originally identified with mAb RR1/1, which elicited with Epstein-Barr virus (EBV)–transformed lymphocytes from a patient deficient in the lymphocyte function–associated antigen-1 (LFA-1) (Maio et al., 1989a).

The mAb P3.58 and MUC18 are two other murine monoclonal antibodies raised against fresh human melanoma tumor tissue that bind to cell-surface molecules involved in cellular adhesion. They were first observed to bind to membrane glycoproteins of 89 and 113 kDa, respectively. When the nucleotide sequences of the complementary DNA (cDNA) clones for these antigens were analyzed, their structural homology with adhesion molecules was revealed. The antigen detected by P3.58 is homologous to ICAM-1, while the integral membrane glycoprotein detected by MUC18 shows extensive sequence similarity with neural cell adhesion molecules (N-CAM) (Johnson et al., 1989). More recently, several reports shed additional light on the structural basis for RGD recognition by integrin $\alpha_v\beta_3$ by identifying the region(s) of the molecule interacting with RGD-containing peptides. Indeed, regions near the NH2 terminus of both the α (residues 139-349) and β (residues 61-302) subunits were shown to be proximal to the RGD binding site. The results implied that the RGD binding pocket of $\alpha_v\beta_3$ involved the NH2 terminal regions of both subunits and that the divalent cation binding domain of α_v plays a direct role in this receptor's capacity to bind ligand (Smith and Cheresh, 1988, 1990). As far as the biosynthesis of integrin $\alpha_v\beta_3$ in melanoma cells is concerned, a number of pulse-chase immunoprecipitation analyses yielded some interesting data regarding the functional roles of the two subunits. Thus, studies with the human melanoma cells M21-L, selected for their inability to produce α_v, indicated that the remaining β_3 subunit could not interact with the RGD affinity matrix. In fact, it was synthesized and rapidly broken down. These data suggested that the α subunit is required for integrin function, as well as transport of the intact heterodimer to the cell surface (Cheresh and Spiro, 1987).

Regarding the functional regulation of $\alpha_v\beta_3$ in the plane of the melanoma cell membrane, evidence from recent studies (Conforti et al., 1990) supported conclusions based on earlier work (Cheresh et al., 1987) that $\alpha_v\beta_3$ is subjected to regulation by other molecules. This is supported by a recent study demonstrating that ligand-binding properties of $\alpha_v\beta_3$ in liposomes depend on the lipid composition of these liposomes. Thus, a change in the receptor's environment could alter its ligand-binding properties. Also, a 50-kDa protein was recently reported to associate with the $\alpha_v\beta_3$ integrin on several cell types, and an antibody directed against this protein modulated the function of $\alpha_v\beta_3$ (Brown et al., 1991). Finally, it was shown that $\alpha_v\beta_3$ on the melanoma cell surface can organize into focal contacts when these cells are attached to fibronectin (Wayner et al., 1991); however, this receptor does not organize into these structures when other ligands attach to the same melanoma cells. Taken together, these data indicate that integrins like $\alpha_v\beta_3$ are able to organize into focal domains on the melanoma cell surface in response to specific ligands; however, the functional significance of these focal contacts remains to be determined.

Another integrin, $\alpha_4\beta_1$, has been reported to be preferentially expressed on certain leukocytes and human melanoma cells. This integrin apparently serves as a receptor for fibronectin that recognizes an alternatively spliced form (CS-1) of this extracellular matrix component (Wayner et al., 1989; Guan and Hynes, 1990). Integrin $\alpha_4\beta_1$ also recognizes the counterreceptor VCAM expressed on activated endothelial cells (Elices et al., 1990). Activation of endothelial cells at the site of injury with cytokines, such as IL-1, aids in supporting leukocyte adhesion (Osborn et al., 1989) and invasion into tissues. Expression of $\alpha_4\beta_1$ may be part of the mechanism for this event, although LFA-1 recognition of ICAM expressed on endothelial cells is also involved in this process (Dustin and Springer, 1988). Analogous to this, $\alpha_4\beta_1$ expression on melanoma cells may potentiate metastatic invasion of these tumor cells into the bloodstream by adding an adhesive substrate to the endothelial cell surface. However, this contention remains to be proven experimentally.

Functional Properties of MAA, Cell-Adhesion Molecules A functional property of the heterodimer adhesion receptor complex identified by mAb LM609 is well delineated by this antibody. Thus, it inhibits the attachment of human endothelial cells and of M21 melanoma cells to such extracellular matrix proteins as fibrinogen, von Willebrand factor, and vitronectin, but has no effect on the attachment of these cells to fibronectin, collagen, or laminin. Monoclonal antibody LM609 also inhibits attachment of these cells to an immobilized peptide containing the RGD sequence. This same antibody was also used to determine for the first time that platelets contain the vitronectin receptor complex (VNR) in addition to glycoprotein IIb/IIIa, its prominent RGD-binding adhesion receptor complex. It has been postulated that RGD recognition may play a significant role in biological events associated with vascular proliferation and with motility and migration of melanoma cells, which are key elements of the metastatic process (Cheresh and Spiro, 1987; Cheresh, 1987).

As far as its biological function is concerned, the ICAM-1 antigen recognized by mAb CL203.4 is highly susceptible to modulation by IFN-γ, interleukin-1 (IL-1) and tumor necrosis factor-alpha (TNF-α). In this regard, it is of considerable interest that by immunohistochemical testing of surgically removed lesions of melanocyte origin, mAb CL203.4 has a markedly lower reactivity with benign lesions than with malignant lesions and stains a higher percentage of metastatic lesions than primary lesions. Melanoma cells isolated from primary lesions acquire reactivity with mAb CL203.4 following a 24-hour in vitro incubation with IFN-γ (100 U/mL), suggesting that such cells are able to synthesize and express ICAM-1. The lack of staining of primary lesions with CL203.4 is thought to reflect insufficient concentration of cytokines, which modulate this antigen. Interestingly, reactivity of CL203.4 with primary lesions removed from patients with stage I melanoma showed a highly significant correlation with stage of disease. Thus, the disease-free interval of patients without detectable reactivity of their primary lesions with mAb CL203.4 was significantly longer ($p = 0.004$) than that of patients whose primary lesions were stained with this antibody (Maio et al., 1989b). Similar observations were made for the antigens defined by P3.58 and MUC18. Expression of both adhesion molecules seems to correlate with increasing vertical thickness, that is, malignancy of melanoma biopsies, and these antigens have therefore been proposed to be directly involved in tumor progression.

Ion Transport and Binding Proteins

Melanotransferrin (p97)

Biochemical and immunological characteristics. A family of antigens of 97 kDa, designated p97, is preferentially expressed on human melanoma cells and tissues. Similar to CSP, the family of p97 glycoproteins is highly immunogenic when human melanoma cells are injected into mice. In initial studies, mAb 4.1 (IgG1) was found to bind significantly to 90% of melanomas tested. Although this monoclonal antibody also reacted in binding assays with 55% of a variety of other tumor cells analyzed, it failed to react with B lymphoblastoid cell lines and cultivated fibroblasts. The target antigen identified by mAb 4.1 proved to be a glycoprotein of 97 kDa (Woodbury et al., 1980) that is encoded by chromosome-3 (Plowman et al., 1983). Although the widespread occurrence of p97 indicates that it was not melanoma-specific, it was evident from studies of normal, adult tissues and melanoma biopsy specimens that normal tissues and nonmelanoma tumors contained p97 in far lesser amounts than melanoma tissues. Antigen p97 was also observed in a number of fetal tissues, such as colon, umbilical cord, lung, and benign nevi (Woodbury et al., 1981).

After immunochemical and molecular characterization of p97, it became evident that several monoclonal antibodies recognized different epitopes on this molecule. Thus, mAb 4.1 and 96.5 reacted with the same antigen epitope, p97a, whereas mAb 118.1 and 8.2 defined epitopes p97b and p97c, respectively. The relatively high frequency of hybridomas secreting antibodies to p97 suggested that this antigen is either particularly immunogenic and/or expressed in larger amounts than other antigens on the melanoma cell lines SK-MEL-28 and K-2, used for immunization. Quantitation by antibody-binding analysis indicated that SK-MEL-28 cells express at least 4×10^5 molecules of p97 per cell, that is, roughly the same number as HLA-ABC determinants identified by anti-HLA mAb W6/32 on these cells. Vastly different amounts of antibodies defining epitopes p97a, b, and c were bound by melanoma, lung carcinoma, as well as by lymphoid B- and T-cell lines. Melanoma cell lines bound from 3.0 to 3.8×10^5 molecules of each antibody per cell, lung carcinoma cell lines bound from

4.0 to 6.2×10^3 molecules per cell, whereas lymphoid B- and T-cell lines bound only from 250 to 1,400 molecules per cell (Brown et al., 1981).

The initial chemical characterization of p97 indicated sialylated carbohydrate chains and a single polypeptide chain with some intrachain disulfide bridges. Partial digestion of p97 with either papain or trypsin resulted in seemingly identical glycosylated fragments of 40 kDa that expressed the p97a, b, and c epitopes. The p97 antigen is functionally related to transferrin and may have evolved from a common ancestor. This was indicated initially by partial amino-terminal amino acid sequence homology between these two molecules, that is, 7 of 12 residues determined were identical, including two of the least common amino acids, tryptophan and cystine. The apparent similarity between p97 and transferrin was further substantiated when p97 was shown to bind iron and an antiserum made to denatured p97 cross-reacted with both denatured transferrin and lactotransferrin. Under reducing conditions, p97 has a molecular weight similar to the transferrin receptor, but the transferrin receptor forms a dimer of 200 kDa on SDS-PAGE under nonreducing conditions, whereas p97 does not. Also, mAb OKT9, which is specific for transferrin receptors, does not immunoprecipitate p97 from radiolabeled human melanoma cells (Brown et al., 1982).

Antigen p97 is one of the relatively few human tumor-associated antigens that had the gene encoding it cloned and its complete nucleotide sequence determined. From this sequence, the amino acid sequence of the 738-residue p97 precursor was deduced. The overall structure of p97 and its possible functional domains, after removal of a 19-residue signal peptide, shows a mature p97 molecule with two extracellular domains of 342 and 352 residues. A possible membrane anchor for p97 is provided by a 25-residue C-terminal stretch of mainly hydrophobic amino acid residues. There is considerable sequence conservation, since each of the extracellular domains contain 14 cystine residues that form seven intradomain disulfide bridges. The p97 molecule has relatively little glycosylation, since the extracellular domain contains only one or two potential N-glycosylation sites. The three antigenic determinants of p97 are protein in nature and are situated on the N-terminal domain. These domains show 46% sequence homology to each other and 39% homology to the corresponding domains of human transferrin. The conservation of the disulfide bridges is thought to create iron binding pockets for p97. Based on the structural homology between p97 and the three members of the transferrin super family, it was suggested that p97 may have diverged from serum transferrin more than 300 million years ago, when mammalian and avian lineages diverged (Rose et al., 1986).

Functional properties. Although p97 has been named melanotransferrin, it binds far less iron than transferrin and its role played in cellular iron metabolism may differ considerably from that played by circulating serum transferrin and its cellular receptors. The anti-p97 mAb is not effective in antibody-dependent cell-mediated cytotoxicity (ADCC) and cannot mediate complement–dependent cytotoxicity (CDC) with human complement. However, since the gene encoding p97 was cloned, an interesting approach was used to favorably modify the immune response of the tumor-bearing host by inducing strong T-cell help and thus produce an immune response against the tumor. Thus, the gene encoding for p97 was introduced into the vaccinia virus genome to produce an antitumor vaccine vp97. This proved effective in producing an immune response against p97 in mice bearing murine tumor, which had been transfected with the p97 gene and subsequently expressed the p97 antigen. The effectiveness of this vaccine remains to be tested and proven in phase I clinical trials (Hellström and Hellström, 1989).

S-100 Protein

Biochemical and functional characteristics. The S-100 proteins are a group of abundant, low-molecular-weight (10–12 kDa) acid proteins that are highly enriched in nerve tissue. The S-100 fraction contains a mixture of hetero- and homodimers of α and β subunits with different amino acid compositions. These proteins contain two Ca^{++} binding regions known as EF hands. Upon calcium binding, such properties of S-100 protein are altered as α-helix and β-sheet structures, absorption and circular dichroism spectra. No enzymatic functions have been shown for S-100 proteins, and they are thought to exert their biological effects by binding to and modulating effector proteins in a manner similar to calmodulin. Thus, the Ca^{++}–dependent changes in the hydrophobicity of S-100 protein are similar to the Ca^{++}–induced changes in calmodulin. This finding is thought to suggest that S-100–effector protein interaction is mediated through exposure of hydrophobic domains upon Ca^{++} binding (Isobe et al., 1978a, 1978b). Interestingly, in all vertebrates studied, the primary amino acid sequences have been >95% conserved. Such a high structural conservation argues for important and conserved biological function for the S-100 proteins. The various proposed and demonstrated effect of S-100 proteins in cell cycle progression, cell-type differentiation, signal transduction, and morphological differentiation are thought to be mediated by the same basic process. Inhibition of cytoskeletal-associated protein phosphorylation by the S-100 proteins is considered key in controlling all of these biological processes (Kligman and Hilt, 1988).

The S-100 proteins, named for their solubility in saturated ammonium sulfate, were first thought to be present only in neural or neural crest-derived tissues; however, S-100 proteins have also been detected in chondrocytes, adipocytes, myoepithelial cells, dendritic cells of lymphoid tissue, Langerhans cells, and T lymphocytes. They are present in a high proportion of malignant melanomas and neurocytic skin nevi. On melanoma cells, the S-100 protein family is the major species of antigens that are only protein in nature (Gaynor et al., 1980). Thus, the S-100 proteins are a particularly good diagnostic marker for secondary, amelanotic melanoma, whose tumor cells resemble those of other tumors. In identifying melanomas that are otherwise doubtful, antiserum to S-100 proteins is often used in combination with monoclonal antibodies to cellular keratin, to common leukocyte antigens, and to MAA. Malignant melanoma cells express S-100 proteins, but neither cytokeratins nor common leukocyte antigens. Melanoma cells can thus be distinguished from carcinoma cells, which express cytokeratins, but contain only small amounts of S-100 protein and common leukocyte antigens, whereas most lymphoma cells express common leukocyte antigens, but are devoid of S-100 proteins and keratins. This approach also serves to detect occult melanoma cells when conventional histology fails to identify single melanoma cells in lymph nodes regional to melanoma (Kligman and Hilt, 1988).

Ganglioside Antigens

Biochemical and Immunological Characteristics A series of carbohydrates can serve as potential antigens on the surface of cells when attached to either a protein or lipid backbone. The specificity and function of these carbohydrate determinants have been addressed with the use of monoclonal antibodies (Hakamori, 1984, 1985; Cheresh et al., 1985). Numerous studies have characterized monoclonal antibodies directed to the carbohydrate portion of glycolipids, particularly those containing one or more sialic acid residues, that is, gangliosides. Recent technological advances have now made it possible to characterize monoclonal antibodies directed against glycolipids mainly by immunostaining individual glycolipid determinants separated on a thin-layer chromatography plate. This technology compares to indirect immunoprecipitation and/or Western blot analysis, which have facilitated the characterization of monoclonal antibodies directed to numerous protein and glycoprotein antigens (Magnani et al., 1980; Cheresh et al., 1984a, 1984b).

One distinct advantage of monoclonal antibodies directed to carbohydrate antigens is their potential use in establishing a structure–function relationship for these determinants on the tumor cell surface, because monoclonal antibodies can recognize a carbohydrate determinant with known sugar composition and anomeric linkages. Thus, by using monoclonal antibodies to define oligosaccharide structures on the tumor cell surface, one can pose questions regarding the functional properties of these structures as they relate to the malignant or metastatic phenotype. This is much more difficult to do with monoclonal antibodies directed to protein or glycoprotein antigens whose epitopes are in most cases structurally ill defined, since they depend on unpredictable conformation and three-dimensional structure, and their complete primary amino acid sequence frequently is not available.

Human melanoma, which is derived from the neuroectoderm, is rich in ganglioside content. A number of reports have described murine monoclonal antibodies directed to the disialoganglioside GD_3, which is similar in structure to GD_2, but lacks a terminal N-acetylgalactosamine. Early studies described mAb R-24 (IgG_3) (Dippold et al., 1980; Pukel et al., 1982) and 4.2 (IgM) (Nudelman et al., 1982), both of which recognize GD_3 specifically on the surfaces of human melanoma cells. The mAb 4.2 was shown to react with melanoma-associated GD_3 by enzymatic degradation and mass spectrometry, which revealed a carbohydrate moiety identical to brain GD_3, yet its ceramide manifested a predominance of longer chain fatty acids than brain GD_3. It has been suggested that because GD_3 in melanoma contains a longer ceramide moiety, its organization in the membrane probably provokes far greater antigenicity than that of GD_3 in normal cell membranes. Thus, GD_3 in normal cells may be cryptic, whereas in the melanoma membrane it is antigenic, since it is highly exposed (Nudelman et al., 1982).

A number of studies have implicated gangliosides expressed on the surfaces of melanoma cells as potentially relevant antigens in man. In this regard, the "AH antigen" was detected during the initial analysis of the humoral immune response of melanoma patients to autologous melanoma cells. Serum from patient AH reacted with a cell surface antigen expressed by cultured autologous melanoma cells, but not by autologous skin fibroblasts or peripheral blood lymphocytes, and was ultimately identified as the GD_2 ganglioside (Watanabe et al., 1983). In other studies, peripheral blood lymphocytes from melanoma patients transformed into B lymphoblastoid cells by EBV were used as an in vitro source to generate monospecific human IgM antibodies of two kinds, one specifically reactive with disialoganglioside GD_2 (OFA-I-2) (Cahan et al., 1982) and another directed to the monosialyated version, that is, GM_2 (OFA-I-1) (Tai et al., 1983). Attempts to produce human monoclonal antibodies with melanoma cells as immunogen essentially produced only antibodies to gangliosides. The rationale for making human monoclonal antibodies was to avoid human antimouse antibody (HAMA) responses that usually occur when patients are injected with murine monoclonal antibodies and also to obtain the type of reagents that could be used to test any humoral responses of patients to tumor antigens. In contrast to murine monoclonal antibodies, all human monoclonal antibodies to ganglioside that were produced thus far are of IgM isotype. Such antibodies are negative in ADCC-type interactions with human effector cells, but effectively fix human complement. Some human monoclonal antibodies such as AbFCM1 (IgM) and AbHJM1 (IgM), which were more recently produced than OFA-I-2 or OFA-I-1, have more diverse reactivity with gangliosides than either of these two human monoclonal antibodies or murine anti-GD_3 mAb R24 (IgG3) and murine anti-GD_2 mAb 3F8 (IgG3), as well as 14.18 (IgG3), and 14.G2a (IgG2a). Thus, AbFCM1 recognizes mainly GM_3, but also several epitopes on GD_3, GD_2, GD_{1a}, and GT_{1b}. Human mAb AbHJM1 recognizes mainly GD_3, but in contrast to murine, anti-GD_3 mAb R24, it also recognizes epitopes of GD_2 and GD_{1b} (Tai et al., 1985). It is evident that at least at this time, there is no clearly documented advantage of human over murine monoclonal antibodies with the exception of fewer HAMA responses being produced in a very limited number of patients studied thus far with human monoclonal antibodies. Of course, it remains to be seen whether this particular advantage of human over murine monoclonal antibodies will be maintained with the current development of quite a number of mouse/human chimeric antibodies by genetic engineering, since such constructs have also shown very few HAMA responses in as yet a rather limited number of patients (LoBuglio et al., 1989). By engineering mouse/human chimeric antibodies with the appropriate human heavy chains, that is, human γ_1, these antibodies can be much more efficient in mediating

ADCC with human effector cells than their murine counterparts. This was shown with a chimeric antibody to GD_2 (ch14.18) on human melanoma target cells (Mueller et al., 1990b).

Another advantage of the recombinant technology used to construct mouse/human chimeric antibodies is that it allows one to further engineer an antibody molecule and, in this way, manipulate its properties and functions. This was accomplished by engineering anti-GD_2 mAb ch14.18 to decrease its serum half-life, reduce its immunogenicity, delete its effector functions, and thereby make it a potentially useful reagent for radioimaging of tumors. Thus, the constant region of the human $\gamma 1$ chain was mutated by deleting the second domain (CH2). The CH2-deleted antibody (ch14.18-ΔCH2) was cleared from the blood of nude mice bearing human melanoma tumor xenografts with the same kinetics as human IgG $F(ab')_2$. In biodistribution experiments, ^{125}I-labeled ch14.18-ΔCH2 targeted specifically to melanoma xenografts more rapidly and with better localization ratios than the intact mAb ch14.18 (Mueller et al., 1990a).

Murine monoclonal antibodies produced in several laboratories have defined at least five melanoma-associated gangliosides: GD_2, GD_3, 9-O-acetylated GD_3, GM_2, and GM_3 (Reisfeld and Cheresh, 1987; Ravindranath and Irie, 1988). Gangliosides GD_2 and GD_3 are also shed by melanoma cells, but usually form micelles in the circulation and have to be extracted with chloroform-methanol before they can be recognized by antiganglioside monoclonal antibodies (Schulz et al., 1984). The ganglioside GD_2, thus determined in extracts of serum of melanoma patients, ranges from 24 to 85 ng/mL of serum, while GD_3 ranges from 10 to 30 ng/mL of serum (Sela et al., 1989). The serum of neuroblastoma patients contains considerably more GD_2, reaching up to >4,000 ng/mL and the appearance of this antigen in the serum correlated with tumor size and stage of disease (Schulz et al., 1984).

In terms of reactivity of antiganglioside, monoclonal antibodies with human melanoma cells and tissues, the use of anti-GD_3 mAb R24 in conjunction with an indirect immunoperoxidase-staining technique on 175 cryopreserved, unfixed human tissue sections, established a striking specificity for malignant melanoma. Thus, 21 of 21 primary and 37 of 37 malignant melanoma tissue sections contained GD_3. Among the numerous normal tissues examined, 9 of 11 nevi were GD_3 positive, and melanocytes in the basal layer of the skin stained weakly. Although GD_3 is heavily expressed on most human melanoma cells examined, it is also present on other cell types derived from the neuroectoderm (Houghton et al., 1985). Another mAb D1.1, that was originally generated against an undifferentiated rat neuronal tumor cell line reacts specifically with a 9-O-acetylated form of the disialoganglioside GD_3. The expression of this antigen is even more restricted to human melanoma cells than that of GD_3, since mAb D1.1 does not react with normal melanocytes, fetal or adult brain tissue, or normal skin (Levine et al., 1984; Cheresh et al., 1984b).

Monoclonal antibodies directed to ganglioside GD_2, such as 126-4 (IgM) (Schulz et al., 1984) and 14.18 (IgG3), 14.G2a (IgG2a) (Mujoo et al., 1987, 1989), and 3F8 (IgG3) (Cheung et al., 1985), generally react well by standard ELISA technique with most cultured human melanoma and neuroblastoma cell, as well as with several glioma and small-cell lung cancer cell lines. These antibodies generally fail to react in this assay with most cell lines derived from other tumors, from T-cell lines and B-lymphoblastoid–cell lines. Tissue reactivity of these antibodies follows along similar lines.

A most comprehensive profile of ganglioside distribution in human melanoma tissues was provided by extensive studies of 80 melanoma specimens, including 52 surgical specimens and 28 cultured cell lines. In this case, ganglioside fractions were isolated and purified from each of these tissues and the amount of each component ganglioside was assessed by thin-layer chromatography. The most commonly expressed gangliosides on these specimens were GM_3, GD_3, GM_2, and GD_2. The distribution of each ganglioside was found to be widely heterogeneous and the total amount of ganglioside ranged from 33 to 302 μg/g wet weight tissue. In this particular study, GM_2 and GD_2 were relatively minor components of biopsied melanomas, but often became major components of cultured melanoma cells; however, alkali-labile gangliosides, such as 9-O-acetylated GD_3, were usually more strongly expressed on biopsied melanomas than on cultured melanoma cells (Tsuchida et al., 1987).

Functional Properties The actual function of glycolipids on the cell surface has not been completely delineated, although several researchers using biochemical and immunochemical approaches have proposed that glycolipids (particularly gangliosides) are involved in cell–substratum interactions. Evidence that some gangliosides may be involved in cell-adhesion processes comes from experiments in which anti-GD_3 mAb MB3.6 and anti-GD_2 mAb 126 localized each of these gangliosides in focal adhesion plaques and on the surfaces of human melanoma cells. Indirect immunofluorescence of human melanoma cells stained with mAb 126 exhibits intense surface fluorescence, as well as specific staining of membrane-associated microprocesses. These structures emanate from the plasma membrane and, in some cases, appear to make contact with the substrate to which these cells are attached. It has also been established that GD_2 and GD_3 are involved in a generalized mechanism of melanoma cell attachment. Thus, anti-GD_2, as well as anti-GD_3, were capable of inhibiting the attachment of human melanoma and neuroblastoma cells to a variety of immobilized extracellular matrix components including fibronectin, vitronectin, collagen, and laminin (Cheresh et al., 1986).

The role of gangliosides in melanoma cell attachment to a more physiological substrate has also been examined. Thus, pretreatment of human melanoma cells with anti-GD_2 antibody resulted in 92% inhibition of attachment to a matrix of bovine endothelial cells laid down on tissue culture plastic. Kinetic analysis of this inhibition suggested that these gangliosides were involved in the initial phases of the cell attachment process. Moreover, these monoclonal antibodies induced cell rounding and loss of attachment by cells preadhered and spread on a fibronectin substrate (Cheresh et al., 1986). This observation was also made with anti-GD_3 mAb R24 (IgG3), which induces similar melanoma cell rounding from tissue culture plastic (Dippold et al., 1984). In contrast, monoclonal antibodies directed to other determinants on the cell surface fail to alter the cells' adhesive properties, indicating that the inhibitory effects observed were not simply due to monoclonal antibody binding to any antigen on the cell surface. Ultrastructural analysis of human melanoma cell attachment using both scanning and transmission immunoelectron microscopy demonstrated that GD_2 gangliosides were preferentially expressed on cell membrane–associated microprocesses in direct contact with the substrate upon which the cells were attached. In fact, an actual gradient of antigen expression could be observed where ganglioside expression increased on the microprocesses as they neared the substrate. Additional evidence suggests that both GD_2 and GD_3 can interact directly with melanoma cell surface glycoprotein receptors for fibronectin or vitronectin; thus, this interaction may potentiate the appropriate receptor configuration leading to optimal cell attachment (Cheresh and Klier, 1986).

A number of anti-GD_2 and GD_3 murine monoclonal antibodies of either IgG3 or IgG2a isotype were shown to effectively mediate ADCC with a variety of effector cells and also mediate complement–dependent cytoxicity with human complement. Some of these same antibodies, that is, anti-GD_3 mAb R24 (IgG3) (Houghton et al., 1985) and ME36.1 (IgG2a) (Sela et al., 1989), produced regressions of melanoma tumors in phase I clinical trials and anti-GD_2 mAb 3F8 (IgG3) did the same in clinical trials with neuroblastoma patients (Cheung et al., 1987). Several mechanisms were proposed that could account for this tumor progression. Initially, humoral immunity was suggested as a mechanism because the monoclonal antibodies used in these phase I clinical trials mediate CDC, and increased amounts of C9 were found in regressing tumor lesions (Houghton et al., 1985). However, more recently, mechanisms of cellular immunity were proposed, since the tumor regression took many weeks and because subpopulations of peripheral T lymphocytes expressed GD_3. Such T cells could be activated in vitro by mAb R24 or its $F(ab')_2$ fragment to proliferate and express interleukin (IL)-2 receptors even when cultures were depleted of macrophages. Another indication that this type of mechanism may have been operative came from the finding that any tumor regression achieved by mAb R24 was dose-limiting and was effective only at lower doses of antibody, since larger doses could putatively kill GD_3-bearing T cells by complement-mediated lysis (Welte et al., 1987). Yet another possible mechanism could be invoked based on the finding that not only some peripheral T lymphocytes express gangliosides (Hersey et al., 1986, 1987), but GD_2 was also expressed on tumor-infiltrating lymphocytes (TIL), which had been shown to be such important factors in melanoma tumor regression when activated ex vivo by IL-2. Whatever the mechanism(s) that will finally be shown as relevant, it is important to realize that murine monoclonal antibodies, directed to gangliosides GD_2 and GD_3, as well as human antibodies to GD_2, are thus far the only antibodies that could achieve measurable tumor regression of tumors in melanoma and neuroblastoma patients.

There seems to be little doubt that gangliosides react more frequently than any other monoclonal antibody–defined MAA with the host immune system. This is evident, as human anti-GD_2 antibodies have been isolated from sera of tumor-bearing patients and human monoclonal antibodies to GD_2, GM_2, and GM_3 have been produced by lymphocytes obtained from melanoma patients (Ravindranath and Irie, 1988). Also, after immunization with melanoma cells, patients developed antibodies to GD_2 and GM_2. Thus, gangliosides may well play a potentially important role in growth regulation and differentiation of melanoma cells, similar to the stimulatory effect of gangliosides on the proliferation of astroglial cells.

Growth Factor Receptors

Growth factor receptors have been found on cultured human tumor cell lines and human tumor tissues. Even though these receptors are not specific for malignant cells, their number can be orders of magnitude higher on tumor cells than on normal cells. A mitogenic effect could be shown for some growth factors on human tumor cells under tissue culture conditions. Some growth factor receptors are homologous to the products of viral oncogenes, e.g., the epidermal growth factor receptor (EGFr) that is coded for by the proto-oncogene *v-erb-B2*. Therefore, it has been speculated that there may be a link between the abundance of these receptor molecules on tumor cells and neoplastic transformation and cell proliferation. Human malignant melanoma cells have been shown to express EGFr, as well as receptors for nerve growth factor (NGFr) and α-melanocyte-stimulating hormone (α-MSH receptor) (Herlyn et al., 1987; Goustin et al., 1986; Herlyn and Koprowski, 1988).

EGFr is a transmembrane mitogenic glycoprotein of 170 kDa with an intracellular tyrosine protein kinase site that is activated by growth factor binding to the extracellular domain. The natural ligands for EGFr are EGF and transforming growth factor-alpha (TGF-α). Monoclonal antibodies to EGFr have been obtained by immunizing mice with the human squamous cell carcinoma cell line A431. Among these antibodies are those that inhibit the binding of EGF to EGFr and some that mimic the mitogenic effect of EGF on tumor cell lines. These anti-EGFr antibodies were used to demonstrate EGFr on the surface of several human melanoma cell lines. While normal melanocytes do not express EGFr, its expression on melanoma cell lines is related to the expression of phenotypic markers of cell differentiation. Less-differentiated melanoma cell lines appearing to be of epithelioid morphology are unpigmented and often express EGFr. In contrast, more highly differentiated, pigmented cell lines with a dendritic morphology do not express EGFr (Real et al., 1986). Whereas EGF has been described to be mitogenic for freshly isolated metastatic melanoma cells, their responsiveness to EGF seems to disappear in long-term tissue culture. In situ, the presence of EGFr has been correlated with malignancy, exhibiting its highest expression on advanced metastatic lesions (Stoscheck and King, 1986; Mendelsohn, 1988).

As far as the expression of EGFr on undifferentiated melanoma cells is concerned, an amelanotic cell line, M24met, expresses 290,000 such molecules per cell. Moreover, EGFr on these highly undifferentiated cells presents a potential target for antibody-mediated therapy. Thus, anti-EGFr mAb 425 was reported to specifically suppress the spontaneous metastasis of human M24met cells to lymph nodes and lungs in mice with severe combined immunodeficiency (Mueller et al., 1991).

Nerve growth factor is of importance for regulating the development of neurons, and NGFr is also expressed by some tumors that are derived from the neural crest. Monoclonal antibodies against NGFr have been raised in mice using human melanoma cell lines such as A875 and WM245 as immunogens. Such antibodies made it possible to detect NGFr in the cytoplasm and on the plasma membrane of human melanoma cells, from where it could be immunoprecipitated as a 75-kDa glycoprotein. Histochemical analysis indicated that although normal melanocytes fail to express NGFr, they are expressed on both common and dysplastic nevi, as well as by primary and metastatic melanoma cells (Ross et al., 1984).

Human melanoma cell lines also produce a number of cytokines and growth factors such as TGF-α and TGF-β, platelet-derived growth factor (PDGF), fibroblast growth factor (FGF), melanoma growth-stimulating activity (MGSA) and interleukin-1 (IL-1). An autocrine function has been proposed for most of these factors, which is thought to influence tumor growth with positive and negative signals. However, an appropriate surface receptor for these growth factors has not yet been described on human melanoma cells (Herlyn et al., 1987).

HLA Class II Antigens

The distribution of HLA class II antigens on human cells is generally more restricted than the occurrence of HLA class I antigens that are expressed on virtually all nucleated cells. The HLA class II antigens are mainly found on lymphocytes and antigen-presenting cells, that is, activated T cell, B cell, monocytes, epidermal Langerhans cells, interdigitating and dendritic reticulum cells, and vascular endothelial cells (Ruiter et al., 1984). However, HLA class II antigens cannot be detected on melanocytes found in tissue sections of normal skin. Cultured melanocytes also fail to express HLA class II and do not contain messenger RNA (mRNA) specific for HLA class II genes, but expression of HLA class II, that is, HLA-DR, DQ, and DP can readily be induced with inteferon (Taramelli et al., 1986). In contrast, approximately 70% of human melanoma cell lines express HLA class II antigens. The expression of these antigens in surgically removed benign and malignant melanoma lesions has been described by many investigators (for review, see Natali et al., 1987). Although HLA class II is rarely observed on melanocytic nevi and detected only by some investigators on dysplastic nevi, it is frequently observed in primary and metastatic lesions. Yet, it is not clear whether the appearance of HLA class II molecules on melanoma cells reflects the stage of differentiation of the melanocytes from which these tumor cells have originated or if it is induced by the malignant process. The level of expression of HLA class II antigens in primary and metastatic melanoma lesions was suggested to correlate with the clinical course of the disease. Thus, the expression of HLA-DR antigen on >20% of tumor cells in a primary lesion correlated with increasing tumor thickness and independent thereof also with an earlier occurrence of metastatic disease (Taramelli et al., 1986; Broecker et al., 1984).

ANTIGEN EXPRESSION DURING MELANOMA TUMOR PROGRESSION

Cutaneous melanoma is both clinically and experimentally one of the best studied solid human tumors. The biological foundation of much of this research has come from studies on tumor progression based on histopathological studies of tumor lesions at six different steps (Clark levels) of tumor progression. Briefly, this starts with the acquired melanocyte nevus, which lacks any architectural or cytological atypia. In step two of this progression, the melanocyte nevus acquires architectural, but no cytological, atypia. Step three features the dysplastic nevus with both architectural and cytological atypia. Both melanocyte and dysplastic nevi are considered precursor lesions of melanoma, although they usually differentiate and disappear. In clear distinction, step four of this tumor progression is represented by the radical growth phase of primary melanoma, which lacks competence for metastasis and its surgical excision usually leads to the cure of cutaneous melanoma. However, during the radical growth phase (RGP), focal lesions may arise that ultimately lead to the vertical growth phase (VGP) of primary melanoma, that is, step five, with acquired competence for metastasis. The incidence of melanoma metastasis is directly related to the thickness of the VGP lesion (Breslow index). Finally, the sixth step of tumor is characterized by the development of extensive metastasis (Herlyn et al., 1987).

It has been a major objective of tumor immunology to identify "tumor-associated" antigens, that is, antigens that may be expressed only on malignant tumors or on particular stages of tumor progression. Such antigens would be useful for tumor diagnosis, and the identification of their biochemical nature might elucidate mechanisms or attribute to a neoplastic phenotype.

As far as the expression of MAA discussed in this article with regard to melanoma tumor progression is concerned, none of the monoclonal antibodies directed against these antigens is exclusively reactive with cells from advanced malignant lesions. Most antigens can be detected on at least a few melanocytic cells in benign lesions, or on normal melanocytes. Among these are the p97 antigen, CSP, and the ganglioside GD_3. While these antigens are not restricted to malignant cells, their expression increases in the malignant process. It should also be noted that these three antigens can be detected on melanoma biopsies of almost all patients. Thus, using immunoperoxidase staining on frozen tissue sections, monoclonal antibodies directed against CSP are not reactive with normal skin melanocytes, but show strong reactivity with essentially 100% of all nevocellular nevi, dysplastic nevi, and melanomas investigated. There is some inconsistency in the literature regarding the expression of these MAA, including GD_3 and 9-O-acetyl GD_3 on melanocytes and nevi cells. This may be due to either using monoclonal antibodies that differ in affinity and avidity or to differences in the sensitivity of the staining method used and also to a different antigen expression in situ versus cultured-skin melanocytes (Herlyn and Koprowski, 1988).

Monoclonal antibodies to other MAA discriminate benign from malignant neoplastic melanocytes. Thus, ganglioside antigen GD_2, HLA-DR, the EGFr, and the adhesion molecules ICAM-1 and N-CAM are found in only a low percentage of nevi and primary melanoma below 0.75 mm thickness. They appear to be mainly restricted to the two latest stages of melanoma progression, VGP primary melanoma and metastatic melanoma. Thus, the average proportion of tumors reactive with either anti-HLA-DR, anti-ICAM-1, or anti-N-CAM is 40% for melanomas between 0.76 and 1.50 mm in thickness, 60% for those between 1.51 and 3.0 mm, and 80% for the group above 3.0 mm. The frequency of melanomas coexpressing various combinations of these three antigens increases in proportion to the tumor thickness. The increase in the number of primary melanomas expressing ICAM-1 or N-CAM according to their thickness is accompanied by an increase in the percentage of positive cells per tumor, whereas HLA-DR is expressed by a fairly constant fraction of tumor cells. These findings imply that expression of different antigen during tumor progression is a quantitative rather than a qualitative phenomenon. It has to be considered that antigens associated with certain stages are present in earlier stages, but below the threshold of detection (Herlyn et al., 1987).

Some MAA are also shed from the tumor cells. Shedding increases with the amount of surface expression. Generally, antigens that are structural compounds of the plasma membrane, like MAA proteoglycan and the ganglioside antigens, are shed to a larger degree than receptor antigens, such as melanotransferrin or EGFr. This observation may have some significance for tumor diagnosis when using MAA as tumor markers or as probes for tumor imaging, where the first requires antigen shed into the bloodstream and the latter should be done preferentially with an antigen that is not shed to any large extent. Also for tumor therapy, monoclonal antibodies against antigens that are not shed may be preferred to obtain better tumor targeting. The practical usefulness of monoclonal antibodies against MAA is determined by the expression of these antigens in tumor progression. Whereas antigens expressed strongly on many or all tumor cells in the advanced stage of melanoma progression should be considered for antibody-directed tumor therapy, expression of ICAM-1 and HLA-DR in primary lesions has been shown to correlate with early occurrence of metastatic disease and may be used as a prognostic marker (Herlyn and Koprowski, 1988).

In summary, MAA and the monoclonal antibodies directed against them have provided, thus far, a basis for an extensive investigation of molecular and cellular mechanisms of tumor invasion and progression that will likely continue well into the next decade. It can only be hoped that this approach will continue to yield basic information that may lead to further advances in cancer research.

PERSPECTIVES

An attempt was made in the preceding discussion to provide a critical appraisal of some of the antigens associated with human cutaneous melanoma whose structure and functional properties have been characterized to some extent by murine monoclonal antibodies directed against these tumor cell-surface markers. It has been pointed out in this discussion that the field of MAA is mainly driven by biological questions;

however, the choice of antigens to be studied depends entirely on the monoclonal antibodies that ultimately emerge as the result of immunizing mice with a given immunogen that usually is either a cultured human melanoma cell, melanoma tissues, or relatively crude extracts obtained from either of these sources. This experimental approach proved to be highly useful and was in the best tradition of the hybridoma technique developed by Köhler and Milstein (1975); however, even this elegant and extremely valuable technology has certain limitations. Thus, when antibody-secreting murine lymphocytes are fused with an immortal myeloma cell line producing hybridomas, one can obtain only a relatively limited number of fused cells ranging from a few hundred to a few thousand. There is also a limit to the number of such cells that can be screened in a reasonable period of time by commonly available technologies. Also, if human monoclonal antibodies are required to possibly define unique antigen epitopes, it has been relatively difficult to produce such reagents with high binding affinity by the Köhler-Milstein approach, since most in vitro immunization procedures have not been optimally effective for this purpose.

The need to produce monoclonal antibodies for cancer therapy that do not evoke an antiisotype, that is, HAMA response, has provided the impetus for the production of chimeric human/mouse antibodies by protein engineering. This has been achieved by either joining the entire immunoglobulin variable (V) domains from mouse monoclonal antibodies to human constant (C) domains (Neuberger et al., 1984; Morrison, 1985; Sahagan et al., 1986; Liu et al., 1987; Sun et al., 1987; Gillies et al., 1989) or by transplanting the complementary-determining regions (CDR) of the mouse monoclonal antibodies into human myeloma proteins (Riechmann et al., 1988). In this manner, the rearranged Ig-V genes provide the starting material for engineering and they have been derived from either genomic DNA or cDNA. This process was made more efficient by designing a set of oligonucleotide primers to amplify the cDNA of mouse immunoglobulin heavy and light chain variable domains by the polymerase chain reaction (PCR) (Orlandi et al., 1989; Ward et al., 1989). This new technology can lead to the cloning of antigenic specificities directly from immunoglobulin genes. Thus, diverse heavy and light chain variable domains (V_H) with good binding affinities could be prepared, for example, 10^7 M^{-1} for lysozyme that can possibly be further improved by site-directed mutagenesis (Ward et al., 1989). A possible disadvantage of these "single domain antibodies" (dAb) is that V_H domains are relatively "sticky," because of hydrophobic surfaces that are usually capped by V_κ or V_λ domains; however, V_H domains with binding activity have been proposed as building blocks for producing Fv fragments or complete antibodies. This is envisioned to be accomplished by coexpressing V_H domains with a repertoire of V_κ domains, derived by PCR amplification of V_κ genes followed by screening for association of the domains and antigen binding (Ward et al., 1989).

Although the novel methods for the production of monoclonal antibodies described by Orlandi et al. (1989) and by Ward et al. (1989) are conceptually exciting and promising for future development, they have some limitations in addition to those already mentioned by these two groups of investigators. Thus, the use of V_H fragments may be further limited, since it is known from available crystal structures of antibody–antigen complexes that there is much contact between antigen and V_L, as well as V_H domains. It is also known from other studies that the V_L domain provides contacts critical to antigen binding (Davies et al., 1988; Wallick et al., 1989). Thus, it is somewhat unlikely that the affinity of V_H fragments will match that of intact antibodies. Furthermore, the large hydrophobic area created on the face of the V_H fragment by the absence of the V_L domain is likely to lead to increased nonspecificity relative to whole antibodies (Ward et al., 1989; Orlandi et al., 1989).

Considering all these limitations, another method was designed to overcome at least some of them and may indeed supersede present-day hybridoma technology. Thus, since individual Fab molecules had already been expressed and assembled in *Escherichia coli* (Better et al., 1988; Skerra and Plückthun, 1988), an approach was developed to mimick antibody diversity in vitro by expressing the repertoires of heavy and light chains in combination (Huse et al., 1989). In this case, a novel bacteriophage lambda vector system was used to express in *E. coli* a large combinatorial library of Fab fragments of the mouse antibody repertoire. This resulted in a large number of monoclonal Fab fragments against a transition state analog hapten, since it was feasible to construct and screen at least three orders of magnitude more of the antibody clones with monospecificity than was previously possible (Huse et al., 1989).

In the last two years, there have been a great number of advances made in developing elegant methods designed to generate many human monoclonal antibodies of interest by repertoire cloning. Thus, combinatorial libraries of antibody heavy and light chains derived from peripheral blood lymphocytes of an individual immunized with tetanus toxoid were expressed in *E. coli* by using phage λ vectors. Screening of such libraries identified a number of human monoclonal Fab fragments specific for tetanus toxoid (Persson et al., 1991). Recently, a very key advance was made by the development of a most effective method based on a phagemid vector with helper phage rescue for the construction and very rapid analysis of antibody Fab libraries (Kang et al., 1991). In this case, antibody genes are expressed in concert with phage morphogenesis, allowing incorporation of functional Fab molecules along the surface of filamentous phage. This new phagemid M13 system now allows one to realize the full power of the combinatorial system. Unlike the λ vector system developed earlier (Huse et al., 1989) that allows for screening of only 0.1% to 1% of library members and generates only monovalent Fab, the new system can screen all the members of a similar-sized library by affinity selection and generates multivalent particles, thereby allowing the capture of a wider range of affinities (Kang et al., 1991).

Based on these advances in technology, one can anticipate in the near future a large number of new monoclonal antibodies that define human tumor-associated antigens with novel functional properties that may contribute to a better understanding of the mechanisms involved in tumor invasion and metastasis. It can only be hoped that such advances will ultimately lead to the development of new and exciting concepts that will truly advance progress in cancer research well into the next century.

ACKNOWLEDGMENTS

The work described in this manuscript was supported by a grant from the National Institutes of Health, CA42508. This is The Scripps Research Institute manuscript number 6349-IMM.

REFERENCES

Better M, Chang CP, Robinson R, et al. *Escherichia coli* secretion of an active chimeric antibody fragment. Science. 1988;240:1041–1043.

Broecker EB, Suter L, Sorg C. HLA-DR antigen expression in primary melanomas of the skin. J Invest Dermatol. 1984;82:244–247.

Brown JP, Nishiyama K, Hellström I, Hellström KE. Structural characterization of human melanoma-associated antigen p97 using monoclonal antibodies. J Immunol. 1981;127:539–546.

Brown JP, Hewick RM, Hellström I, Hellström KE, Doolittle RF, Dreyer WJ. Human melanoma-associated antigen p97 is structurally and functionally related to transferrin. Nature. 1982;296:171–173.

Brown E, Hooper L, Ho T, Gresham H. Integrin-associated protein: a 50 kDa plasma membrane antigen physically and functionally associated with integrins. J Cell Biol. 1991, in press.

Bumol TF, Reisfeld RA. A unique glycoprotein-proteoglycan complex defined by monoclonal antibody on human melanoma cells. Proc Natl Acad Sci USA. 1982;79:1245–1249.

Bumol TF, Walker LE, Reisfeld RA. Bio-synthetic studies of proteoglycans on human melanoma cells with a monoclonal antibody to a core glycoprotein of chondroitin sulfate proteoglycans. J Biol Chem. 1984;259:12733–12739.

Cahan LD, Irie RF, Singh R, Cassidenti A, Paulson JC. Identification of a human neuroectodermal tumor antigen (OFA-I-2) as ganglioside GD_2. Proc Natl Acad Sci USA. 1982;79: 7629–7633.

Chattopadhey P, Kavery S-V, Byan N, et al. Human high molecular weight-melanoma associated antigen mimicry by an anti-idiotypic antibody: characterization of the immunogenicity and the immune response to the mouse monoclonal antibody IMEL-1. Cancer Res. 1991; 51:6045–6051.

Cheresh DA, Harper JR, Schulz G, Reisfeld RA. Localization of the gangliosides GD_2 and GD_3 in adhesion plaques and on the surface of human melanoma cells. Proc Natl Acad Sci USA. 1984a;81:5767–5881.

Cheresh DA, Reisfeld RA, Varki AP. O-acetylation of disialoganglioside GD_3 by human melanoma cells creates a unique antigenic determinant. Science. 1984b;225:844–846.

Cheresh DA, Honsik CJ, Staffileno LK, Jung G, Reisfeld RA. Disialoganglioside GD3 on human melanoma cell serves as a relevant target antigen for monoclonal antibody-induced cytotoxicity in vitro and immunotherapy in vivo. Proc Natl Acad Sci USA. 1985;82:5155–5159.

Cheresh DA, Herzig M, Pierschbacher MD, Mujoo K. Disialogangliosides GD_2 and GD_3 are involved in the binding of human melanoma and neuroblastoma cells to extracellular matrix proteins. J Cell Biol. 1986;102:688–698.

Cheresh DA, Klier FG. Disialoganglioside GD_2 distributes preferentially into substrate-associated microprocesses of human melanoma cells during their attachment to fibronectin. J Cell Biol. 1986;102:1887–1897.

Cheresh DA. Human endothelial cells synthesize and express an Arg-Gly-Asp directed adhesion receptor involved in attachment to fibrinogen and von Willebrand factor. Proc Natl Acad Sci USA. 1987;84:6471–6475.

Cheresh DA, Pytela R, Klier FG, et al. An Arg-Gly-Asp-directed receptor on the surface of human melanoma cells exists in a functional complex with the disialoganglioside GD2. J Cell Biol. 1987;105:1163–1173.

Cheresh DA, Spiro RC. Biosynthetic and functional properties of an Arg-Gly-Asp-directed receptor involved in human melanoma cell attachment to vitronectin, fibrinogen, and von Willebrand factor. J Biol Chem. 1987;262:17703–17711.

Cheung NKV, Saarinen UM, Neely J, Landmeier B, Donovan D, Coccia PF. Monoclonal antibodies to a glycolipid antigen on human neuroblastoma cells. Cancer Res. 1985;45:2642–2649.

Cheung NKV, Lazarus H, Miraldi FD, et al. Ganglioside GD_2 specific monoclonal antibody 3F8: A phase I study in patients with neuroblastoma and malignant melanoma. J Clin Oncol. 1987;5:1430–1440.

Conforti G, Zanetti A, Pasquali-Ronchetti I, et al. Modulation of vitronectin receptor binding by membrane lipid composition. J Biol Chem. 1990;265:4011–4019.

Davies DR, Sheriff S, Padlan EA. Antibody–antigen complexes. J Biol Chem. 1988;263: 10541–10544.

Dippold WG, Lloyd KO, Li LTC, Ikeda H, Oettgen HF, Old LJ. Cell surface antigens of human malignant melanoma: definition of six antigenic systems with mouse monoclonal antibodies. Proc Natl Acad Sci USA. 1980;77:6114–6118.

Dippold WG, Knuth A, Meyer zum Büschenfeld KH. Inhibition of human melanoma cell growth in vitro by monoclonal anti-GD_3 ganglioside antibody. Cancer Res. 1984;44:806–813.

Dustin ML, Springer TA. Lymphocyte function-associated antigen-1 (LFA-1) interaction with intercellular adhesion molecule-1 (ICAM-1) is one of at least three mechanisms for lymphocyte adhesion to cultured endothelial cells. J Cell Biol. 1988;107:321–331.

Elices MJ, Osborn L, Takada Y, et al. VCAM-1 on activated endothelium interacts with the leukocyte integrin VLA-4 at a site distinct from the VLA-4/fibronectin binding site. Cell. 1990;60:577–584.

Gaynor R, Irie R, Morton D, Herschman HR. S100 protein is present in cultured human malignant melanomas. Nature. 1980;286:400–401.

Gillies SD, Lo KM, Wesolowski T. High level expression of chimeric antibodies using adapted cDNA variable region cassettes. J Immunol Methods. 1989;125:191–202.

Goustin AS, Leof EB, Shipley GD, Moses HL. Growth factors and cancer. Cancer Res. 1986;46:1015–1029.

Guan J-L, Hynes RO. Lymphoid cells recognize an alternatively spliced segment of fibronectin via the integrin receptor $\alpha4\beta1$. Cell. 1990;60:53–61.

Hakamori SI. Tumor-associated carbohydrate antigens. Annu Rev Immunol. 1984;2:103–126.

Hakamori SI. Aberrant glycosylation in cancer cell membranes as focused on glycolipids: overview and perspectives. Cancer Res. 1985;45:2405–2414.

Harper JR, Bumol TF, Reisfeld RA. Serological and biochemical analyses of monoclonal antibodies to human melanoma-associated antigens. Hybridoma. 1982;14:423–427.

Harper JR, Reisfeld RA. Inhibition of anchorage-independent growth of human melanoma cells by a monoclonal antibody to a chondroitin sulfate proteoglycan. J Natl Cancer Inst. 1983; 71:259–262.

Harper JR, Quaranta V, Reisfeld RA. Biosynthesis and intracellular transport of proteoglycan coreprotein by human melanoma cells: involvement of low-pH mechanisms. In: Reddi AH, ed. Extracellular matrix: structure and function. New York, NY: Alan R Liss, Inc.; 1985: 367–372.

Harper JR, Quaranta V, Reisfeld RA. Ammonium chloride interferes with a distinct step in the biosynthesis and cell surface expression of human melanoma-type chondroitin sulfate proteoglycan. J Biol Chem. 1986;261:3600–3606.

Hellström KE, Hellström I. Immunological approaches to tumor therapy: monoclonal antibodies, tumor vaccines, and anti-idiotypes. In: Quash GA, Rodwell JD, eds. Covalently modified antigens and antibodies in diagnosis and therapy. New York, NY: Marcel Dekker, Inc.; 1989:1–39.

Herlyn M, Clark WH, Rodeck U, Mancianti ML, Jambrosic J, Koprowski H. Biology of tumor progression in human melanocytes. Laboratory Inv. 1987;56:461–465.

Herlyn M, Koprowski H. Melanoma antigens: immunological and biological characterization and clinical significance. Annu Rev Immunol. 1988;6:283–308.

Hersey P, Schibeci SD, Townsend P, Burns P, Cheresh DA. Potentiation of lymphocyte responses by monoclonal antibodies to the ganglioside GD3. Cancer Res. 1986;46:6083–6090.

Hersey P, Townsend P, Burns C, Cheresh DA. Enhancement of cytotoxic and proliferative responses of lymphocytes from melanoma patients by incubation with monoclonal antibodies against ganglioside GD_3. Cancer Immunol Immunother. 1987;24:144–150.

Houghton AN, Mintzer D, Cordon-Cardo C, Welt S, Fliegel B, Vadham S, et al. Mouse monoclonal IgG3 antibody detecting GD_3 ganglioside—a phase I trial in patients with malignant melanoma. Proc Natl Acad Sci USA. 1985;82:1242–1246.

Huse WD, Sastry L, Iverson SA, et al. Generation of a large combinatorial library of the immunoglobulin repertoire in phage lambda. Science. 1989;24:1275–1281.

Imai K, Ng AK, Ferrone S. Characterization of monoclonal antibodies to human melanoma-associated antigens. J Natl Cancer Inst. 1981;66:489–496.

Isobe T, Tsugita A, Okuyama T. The amino acid sequence and the subunit structure of bovine brain S100 protein (PAP1-b). J Neurochem. 1987a;30:921–923.

Isobe T, Okuyama T. The amino-acid sequence of S100 protein (PAP1-b protein) and its relation to the calcium-binding proteins. Eur J Biochem. 1987b;89:379–388.

Johnson JP, Stade BG, Holzmann B, Schwable W, Riethmuller G. De novo expression of intercellular-adhesion molecule 1 in melanoma correlates with increased risk of metastasis. Proc Natl Acad Sci USA. 1989;86:641–645.

Kang AS, Barbas CF, Janda KD, et al. Linkage of recognition and replication functions by assembling combinatorial Fab libraries along phage surfaces. Proc Natl Acad Sci USA. 1991;88:4363–4366.

Kantor RRS, Ng AK, Giacomini P, Ferrone S. Analysis of the NIH workshop monoclonal antibodies to human melanoma antigens. Hybridoma. 1982;1:473–482.

Kligman D, Hilt DC. The S-100 protein family. Trends Biochem Sci. 1988;11:437-439.

Köhler G, Milstein C. Continuous cultures of fused cells secreting antibody of predefined specificity. Nature. 1975;256:495–498.

Levine JM, Beasley L, Stallcup WB. The D1.1 antigen: a cell surface marker for germinal cells of the central nervous system. J Neurosci. 1984;4:820–831.

Liu AY, Robinson RR, et al. Chimeric mouse-human IgG1 antibody that can mediate lysis of cancer cells. Proc Natl Acad Sci USA. 1987;84:3439–3443.

LoBuglio AF, Wheeler RH, Trang J, et al. Mouse/human chimeric monoclonal antibody in man: kinetics and immune response. Proc Natl Acad Sci USA. 1989;86:4220–4224.

Magnani JL, Smith DF, Ginsburg V. Detection of gangliosides that bind cholera toxin: direct binding of ^{125}I-labeled toxin to thin layer chromatograms. Anal Biochem. 1980;109:399–402.

Maio M, Tessitori G, Pinto A, Temponi M, Colombalti A, Ferrone S. Differential role of distinct determinants of intercellular adhesion molecule-1 in immunologic phenomena. J Immunol. 1989a;143:181–188.

Maio M, Gulwani B, Tombessi S, Ferrone S. Modulation by cytokines of HL-A antigen, intracellular adhesion molecule 1 and high molecular weight melanoma antigen expression and of immune lysis of clones derived from the melanoma cell line MEM 50-10. Cancer Immunol Immunother. 1989b;30:34–42.

Mendelsohn J. Growth factor receptors as targets for antitumor therapy with monoclonal antibodies. In: Waldman H, ed. Monoclonal antibody therapy progress in allergy. Basel: Karger; 1988:147–160.

Morgan Jr AC, Galloway DR, Reisfeld RA. Production and characterization of monoclonal antibody to a melanoma specific glycoprotein. Hybridoma. 1981;11:27–32.

Morrison SL. Transfectomas provide novel chimeric antibodies. Science. 1985;229:1202–1204.

Mueller BM, Reisfeld RA, Gillies SD. Serum half-life and tumor localization of a chimeric antibody deleted of the CH2 domain and directed against disialoganglioside GD2. Proc Natl Acad Sci USA. 1990a;87:5702–5705.

Mueller BM, Romerdahl CA, Gillies SD, Reisfeld RA. Enhancement of antibody-dependent cytotoxicity with a chimeric anti-GD2 antibody. J Immunol. 1990b;144:1382–1386.

Mueller BM, Romerdahl CA, Trent JM, Reisfeld RA. Suppression of spontaneous melanoma metastasis in scid mice with an antibody to the epidermal growth factor receptor. Cancer Res. 1991;51:2193–2198.

Mujoo K, Cheresh DA, Yang HM, Reisfeld RA. Disialoganglioside GD2 on human neuroblastoma cells: a target antigen for monoclonal antibody–mediated cytolysis and suppression of tumor growth. Cancer Res. 1987;47:1098–1104.

Mujoo K, Kipps TJ, Yang HM, et al. Functional properties and effect of growth suppression of human neuroblastoma tumors by isotype switch variants of monoclonal antiganglioside GD2 antibody 14.18. Cancer Res. 1989;49:2857–2864.

Natali P, Bigotti A, Cavaliere R, Ruiter DJ, Ferrone S. HLA class II antigens synthesized by melanoma cells. Cancer Res. 1987;9:1–5.

Neuberger M, Williams GT, Fox RO. Recombinant antibodies possessing novel effector function. Nature. 1984;312:604–608.

Nudelman E, Hakomori S, Kannagi R, et al. Characterization of a human melanoma-associated ganglioside antigen defined by a monoclonal antibody. J Biol Chem. 1982;257:12752–12756.

Orlandi R, Gussow DH, Jones PT, Winter G. Cloning immunoglobulin variable domains for expression by the polymerase chain reaction. Proc Natl Acad Sci USA. 1989;86:3833–3837.

Osborn L, Hession C, Tizard C, et al. Direct expression cloning of vascular cell adhesion molecule 1, a cytokine-induced endothelial protein that binds to lymphocytes. Cell. 1989; 59:1203–1211.

Persson MA, Caothien RH, Burton DR. Generation of diverse high affinity human monoclonal antibodies by repertoire cloning. Proc Natl Acad Sci USA. 1991;88:2432–2436.

Plowman GD, Brown JP, Enns CA, et al. Assignment of the gene for human melanoma-associated antigen p97 to chromosome 3. Nature. 1983;303:70–73.

Pukel CS, Lloyd KO, Trabassos LR, Dippold WG, Oettgen HF, Old LJ. GD_3, a prominent ganglioside antigen of human melanoma, detection and characterization by mouse monoclonal antibody. J Exp Med. 1982;155:1133–1147.

Ravindranath MH, Irie RF. Gangliosides as antigens of human melanoma. In: Nathanson L, ed. Malignant melanoma: biology, diagnosis and therapy, pp. 17–43, Boston: Kluwer Academic Publishers; 1988:17–43.

Real FX, Rettig WJ, Chesa PG, Melamed MR, Old LJ, Mendelsohn J. Expression of epidermal growth factor receptor in human cultured cells and tissues: relationship to cell lineage and stage of differentiation. Cancer Res. 1986;46:4726–4731.

Reisfeld RA, Cheresh DA. Human tumor antigens. Adv Immunol. 1987;40:323–377.

Rettig WJ, Real FX, Spengler BA, Biebler JL, Old LJ. Human melanoma proteoglycan: expression of hybrids controlled by intrinsic and extrinsic signals. Science. 1986;231:1281–1284.

Riechmann L, Clark M, Waldmann H, Winter G. Reshaping human antibodies for therapy. Science. 1988;332:323–327.

Rose TM, Plowman GD, Teplow DB, Dreyer WJ, Hellström KE, Brown JP. Primary structure of the human melanoma-associated antigen p97 (melanotransferrin) deduced from the mRNA sequence. Proc Natl Acad Sci USA. 1986;83:1261–1265.

Ross AH, Grod P, Bothwell M, et al. Characterization of nerve growth factor receptor in neural crest tumors using monoclonal antibodies. Proc Natl Acad Sci USA. 1984;81:6681–6685.

Ruiter DJ, Bergman W, Welvaart K, et al. Immunohistological analysis of malignant melanomas and nevocellular nevi with monoclonal antibodies to distinct monomorphic determinants of HLA antigens. Cancer Res. 1984;44:3930–3935.

Sahagan BG, Dorai H, Saltzgaber-Muller J, et al. A genetically engineered murine/human chimeric antibody retains specificity for human tumor associated antigen. J Immunol. 1986; 137:1006–1008.

Schulz G, Cheresh DA, Varki MN, Yu A, Staffileno LK, Reisfeld RA. A murine monoclonal antibody detects ganglioside GD_2 in tumor tissues and sera of neuroblastoma patients. Cancer Res. 1984;44:5914–5920.

Sela BA, Iliopoulos D, Gerry D, Herlyn D, Koprowski H. Levels of disialogangliosides in sera of melanoma patients monitored by sensitive thin-layer chromatography and immunostaining. J Natl Cancer Inst. 1989;81:1489–1491.

Skerra A, Plückthun A. Assembly of a functional immunoglobulin Fv fragment in *Escherichia coli*. Science. 1988;240:1038–1040.

Smith JW, Cheresh DA. The RGD binding domain of the vitronectin receptor: photoaffinity crosslinking implicates residues 61-203 of the β subunit. J Biol Chem. 1988;263:18726–18731.

Smith JW, Cheresh DA. Integrin (αvβ3)-ligand interaction: identification of a divalent cation-dependent, heterodimeric RGD binding site on the vitronectin receptor. J Biol Chem. 1990; 256:2168–2172.

Spiro RC, Parsons WG, Perry SK, et al. Inhibition of post-translational modification and surface expression of a melanoma-associated chondroitin sulfate proteoglycan by diethyl-carbamazine or ammonium chloride. J Biol Chem. 1986;261:5121–5126.

Steplewski Z. Antigens of human melanoma as defined by monoclonal antibodies. Hybridoma. 1982;1:379–482.

Stoscheck CM, King LE. Role of epidermal growth factor in carcinogenesis. Cancer Res. 1986;46:1030–1037.

Sun LK, Curtis P, Rakowicz-Szulczynska E, et al. Chimeric antibody with human constant regions and mouse variable regions directed against carcinoma-associated antigen 17-1A. Proc Natl Acad Sci USA. 1987;84:214–218.

Tai T, Paulson JC, Cahan CD, Irie RF. Ganglioside GM_2 as a human tumor antigen (OFA-I-1). Proc Natl Acad Sci USA. 1983;80:5392–5396.

Tai T, Cahan LD, Tsuchida T, Morton DL, Irie RF. Immunogenicity of melanoma-associated gangliosides in cancer patients. Int J Cancer. 1985;35:607–612.

Taramelli D, Fossati G, Mazzocchi A, Delia D, Ferrone S, Parmiani G. Classes I and II HLA and melanoma-associated antigen expression and modulation on melanoma cells isolated from primary and metastatic lesions. Cancer Res. 1986;46:433–439.

Tsuchida T, Saxton RE, Irie RF. Gangliosides of human melanoma: GM_2 and tumorigenicity. J Natl Cancer Inst. 1987;78:55–60.

Wallick SC, Kabat EA, Morrison SL. The effect of isotype and the J_κ region on antigen binding and idiotype expression by antibodies binding $\alpha(16)$ dextran. J Immunol. 1989;142:1235–1238.

Ward SE, Güssow D, Griffith AD, Jones PT, Winter G. Binding activities of a repertoire of single immunoglobulin variable domains secreted from *Escherichia coli*. Nature. 1989;341: 544–546.

Watanabe T, Pukel CS, Takeyama H, et al. Human melanoma antigen AH is an autoantigenic ganglioside related to GD2. J Exp Med. 1983;156:1884–1889.

Wayner EA, Garcia-Pardo A, Humphries MJ, et al. Identification and characterization of the T lymphocyte adhesion receptor for an alternate attachment domain (CS-1) in plasma fibronectin. J Cell Biol. 1989;109:1321–1330.

Wayner EA, Orlando RA, Cheresh DA. Integrins $\alpha v\beta 3$ and $\alpha v\beta 5$ contribute to cell attachment to vitronectin but differentially distribute on the cell surface. J Cell Biol. 1991;113:919–929.

Welte K, Miller G, Chapman PB, et al. Stimulation of T lymphocyte proliferation by monoclonal antibodies against GD_3 ganglioside. J Immunol. 1987;139:1763–1768.

Woodbury RG, Brown JP, Yeh MY, Hellström I, Hellström KE. Identification of a cell surface protein, p97, in human melanomas and certain other neoplasms. Proc Natl Acad Sci USA. 1980;77:2183–2186.

Woodbury RG, Brown JP, Loop SM, Hellström KE, Hellström I. Analysis of normal and neoplastic human tissues for the tumor-associated protein p97. Int J Cancer. 1981;27:145–149.

CHAPTER 7

BIOMODULATION WITH NETWORK EPITOPES

Darrell R. Anderson
Heinz Köhler
Sybille Müller

Niels Jerne's (1974) network hypothesis in immunology states certain principles that are attractive for immunological intervention in disease. Consequently, the application of anti-idiotypes for therapy of human cancer has precipitated an impressive number of reports in the experimental field of idiotypy. In particular, the early work on using anti-idiotypes as surrogate antigens (Kohler, 1984; Kohler et al., 1985; Nissonoff and Lamoyi, 1981; Eichmann and Rajewski, 1975) testifies to the validity of the concept for human tumor therapy.

Initial findings of anti-idiotypic antibodies as biomodulators have been reported in clinical settings of malignant tumors and are particularly interesting in those situations where conventional approaches such as surgery and chemotherapy have failed. While the armamentarium of cancer therapies is impressive, very few cures are achieved and almost all modalities suffer from severe side effects. As cancer persists as a chronic disease despite a variety of therapeutic measures, the question of quality of life of the patient during treatment gains significance. These reasons are sufficient for continuing development of alternative approaches to the management of human tumors by means of improved molecular immunoregulators. The limited known clinical experience in the anti-idiotype therapy (Herlyn et al., 1987b; Kageshita et al., 1988) suggests that side effects are minimized under this therapy and give cancer patients an alternative therapy that provides for a higher quality of life.

In this chapter, we will discuss the current data on experimental therapy in both human and animal models. This work is considered as the basis for a rational approach in anti-idiotype therapy of human cancer.

CONVENTIONAL IMMUNOTHERAPY

Human and animal tumors express tumor-associated antigens (TAA), which may be exploited as targets for immunotherapeutic attack. Numerous attempts have been made to isolate these antigens in pure form. It has proven difficult to isolate many of these antigens in a form suitable for widespread clinical use. In some instances, the native forms of these antigens have not been effective in eliciting immune responses that result in tumor regressions, thus requiring new strategies (Livingston et al., 1985, 1987a). In 1984, Chanock (1984) outlined eight new strategies for constructing novel immune-based therapies. Those strategies specifically addressing the nonreplicating antigen category included anti-idiotype antibodies as a means for dealing with antigens synthesized through complex metabolic or enzymatic pathways.

As early as 1981, investigators (Nissonoff and Lamoyi, 1981; Roitt et al., 1981) proposed using anti-idiotype antibodies as immunomodulators to program the immune systems of diseased individuals as a means of enhancing a specific response to tumor antigens. This phenomenon plays a natural role in immune-system regulation, apparently having a normal function as a "dampening" mechanism. The proposals were made on the assumption that Jerne's network hypothesis offers an approach to transform epitope structures of TAA into idiotypic determinants (idiotypes) (Eichmann and Rajewski, 1975). This transformation would not only provide a "surrogate" antigen (Sharpe et al., 1984), but may add extra dimensions of effectors in the form of different helper T-cell responses and antigenic presentations with an overall upregulation of a specific antitumor response.

The use of anti-idiotypic immunotherapies for cancer is appealing for a number of reasons. Anti-idiotypes used as active therapeutic agents should have relatively low toxicity and not be associated with the severe myelosuppression that accompanies cytotoxic chemotherapy. Their modes of action in promoting antitumor effects are quite different from chemotherapy agents. Tumor cells resistant to chemotherapy would still be susceptible to anti-idiotype therapy provided that patients are not severely immunosuppressed at the time of treatment.

Additionally, anti-idiotype immunotherapeutic agents provide several advantages over synthetic or extracted tumor antigens or antigens prepared by recombinant DNA techniques. Conventional methods usually require lengthy synthetic routes or extraction and extensive purification of TAA, while recombinant DNA techniques are limited to protein antigens and cannot be employed to generate carbohydrate or lipid epitopes, which are inherently limited in the types of immune responses they alone can provoke. Also, many of the protein antigens may be difficult to characterize to the extent needed to employ other technologies.

ANIMAL TUMOR MODELS

Solid Tumors

A number of important tumor immunotherapy models have been reported using anti-idiotype antibodies as network modulators. Forstrom et al. (1983) were the first to demonstrate a potential role of anti-idiotype antibodies in tumor immunity. The model employed a putative anti-idiotype antibody 4.72 derived from a mouse that was hyperimmunized with mouse sarcoma tumor cells. This antibody lacked sufficient proof of its anti-idiotypic nature; however, failure to bind to the tumor cells and the ability to elicit a tumor-specific, delayed-type hypersensitivity (DTH) reaction provides indirect evidence.

Polyclonal anti-idiotypic antibodies were generated in rabbits by Nepom et al. (1984) against the antihuman melanoma antibody 8.2. When mice were immunized with these antibodies, they developed a sensitivity against human melanoma-associated antigens.

Kennedy et al. (1985) treated mice with two anti-idiotype antibodies derived from two monoclonal antibodies (mAB) directed against two different regions of the SV40 virus. It was demonstrated that the anti-idiotypes could induce tumor-specific immunity against SV40-transformed cells.

The first detailed study of anti-idiotype antibodies and their biological effect in tumor immunotherapy was that of Raychaudhuri et al. (1986, 1987a, 1987b). In this study, the tumor-specific immune response induced by irradiated tumor cells (L1210/GZL) and by anti-idiotype antibodies was compared. The anti-idiotype antibodies (Ab2) were made against the paratope of a monoclonal antitumor antibody (11C1) that recognizes a TAA corresponding to the mouse mammary tumor virus envelope glycoprotein 52. The two Ab2 (2F10 and 3A4) induced idiotypes (Ab3) expressed by the monoclonal antitumor antibody 11C1. Cytotoxic T cells obtained from the immunization with irradiated tumor cells were capable of lysing hybridoma cells expressing surface antibody bearing the idiotypes of 2F10 and 3A4. Immunization with Ab2 included tumor-specific cytotoxic T lymphocytes (CTL). The frequency of tumor-reactive CTL was found to be equivalent in mice immunized with Ab2 or irradiated tumor cells when examined at the precursor level. However, only 2F10 induced protective immunity against the growth of L1210/GZL tumor cells. The success of 2F10 and failure of 3A4 have been linked to components within the T-cell population and to the presence of a protective idiotope unique to 2F10 (Chen and Köhler, 1990). The role of T cells in tumor immunotherapy and idiotype matching will be discussed below in a separate section.

Lymphoma/Leukemia Tumors

Several groups have reported encouraging results with mouse lymphoma models. The B-cell lymphomas represent a particularly well-suited class of tumors for anti-idiotype therapy due to the presence of surface Ig-bearing idiotypes that serve as unique tumor-specific antigens.

A number of murine lymphoma models have provided important information supporting the feasibility of a therapeutic approach to management of human B-cell lymphoma. Levy and colleagues (Campbell et al., 1987) examined the immunity generated by vaccination with free idiotype derived from IgM (38C-id) that was expressed on the surface of the carcinogen-induced B-cell tumor line 38C13. They demonstrated that idiotype was capable of inducing both humoral and cellular immune responses in the syngeneic host, which provided significant protection against a subsequent lethal tumor cell challenge. Other studies using idiotypic determinants as immunogens against tumor were conducted by Stevenson and co-workers (George et al., 1987, 1988). Immunization of BALB/c mice with idiotypic IgM rescued by hybridization from mouse lymphoma cells produced a specific protective response against challenge with tumor cells. Passive transfer studies demonstrated a major role for antibody in humoral protection with minimal enhancement by cytotoxic T cells.

Kohler and co-workers (Bhattacharya-Chatterjee et al., 1987) produced anti-idiotype antibodies with a potential to treat human T-cell leukemia and have tested the ability of the antibodies to elicit an antitumor immune response in a mouse system. Two Ab2 (4EA2 and 4DC6) were produced against a murine monoclonal antitumor antibody (SN2) that defines a unique cell-surface glycoprotein (gp37, Mol. wt. 37,000). The anti-idiotypes were shown to be paratope-specific by inhibition of binding of SN2 to the tumor (MOLT-4) membrane. The purified Ab2 was used to immunize syngeneic mice and was shown to induce antibody binding to MOLT-4 cells or gp37.

HUMAN TUMOR SYSTEMS

Target Antigens for Tumor Immunotherapy

Cancer cells express relatively few specific TAA. Consequently, they are often able to masquerade as normal tissues and escape immune surveillance. Moreover, many malignant cells are unstable and rapidly become heterogeneous with variable antigen expression (Thurin et al., 1986; Harper et al., 1976). Several cancers, however, do express a number of TAA that can serve as appropriate targets for immunotherapy. These TAA may be common to normal tissues, but are generally restricted to tissue type or characterized by relatively low surface distribution on normal cells.

As early as 1976, it was determined that many tumor cells carry antigens that are distinguishable by host immune systems (Carey et al., 1976). Sera of patients gave mixed responses to autologous tumors, yet significant evidence for unique antigens was subsequently provided by monoclonal antibody technology.

Many of these antigens may serve as foci for humoral and cellular immune responses if a proper stimulus is applied. The major difficulty arises from the general nonimmunogenic nature of a large portion of these antigens in the host immune system. Other problems include the shedding or excretion of large amounts of immunoreactive antigen into the circulation resulting in neutralization of antibodies within nonproductive immune complexes (Herlyn et al., 1987a). In some instances TAA may not be directly or strongly associated with vulnerable surface portions of the integral tumor cell membrane. Immunoreactive epitopes may be located within subsurface components (Fukaya et al., 1986) or on distal surface structures such as proteoglycans (Kantor et al., 1986), which may not be in sufficient contact with the membrane bilayer to effectively target humoral or cellular cytotoxic events to the surface of the malignant cell.

Malignant Melanoma as Target for Anti-idiotype Therapy

Significant progress in the understanding of the epidemiology, genetics, and pathobiology of melanoma during the last decade has provided new concepts for the management of the disease (Ho and Sober, 1990). Although many new methods are under investigation, few have proven to be effective agents without the presence of significant side effects.

Several antigens associated with melanoma and carcinoma are reasonably well characterized and reported in the literature. A number of these are of considerable interest as target antigens for tumor immunotherapy. These TAA may be classified as peptide or carbohydrate TAA, depending on the nature of the epitope that is expressed on a glycoprotein, proteoglycan, glycolipid, or mucin. Highly specific humoral immune responses can be elicited against either the lipid, peptide, or carbohydrate portion or a combination thereof (Viale et al., 1989). The latter case may result in a more successful therapy because a particular combination may be more immunogenic and unique to the tumor. Cellular responses are generally limited to the presence of T-cell epitopes and, at present, appear to be highly restricted to the peptide moiety (Abbas, 1988; Milich, 1988).

At least two melanoma-related glycoproteins have been identified in an estimated 30% to 40% of the patient groups studied (Dippold et al., 1980; Saxton et al., 1982). Some antibodies have been produced against these antigens and have served to identify them as 96- to 97-kDa and 125- to 150-kDa components. These antigens, being T cell–dependent, could provide a means for a recombinant product that would provoke a melanoma-specific cytotoxic response by both humoral- and cell-mediated mechanisms.

Glycolipids are of major interest as target antigens for tumor immunotherapy (Natoli et al., 1986; Pukel et al., 1982; Cheresh et al., 1984b). They are widely distributed over the patient populations to an estimated 90% or greater and remain present throughout most stages of the disease (Kantor et al., 1986; Tsuchida et al., 1987). Related glycolipids are less common on the surfaces of some carcinomas, appearing to the extent of an estimated 15% to 30% (Brezicka et al., 1989). The lipophilic portion of the molecule prevents excessive shedding and secretion into the circulation outside of lipophilic complexes. Their externally oriented, hydrophilic glycosylated structures show good immunogenicity when presented to xenogeneic or allogeneic individuals on the surface of intact tumor cells (Natoli et al., 1986). In addition, there have been no reported side effects from antibodies found in patients or from animal models (Livingston et al., 1987a; Cheresh et al., 1985).

Proteoglycans are also considered to be good target antigens. They are estimated to be expressed by >80% over the patient population and generally remain closely associated with the tumor mass. They are perhaps more suitable targets for antigen-specific T-cell recognition than glycolipids, due to the presence of some T cell–dependent epitopes (Morgan et al., 1981).

Other Human Solid Tumors as Targets for Anti-idiotype Therapy

Unique epitopes have been identified in complex mucins associated with human colon carcinoma (Gendler et al., 1988). A number of monoclonal antibodies have been produced to various epitopes of the TAG 72 mucin (Herlyn et al., 1987a). Tumor-specific altered mucins are reported on 50% to 75% of colon and breast carcinomas.

Carcinoembryonic antigen (CEA) has some potential as a glycoprotein target antigen. Several antibodies against epitopes on this determinant have been produced. It is estimated that up to 75% of colon carcinoma patients express this antigen. It is limited in its tissue distribution to low amounts on colonic mucosa; however, it is also produced in significant amounts and excreted in a soluble form (Herlyn et al., 1987a).

All of the antigens described above have unique limitations as potential immunotherapeutic targets. To purify and apply them directly would not be economically feasible. Methods and means for reproducing the antigenic structures in glycoproteins can be achieved through recombinant DNA or organic peptide synthesis as long as the epitopes can be identified and sequenced. The small number of antigens meeting this criterion severely limits the applications of the technology. While some antigens may be derived from a template, they may be difficult to characterize to the extent needed for sequencing. Anti-idiotype technology has effectively demonstrated that it can provide a suitable alternative under these conditions (Kantor et al., 1986).

HUMAN TUMOR IMMUNOTHERAPY

Anti-idiotype immunotherapy in animal models is now being expanded to human disease. While the number of clinical trials completed or in progress remains small and the patient population somewhat low for statistically relevant conclusions, initial studies have shown encouraging results. A number of questions remain to be answered concerning optimal dose levels and formulations that, hopefully, will improve as more trials are completed.

Lymphoma

One of the most recent reported studies done in humans with anti-idiotype immunotherapy was a passive lymphoma trial conducted by Levy et al. (Brown et al., 1989). Eleven patients with B-cell lymphoma were treated with mouse monoclonal anti-idiotype antibodies. All but one of these patients had been previously treated with conventional lymphoma therapy and had shown no response. All antibodies were prepared against, and were uniquely reactive with, each patient's individual tumor. Six of the patients showed significant antitumor responses, with one remaining disease-free in excess of 42 months. Toxicity and side effects were minimal. This therapy shows promise as an alternative to toxic chemotherapy and radiation treatments. Further studies are needed, which should lead to significantly improved clinical results. Miller et al. (1989) have generated a large panel of murine anti–B-cell lymphoma anti-idiotypes and have recently shown that a fraction of these anti-idiotypes detect idiotypes present in sera of normal individuals and in nonlymphoma patients. The occurrence of shared idiotypes on antibodies derived from normal or nonlymphoma individuals emphasizes the close overlap of the idiotypic network in physiological and pathological states in an allogeneic situation. This can be utilized by generating anti-idiotypic antibodies detecting shared idiotypes on antibodies derived from different individuals at the same disease stage. These "shared" anti-idiotypes (SID) would obviate the manufacturing of "custom-made," individual anti-idiotypic antibodies derived from, and for, one single patient.

Solid Tumors

Limited human cancer trials using anti-idiotype immunotherapy on solid tumors such as melanoma and carcinoma have also shown guardedly optimistic results. The preliminary results emphasize the need for additional studies to determine optimum methods of administration as is indicated from the lymphoma studies described above.

Thirty patients with advanced colorectal carcinoma (CRC) were treated with Ab2 produced as a polyclonal antiserum in goats (Herlyn et al., 1987b; Kropowski et al. 1984). The Ab2 was produced against a monoclonal anti-CRC antibody, CO17-11A. The goat Ab2 was administered to patients with advanced CRC (Dukes D stage). All patients had their primary tumor surgically resected, and at the time of the trial, all had progressive forms of liver metastases. Fifteen of the patients had unsuccessful chemotherapy. Six patients showed partial clinical remission, and seven patients showed arrest of metastases following immunotherapy. A number of human monoclonal Ab2 antibodies made against the same Ab1 were obtained from Epstein-Barr virus (EBV) transformed lymphocytes derived from patients treated with 17-1A in a passive immunotherapy trial (Steinitz et al., 1988). These anti-idiotypes have not yet been evaluated as active antitumor immunomodulators; however, peripheral blood mononuclear cells (PBMC) taken from these patients and stimulated with Ab2 in vitro produced Ab3 populations that shared idiotopes and tumor binding specificities with the Ab1 (Wetlendorf et al., 1989). It was suggested that these Ab3 responses may underlie delayed clinical responses often seen in cancer patients receiving monoclonal antibody treatments.

Intralesional administration of human monoclonal antibodies in melanoma patients has met with some success in two clinical studies by Irie and colleagues (Irie et al., 1989; Ravindranath et al., 1989). Although the number of patients in the experimental group was small, the results optimistically support passive immunotherapy in combination with surgical removal of primary lesions as a method for management of melanoma. The most recent study (Irie et al., 1989) also reported significant production of anti-idiotype antibodies within the patients with well-stabilized forms of the disease beginning at about day 12 after initial treatment with mAb L72 and peaking at day 62. The mAb L72 specifically binds to the melanoma TAA glycolipid GD_2. As a result of the Ab2 response, a corresponding Ab3 response was detected beginning at about day 50 and peaking on day 137. The anti-GD_2 antibodies detected appear to be a result of Ab2 idiotype–directed, B-lymphocyte activation due to the absence of IgM isotypes normally derived from direct GD_2 antigenic responses. The presence of these new isotypes may have important implications in stabilization and management of patients over long-term intervals.

Role of Helper T Cells in Tumor Immunotherapy

The results of Raychaudhuri et al. (1987b), introduced previously in the discussion of animal models, provided evidence of a role of regulatory T cells in the expression of effective antitumor immunity. Two Ab2 (2F10 and 3A4), when used to immunize mice, induced tumor-specific CTL. The frequency of tumor-reactive CTL was found to be similar in mice immunized with Ab2 or irradiated tumor cells when examined at the precursor T-cell level. However, only 2F10 was capable of inducing protective immunity against a challenge of L1210/GZL cells. The depletion of (CD4) $L3T4^+$ T-cell populations for 2F10-immune mice was found to enhance the effectiveness of transferred T cells in the inhibition of tumor growth. The inability of the other Ab2 (3A4) to induce protection could be linked to the presence of a population of $Lyt2^+$ regulatory T cells. These results together demonstrate the existence of a regulatory network controlling the expression of effective tumor immunity.

In an extension of this work, Saeki and colleagues (1988, 1989) have cloned helper cells from mice immunized with protective and nonprotective Ab2. The Ab2 have been shown to require intracellular antigen processing before effective presentation to the anti-idiotype–specific T-cell clones can take place. Preliminary experiments have given evidence that adoptive transfer of the T-cell clones induces immunity against the L1210/GZL tumor (Kohler et al., unpublished).

Combination Therapy

Several investigators have attempted to develop antitumor therapies by combining chemotherapy with immunotherapy (Brown et al., 1989; Releveld et al., 1987; Kataoki et al., 1978). Although most chemotherapeutic agents tend to suppress the immune system, it has been reported that certain drugs under restricted conditions are able to augment the host antitumor response.

One example of combined therapy is the use of nonspecific immunostimulants such as the strain bacillus Calmette-Guérin (BCG) or other adjuvants (Kataoki et al., 1978; Allison and Byars, 1986) in the presence of partially purified tumor extracts or recombinant products. Several investigators have reported limited success with cyclophosphamide pretreatment in conjunction with whole-cell or partially purified tumor extracts (Mokyr et al., 1982; Mokyr and Dray, 1983; Campbell et al., 1988; Livingston et al., 1983).

Chen et al. (1989) investigated optimal stimulatory anti-idiotype therapy with cyclophosphamide in a mouse tumor model. They reported significant dose dependence on optimal tumor growth and survival times. These results did show synergistic effects and may provide guidelines for developing clinical protocols for cancer patients using combination therapy. Other types of cytostatic drugs have been tried in limited quantities with varying degrees of success (Morikawa et al., 1985; Mokyr and Barker, 1986; Kataoki et al., 1978). Clearly, additional trials will provide needed information on mechanisms associated with the observations as many of these studies require more clarifications.

Idiotype Matching

Recently, anti-idiotype antibodies have been used in active immunization protocols in human cancer patients (Herlyn et al., 1987b; Kageshita et al., 1988). The clinical response of these patients was inconsistent and unpredictable. Studies by Kahn et al. (1989) with human antigen transfected into a mouse melanoma model suggest that some epitopes may not be suitable targets. Clearly, a better understanding of the effective mechanisms is needed for therapeutically applied anti-idiotype antibodies. More recent studies provided by Chen et al. (1990) have begun to address these questions in a reasonably well-characterized animal model system. This study suggests that it is necessary to match a prospective therapeutic anti-idiotype with the tumor host to maximize the antitumor response. This approach is based on the assumption that the effective anti-idiotype antibody must identify idiotopes expressed in the tumor host that correlate with tumor regression. This study identified an idiotope (2F10) that is preferentially associated with antibodies involved in tumor regression. The trend in 2F10 expression correlated better with survival than did the changes in tumor-binding antibodies. In other words, antitumor antibodies that do not express the 2F10 idiotope do not correlate with survival, while those that express the idiotope do correlate. It is not clear if this idiotope remains protective across species lines.

Summary of Idiotype Therapy

Anti-idiotype immunotherapeutic agents provide several advantages over synthetic or extracted tumor antigens or antigens prepared by recombinant DNA techniques. Conventional methods usually require lengthy synthetic routes or extraction and extensive purification of TAA, while recombinant DNA techniques are limited to protein and cannot be employed to generate several carbohydrate or lipid TAA of interest for tumor immunotherapy. Reproduction of the peptide antigenic structures in glycoproteins can be accomplished through recombinant DNA or chemical methods only when relevant, target peptide epitopes can be identified, sequenced, and synthesized in immunogenic form. The identification of the relevant protective epitope for immunotherapy and its production in a form that maintains the conformational "fidelity" of the native epitope severely limits some applications of the technology. Many other protein antigens may be difficult to characterize to the extent needed for amino acid sequencing. Anti-idiotype technology can provide suitable "network" or internal image antigens in these cases.

A very large portion of the remaining TAA belongs to subclasses of antigens that cannot be made by recombinant techniques or by peptide synthesis. Their relative complexity prevents effective duplication by other biochemical means. Purification of many of these structures or related precursors from tissue extracts provides only small amounts, and these materials tend to be less immunogenic when used in purified form with no additional modification.

By contrast, the ability to "mimic" defined chemical structures with anti-idiotypes dramatically increases the potential repertoire of agents for tumor immunotherapy. In bioreactors, large quantities of clinical grade anti-idiotype TAA network antigens can be produced under controlled and reproducible good manufacturing practices (GMP) conditions. A single manufacturing technology can be used to produce all anti-idiotype network antigens and would not be subject to limitations imposed by the biochemical nature of the native target TAA.

Anti-idiotype technology also offers exploitation, through the network, of certain antigens that are impossible to completely characterize due to limited amounts of starting material or other complexities such as microheterogeneity (Anderson and Grimes, 1982). Theoretically, it is also possible for anti-idiotype surrogates to mimic "combination epitopes" composed of both glycosyl-lipid or glycosyl-peptide structures (Viale et al., 1989). Finally, anti-idiotypes could be utilized to stimulate immune responses to weakly immunogenic or tolerized antigens and thus may be used to enhance immune responses to TAA that are poor immunogens or in which a state of immune tolerance has developed.

Glycoconjugate Modulators

A large number of defined tumor antigens appear to be glycosylated. Anti-idiotype surrogates of carbohydrate structures have been reported to alter certain disease states with demonstrated efficacy (Sacks et al., 1985). However, it is not clear if all glycosylated structures for which modulation may be beneficial can be supplied with this technology. In general, the successful transition from carbohydrate epitope to network antigen appears to be restricted. For example, it has been extremely difficult to generate network responses against carbohydrate antigens through anti-idiotypes derived from Ab1 idiotypes linked to a γ3 isotype. There has been only a single example recently reported (Chapman and Houghton, 1991), where significant IgG Ab3 ganglioside responses have been induced from an Ab2 derived from Ab1 of this subclass. This isotype is a predominant isotype, generated in response to carbohydrate antigens. All other successful antitarget Ab3 network responses have come through other γ isotype subclasses or from IgM. This may be due to involvement of a certain class or the lack of helper T cells or perhaps a clonal restriction in carbohydrate-specific hypervariable region gene families. Another explanation is that many anticarbohydrate antibodies may derive from precursor-cell populations as defined by Linton et al. (1990). One would speculate that anticarbohydrate antibodies originate within the primary antibody-forming clones, but are somehow not accessible to network modulation through the secondary B-cell population and remain difficult to activate. It is empirically suggestive that anti-idiotypes capable of impersonating carbohydrate structures are exceedingly more difficult to produce than from peptide epitope sources.

For those glycoconjugate antigens not accessible to network modulators, it may be possible to chemically synthesize and modify the inherent structures to produce a more immunogenic form (Kjeldsen et al., 1988; Fung et al., 1990). These groups of compounds are beginning to play a larger role in biomodulation of cancer as well as many other forms of disease. As chemical methods for characterizing glycosylated structures become more sophisticated, it is anticipated that a new group of biomodulators will be added as therapeutics. Many of these compounds may already be available, but are awaiting the assignment of a functional role. Some may function by stimulating immune responses through classical humoral pathways (Boros and Rapp, 1970) or by synergistic combinations such as complement mediation coupled with alternative pathway activation (Michalek et al., 1988a, 1988b). Others may act to modulate cell-surface receptors linked with control of cell growth by interacting with the receptors for growth hormones and cytokines (Bremer et al., 1984, 1985), or perhaps by blocking integrins and other adhesion-type molecules and/or their receptors (Rice and Bevilacqua, 1989). Yet other structures may eventually be identified as playing regulatory roles in the activation of T cells and other cellular immune components.

Immunohistology of Tumor Antigens

It is important to bear in mind that immunotherapeutics developed against tumor antigens may not be totally without side effects. Immunohistochemical data have repeatedly emphasized that it is unlikely there will ever be discovered a true "tumor specific antigen." There will probably always be some expression on certain normal tissues. Physicians and tumor immunologists must weigh the consequences against the possible beneficial effect when employing a biomodulator of the immune system. The nature of the modulation mechanism should be carefully considered. In some instances, a humoral response may have few or no toxic side effects. In other cases, activation of cellular mechanisms could open a cascade leading to autoimmunity. It is expected that all agents will have been thoroughly evaluated prior to their availability as a therapeutic, with contraindications well documented. The major point to consider is whether limited, or in some cases major, side effects can be acceptable under the circumstances. If approval of these agents is viewed in the same manner as most chemotherapeutics now available, it is likely that they will be less toxic overall and therefore acceptable.

CONCLUSION

Among the modern biotechnology approaches in immunotherapy that take advantage of gene technologies and sophisticated cell biology, the anti-idiotype concept is rooted in basically simple and general immunobiology. The concept of classical immunobiologists who characterize and analyze the immune response to well-defined antigen is moved up in the immune system one order of complexity. Like their colleagues in classical immunology, anti-idiotype therapists select an anti-idiotype and perform test immunizations in relevant animal models. If the response data are convincing enough, human phase trials can be initiated.

However, there are several problems with the current method. The most important undefined parameter is the unpredictable nature of the response to anti-idiotype immunization. Because anti-idiotypes induce complicated cascade responses, which Jerne had initially predicted in 1974 and described as parallel idiotypic circuits, one basically deals with a "black box" phenomenon (Eichmann and Rajewski, 1975). It is the challenge for the next decade to gain a much deeper understanding of regulatory events in the immune response, in particular, as they vary in different idiotypic repertoires. For example, is it not an oversimplification to predict the patient's response on the basis of data in animal models? Which animal model best mimics the idiotypic repertoire of humans? How much variation exists among individuals within one species? Do we need to type the idiotypes of patients in order to predict the future disease course or the therapeutic response? Can we somehow predict the patient's response to anti-idiotype therapy by test therapy of human severe combined immune deficiency (SCID) mice established from patients scheduled to receive anti-idiotype therapy? Preliminary results indicate that SCID mice reconstituted with PBMC from patients with malignant melanoma immunized previously with IMel PG 1 (a murine monoclonal anti-idiotypic antibody carrying the internal image of the melanoma antigen MPG) had higher anti-idiotype titers than SCID mice reconstituted with PBMC from patients not treated with IMel PG 1. Therefore, SCID mice reconstituted with lymphocytes from patients can serve as a model to analyze the human immune response to anti-idiotype immunotherapy (Norton et al., 1990a, 1990b).

It is clear that these questions will continue to challenge immunologists dedicated to developing novel immunotherapy concepts. The anti-idiotype approach is at the beginning of its exploration. It aims at the entire immune system by attempting to change and redirect certain immune responses that normally occur during a disease process. The anti-idiotype approach distinguishes itself from the majority of other immunotherapies by attempting to be selective and specific. The results achieved so far are encouraging and warrant being continued.

REFERENCES

Abbas AK. A reassessment of the mechanisms of antigen-specific T-cell dependent B cell activation. Immunol Today. 1988;9:89–94.

Allison AC, Byars NE. An adjuvant formulation that selectively elicits the formation of antibodies of protective isotypes and of cell-mediated immunity. J Immunol Methods. 1986; 95:157–168.

Anderson DR, Grimes WJ. Heterogeneity of aspargine-linked oligosaccharides of five glycosylation sites on immunoglobulin M heavy chain from mineral oil plasmacytoma 104E. J Biol Chem. 1982;257:14858–14864.

Bhattacharya-Chatterjee M, Pride MW, Seon BK, Köhler H. Idiotype vaccines against human T cell acute lymphoblastic leukemia I: generation and characterization of biologically active monoclonal anti-idiotypes. J Immunol. 1987;139:1354–1360.

Borsos T, Rapp HJ. The molecular basis of complement action. New York, NY: Appleton Century Crofts; 1970.

Bremer EG, Hakomori S, Bowen-Pope DF, Raines E, Ross R. Ganglioside-mediated modulation of cell growth, growth factor binding and receptor phosphorylation. J Biol Chem. 1984;259:6818.

Bremer EG, Schlessinger J, Hakomori S. Ganglioside-mediated modulation of cell growth. J Biol Chem. 1985;261:2434–2440.

Brezicka F-T, Olling S, Nilsson O, et al. Immunohistological detection of fucosyl-Gm1 ganglioside in human lung cancer and normal tissues with monoclonal antibodies. Cancer Res. 1989;49:1300–1305.

Brown SL, Miller RA, Horning SJ, et al. Treatment of B-cell lymphomas with anti-idiotype antibodies alone and in combination with alpha interferon. Blood. 1989;73:651–661.

Campbell MJ, Carrol W, Kon S, et al. Idiotype vaccination against murine B cell lymphoma. J Immunol. 1987;139:2825–2833.

Campbell MJ, Esserman L, Levy R. Immunotherapy of established murine B cell lymphoma. Combination of idiotype immunization and cyclophosphamide. J Immunol. 1988;141:3227–3233.

Carey TE, Takahashi T, Resnick LA, Oettgen HF, Old LJ. Cell surface antigens of human malignant melanoma: mixed hemadsorption assays for humoral immunity to cultured autologous melanoma cells. Proc Natl Acad Sci USA. 1976;73:3278–3282.

Chanock RM. Summary: molecular and chemical basis of virus virulence and immunogenicity. In: Chanock RM, Lerner RA, eds. Modern approaches to vaccines. Cold Spring Harbor Laboratory; 1985;439–446.

Chapman PB, Houghton AN. Induction of IgG antibodies against GD3 ganglioside in rabbits by an anti-idiotypic monoclonal antibody. J Clin Invest. 1991;88:186–192.

Chen J-J, Saeki Y, Shi L, Kohler H. Tumor idiotype vaccines VI: synergistic anti-tumor effects with combined "internal image" anti-idiotypes and chemotherapy. J Immunol. 1989;143: 1053–1057.

Chen J-J, Saeki Y, Köhler H. Idiotype matching: correlation of expression of protective idiotype in sera with survival of tumor mice. J Immunol. 1990;144:759–764.

Cheresh DA, Reisfeld RA. O-Acetylation of disialoganglioside GD3 by human melanoma cells creates a unique antigenic determinant. Science. 1984;225:844–846.

Cheresh DA, Harper JR, Schultz G, Reisfeld RA. Localization of the gangliosides GD2 and GD3 in adhesion plaques and on the surface of human melanoma cells. Proc Natl Acad Sci USA. 1984;81:5767–5771.

Cheresh DA, Honsik CJ, Staffileno LK, Jung G, Reisfeld RA. Disialoganglioside GD3 on human melanoma serves as a relevant target antigen for monoclonal antibody-mediated tumor cytolysis. Proc Natl Acad Sci USA. 1985;82:5155–5159.

Dippold WG, Lloyd KO, Li LTC, Ikeda H, Oettgen HF, Old LJ. Cell surface antigens of human malignant melanoma: definition of six antigenic systems with mouse monoclonal antibodies. Proc Natl Acad Sci USA. 1980;77:6114–6118.

Eichmann K, Rajewski K. Induction of T and B cell immunity by anti-idiotypic antibody. Eur J Immunol. 1975;5:661–666.

Forstrom JW, Nelson KA, Nepom GT, Hellstrom I, Hellstrom KE. Immunization to a syngeneic sarcoma by a monoclonal auto-anti-idiotypic antibody. Nature. 1983;303:627–629.

Fukaya T, Hashimoto K, Eto H, Mehregan A. Mouse monoclonal antibody (FKH1) detecting human melanoma-associated antigens. Cancer Res. 1986;46:5195–5200.

Fung PS, Madej M, et al. Active specific immunotherapy of a murine mammary adenocarcinoma using a synthetic tumor-associated glycoconjugate. Cancer Res. 1990;50:4308–4314.

Gendler S, Taylor-Papadimitriou J, Duhig T, Rothbard J, Burchell JJ. A highly immunogenic region of a human polymorphic epithelial mucin expressed by carcinomas is made up of tandem repeats. J Biol Chem. 1988;263:12820–12823.

George AJT, Tutt AL, Stevenson FK. Anti-idiotypic mechanisms involved in suppression of a mouse B cell lymphoma, BCL1. J Immunol. 1987;138:628–634.

George AJT, Spellerberg MB, Stevenson FK. Idiotype vaccination leads to the emergence of a stable surface Ig-negative variant of the mouse lymphoma BCL1 with different growth characteristics. J Immunol. 1988;140:1695–1701.

Harper JR, Bumol TF, Reisfeld RA. Serological and biochemical analyses of monoclonal antibodies to human melanoma-associated antigens. Hybridoma. 1982;1:423–432.

Herlyn D, Rodeck U, Koprowski H. Shedding of human tumor-associated antigens in vitro and in vivo. Adv Cancer Res. 1987a;49:189–221.

Herlyn D, Wettendorf M, Schmoll E, et al. Anti-idiotype immunization of cancer patients: modulation of the immune response. Proc Natl Acad Sci USA. 1987b;84:8055–8059.

Ho VC, Sober AJ. Therapy for cutaneous melanoma: an update. J Am Acad Dermatol. 1990;22:159–176.

Irie RF, Matsuki T, Morton DL. Human monoclonal antibody to ganglioside GM2 for melanoma treatment. Lancet. 1989;8:786–787.

Jerne NK. Towards the network theory of the immune system. Ann Immunol (Paris). 1974; 125C:373–389.

Kageshita T, Chen ZJ, Kim J-W, et al. Murine anti-idiotypic monoclonal antibodies to syngeneic anti-human high molecular weight-melanoma associated antigen monoclonal antibodies: development, characterization, and clinical application. Pigment Cell Res. 1988;1:185–191.

Kahn M, Hellstrom I, Estin CD, Hellstrom KE. Monoclonal anti-idiotypic antibodies related to the p97 human melanoma antigen. Cancer Res. 1989;49:3157–3162.

Kantor RRS, Ng AP, Ferrone S. Biosynthesis and intracellular processing of four human melanoma associated antigens. Cancer Res. 1986;46:5223–5228.

Kataoki T, Hobayashi H, Sakurai Y. Potentiation of concanavalin A-bound L1210 vaccine in vivo by chemotherapeutic agents. Cancer Res. 1978;38:1202–1207.

Kennedy RC, Dreesman GR, Butel JS, Lanford RE. Suppression of in vivo tumor formation induced by simian virus 40–transformed cells in mice receiving anti-idiotypic antibodies. J Exp Med. 1985;161:1432–1449.

Kjeldsen T, Clausen H, Hirohashi S, Ogawa T, Iijima H, Hakomori S. Preparation and characterization of monoclonal antibodies directed to the tumor-associated O-linked sialosyl-2 6 a*N*-acetylgalactosaminyl (sialosyl-In) epitope. Cancer Res. 1988;48:2214–2220.

Köhler H. The immune network revisited. In: Köhler H, Cazenave P, Urbain J, eds. Idiotypy in biology and medicine. New York, NY: Academic Press; 1984.

Köhler H, Muller S, Bona C. Internal idiotype antigens. Proc Soc Exp Biol Med. 1985;178:189–195.

Koprowski H, Herlyn D, Lubeck M, DeFreitas E, Sears H. Human anti-idiotype antibodies in cancer patients: is the modulation of the immune response beneficial for the patient? Proc Natl Acad Sci USA. 1984;81:216–219.

Linton P-J, Decker DJ, Klinman NR. Primary antibody-forming cells and secondary B cells are generated from separate precursor cell subpopulations. Cell. 1990;59:1049–1059.

Livingston PO, Deleo AB, Jones M, Oettgen HF. Comparison of approaches for augmenting the serologic response to the individually specific methylcholanthrene-induced sarcoma-meth A: pretreatment with cyclophosphamide is most effective. J Immunol. 1983;131:2601–2605.

Livingston PO, Old LJ, Oettgen HF. Approaches to augmenting the immunogenicity of tumor antigens. In: Monoclonal antibodies and cancer therapy. New York, NY: Alan R Liss; 1985:537–548.

Livingston PO, Calves MJ, Natoli EJ Jr. Approaches to augmenting the immunogenicity of the ganglioside GM2 in mice: purified GM2 is superior to whole cells. J Immunol. 1987a; 138:1524–1529.

Livingston PO, Natoli EJ, Calves MJ, Stockert E, Oettgen HF, Old LJ. Vaccines containing purified GM2 ganglioside elicit GM2 antibodies in melanoma patients. Proc Natl Acad Sci USA. 1987b;84:2911–2915.

Michalek MT, Bremer EG, Mold C. Effect of gangliosides on activation of the alternative pathway of human complement. J Immunol. 1988a;140:1581–1587.

Michalek MT, Mold C, Bremer EG. Inhibition of the alternative pathway of human complement by structural analogues of sialic acid. J Immunol. 1988b;140:1588–1594.

Milich DR. T- and B-cell recognition of hepatitis B viral antigens. Immunol Today. 1988;9:380–386.

Miller RA, Hart S, Samoszuk M, et al. Shared idiotypes expressed by human B-cell lymphomas. New Engl J Med. 1989;321:851–857.

Mokyr MB, Dray S. Some advantages of curing mice bearing a large subcutaneous MOPC-315 tumor with a low dose rather than a high dose of cyclophosphamide. Cancer Res. 1983; 43:3112–3119.

Mokyr MB, Hengst JCD, Dray S. Role of anti-tumor immunity in cyclophosphamide-induced rejection of subcutaneous nonpalpable MOPC-315 tumors. Cancer Res. 1982;42:974–979.

Mokyr MB, Barker E. Specificity of the generation and expression of enhanced anti-plasmacytoma immunity by spleen cells from melphalan-treated MOPC-315 tumor bearers. Cancer Immunol Immunother. 1986;23:11–19.

Morgan AC Jr, Galloway DR, Reisfeld RA. Production and characterization of monoclonal antibody to a melanoma specific glycoprotein. Hybridoma. 1981;1:27–36.

Morikawa K, Hosokawa M, Hamada J-I, Sugawara M, Kobayashi H. Host-mediated therapeutic effects produced by appropriately timed administration of bleomycin on a rat fibrosarcoma. Cancer Res. 1985;45:1502–1506.

Natoli EJ Jr, Livingston PO, Weigandt H, Szalay J, Oettgen HF, Old LJ. A murine monoclonal antibody detecting N-acetyl and N-glycolyl GM2: characterization of cell surface reactivity. Cancer Res. 1986;46:4116–4120.

Nepom GT, Nelson KA, Holbek SL, Hellstrom I, Hellstrom KE. Proc Natl Acad Sci USA. 1984;81:2864–2867.

Nissonoff A, Lamoyi E. Implications of the presence of an internal image of the antigen in anti-idiotypic antibodies, possible applications to vaccine production. Clin Immunol Immunopathol. 1981;21:357–406.

Norton FL, Shuey S, Morton D, et al. Response to anti-idiotype in SCID mice reconstituted with lymphoid cells from melanoma patients. In: Finn O, ed. Cellular immunity and the immunotherapy of cancer. New York, NY: Wiley-Liss, Inc. 1990:360–369.

Pukel CS, Lloyd KO, Travassos LR, Dippold WG, Oettgen HF, Old LJ. GD3. A prominent ganglioside of human melanoma. J Exp Med. 1982;155:1133–1147.

Ravindranath MH, Paulson JC, Irie RF. Human melanoma antigen O-acetylated ganglioside GD3 is recognized by cancer antennarius lectin. J Biol Chem. 1988;263:2979–2986.

Ravindranath MH, Morton DL, Irie RF. An epitope common to gangliosides O-acetyl-GD_3 and GD_3 recognized by antibodies in melanoma patients after active specific immunotherapy. Cancer Res. 1989;49:3891–3897.

Raychaudhuri S, Saeki Y, Fuji H, Köhler H. Tumor-specific idiotype vaccines. I. Generation and characterization of internal image tumor antigen. J Immunol. 1986;137:1743–1749.

Raychaudhuri S, Saeki Y, Chen J-J, Iribe H, Köhler H. Tumor specific idiotype vaccines II. Analysis of the tumor-related network response induced by the tumor and by internal image antigens (Ab2β). J Immunol. 1987a;139:271–278.

Raychaudhuri S, Saeki Y, Chen J-J, Köhler H. Tumor-specific idiotype vaccines III. Induction of T helper cells by anti-idiotype and tumor cells. J Immunol. 1987b;139:2096–2102.

Releveld EH, Bizzini B, Ophir R, Shlomo B-E. Synergy between low-dose chemotherapy and immunotherapy in mouse L1210 leukemia. Cancer Treat Rep. 1987;71:241–246.

Rice GE, Bevilacqua MP. An inducible endothelial cell surface glycoprotein mediates melanoma adhesion. Science. 1989;246:1303–1306.

Roitt IM, Male DK, Guarnotta G, et al. Idiotypic networks and their possible exploitation for manipulation of the immune response. Lancet. 1981;1:1041–1045.

Sacks DL, Kirchoff LV, Hieny S, Sher A. Molecular mimicry of a carbohydrate epitope on a major surface glycoprotein of *Trypanasoma cruzi* by using anti-idiotypic antibodies. J Immunol. 1985;135:4155–4159.

Saeki Y, Chen J-J, Shi L, Kohler H. Idiotypic intramolecular help. J Immunol. 1988;142:2629–2634.

Saeki Y, Chen J-J, Shi L, Raychaudhuri S, Kohler H. Characterization of "regulatory" idiotope-specific T cell clones to a monoclonal anti-idiotypic antibody mimicking a tumor associated antigen (TAA). J Immunol. 1989;142:1046–1052.

Saxton RE, Mann BD, Morton DL, Burk MW. Monoclonal antibodies to 125 kd and 95 kd proteins on human melanoma cells: comparison with other monoclonal defined melanoma antigens. Hybridoma. 1982;1:433–444.

Sharpe AH, Gaulton GN, McDade KK, Fields BN, Greene MI. Syngeneic monoclonal anti-idiotype can induce cellular immunity to reovirus. J Exp Med. 1984;160:1195–1205.

Steinitz M, Tamir S, Frodin J-E, Lefvert A-K, Mellstedt H. Human monoclonal anti-idiotypic antibodies: I. Establishment of immortalized cell lines from a tumor patient treated with mouse monoclonal antibodies. J Immunol. 1988;141:3516–3522.

Thurin J, Thurin M, Herlyn M, et al. GD_2 ganglioside biosynthesis is a distinct biochemical event in human melanoma tumor progression. FEBS letter. 1986;208:17–22.

Tsuchida T, Saxton RE, Morton DL, Irie RF. Gangliosides of human melanoma. J Natl Cancer Inst. 1987;78:45–53.

Viale G, Flamini G, Grassi F, et al. Idiotypic replica of an antihuman tumor-associated antigen monoclonal antibody. J Immunol. 1989;143:4338–4344.

Wettendorf M, Iliopoulos D, Tempero M, et al. Idiotypic cascades in cancer patients treated with monoclonal antibody Co 17-1A. Proc Natl Acad Sci USA. 1989;86:3787–3791.

CHAPTER **8**

BIOLOGICAL THERAPY FAILURES: SANCTUARIES FOR TUMORS

Elizabeth A. Grimm

As of 1990, one of the critical problems to be resolved in cancer therapy is that of oncolytic agent delivery. It is well known that most therapeutic agents, including biologics, can induce regression of some lesions in a cancer patient, while other lesions in the same patient are unaffected or continue to progress. For the purposes of this chapter, I hypothesize that such failures are not simply a result of ineffective dose administered to the patient, but rather ineffective dose to individual tumor cells. Currently, delivery of biologics to tumor cells is unpredictable. The factors involved in incomplete access or otherwise ineffective delivery are probably due to an aggregate of conditions, including many of tumor origin. It has been suggested that tumors manifest mechanisms to deflect as well as resist immigration of biological agents, thus producing sanctuaries for self-perpetuation. In addition to the physiological influence of the local tumor environment, physical barriers such as the blood–brain barrier (BBB) of the central nervous system (CNS) also can selectively permit immigration of some tumor cells, but not therapeutic agents. An example of combined physiological and physical resistance to biological therapy is probably best represented by the recent report of complete regression of all peripheral melanoma in a series of six patients, all of whom later recurred in the CNS only (Mitchell, 1989). As the peripheral systemic therapies improve, tumor recurrence in the CNS will increase as a clinical problem. An autopsy review of over 2,000 cancer patients at Memorial Sloan-Kettering revealed an 18% incidence of clinically occult intracranial metastases (Cairncross and Posner, 1983). Considering over 300,000 new cases per year of patients with tumors known to metastasize to the CNS (most from lung, breast, melanoma, and renal), we extrapolate that better peripheral systemic therapies could result in 45,000 to 50,000 more patients per year presenting with CNS metastases.

The concept of solid tumors spawning their own sanctuaries to resist therapy must be considered from two perspectives: (1) the physiological tumor-generated aura, which includes immunosuppressive factors, acidic pH, local pressure gradients emanating from tumors, abnormal glycocalyx tumor cell coats, and shed antigens and (2) constitutive physical barriers represented by the highly regulated tight junctions of the CNS, eye, testis, and placenta. Because of the excellent recent review of the physiological tumor-generated barrier(s) by Rakesh Jain (1989), this first topic will be addressed only in combination with approaches to overcome the physical barriers, as our current research directly addresses this issue. A summary of the present understanding of these situations, as well as research in progress to overcome the barriers, is included here. Further therapeutic attempts must not only provide tumoricidal agents, but must also attempt to provide means for biological component–access into tumor sanctuaries.

CONSTITUTIVE BARRIERS TO BIOLOGICAL THERAPY

The proclivity of certain tumors to metastasize into the CNS results in tumor growth usually unaffected by systemic manipulations. Survival of patients with CNS metastases from lung, breast, or melanoma is measured in months (Jacobs et al., 1986a; Shapiro et al., 1977; Wasserstrom et al., 1982; Cairncross and Posner, 1983). The physical barriers provided by the tight junctions at the BBB and in the testes, placenta, and eye are impediments to systemic treatments with even very small drugs. These areas, and especially the CNS, provide physical sanctuaries not only for primary and metastatic tumors, but also for many types of viruses.

BYPASSING PHYSICAL BARRIERS BY INTRALESIONAL THERAPY

Active research is in progress to determine means by which biologics can be delivered into the sites of the body protected by tight junctions. The most simplistic approach for overcoming the physical barriers protecting tumors from biological therapies is that of direct intralesional injection. In the brain, this approach has recently been used for injection of normal lymphocytes, as well as activated ones, with additional cytokines (Neuwelt et al., 1978; Merchant et al., 1988a, 1988b; Jacobs et al., 1985, 1986b, 1986c). Although probably impractical on a large scale, direct intraoperative–intralesional injection of agents is still considered valuable from the view that we do not yet know which agent(s) may be best in vivo for tumor regression. This approach has been used recently for lymphokine-activated killer (LAK) cell and interleukin (IL)-2 biological therapy of malignant glioma, and dose-limiting toxicity reached by the studies of Barba et al. (1989). At lower doses of LAK cells and IL-2 or of IL-2 alone, varying responses are published (Jacobs et al., 1986c, 1986d; Ingram et al., 1987; Merchant et al., 1988a, 1988c).

The LAK cell and IL-2 method is not yet optimized, but already appears limited, as the LAK cells may not migrate throughout the entire tumor area (Sasaki et al., 1989). Testing of combinations of biologics, especially those stimulating lymphocyte motility, or well-defined cellular subpopulations should be considered for future trials. The direct injection approach is very useful to test the toxicity of agent(s) in the tumor site, as delivery to the organ is guaranteed. However, direct access to individual tumor cells, especially those tumor cells such as in the brain along nerve tracts or in cases of metastatic disease, may not contact small lesions some distance from the injection site. Until cell migration can be regulated, direct intralesional injection of biologics to avoid physical barriers may have its major application in solitary or encapsulated lesions.

BIOLOGICAL REGULATION OF THE BLOOD–BRAIN BARRIER

It is well known that the CNS is devoid of lymphatics and normal immune surveillance; however, in some CNS disease states (encephalitis, multiple sclerosis), effector lymphocytes are documented to cross the BBB (Santoli et al., 1984). Furthermore, because certain histologic tumor types demonstrate a predilection for crossing the BBB, we hypothesize that definite mechanisms do exist for cell entry into the CNS. It is known that effector components of the immune system, especially $CD4^+$ lymphocytes do cross the BBB (Santoli et al., 1984). Whenever the biological mechanisms of cellular (tumor or immune-system cell) migration through the BBB opening are elucidated, perhaps selective opening could be employed for tumor therapy. Research in this area involves studies of brain tumor–derived endothelial cell responses and the use of lymphocyte-derived cytokines to open the BBB (Watts et al., 1989).

Possible exploitation of the normal adrenal–pituitary regulation of BBB integrity is suggested by the work of Long and Holaday (1989), whose data indicated that the tight junctions of the BBB are hormonally regulated under normal circumstances. Complete adrenelectomy, but not adrenal demullation of rats, resulted in significant permeability of albumin into the brain. Positive identification of the adrenal cortical factor(s) that mediate BBB opening is another area of active investigation.

Additional means to perturb the BBB biologically are suggested by the vasodilatory and "leaky" capillary syndrome resulting from intravenous IL-2 administration in cancer patients (Lotze et al., 1986). Ellison et al. (1987) specifically monitored the effects of systemic recombinant IL-2 (rIL-2) on the BBB in cats. Their results of numerous endothelial lesions and disrupted neuronal and glial processes indicate that local IL-2 concentrations can be modulatory toward BBB function. In a series of 12 humans receiving intravenous IL-2, Saris et al. (1988) sampled the cerebrospinal fluid (CSF) by lumbar puncture and documented 3 to 9 units/mL of IL-2 within the first 4 to 6 hours, suggesting that IL-2 can cross the BBB. Two of these patients also exhibited albumin in their CSF, indicative of BBB disruption. The role of IL-2 in directly mediating BBB opening is controversial. One likely explanation for this discrepancy is via variable production of the IL-2–induced secondary cytokine, tumor necrosis factor-alpha (TNF-α). The TNF-α is produced by many cell types, including monocytes and T lymphocytes (Owen-Schaub et al., 1989). The TNF-α is proposed to interact with vascular endothelia and facilitate extravasation of blood cells (Sherry and Cerami, 1988). The observations that vascular leak in endotoxin shock could be blocked by anti–TNF-α antibodies further support this hypothesis (Tracey et al., 1986, 1987). Direct evidence of a role for TNF-α and also of IL-1 inducing cellular migration through non-CNS vascular endothelia in vitro is known (Furie and McHugh, 1989) and is consistent with the preliminary results of this author's own laboratory findings (Belloni, Köppen, and Grimm, unpublished). While TNF regulation of vascular permeability data is consistent and generally accepted, the role of IL-2 is suggested and has yet to be resolved.

ACCESS OF CURRENTLY AVAILABLE BIOLOGICS TO CNS

It is generally unappreciated that the BBB at tumor sites is not especially tight (Groothuis et al., 1982; Blasberg et al., 1981, 1985, 1984). As the tumor-generated angiogenesis proceeds, initiation of the tumor–vascular network occurs; however, the BBB tight junctions do not mature, and tumor vasculature is believed to remain incomplete and "leaky." Selective advantage of this observation seems possible, and the documented responses of malignant glioma to intravenous interferon-beta (IFN-β) may indicate that IFN does reach the tumor. Two reported responses (27% to 30% range) of glioblastoma patients to systemic IFN-β are notable, although no attempt to document evidence of the IFN-β itself crossing the BBB was provided (Yung et al., 1990; Nagai et al., 1989). As secondary cytokines appear to be involved in IL-2 effects in the CNS, an equally likely scenario is that IFN-β causes production of secondary mediators that result in the therapeutic responses in the brain. Irrespective of the mechanism, systemic administration of IFN-β somehow resulted in biological therapy products effecting glioblastoma tumor regression in the brain parenchyma.

ATTRACTION OF IMMUNE SYSTEM CELLS INTO PRIVILEGED AREAS

Means to induce immigration of immune-system cells into tumors spaces, particularly into the CNS, are indicated by our recent results testing the effects of intraventricular recombinant IL-2. These studies were initiated to provide IL-2 half-life and toxicity data as a prelude to LAK cell adoptive therapy for leptomeningeal carcinomatosis. Surprisingly, administration of IL-2 alone via injection into an Ommaya reservoir (in communication with the ventricular system) resulted in a pronounced leukocytosis, secondary cytokine elaboration, and CSF-tumor regression (Grimm et al., 1989; Steuer et al., 1990). Apparently, IL-2 administration directly into the tumor environment initiated a cascade of events that resulted in polymorphonuclear neutrophil leukocyte (PMN) and lymphocyte invasion, concurrent with tumor regression in 7 of 9 cases. Both TNF-α and IFN-γ were detected in the CSF, indicating endogenous production. The source of these secondary cytokines is not known, but because of the minimal systemic toxicities observed, we hypothesize that they are of CNS origin. The use of the human CNS as a model to elucidate factors that are ultimately responsible for emigration of effector cells into tumor sites should lead to application of such mechanisms to tumors elsewhere.

Recent studies in a rat model by Watts et al. (1989) addressed the kinetics and pathophysiology of single intracerebral injections of IL-2. The rats routinely showed increased cerebrovascular permeability as evidenced by horseradish peroxidase entry into the brain. Most interesting was the increased lymphocytic infiltration into the injection site, perivascular cuffing, and localized edema. The lymphocyte infiltration is consistent with our observations in the CSF.

PHYSICAL MANIPULATIONS FOR BBB OPENING

Physical means to open the BBB and provide biological-agent access to the entire CNS, irrespective of the possible increased access to tumor margins, has been studied extensively by Neuwelt and colleagues (Neuwelt and Rapoport, 1984; Neuwelt et al., 1988). Intracarotid infusion of hyperosmotic mannitol was initially used to increase chemotherapeutic drug delivery (Neuwelt and Rapoport, 1984). Currently, the mechanism(s) of hyperosmotic BBB opening are not known, but this approach has been applied to monoclonal antibody delivery (Neuwelt et al., 1988). In a rat model, Fab and whole IgG were administered via the carotid artery after hyperosmotic mannitol, and a significant increase of antibody delivery was documented $P < 0.0001$. The Fab cleared more rapidly, decreasing 50% within 4.5 hours, compared to 25.5 hours for IgG. In a pilot study, this approach was applied in three melanoma patients. No uptake was observed after intravenous injection of the antibody, but after unilateral BBB disruption, a marked increase was observed in the disrupted hemisphere as determined by a radiolabel tracer. Immunohistologic studies indicated that only a fraction of the antigen binding sites on the tumor cells were bound with antibody, which was attributed to the possibility of an inadequate dose of antibody (Neuwelt et al., 1987). Studies are continuing in the area of BBB opening, to optimize the method and to improve its application for use with appropriate biological agents.

IMMUNE CELL MIGRATION INTO THE BRAIN

A series of recent studies examining tumor-infiltrating lymphocytes (TIL) trafficking into primary and metastatic brain tumors indicates that lymphocytes do indeed infiltrate the local tumor area. Because of the absence of brain lymphatics, it seems plausible that brain-tumor TIL represent more specific immune responses to the tumor than TIL elsewhere and that these TIL possess mechanisms to cross the BBB. Recently, we initiated a phase I trial to determine whether TIL from primary or metastatic brain tumors might traffic to the sites of recurrence. Using TIL generated by initiation with OKT3 (10 ng/mL for 2 days) and cultured further in IL-2 only (Hoffmann-La Roche), homing of TIL into the tumor area was observed in three of five attempts (Fig. 8-1).

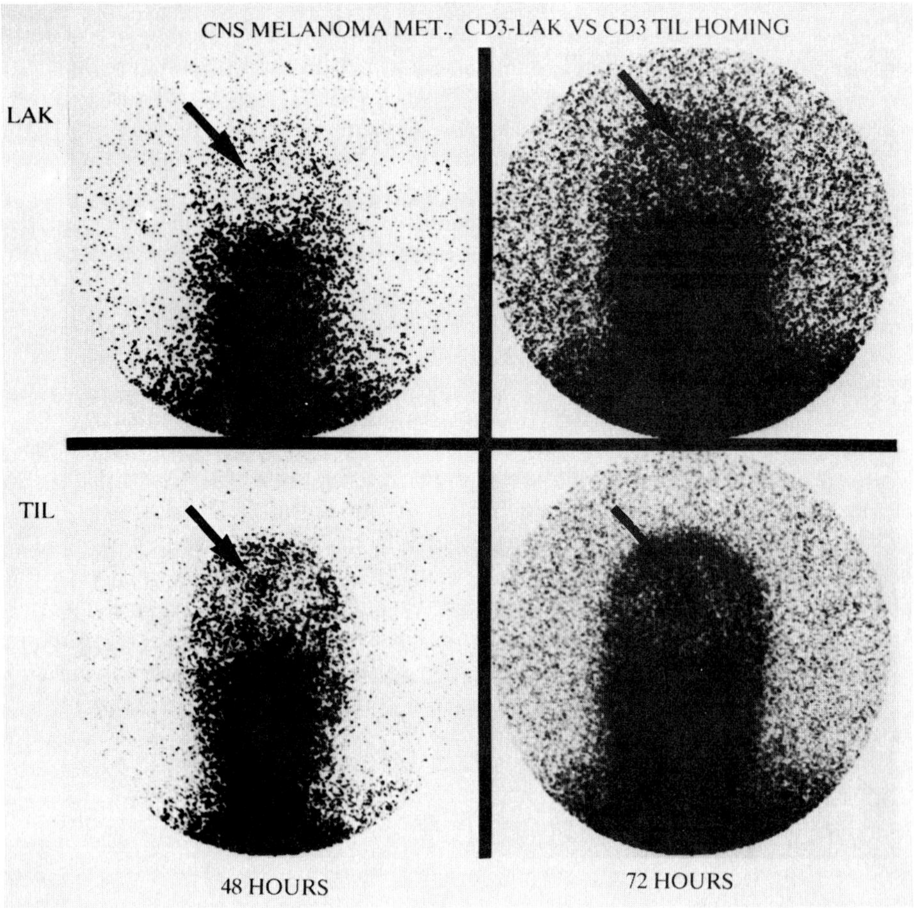

FIGURE 8-1
LAK cells and TIL homing into central brain melanoma metastases. Melanoma metastases to the brain were debulked surgically, and the TIL stimulated to grow by use of anti-CD3 (OKT3, Ortho) monoclonal antibody, followed by IL-2 for 4 weeks. The resultant TIL were then radiolabeled with 111-Indium and injected intravenously. Gamma counter imaging was performed at various times. Localization is evident in the central portion, coincident with an area of tumor recurrence documented by computerized tomography (CT). Next, peripheral blood mononuclear cells (PBMC) from this same patient were stimulated identically to produce CD3-LAK cells or LAK cells. These LAK cells were grown for the same length of time, were labeled with 111-Indium, and then the trafficking pattern was likewise followed. There is little evidence of LAK cell homing, suggesting that the TIL may possess tumor-recognition properties and cross the BBB into the tumor site.

A digital gamma camera was used to obtain spot views at 2, 24, 48, and 72 hours post–intravenous TIL injection. As a control for nonspecific vascular trapping of activated lymphocytes, OKT3-initiated autologous LAK cells were tested in two of these five cases. The tumor (T):background (B) ratio increased from 1.36 ± 0.1 to 1.9 ± 0.2 (mean ± SEM) from 2 to 72 hours postinjection with TIL. With the LAK cells, the T:B were 1.07 ± 0.04 to 1.2 ± 1.3. Therefore, while the density of localization of LAK cells appeared above the background of "normal" brain, the TIL localization was more pronounced (Grimm et al., 1989). Although much more work is needed to define the specific cells that home to the CNS tumors and to optimize their potential therapeutic value, these observations of putative TIL homing provide hope that the cellular mechanisms for immigration into the tumors of the CNS may someday be elucidated.

As the peripheral systemic therapies improve, an increase in the number of patients presenting with (previously occult) CNS metastases is expected. This prediction is dramatically supported by the recent data from Mitchell (1989), in which all six of his most successfully treated melanoma patients in prolonged remission presented with CNS relapse, even as the peripheral remission remained. It was likely that the melanoma had previously migrated into the brain and had been growing continuously during the period of peripheral tumor remission. Curiously, four of the six patients exhibited a single lesion, which is unusual for metastases. It is tempting to speculate that perhaps the systemic therapy did reduce some of the blood-borne tumor even in the CNS. Further follow-up on these patients and confirmation by other groups are required to resolve this speculation.

SUMMARY—PROSPECTS FOR THE FUTURE

Both biological (IL-2, TNF-α, others including endocrine ones, and those yet to be examined) and physical manipulations (hyperosmotic mannitol) are regulatory for the BBB and probably other areas of tight junctions. These mechanisms may be optimized for generalized opening and access to tumors of the CNS. In the future, eludicating the interactions used by tumor cells or TIL to enter the brain appears even more exciting, as they provide the rationale for specific delivery via mechanisms as yet not known.

REFERENCES

Barba D, Saris SC, Holder C, Rosenberg SA, Oldfield EH. Intratumoral LAK cell and interleukin-2 therapy of human gliomas. J Neurosurg. 1989;70:175–182.

Blasberg RG, Groothuis D, Molnar P. Application of quantative autoradiographic measurements in experimental brain tumor models. Semin Neurol. 1981;1:203–223.

Blasberg RG, Molnar P, Groothuis D, Patlak CS, Owens E, Fenstermacher JD. Concurrent measurements of blood flow and transcapillary transport in ASV-induced experimental brain tumors: implications for brain tumor chemotherapy. J Pharmacol Exp Ther. 1984;231:724–735.

Blasberg RG, Horowitz M, Strong J, et al. Regional measurements of C-misonidazole distribution and blood flow in subcutaneous RT-9 experimental tumors. Cancer Res. 1985; 45:1692–1701.

Cairncross JG, Posner JB. The management of brain metastasis. In: Walker MD, ed. Oncology of the nervous system, Boston, Mass: Martinus Nijhof; 1983:341–377.

Ellison MD, Povlishock JT, Merchant RE. Blood–brain barrier dysfunction in cats following recombinant interleukin-2 infusion. Cancer Res. 1987;47:5765–5770.

Furie MB, McHugh DD. Migration of neutrophils across endothelial monolayers is stimulated by treatment of the monolayers with interleukin-1 or tumor necrosis factor-alpha. J Immunol. 1989;143:3309–3317.

Grimm EA, Moser RP, Blacklock JB, Loudon W, Carinhas J. Interleukin-2 and cytotoxic lymphocyte therapy of primary and metastatic brain tumors. In: Johanssen B, Widner H, eds. Pathophysiology of the blood brain barrier. Amsterdam: Elsevier Science; 1989:527–538.

Groothuis DR, Fisher JM, Lapin G, Bigner DD, Vick NA. Permeability of different brain tumor models to horseradish peroxidase. J Neuropathol Exp Neurol. 1982;41:164–185.

Ingram M, Shelden CH, Jacques S, et al. Preliminary clinical trial of immunotherapy for malignant glioma. J Biol Resp Mod. 1987;6:489–498.

Jacobs SK, Kornblith PI, Wilson DJ, Grimm EA. Studies on the immunotherapy of human gliomas using autologous lymphokine-activated killer cells. Surg Forum. 1985;36:504–506.

Jacobs SK, Wilson DJ, Kornblith PI, Grimm EA. In vitro killing of human glioblastoma by interleukin-2 activated autologous lymphocytes. J Neurosurg. 1986a; 64:114–117.

Jacobs SK, Wilson DJ, Melin G, et al. Clinics and experimental studies of IL-2 and IL-2 activated (LAK) cells. In: Urushizaki I, Aoki T, Tsubura E, eds. Host defense mechanisms against cancer. Amsterdam: Excerpta Medica; 1986b:36–46.

Jacobs SK, Wilson DJ, Kornblith PI, Grimm EA. Interleukin-2 or autologous lymphokine-activated killer cell treatment of malignant glioma. Phase I trial. Cancer Res. 1986c; 46:2101–2104.

Jacobs SK, Wilson DJ, Melin J. Interleukin-2 and lymphokine-activated killer (LAK) cells in the treatment of malignant glioma: clinical and experimental studies. Neurosci Res. 1986d; 8:81–87.

Jain RK. Delivery of novel therapeutic agents in tumors: physiological barriers and strategies. J Natl Cancer Inst. 1989;81:570–576.

Long JB, Holaday JW. Blood–brain barrier: endogenous modulation by adrenal-cortical function. Science. 1989;227:1580–1583.

Lotze MT, Chang AE, Seipp CA, Simpson C, Vetto JT, Rosenberg SA. High dose recombinant interleukin-2 in the treatment of patients with disseminated cancer. JAMA. 1986;256:3117–3124.

Merchant RE, Grant AJ, Merchant LH, Young HF. Adoptive immunotherapy for recurrent glioblastoma multiforme using lymphokine activated killer cells and recombinant interleukin 2. Cancer. 1988a;62:665–671.

Merchant RE, Merchant LH, Cook SHS, McVicar DW, Young HF. Intralesional infusion of lymphokine-activated killer (LAK) cells and recombinant interleukin-2 (rIL-2) for the treatment of patients with malignant brain tumor. Neurosurgery. 1988b;23(6):725–732.

Mitchell MS. Relapse in the central nervous system in melanoma patients successfully treated with biomodulators. J Clin Oncol. 1989;7(11):121–129.

Nagai M, Arai T, Watanabe K. Treatment of malignant brain tumors with interferons—with special reference to the combination therapy and the maintenance therapy. In: Kawade Y, Kobayashi S, eds. The biology of the interferon systems. Boston: Kluwer Academic Publishers; 1989:207–212.

Neuwelt EA, Rapoport SI. Modification of the blood–brain barrier in the chemotherapy of malignant brain tumors. Fed Proc. 1984;43(2):214–219.

Neuwelt EA, Clark K, Kirkpatrick JB, Toben H. Clinical studies of intrathecal autologous lymphocyte infusions in patients with malignant glioma: a toxicity study. Ann Neurol. 1978; 4:307–312.

Neuwelt EA, Specht HD, Barnett PA, et al. Increased delivery of tumor specific monoclonal antibodies to brain after osmotic blood–brain barrier modification in patients with melanoma metastatic to the CNS. Neurosurgery. 1987;20:885–895.

Neuwelt EA, Barnett PA, Hellstrom I, et al. Delivery of melanoma-associated immunoglobulin monoclonal antibody and Fab fragments to normal brain utilizing osmotic blood–brain barrier disruption. Cancer Res. 1988;48:4725–4729.

Owen-Schaub LB, Crump WL, III, Morin GI, Grimm EA. Regulation of lymphocyte tumor necrosis factor receptors by IL-2. J Immunol. 1989;143:2236–2241.

Santoli D, Defreitas EC, Sandberg-Wollheim M, Francis MK, Koprowski H. Phenotypic and functional characterization of T cell clones derived from the cerebrospinal fluid of multiple sclerosis patients. J Immunol. 1984;132(5):2386–2392.

Saris SC, Rosenberg SA, Friedman RB, Rubin JT, Barba D, Oldfield EH. Penetration of recombinant interleukin-2 across the blood–cerebrospinal fluid barrier. J Neurosurg. 1988; 69:29–34.

Sasaki A, Jain RK, Maghazachi AA, Goldfarb RH, Herberman RB. Low deformability of lymphokine-activated killer cells as a possible determinant of in vivo distribution. Cancer Res. 1989;49:3742–3746.

Shapiro WR, Posner JB, Ushio Y. Treatment of meningeal neoplasms. Cancer Treat Rep. 1977;61:733–743.

Sherry B, Cerami A. Cachetin/tumor necrosis factor exerts endocrine, paracrine, and autocrine control of inflammatory responses. J Cell Biol. 1988;107:1269–1277.

Steuer MR, Moser RP, Blacklock JB, Crump W, Grimm EA. Cytokines in the cerebrospinal fluid following intraventricular injection of interleukin-2 in patients with leptomeningeal. In: Powander et al., eds. Molecular and cellular biology of cytokines. New York, NY: Alan R. Liss; 1990:49–54.

Tracey KJ, Beutler B, Lowry SF, et al. Shock and tissue injury induced by recombinant human cachectin. Science. 1986;234:470–474.

Tracey KJ, Fong Y, Hesse DG, et al. Anticachectin/TNF monoclonal antibodies prevent septic shock during lethal bacteraemia. Nature. 1987;330:662–664.

Wasserstrom WR, Glass KP, Posner JB. Diagnosis and treatment of leptomeningeal metastases from solid tumors: experience with 90 patients. Cancer. 1982;49:759–772.

Watts RG, Wright JL, Atkinson LL, Merchant RE. Histopathological and blood–brain barrier changes in rats induced by an intracerebral injection of human recombinant interleukin 2. Neurosurgery. 1989;25(2):202–208.

Yung WKA, Castellanos AM, Vantessel P, Moser RP, Marcus ST. A pilot phase II study of rIL-2-beta in patients with recurring glioma. J Neuro-Oncol. 1990;9:29–34.

CHAPTER **9**

HIV-INDUCED IMMUNE DYSFUNCTION AND AIDS-ASSOCIATED NEOPLASMS

Otoniel Martínez-Maza

The acquired immunodeficiency syndrome (AIDS) is an epidemic, transmissible form of secondary acquired immune deficiency, first described in 1981 (Gottlieb et al., 1983; Lane and Fauci, 1985; Krowka et al., 1989). More than 100,000 people have died from AIDS, and from 1–2 $\times$ 10^6 people are infected with human immunodeficiency virus (HIV), in the United States. AIDS is caused by infection with a retrovirus, HIV (Lane and Fauci, 1985; Krowka et al., 1989; Gallo, 1988). This review will focus on changes in the human immune system that are associated with AIDS and HIV infection and on how these immune system changes might play a role in the development of AIDS-associated malignancies, particularly Kaposi's sarcoma (KS) and B-cell lymphoma.

IMMUNE DEFECTS IN AIDS AND HIV INFECTION

Various immune system defects and abnormalities are associated with AIDS and HIV infection. The most pronounced and consistent change seen in the immune system of people with AIDS is a numerical and functional deficiency in $CD4^+$ (helper/inducer) T cells (Lane and Fauci, 1985; Krowka et al., 1989). Healthy donors, not infected with HIV, typically have 400 to 1400 $CD4^+$ T cells per mm^3 of circulating blood, a number that represents approximately 50% of circulating lymphocytes. Individuals with AIDS typically have greatly reduced numbers of peripheral blood $CD4^+$ T cells, but in any given person with AIDS, $CD4^+$ T-cell numbers in blood can range from the levels seen in healthy, uninfected donors to no detectable $CD4^+$ cells. This decreased CD4$^+$ T-cell number results in the decreased CD4:CD8 ratio characteristically seen in AIDS. The CD4$^+$ T-cell number was seen to be very significantly related to prognosis (Taylor et al., 1986; Fahey et al., 1986; Detels et al., 1988); for instance, low CD4$^+$ T-cell number correlated with a shorter time to death in patients with AIDS.

The CD8$^+$ (suppressor T/cytotoxic) cell numbers are not typically decreased in AIDS, and in a given person with AIDS can be within, above, or below the expected range for healthy adult donors. In fact, CD8$^+$ cell numbers are often significantly elevated in AIDS and in HIV infection, at times resulting in a decreased CD4:CD8 ratio, even though CD4$^+$ cell numbers might not be markedly decreased. The CD8 cell number is often elevated in other acute viral infections, such as infection with Epstein-Barr virus (EBV), cytomegalovirus (CMV), or other herpesviruses (Blomberg and Schooley, 1985).

Many T cell–mediated immune functions such as response to mitogens or antigens are deficient in people with AIDS (Lane and Fauci, 1985; Lane et al., 1985). Proliferation of peripheral blood mononuclear cells (PBMC) to T-cell mitogens is often subnormal in AIDS (Lane and Fauci, 1985; Krowka et al., 1989; Lane et al., 1985). However, HIV-infected donors without AIDS often show no decrease in mitogen-induced PBMC proliferation. A more consistent functional defect in AIDS is the markedly impaired ability of PBMC isolated from AIDS patients to proliferate in response to soluble antigens (Lane et al., 1985). The mechanism for this defect in antigen-specific responsiveness has not been defined. Enriched CD4$^+$ cell preparations, isolated from AIDS PBMC, did not effectively respond to antigen (Lane et al., 1985), indicating that this defect in antigen-specific responsiveness is not due principally to the numerical depletion of CD4$^+$ T cells. Perhaps infection of CD4$^+$ T cells with HIV and/or the production of suppressive factors by HIV-infected cells (Krowka et al., 1989), or the selective depletion of antigen-reactive CD4$^+$ clones are responsible for this defect. Defects in major histocompatibility complex (MHC)-restricted and allo-reactive cytotoxic T-cell responses also are seen in AIDS (Lane and Fauci, 1985; Krowka et al., 1989). These defects in cell-mediated immunity might result from either poor cytokine production and/or the loss of the ability to respond to cytokines, since defects in both interleukin-2 (IL-2) production and response have been reported (Lane and Fauci, 1985; Krowka et al., 1989; Murray et al., 1985; Ebert et al., 1985; Prince et al., 1984). It is also possible that HIV infection results in direct or indirect suppression of host immune responses (Lane et al., 1985; Krowka et al., 1989; Benveniste et al., 1983; Laurence et al., 1983; Hoffman et al., 1986).

In HIV infection, T-cell proliferative responses to HIV-encoded antigens appear to be variable. However, it is clear that PBMC isolated from HIV seropositive, asymptomatic donors or HIV-seropositive donors with less advanced disease can at times proliferate in response to HIV gp120 and/or p24 proteins, while patients with AIDS have a severely impaired anti-HIV proliferative response (Krowka et al., 1989). Also, the often dramatic increase in CD8$^+$ cell number seen in association with HIV infection in asymptomatic donors suggests that an increased cytotoxic T-cell response might occur in response to HIV early in the course of infection. Whether these anti-HIV T-cell responses are beneficial, in terms of controlling or slowing HIV infection, is not known. While these immune responses might play an important role in controlling HIV infection, it is possible that induction of T cell–mediated responses could contribute to the accelerated destruction of the host immune system, since activation of T cells is required for HIV entry into $CD4^+$ cells (Gowda et al., 1989). Also, cytotoxic anti-self responses could lead to $CD4^+$ T-cell depletion. However, some reports indicate that $CD8^+$ T cells can play an important role in the control of HIV production by HIV-infected, autologous $CD4^+$ cells (Krowka et al., 1989; Walker et al., 1986). The specific mechanisms by which these $CD8^+$ cells control HIV production by infected T cells are not known.

Many other immune system changes are seen to accompany HIV infection and AIDS, in addition to the characteristic decrease in $CD4^+$ T-cell number and T-cell function. These include changes in B-cell, monocyte, and natural killer (NK)-cell function and phenotype (Lane and Fauci, 1985; Krowka et al., 1989; Sirianni et al., 1990). Recently, much attention has focused on the role of monocytes in HIV infection and AIDS. Human immunodeficiency virus can bind to monocytes, and monocytes can host productive infection with HIV (Meltzer et al., 1990; Gartner et al., 1986; Ho et al., 1986; Koyanagi et al., 1987). A substantial proportion of circulating monocytes are $CD4^+$. Therefore, entry of HIV into monocytes might be mediated by specific binding to this molecule. Alternatively, monocytes might ingest HIV by phagocytosis. Interestingly, monocytotropic HIV strains have been described (Koyanagi et al., 1987). The relative role of monocyte infection with HIV in the pathogenesis of AIDS and related conditions has yet to be determined. However, it is clear that HIV-infected monocytes have the potential to be a significant source of in vivo virus production. Also, exposure of monocytes to HIV or HIV-encoded proteins might result in responses that contribute to the pathogenesis of HIV-associated disease. For example, the aberrant overproduction of cytokines (tumor necrosis factor [TNF], interleukin-1 [IL-1], interleukin-6 [IL-6]) by HIV-exposed monocytes (Nakajima et al., 1989a; Wright et al., 1988; Clouse et al., 1989) could potentially contribute to increased virus production and, thereby, accelerate HIV-induced disease progression, since HIV-infected cells show increased virus production in response to TNF and/or IL-6 (Poli et al., 1990).

Interestingly, many other signs of immune system hyperactivation also are seen in HIV infection. For example, phenotypic changes indicative of cellular activation have been described in the $CD8^+$ T-cell subpopulation (Salazar-Gonzalez et al., 1985); B-cell hyperactivation is characteristically seen in AIDS and HIV infection (Lane et al., 1983; Martínez-Maza et al., 1987a). Hyperimmunoglobulin (hyper-Ig) production, particularly elevated IgG and/or IgA overproduction, is often seen in AIDS, as evidenced by hypergammaglobulinemia, as well as by elevated levels of circulating, spontaneous Ig-secreting cells (Lane et al., 1983). Also, increased levels of activated B cells (CD20 and transferrin double-receptor-positive cells) are often found in the circulation of HIV-infected people and people with AIDS (Martínez-Maza et al., 1987a). Evidence of B-cell hyperactivation can also be found in the high frequency of B-cell malignancies associated with HIV infection (Ziegler and Levy, 1985).

In addition to these phenotypic and functional changes, HIV infection results in increased levels of various soluble serum molecules and cytokines associated with immune system activation. These include elevated levels of neopterin, β_2 microglobulin C-reactive protein (CRP), IL-6, and soluble IL-2 receptor (sIL-2R) (Krowka et al., 1989; Poli et al., 1990; Fahey et al., 1990; Hofmann et al., 1990; Rosenberg and Fauci, 1990; Breen et al., 1990), as well as elevated levels of IgG and IgA. Since some of these molecules such as IL-6 and TNF are potent, pleiotropic growth and/or differentiation factors, it is possible that the overproduction of these factors could contribute directly to the immunopathology of AIDS and related conditions, by increasing cellular proliferation, autoimmune responses, and virus production, ultimately resulting in increased or accelerated $CD4^+$ T-cell destruction. In fact, recent work indicates that cytokines such as TNF and IL-6, whose production can be induced by HIV (Nakajima et al., 1989a; Wright et al., 1988), can lead to elevated levels of HIV production by virus-infected cells (Poli et al., 1990; Rosenberg and Fauci, 1990). Interestingly, in a recent report (Roederer et al., 1990), N-acetyl-L-cysteine was seen to inhibit cytokine-induced HIV replication, suggesting that this drug might be useful as a possible therapeutic agent in AIDS.

B-CELL MALIGNANCIES IN AIDS AND HIV INFECTION

An elevated frequency of B-cell malignancies, especially non-Hodgkin's lymphoma, is seen in association with HIV infection and in AIDS (Ziegler and Levy, 1985; Ziegler et al., 1984; Knowles and Chadburn, 1990; Riggs and Hagemeister, 1988; Hersh and Miller, 1988). In fact, non-Hodgkin's lymphoma is the second most common AIDS-associated malignancy, after Kaposi's sarcoma. The risk for developing non-Hodgkin's lymphoma is about 60 times greater in people with AIDS than in the general population (Beral et al., 1991). Hodgkin's disease also is seen in association with AIDS and HIV infection (Knowles and Chadburn, 1990; Riggs and Hagemeister, 1988; Hersh and Miller, 1988; Mitsuyasu et al., 1986). It has been estimated that between 8% and 27% of non-Hodgkin's lymphoma cases that occur in the United States in 1992 will be associated with HIV infection (Gail et al., 1991).

Interestingly, some reports document an increasing incidence of AIDS-associated lymphoma seen in association with the use of effective antiretroviral therapy with zidovudine (AZT) (Pluda et al., 1990; Moore et al., 1991). Presumably, this is due to an antiretroviral treatment–induced increase in the life span of severely immunosuppressed individuals who are at particularly great risk for the development of AIDS-associated B-cell lymphoma (Pluda et al., 1990). Although the possibility that zidovudine treatment might more directly facilitate the development of AIDS-associated lymphoma cannot be excluded at this time, the results of a placebo-controlled study of zidovudine therapy in asymptomatic HIV-infected people suggest that zidovudine use was not associated with an increased incidence of AIDS-associated lymphoma in this study population (Volberding et al., 1990). Clearly, further studies are needed to define the role, if any, of zidovudine therapy in the pathogenesis of AIDS-associated lymphoma.

Non-Hodgkin's lymphoma has been seen in all groups at risk for AIDS, including children with hemophilia, children of HIV-infected mothers, recipients of HIV-infected blood or blood products, and the heterosexual partners of HIV-infected people (Knowles and Chadburn, 1990). A majority of AIDS-associated non-Hodgkin's lymphoma cases are seen in homosexual and/or bisexual men and in intravenous (IV) drug users. In a study by Ziegler and co-workers (1984), the development of lymphoma was the first sign of HIV-associated disease in nearly 20% of the study subjects, with the diagnosis of AIDS preceding the development of lymphoma in approximately half of cases. Nearly all AIDS-associated lymphomas are B-cell lymphomas (Ziegler and Levy, 1985; Ziegler et al., 1984; Knowles and Chadburn, 1990; Riggs and Hagemeister, 1988). One third to one half of patients have a history of persistent, generalized lymphadenopathy prior to the development of non-Hodgkin's lymphoma (Knowles and Chadburn, 1990). Many patients with AIDS-associated lymphoma develop opportunistic infections and/or KS during the course of their disease (Ziegler and Levy, 1985; Knowles and Chadburn, 1990; Riggs and Hagemeister, 1988).

AIDS-associated non-Hodgkin's lymphoma generally follows a more aggressive course of disease than non-Hodgkin's lymphoma not associated with immune deficiency, with a shorter survival time than non-Hodgkin's lymphoma not associated with AIDS (Knowles and Chadburn, 1990; Riggs and Hagemeister, 1988). A majority of patients have widely disseminated disease, with an especially high frequency of extranodal involvement (Ziegler and Levy, 1985; Ziegler et al., 1984; Knowles and Chadburn, 1990; Riggs and Hagemeister, 1988). Extranodal sites of involvement in AIDS-associated non-Hodgkin's lymphoma include the central nervous system (CNS), the gastrointestinal tract, the heart, and the liver, sites that are not uncommon in non-Hodgkin's lymphoma not associated with immune deficiency. Patients infected with HIV can develop non-Hodgkin's lymphoma of the anorectum or esophagus, extranodal sites that are particularly rare in the general population (Riggs and Hagemeister, 1988). About 20% of patients also have bone marrow involvement.

AIDS-associated non-Hodgkin's lymphoma falls into three histopathological categories: large noncleaved cell lymphoma, small noncleaved cell lymphoma, and large-cell immunoblastic plasmacytoid lymphoma (Knowles and Chadburn, 1990). Response to therapy and survival time correlate with histopathological category: a lower response rate and shorter mean survival have been seen for immunoblastic plasmacytoid lymphoma, with a relatively better response rate and survival time for small-cell noncleaved lymphoma and large-cell noncleaved lymphoma. Also, clinical stage and the involvement of certain extranodal sites have been seen to correlate with histopathological stage in AIDS-associated non-Hodgkin's lymphoma, with a much greater percentage of patients with small noncleaved cell lymphoma showing bone marrow involvement than those with large-cell immunoblastic plasmacytoid lymphoma, with no patients with large noncleaved cell lymphoma showing bone marrow involvement (Knowles and Chadburn, 1990). In contrast, many patients with large-cell immunoblastic plasmacytoid or large noncleaved cell lymphoma had disease that involved the gastrointestinal tract, while a relatively small percentage of patients with small noncleaved cell lymphoma showed such involvement. Knowles and Chadburn (1990) have concluded from these observations that AIDS-associated small-cell noncleaved lymphoma appears to originate in lymph nodes and disseminate to other nodes, to bone marrow, and to extranodal sites, while immunoblastic plasmacytoid and large-cell noncleaved lymphoma may originate in extranodal sites and then grow to involve regional lymph nodes and disseminate.

Most AIDS-associated B-cell lymphomas display clonal Ig gene rearrangements, with some evidence for additional B-cell clones in addition to the predominant tumor clone (Hersh and Miller, 1988). A recent study suggests that a significant fraction of cases of HIV infection–associated B-cell lymphoma are multiclonal and not predominantly monoclonal (Herndier et al., 1990).

A majority of AIDS-associated lymphomas show rearrangement of the c-*myc* oncogene, an event that is thought to be important in the generation of Burkitt's lymphoma (Knowles and Chadburn, 1990; Pelicci et al., 1986; Subar et al., 1988; Klein, 1987). However, unlike endemic African Burkitt's lymphoma (which is typically associated with EBV infection) and sporadic Burkitt's lymphoma (which is usually not associated with EBV infection), AIDS-associated lymphoma is associated with EBV in about 40% of cases (Subar et al., 1988). A recent report indicates that EBV may play an important role in the pathogenesis of AIDS-associated primary CNS lymphoma (MacMahon et al., 1991). In this study, 100% of AIDS-related primary CNS lymphoma specimens expressed short, noncoding EBV transcripts, as well as EBV latent membrane protein (MacMahon et al., 1991). These results suggest that the pathogenesis of AIDS-associated CNS lymphoma may differ from that of systemic lymphoma.

Several immunodeficiency states, in addition to AIDS and related conditions, are associated with an elevated frequency of B-cell malignancies (Knowles and Chadburn, 1990; Riggs and Hagemeister, 1988). These include the immune deficiency associated with *Plasmodium falciparum* malaria, and immunodeficiency induced by treatment with immunosuppressive agents, such as cyclosporine or cyclophosphamide, or congenital or acquired immunodeficiency syndromes (Riggs and Hagemeister, 1988; Whittle et al., 1984; Epstein, 1984; Martínez-Maza et al., 1987b). For instance, while non-Hodgkin's lymphoma represents only a small fraction of the cancers seen in non-immunosuppressed people, non-Hodgkin's lymphoma is a common malignancy in immunosuppressed transplant recipients (Riggs and Hagemeister, 1988). As is seen in AIDS-associated lymphoma, non-Hodgkin's lymphoma in immunosuppressed people often follows a more aggressive clinical course, with a poorer prognosis, than non-Hodgkin's lymphoma in non-immunosuppressed donors (Knowles and Chadburn, 1990; Riggs and Hagemeister, 1988).

B-Cell Hyperactivation and AIDS-Associated Lymphoma

Possibly, the development of B-cell lymphomas associated with AIDS and other immune deficiencies follows the chronic, polyclonal stimulation of B cells in an environment devoid of normal T cell–mediated immunoregulation (Fig. 9-1). In these situations, polyclonal or oligoclonal B-cell activation could be induced by agents such as EBV, HIV, malarial molecules, chronic antigenic stimulation, and/or the inappropriate production of B cell–stimulating molecules. This ongoing, uncontrolled, chronic B-cell proliferation and differentiation allow a greatly elevated risk for a genetic error; the chromosomal translocation that places an oncogene (c-*myc*) in juxtaposition with an Ig gene, which results in the generation of a B-cell malignancy (Klein, 1987). Therefore, chronic polyclonal B-cell activation and T-cell immune deficiency are two

FIGURE 9-1
Immunopathogenesis of B-cell lymphoma associated with HIV infection. Chronic activation of B cells can be induced by: polyclonal activation by EBV or HIV, antigenic stimulation with HIV, lack of effective T-cell immunoregulation, and/or by the HIV-induced overproduction of IL-6 by monocytes. This chronic B-cell hyperstimulation results in an increase in the size of the target pool of B cells susceptible to c-*myc* chromosomal translocation, thereby resulting in B-cell lymphoma. HIV, human immunodeficiency virus; EBV, Epstein-Barr virus; IL-6, interleukin-6.

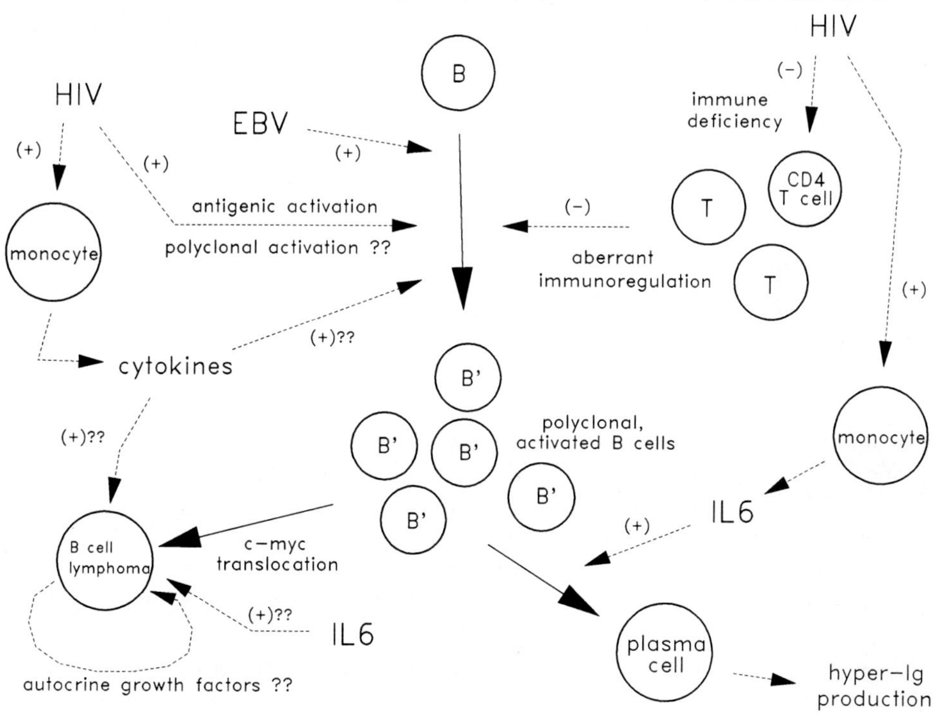

important characteristics of disease situations associated with an increased risk of the development of B-cell lymphoma.

Paradoxically, the severe T-cell immune deficiency seen in AIDS is characteristically accompanied by B-cell hyperactivity, including an elevated level of Ig-secreting cells, elevated spontaneous B-cell proliferation, and elevated levels of serum Ig, as well as a high frequency of B-cell malignancies (Lane and Fauci, 1985; Lane et al., 1983; Martínez-Maza et al., 1987a; Modlin et al., 1983). For example, patients with AIDS and HIV-seropositive donors had an increased fraction of activated (transferrin-receptor-positive) circulating B cells, along with greatly elevated levels of spontaneous Ig secretion (Martínez-Maza et al., 1987a). This increase in the fraction of circulating B cells with an activated phenotype was accompanied by decreased levels of resting, mature (Leu 8^+) B cells. Surprisingly, patients with AIDS also had elevated levels of circulating, immature phenotype, CD10 common acute lymphoblastic leukemia antigen $(CALLA)^+$ B cells (Martínez-Maza et al., 1987a). Therefore, in vivo infection with HIV results in an increase in both activated and apparently immature B cells, an increase in terminally differentiated Ig-secreting cells, and a decrease in the pool of resting, mature B cells. It is possible that the CD10 $CALLA^+$ B cells represent a preneoplastic subset, since nearly 90% of AIDS-associated non-Hodgkin's lymphoma are at least partially CD10 $CALLA^+$ (Knowles and Chadburn, 1990).

There are several possible sources for the excessive B-cell activation seen in association with AIDS and HIV infection (Fig. 9-1). Infection with HIV might functionally impair the T-cell subsets responsible for controlling B-cell activation induced by common activating agents such as EBV (Bird and Britton, 1979; Birx et al., 1986). Human immunodeficiency virus itself could induce polyclonal B-cell activation; several reports indicate that HIV is a polyclonal B-cell activator (Pahwa et al., 1985, 1986; Schnittman et al., 1986; Yarchoan et al., 1986). However, these differ in several important details regarding the putative activation of B cells by HIV, specifically on the need for "live," biologically active virus, and on the role of T cells in this process. A third possible source of B-cell activation in AIDS is the overproduction of B-cell stimulatory factors by HIV-infected cells. Finally, antigenic stimulation by HIV antigens might result in a substantial level of chronic B-cell activation (Amadori et al., 1989).

Immunoregulatory Defects and AIDS-Associated B-Cell Hyperactivation

Immunoregulation of EBV-induced B-cell activation is defective in AIDS (Birx et al., 1986; Tsokos, 1986). In previous work (Tsokos, 1986; Palacios and Martínez-Maza, 1983), it was found that $CD4^+$ T cells play an important immunoregulatory role (suppression of Ig secretion) if they are present early in the course of the in vitro polyclonal activation of B cells induced by EBV. The suppressive effect of CD4 cells could be replaced by the addition of interferon-gamma (IFN-γ) early (<24 hours) after exposure of B cells to EBV (Palacios and Martínez-Maza, 1983; Martínez-Maza et al., 1984; Andersson et al., 1984; Lotz et al., 1985). When $CD4^+$ T-cell number,

PHA-induced IFN-γ secretion, and spontaneous Ig secretion were concurrently measured in patients with AIDS, a significant linear correlation was seen between decreased CD4$^+$ cell number, decreased in vitro IFN-γ secretion, and elevated spontaneous Ig secretion (Martínez-Maza et al., 1987c). A significant correlation between increased B-cell hyperactivation and decreased CD4$^+$ T-cell number also has been described by others (Mizuma et al., 1988). Together, these results suggest that immune functions that are known to play a role in the immunoregulation of EBV-activated B cells are defective in AIDS and HIV infection, allowing chronically activated B cells to excessively proliferate and differentiate.

Polyclonal Activation of B Cells by HIV

Several published reports (Pahwa et al., 1985, 1986; Schnittman et al., 1986; Yarchoan et al., 1986) have indicated that HIV is a B-cell polyclonal activator, although these differ regarding the need for T cells and/or "live" HIV for this B-cell activation to occur. Schnittman and co-workers (1986) have reported that HIV-containing supernatants can activate B cells to secrete Ig, in a direct, T cell–independent fashion, and Pahwa et al. (1985) that inactivated HIV can activate B cells. Yarchoan et al. (1986) have found HIV to be a T cell–dependent B-cell activator. However, exposure of purified B cells (T and monocyte-depleted, PBMC lymphocytes) to live, disrupted, or inactivated HIV preparations did not consistently result in cellular proliferation or Ig production (Breen and Martínez-Maza, unpublished observations). B-cell activation markers—CD25 (IL-2 receptor) (IL-2R), transferrin receptor, and MHC class II antigens: HLA-DR—were examined after exposure of PBMC to HIV preparations by two-color flow cytometry. No HIV-induced changes in the expression of B-cell surface markers were noted after 24 or 48 hours of exposure to HIV preparations, while 24 hours of in vitro exposure to pokeweed mitogen (PWM) resulted in an increase in CD25 (IL-2R)$^+$ B (CD20) cells from not detectable ($<2\%$) to 30% to 70% positive, with a rise in transferrin-receptor positive B cells from not detectable ($<2\%$) to 7% to 15% positive (Martínez-Maza, unpublished observations). The HLA-DR antigen is found on virtually all B cells; however, the density of HLA-DR antigen was found to increase about 30% following exposure to PWM, but did not change following HIV exposure. No changes were seen in the expression of these markers on B cells exposed to media for 24 hours.

In other experiments, the binding of HIV to B cells was examined by flow cytometry, using betapropiolactone-inactivated HIV (iHIV), biotinylated anti-HIV serum, and avidin-fluorescein isothioyanate (FITC). With this system, approximately 50% of control CD4$^+$ T cells (CEM cells) were seen to bind virus, with no binding without added iHIV. When the ability of several B-cell lines to bind iHIV was examined, none of these cells showed detectable iHIV binding (Martínez-Maza, unpublished observations). Similar results were seen when PBMC were studied by two-color flow cytometry: most CD4$^+$ cells were seen to bind iHIV, while few or no B cells bound iHIV. Admittedly, this system would not detect a low level of binding of HIV to B cells. However, it is safe to conclude that the level of HIV binding to B cells is not of the same magnitude as is seen in $CD4^+$ T cells, since iHIV binding to $CD4^+$ T cells is clearly detected in this system.

These results suggest that HIV is not a direct B-cell activator. Therefore, other mechanisms, including the induction of B cell–stimulating factors by HIV, may be involved in the polyclonal B-cell activation seen in AIDS and HIV infection.

HIV-Induced B-Cell Stimulating Factor Production

Rather than directly activating B cells, HIV infection could result in hyper-Ig production by inducing the production of B cell–stimulating factors by T cells, B cells, or monocytes or other nonlymphoid cells.

The role of IL-6 in AIDS-associated B-cell hyperactivation was examined, since IL-6, also known as B cell–stimulating factor type 2 (BSF-2), has B-cell differentiation-inducing effects. Interleukin-6, a 26-kDa glycoprotein, is a pleiotropic cytokine with a wide range of biological effects on a variety of cell types (Kishimoto, 1989; Kishimoto and Hirano, 1988). Originally, IL-6 was described independently by various investigators as: BSF-2, plasmacytoma/hybridoma growth factor, interferon-beta-2 (IFN-β_2), 26-kDa protein, and hepatocyte stimulatory factor (Kishimoto and Hirano, 1988; Gauldie et al., 1987; Sehgal et al., 1987). The biological activities that have been described for IL-6 include induction of differentiation of activated B cells, support of plasmacytoma and myeloma growth, induction of acute phase reactants and stimulation of hepatocytes, nerve growth factor–like activity, induction of cytotoxic T cells, and support of hematopoietic differentiation (Kishimoto, 1989; Kishimoto and Hirano, 1988). The gene for IL-6 has been cloned and sequenced, and the structure of the IL-6 gene described (Hirano et al., 1986). The receptor for IL-6 is composed of two polypeptides: an IL-6–binding protein, which is associated on IL-6 binding to a second signal-transducing molecule (Yamasaki et al., 1988). Interleukin-6 can be produced by several types of cells, including T lymphocytes, monocyte/macrophages, fibroblasts, certain tumor cells, epithelial cells, and endometrial cells (Kishimoto, 1989; Kishimoto and Hirano, 1988; Luger et al., 1989; Kernbauer et al., 1989; Tabibzadeh et al., 1989). It appears that monocytes are the primary source of IL-6 produced by PBMC (Kishimoto, 1989). The production of IL-6 by monocytes is readily induced by different activators, including viruses, other lymphokines (IL-1 and TNF), and bacterial endotoxins (Nakajima et al., 1989a; Kishimoto, 1989).

Recent work indicates that in vitro exposure of PBMC (isolated from healthy, HIV-seronegative donors) to HIV led to the rapid production of IL-6 messenger RNA (mRNA) and secreted IL-6 (Nakajima et al., 1989a, 1989b). Lipopolysaccharide (LPS) or HIV led to detectable IL-6 mRNA in PBMC within 2 hours of exposure, with peak levels of IL-6 secretion detected at <24 hours post-HIV exposure (Nakajima et al., 1989a). Monocyte/macrophages were the primary cell type involved in producing IL-6 on exposure to HIV (Nakajima et al., 1989a), although other cell types, including T cells, can produce IL-6 when other stimuli are used. Interestingly, inactivated, noninfectious HIV induced IL-6 production as effectively as live virus, indicating that infection with HIV is not necessary for the induction of IL-6 gene expression in human monocytes (Nakajima et al., 1989a). In preliminary studies, the THP-1 human monocyte-cell line was seen to be induced to secrete IL-6 by HIV exposure (Rezai et al., in preparation). The use of this cell line should lead to new information on the mechanisms by which HIV leads to IL-6 gene expression in human monocytes.

In another study, elevated in vivo levels of IL-6 were seen in HIV-infected donors, as determined by measurement of plasma IL-6, spontaneously secreted IL-6, and IL-6 mRNA production in PBMC (Breen et al., 1990). The observation that elevated IL-6 levels are associated with HIV infection has been confirmed by other studies (Birx et al., 1990; Honda et al., 1990; Lafeuillade et al., 1991; Rautonen et al., 1991). Although elevated IL-6 levels were seen to correlate with HIV infection, no correlation was seen between the presence or absence of coinfections, or the severity of HIV-induced disease, and plasma IL-6 levels (Breen et al., 1990). However, since a relatively small number of subjects were examined in this study, further work will be required to establish the relationship between elevated plasma IL-6 levels and the severity of HIV-induced disease. Elevated plasma levels of C-reactive protein, an acute-phase reactant whose production is induced by IL-6, also were seen in HIV-infected donors (Breen et al., 1990).

Chronic B-Cell Activation in Response to HIV Antigens

Initial work examining the antigen specificity of activated B cells in AIDS and HIV infection suggested that a relatively small fraction of activated B-cell clones were responding to HIV-encoded antigens. A recent report indicates that a much greater fraction of activated B-cell clones may be responding to HIV-encoded antigens (Amadori et al., 1989). However, even in this more recent study, a majority of activated B-cell clones appear not to be producing anti-HIV antibodies. Clarification of the relative contribution of anti-HIV B-cell responses to the B-cell hyperactivation seen in AIDS and HIV infection awaits further study.

Summary

At this time there is not sufficient information to determine precisely what immune defects and mechanisms result in B-cell hyperactivation in AIDS and HIV infection, although several possible immune defects could play a role in this hyperactivation (Fig. 9-1). While published reports indicate that HIV is a direct B-cell activator, other work indicates that this may not be the case. Therefore, it is not clear whether direct B-cell activation by HIV contributes significantly to the polyclonal B-cell activation seen in AIDS. However, HIV-induced cytokines, including the overproduction of IL-6 induced by HIV (Nakajima et al., 1989a, 1989b; Breen et al., 1990), could lead directly to polyclonal B-cell activation. Also, chronic, antigen-specific (anti-HIV) B-cell responses might contribute to B-cell hyperactivation in HIV infection (Amadori et al., 1989), as could defective T cell–mediated immunoregulation of activated B cells.

Regardless of the source(s) of B-cell hyperactivation, chronic B-cell stimulation in HIV infection, in association with various immunoregulatory defects, probably plays an important role in the genesis and/or development of B-cell neoplasms in AIDS and HIV infection. Chronic B-cell hyperstimulation could contribute to the development of lymphoma directly, by chronically stimulating a large number of B-cell clones in an uncontrolled fashion, in an environment depleted of effective T-cell immunoregulatory influences. Also, B-cell hyperactivation could contribute to the development of lymphoma by increasing the size of the target pool of B cells susceptible to transformation by undergoing the c-*myc*/Ig gene chromosomal translocation.

AIDS-ASSOCIATED KAPOSI'S SARCOMA

AIDS-associated KS (AIDS-KS), a multifocal endothelial lesion that is often seen in HIV-infected individuals, is the most common AIDS-related malignancy (Knowles and Chadburn, 1990; Centers for Disease Control, 1981; Mitsuyasu, 1988; Friedman-Kien, 1988; Volberding, 1989; Hymes, 1987; Schüpbach, 1988). The first cases of AIDS-KS were reported in 1981 (Centers for Disease Control, 1981). A form of KS, not associated with HIV infection, was first described in 1872 (Kaposi, 1872; Safai and Good, 1980). This classic, or traditional, form of KS is seen in the developed countries of Europe and North America as a rare, relatively benign, localized cutaneous tumor of the lower extremities in older men, primarily those of Mediterranean origin, which generally runs an indolent course over several years (Safai and Good, 1980). Another form of KS is seen in sub-Saharan Africa, with an indolent course of disease in older men similar to that seen in classic KS, but with much more aggressive disease in younger men, often spread to lymph nodes and other sites (Riggs and Hagemeister, 1988; Friedman-Kien, 1988; Hymes, 1987). This form of KS is one of the most common and endemic tumors seen in sub-Saharan Africa. A third, non–HIV-associated form of KS is seen in association with immunosuppressed states, such as those induced by treatment with immunosuppressive drug therapy in organ transplant recipients to prevent graft rejection (Riggs and Hagemeister, 1988; Friedman-Kien, 1988).

Earlier in the history of the AIDS epidemic, as many as 35% of AIDS patients developed KS (Knowles and Chadburn, 1990). However, more recently, the overall incidence of AIDS-KS has been decreasing; currently about 20% of AIDS patients develop KS (Knowles and Chadburn, 1990; Mitsuyasu, 1988; Safai et al., 1987; Beral et al., 1990). Many AIDS patients are found to have KS at the time of autopsy, indicating that the incidence of AIDS-KS may be somewhat higher than reflected by the frequency of AIDS patients that develop clinically apparent AIDS-KS (Moskowitz et al., 1985; Niedt and Schinella, 1985). Generally, AIDS-KS is seen in younger people than the classical form of KS (Beral et al., 1990). Also, AIDS-KS is seen more frequently in homosexual men than in patients belonging to other risk groups, such as IV drug users or hemophiliacs (Knowles and Chadburn, 1990; Friedman-Kien, 1988; Volberding, 1989; Beral et al., 1990; Centers for Disease Control, 1984; Ziegler, 1988). It appears that AIDS-KS is seen more frequently in people who have acquired HIV infection by sexual contact, rather than by IV drug use, transfusion, or parenteral use of infected blood products (Beral et al., 1990). Women with AIDS are more likely to have AIDS-KS if their sexual partner is a bisexual man, rather than an IV drug user (Beral et al., 1990). Also, there is a bias in the geographic distribution of AIDS-KS within the United States, with a greatly elevated percentage of homosexual/bisexual men developing AIDS-KS in California or New York, compared to midwestern states (Beral et al., 1990).

The discovery of one or more KS skin lesions often is the first sign of AIDS seen in apparently healthy individuals (Friedman-Kien, 1988). The AIDS-KS lesions are purplish, erythematous patches, which can be located on skin, mucous membranes, or in lymphatic tissue (lymph nodes and spleen) (Knowles and Chadburn, 1990; Mitsuyasu, 1988; Friedman-Kien, 1988; Volberding, 1989; Hymes, 1987). In contrast to classic KS, in which lesions are generally located on the lower extremities, AIDS-KS lesions are found on the trunk, head, arms, face, and on internal organs (including the gastrointestinal tract) in a multifocal pattern of distribution. At autopsy, nearly every organ can be involved with KS, although brain involvement is uncommon (Mitsuyasu, 1988). Patients with AIDS-KS, in the absence of the other infectious or neoplastic diseases associated with AIDS, generally have a longer life expectancy than those presenting with opportunistic infection or AIDS-related lymphoma (Friedman-Kien, 1988). Rarely is AIDS-KS the cause of death in AIDS. Although AIDS-KS tends to be debilitating and not fatal, pulmonary KS is rapidly and uniformly fatal (Mitsuyasu, 1988). A clinical staging system for AIDS-KS has been developed by Mitsuyasu and co-workers (Mitsuyasu, 1988; Mitsuyasu and Groopman, 1984).

Histopathologically, AIDS-KS is characterized by the presence of anastomosing vascular spaces and by spindle-cell morphology (Knowles and Chadburn, 1990). The cell of origin for AIDS-KS cells is not known, although it is believed that KS originates from vascular endothelium or from lymphatic endothelium (Knowles and Chadburn, 1990; Rutgers et al., 1986; Scully et al., 1988; Beckstead, et al., 1985; Dorfman, 1988). The presence of KS lesions along the lines of lymphatic vessels in the skin and gastrointestinal tract and the development of lymphedema in many patients suggest a lymphatic origin for AIDS-KS cells. However, cell-surface-marker expression indicates that AIDS-KS cells display a phenotype reminiscent of vascular endothelial cells.

The pathogenesis of AIDS-associated KS is not well understood. The epidemiology of AIDS-KS has been interpreted by some investigators as suggesting the involvement of an infectious agent, including an as yet unidentified agent, in the development of this tumor (Beral et al., 1990). Certainly, the observation that AIDS-KS is seen more frequently in homosexual men than in other AIDS risk group members suggests that a sexually transmitted agent may be involved in the genesis of AIDS-KS. Also, the finding that KS can occur in homosexual men with no serologic evidence for HIV infection suggests that a sexually transmitted agent other than HIV is involved in the pathogenesis of KS (Afrasiabi et al., 1986). The malignant transformation of AIDS-KS cells does not appear to involve the direct infection of these cells with HIV

(Groopman, 1987). An epidemiologic association between the development of AIDS-KS and CMV infection in AIDS has been noted, and CMV DNA has been detected in AIDS-KS lesions (Chadburn and Knowles, 1990; Mitsuyasu, 1988; Friedman-Kien, 1988; Volberding, 1989; Hymes, 1987; Schüpbach, 1988; Grody et al., 1988; McDougall et al., 1987). However, CMV infection is common in the general adult population, and no direct evidence connecting CMV infection to the development of AIDS-KS has been presented. Certainly, it is possible that the presence of CMV DNA in AIDS-KS lesions is due to the coinfection of these cells due disseminated CMV infection associated with AIDS and is unrelated to the pathogenesis of AIDS-KS.

Some workers have suggested that KS is not a malignant tumor, but represents instead a hyperplastic growth, induced by an infectious agent and/or by the inappropriate production of growth factors (Ziegler, 1988; Brooks, 1986). There is some evidence to support the belief that KS is an angioproliferative lesion, since KS cells are diploid and since the regression of KS has been seen following the discontinuation of immunosuppressive drug treatment in KS associated with organ transplantation (Sanchez et al., 1985; Wijnveen et al., 1987).

Therefore, AIDS-KS may be a nonmalignant proliferative lesion of endothelial cells that occurs in the setting of immune suppression. The cell of origin (a mesenchymal cell, possibly a lymphatic endothelial cell) for AIDS-KS may grow in response to one or several growth factors (Miles et al., 1990; Marx, 1990; Ensoli et al., 1989) or directly in response to HIV products, in particular the HIV *tat* gene product (Ensoli et al., 1990) (Fig. 9-2).

The Role of Cytokines in the Development and Growth of AIDS-KS

The AIDS-KS–derived cell lines (Nakamura et al., 1988; Salahuddin et al., 1988) produce several defined cytokines and growth factors including IL-1 β, GM-CSF, and basic fibroblast growth factor (bFGF), a potent angiogenic growth factor (Marx, 1990). Addition of anti–IL-1 β or anti-bFGF sera to AIDS-KS cell lines resulted in decreased cellular proliferation, indicating that these factors might be operating as autocrine or paracrine growth factors for AIDS-KS cells (Marx, 1990). Also, AIDS-KS cells produce and respond to an as yet unidentified growth factor; the growth of AIDS-KS cell lines can be increased by culturing them in the presence of conditioned medium from human T-cell leukemia virus (HTLV)-I–infected or HTLV-II–infected $CD4^+$ T-cell lines (Nakamura et al., 1988; Salahuddin et al., 1988), suggesting that a soluble factor produced by these retrovirus-infected T cells augments their growth. A 28- to 30-kDa AIDS-KS growth factor has been isolated from these $CD4^+$ T-cell supernatants and is also produced by AIDS-KS cell lines (Marx, 1990). This growth factor has autocrine and paracrine properties for AIDS-KS cells in vitro, and its altered regulation in vivo may play a role in the development of AIDS-KS.

A cytokine with properties that are reminiscent of those attributed to this AIDS-KS growth factor is IL-6 (Kishimoto, 1990; Kishimoto and Hirano, 1988). Cytokines produced by AIDS-KS cells, including IL-1 β, are known to induce IL-6 secretion by

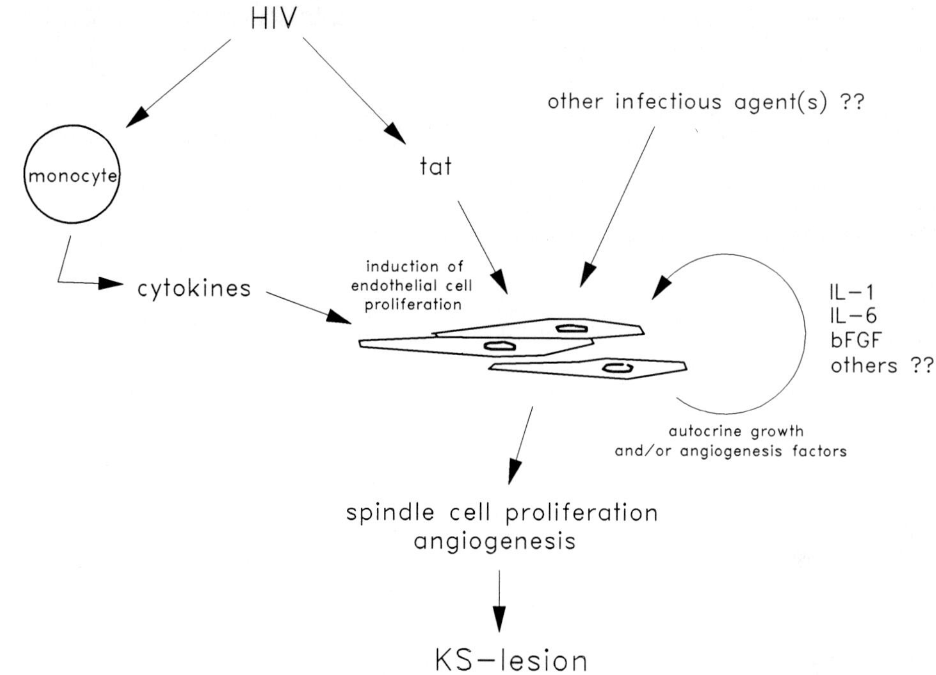

FIGURE 9-2
Immunopathogenesis of AIDS-associated Kaposi's sarcoma (KS). Infection with HIV results in the over-production of cytokines, such as IL-6, and of HIV products, such as *tat,* that can stimulate the growth of endothelial cells. An as yet undefined infectious agent could also play a role in this process. These endothelial spindle cells also produce several cytokines that result in their increased proliferation (autocrine function) and in other biological effects, such as angiogenesis. This continued stimulation could then result in the development of KS lesions. HIV, human immunodeficiency virus; IL-1, interleukin-1; IL-6, interleukin-6; bFGF, basic fibroblast growth factor.

various types of cells, including normal human umbilical vein and primary bovine aortic endothelial cell cultures (Podor et al., 1989). In previous studies, we found that exposure of human monocytes to HIV results in rapid IL-6 gene expression and in IL-6 secretion by these cells (Nakajima et al., 1989a). Also, we have seen that HIV infection is accompanied by elevated plasma IL-6 levels and elevated levels of IL-6 mRNA expression in PBMC in vivo and by elevated levels of IL-6 production in vitro by cultured monocytes isolated from HIV-infected donors (Breen et al., 1990). These findings led to the examination of the role of IL-6 as a growth factor in AIDS-KS.

In recent work, AIDS-KS cells lines were seen to produce and respond to IL-6 (Miles et al., 1990). Two AIDS-KS–derived cell lines, N521J (Nakamura et al., 1988) and EKS3, were seen to secrete substantial amounts of IL-6 (apparently constitutively), to contain intracellular IL-6 by immunoperoxidase staining, and to display high levels of IL-6 mRNA (Miles et al., 1990). The IL-6 produced by these cells is biologically active; the diluted supernatant of these AIDS-KS cell lines can support the growth of an IL-6–dependent cell line (Miles et al., 1990).

When the IL-6 receptor is simultaneously expressed in IL-6–producing cells, IL-6 can act as an autocrine growth factor, as is seen in human multiple myeloma (Kawano et al., 1988) or renal cell carcinoma (Miki et al., 1989). The AIDS-KS cell lines have high constitutive levels of IL-6 receptor mRNA expression (Miles et al., 1990). An AIDS-KS biopsy taken shortly after death from a person with AIDS-KS was seen to show substantial overexpression of IL-6 receptor mRNA, in comparison to noninvolved epithelium isolated from the same donor (Miles et al., 1990).

Exposure of AIDS-KS cells to IL-6 antisense oligodeoxynucleotides leads to decreased IL-6 production by these cells and dramatically inhibits their growth (Miles et al., 1990). The antiproliferative effect of IL-6 antisense oligonucleotides on AIDS-KS cells is reversed by the addition of exogenous recombinant human IL-6 (Miles et al., 1990). These results suggest that IL-6 is an autocrine growth factor for AIDS-KS cells. It is interesting to note that recent work suggests that IL-6 also has angiogenic properties (Motro et al., 1990), indicating that IL-6 production by AIDS-KS spindle cells might help induce the characteristic vascularization seen in KS lesions.

In preliminary work, exposure of AIDS-KS cell lines to various recombinant human cytokines, including IFN-γ, TNF, and IL-1 β, has been seen to lead to the upregulation of IL-6 production and of cellular proliferation by these cells (Miles et al., in preparation). Therefore, the aberrant induction of cytokine production associated with HIV infection (Wright et al., 1988; Rosenberg and Fauci, 1990; Breen et al., 1990), which has been proposed to contribute directly to the immunopathogenesis of AIDS by leading to increased levels of virus production by HIV-infected monocytes and T cells (Poli et al., 1990; Rosenberg and Fauci, 1990), may also lead to, or enhance, the generation and growth of AIDS-KS, possibly by upregulating the production of, or responsiveness to, IL-6 by these cells.

In recent studies by Miles and co-workers (submitted for publication), oncostatin-M, another cytokine with properties reminiscent of the 28- to 30-kDa AIDS-KS growth factor, was seen to act as a potent growth factor for AIDS-KS–derived cells. Oncostatin-M, a 28- to 36-kDa cytokine that is produced by activated lymphoid cells and can regulate the growth and differentiation of a number of tumor cells, was seen to act as a mitogen for AIDS-KS cells, as well as to induce a spindle morphology and IL-6 production by these cells (Miles et al., submitted for publication). Also, AIDS-KS cells were seen to produce oncostatin-M (Miles and co-workers, submitted for publication). These results suggest that oncostatin-M can act as a paracrine/autocrine growth and differentiation factor for AIDS-KS cells and that this cytokine may play a role in the pathogenesis of AIDS-KS.

The Role of HIV-Encoded Products in the Development and Growth of AIDS-KS

Recently, much attention has been directed to the examination of the possible role of HIV-encoded products, especially HIV *tat,* in the development and growth of AIDS-

KS. Mice, transgenic for HIV *tat,* have been seen to develop KS-like lesions, of mouse cell origin (Vogel et al., 1988), suggesting that the HIV *tat* gene product could, directly or indirectly, induce the abnormal proliferation of a KS–precursor cell.

More recently, recombinant HIV *tat* has been shown to induce the proliferation of AIDS-KS cells (Ensoli et al., 1990). However, the mechanisms by which HIV *tat* stimulates the growth of AIDS-KS cells has not been determined. The AIDS-KS cell growth-inducing effect of HIV *tat* could be a direct effect, or, alternatively, could operate indirectly, via the induction of cytokine production by AIDS-KS cells or surrounding cells and/or via the upregulation of growth factor–receptor expression by AIDS-KS cells. Recent studies indicate that exposure of AIDS-KS cells to HIV *tat* leads to increased IL-6 production and proliferation by these cells (Rezai et al., submitted for publication). Inhibition of HIV *tat*-induced IL-6 production by AIDS-KS cells, using an IL-6 antisense oligonucleotide, results in the inhibition of this HIV *tat*-induced KS-cell proliferation (Rezai et al., submitted for publication).

Summary

The immune system alterations that are seen in HIV infection and AIDS provide aberrant regulation of growth factor and growth factor–receptor production, in the setting of immune system suppression and inadequate immune surveillance. Also, HIV infection results in the production and circulation of HIV-encoded molecules such as *tat.* Independently or together, cytokines such as IL-1 β, IL-6, and/or oncostatin-M and HIV *tat* could result in the disordered, hyperplastic growth of spindle cells of endothelial origin, which would then produce angiogenesis-inducing and/or proliferation-inducing factors (bFGF, IL-1, GM-CSF, IL-6), ultimately resulting in the formation of an AIDS-KS lesion (Fig. 9-2). Perhaps, an unknown, sexually transmitted pathogen cofactor is also involved in the development of AIDS-KS, operating either by direct stimulation and/or infection of KS spindle cells and/or by inducing aberrant cytokine production.

It remains to be determined whether the growth-inducing effects of HIV *tat,* or of Il-1 β, bFGF, IL-6, oncostatin-M, or TNF on AIDS-KS cells operate by independent mechanisms or via the induction of the production of one pivotal cytokine, such as IL-6. Also, any synergistic effects of these cytokines on the growth and development of KS remain to be elucidated.

Although many unanswered questions remain regarding the etiology and immunopathogenesis of AIDS-KS, it appears that abnormal growth factor production and/or responsiveness can play an important role in the growth of AIDS-KS.

ACKNOWLEDGMENTS

This work was supported by NIH grants AI24691, CAO1588, CA57152, and AI72631, by funds provided by the state of California and allocated on the recommendation of the Universitywide Task Force on AIDS (86LA012, 91LA149), and by a grant from the American Cancer Society JFRA-165.

REFERENCES

Afrasiabi R, Mitsuyasu R, Nishanian P, Schwartz K, Fahey JL. Characterization of a distinct subgroup of high risk persons with Kaposi's sarcoma and a good prognosis who present with normal T4 cell number and T4:T8 ratio and negative HTLV-III/LAV serologic test results. Am J Med. 1986;81:969–973.

Amadori A, Zamarchi R, Ciminale V, et al. HIV-1-specific B-cell activation: a major constitutent of spontaneous B cell activation during HIV-1 infection. J Immunol. 1989;143:2146–2152.

Andersson JP, Andersson UG, Ernberg IT, Britton SF, DeLey M. Effects of pure interferon on Epstein-Barr virus infection in vitro. J Virol. 1984;54:615–618.

Beckstead JH, Wood GS, Fletcher V. Evidence for the origin of Kaposi's sarcoma from lymphatic endothelium. Am J Pathol. 1985;119:294–300.

Benveniste E, Schroff R, Stevens RH, Gottlieb MS. Immunoregulatory T cells in men with a new acquired immune deficiency syndrome. J Clin Immunol. 1983;3:359–367.

Beral V, Peterman TA, Berkelman RL, Jaffe HW. Kaposi's sarcoma among persons with AIDS: a sexually transmitted infection? Lancet. 1990;335:3–128.

Beral V, Peterman T, Berkelman R, Jaffe H. AIDS-associated non-Hodgkin lymphoma. Lancet. 1991;337:805–809.

Bird AG, Britton S. A new approach to the study of human B lymphocyte function using an indirect plaque assay and a direct B cell activator. Immunol Rev. 1979;45:41–66.

Birx DL, Redfield RR, Tosato G. Defective regulation of Epstein-Barr virus infection in patients with acquired immunodeficiency syndrome (AIDS) or AIDS-related disorders. New Engl J Med. 1986;314:874–879.

Birx DL, Redfield RR, Tencer K, et al. Induction of interleukin-6 during human immunodeficiency virus infection. Blood. 1990;76:2303–2310.

Blomberg RS, Schooley RT. Lymphocyte markers in infectious diseases. Semin Hematol. 1985;22:81–114.

Breen EC, Rezai AR, Nakajima K, et al. Infection with HIV is associated with elevated IL-6 levels and production. J Immunol. 1990;144:480–484.

Brooks J. Kaposi's sarcoma: a reversible hyperplasia. Lancet. 1986;2:1309–1311.

Centers for Disease Control. Kaposi's sarcoma and pneumocystic pneumonia among homosexual men—New York City and California. MMWR. 1981;30:305–308.

Centers for Disease Control. Update: acquired immunodeficiency syndrome (AIDS) in persons with hemophilia. MMWR. 1984;33:589–591.

Clouse KA, Powell D, Washington G, et al. Monokine regulation of human immunodeficiency virus-1 expression in a chronically infected human T cell clone. J Immunol. 1989;142:431–438.

Detels R, English PA, Giorgi JV, et al. Patterns of $CD4^+$ cell changes after HIV-1 infection indicate the existence of a codeterminant of AIDS. J Acquir Immune Defic Syndr. 1988; 1:390–395.

Dorfman RF. Kaposi's sarcoma: evidence supporting its origin from the lymphatic system. Lymphology. 1988;21:45–52.

Ebert EC, Stoll DB, Cassens BJ, Lipshutz WH, Hauptman SP. Diminished interleukin 2 production and receptor generation characterize the acquired immunodeficiency syndrome. Clin Immunol Immunopathol. 1985;37:283–297.

Ensoli B, Nakamura S, Salahuddin SZ, et al. AIDS-Kaposi's sarcoma–derived cells express cytokines with autocrine and paracrine growth effects. Science. 1989;243:223–226.

Ensoli B, Barillari G, Salahuddin SZ, Gallo RC, Wong-Staal F. *Tat* protein of HIV-1 stimulated growth of cells derived from Kaposi's sarcoma lesions of AIDS patients. Nature. 1990; 345:84–86.

Epstein MA. Clues to the role of malaria. Nature. 1984;312:398.

Fahey JL, Taylor JMG. Korns E, Nishanian P. Diagnostic and prognostic factors in AIDS. Mt Sinai J Med. 1986;53:657–663.

Fahey JL, Taylor JMG, Detels R, et al. The prognostic value of cellular and serologic markers in infection with human immunodeficiency virus type 1. New Engl J Med. 1990;322:166–172.

Friedman-Kien AE. AIDS-related Kaposi's sarcoma. In: Schmid L, Senn H-J, eds. AIDS-related neoplasias. New York, NY: Springer-Verlag; 1988:27–36.

Gail MH, Pluda JM, Rabkin CS, et al. Projections of the incidence of non-Hodgkin's lymphoma related to acquired immunodeficiency syndrome. J Natl Cancer Inst. 1991;83:695–701.

Gallo RC. HIV—the cause of AIDS: an overview on its biology, mechanisms of disease induction, and our attempts to control it. J Acquir Immune Defic Syndr. 1988;1:521–535.

Gartner S, Markovitz P, Markovitz DM, Kaplan MH, Gallo RC, Popovik M. The role of mononuclear phagocytes in HTLV-III/LAV infection. Science. 1986;233:215–219.

Gauldie J, Richards C, Harnish D, Lansdorp P, Baumann H. Interferon β_2/B cell stimulatory factor type 2 shares identity with monocyte-derived hepatocyte-stimulating factor and regulates the major acute phase protein response in liver cells. PNAS. 1987;84:7251–7255.

Gottlieb MS, Groopman JE, Weinstein WM, Fahey JL, Detels R. The acquired immunodeficiency syndrome. Ann Intern Med. 1983;99:208–220.

Gowda SD, Stein BS, Mohagheghpour N, Benike CJ, Engleman EG. Evidence that T cell activation is required for HIV-entry in $CD4^+$ lymphocytes. J Immunol. 1989;142:773–780.

Grody WW, Lewin KJ, Naeim F. Detection of cytomegalovirus DNA in classic and epidemic Kaposi's sarcoma by in situ hybridization. Hum Pathol. 1988;19:524–528.

Groopman JE. Biology and therapy of epidemic Kaposi's sarcoma. Cancer. 1987;59:633–637.

Herndier B, Shiramizu B, Sanchez H, Kaplan L, Meeker T, McGrath M. Multisite molecular analysis of AIDS-associated lymphomas. Sixth Int Cong AIDS. 1990;Th.A.329. Abstract.

Hersh EM, Miller TP. Malignant lymphomas in patients with human immunodeficiency virus infection. Recent Results Cancer Res. 1988;112:54–62.

Hirano T, Yasukawa K, Harade H, et al. Complementary DNA for a novel human interleukin (BSF-2) that induces B lymphocytes to produce immunoglobulin. Nature. 1986;324:73–76.

Ho DD, Rota TR, Hirsh MS. Infection of monocyte/macrophages by human T lymphotropic virus type III. J Clin Invest. 1986;77:1712–1714.

Hoffman B, Odum N, Jakobsen BK, et al. Immunological studies in the acquired immunodeficiency syndrome: II. Active suppression or intrinsic defect investigated by mixing AIDS cells with HLA-DR identical normal cells. Scand J Immunol. 1986;23:669–678.

Hofmann B, Wang Y, Cumberland WG, Detels R, Bozorgmehri M, Gahey JL. Serum beta$_2$-microglobulin level increases in HIV infection: relation to seroconversion, CD4 T-cell fall and prognosis. AIDS 1990. 1990;4:207–214.

Honda M, Kitamura K, Mizutani Y, et al. Quantitative analysis of serum IL-6 and its correlation with increased levels of serum IL-2R in HIV-induced diseases. J Immunol. 1990;145:4059–4064.

Hymes KB. Kaposi's sarcoma in AIDS. In: Wormser GP, Stahl RE, Bottone EJ, eds. AIDS and other manifestations of HIV infection. Park Ridge, NJ: Noyes Publications; 1987:747–766.

Kaposi M. Idiopathisches multiples Pigment-Sarkom der Haut. Arch Dermatol Syphil. 1972; 4:265–272.

Kawano M, Hirano T, Matsuda T, et al. Autocrine generation and requirement of BSF-2/IL-6 for human multiple myelomas. Nature. 1988;332:83–85.

Kernbauer R, Kock A, Schwarz T, et al. IFN-β2, B cell differentiation factor 2, or hybridoma growth factor (IL-6) is expressed and released by human epidermal cells and epidermoid carcinoma cell lines. J Immunol. 1989;142:1922–1928.

Kishimoto T. The biology of interleukin-6. Blood. 1989;74:1–10.

Kishimoto T, Hirano T. Molecular regulation of B lymphocyte response. Annu Rev Immunol. 1988;6:485–512.

Klein G. In: Melchers F, Potter M, eds. Mechanisms of B cell neoplasia 1987. Basel: Editiones Roche; 1987:225.

Knowles DM, Chadburn A. The neoplasms associated with AIDS. In: Joshi VV, ed. Pathology of AIDS and other manifestations of HIV infection. New York, NY: Igaku-Shoin; 1990:83–120.

Koyanagi Y, Miles S, Mitsuyasu RT, Merrill J, Vinters HV, Chen ISY. Dual infection of the central nervous system by AIDS viruses with distinct cellular tropisms. Science. 1987; 236:819–822.

Krowka JF, Moody DM, Stites DP. Immunological effects of HIV infection. In: Levy JA, ed. AIDS pathogenesis and treatment. New York, NY: Marcel Dekker; 1989:257–303.

Lafeuillade A, Poizotmartin I, Quilichini R, et al. Increased interleukin-6 production is associated with disease progression in HIV infection. AIDS. 1991;5:1139–1140.

Lane HC, Fauci AS. Immunologic abnormalities in the acquired immune deficiency syndrome. Annu Rev Immunol. 1985;3:477–500.

Lane HC, Masur H, Edgar LC, Whalen G, Rook AH, Fauci AS. Abnormalities of B-cell activation and immunoregulation in patients with the acquired immunodeficiency syndrome. New Engl J Med. 1983;309:453–458.

Lane HC, Depper JM, Greene WC, Whalen G, Waldmann TA, Fauci AS. Qualitative analysis of immune function in patients with the acquired immunodeficiency syndrome: evidence for a selective defect in soluble antigen recognition. New Engl J Med. 1985;313:79–84.

Laurence J, Gottlieb AB, Kunkel HG. Soluble suppressor factors in patients with acquired immune deficiency syndrome and its prodrome. J Clin Invest. 1983;72:2072–2081.

Lotz M, Tsoukas CD, Fong S, Carson DA, Vaughan JH. Regulation of Epstein-Barr virus infection by recombinant interferons. Selected sensitivity to interferon-γ. Eur J Immunol. 1985;15:520–525.

Luger TA, Schwartz T, Krutmann J, et al. Interleukin-6 is produced by epidermal cells and plays an important role in the activation of human T-lymphocytes and natural killer cells. Ann NY Acad Sci. 1989;557:405–414.

MacMahon EME, Glass JD, Hayward SD, et al. Epstein-Barr virus in AIDS-related primary central nervous system lymphoma. Lancet. 1991;338:969–973.

Martínez-Maza O, Andersson U, Andersson J, Britton S, De Ley, M. Spontaneous production of interferon-γ in adult and newborn humans. J Immunol. 1984;132:251–255.

Martínez-Maza O, Crabb E, Mitsuyasu RT, Fahey JL, Giorgi JV. Infection with the human immunodeficiency virus (HIV) is associated with an in vivo increase in B lymphocyte activation and immaturity. J Immunol. 1987a;138:3720–3724.

Martínez-Maza O, Moody, DJ, Rezai AR, et al. Increased spontaneous immunoglobulin secretion associated with cyclophosphamide-induced immune suppression. J. Clin Immunol. 1987b;7:107–113.

Martínez-Maza O, Salazar-Gonzalez JF, Rezai AR, Mitsuyasu RT, Fahey JL. B cell activation in AIDS and HIV-infection: role of decreased CD4 number and IFN-γ production. 2nd Ann Conf Clin Immunol. 1987c; Abstracts.

Marx J. Kaposi's sarcoma puzzle begins to yield. Science. 1990;248:442–443.

McDougall JK, Olson KA, Smith PP, Collier AC. Detection of cytomegalovirus and AIDS-associated retrovirus in tissues of patients with AIDS, Kaposi's sarcoma and persistent lymphadenopathy. Antibiot Chemother. 1987;38:99–112.

Meltzer MS, Skillman DR, Hoover DL, et al. Macrophages and the human immunodeficiency virus. Immunol Today. 1990;11:217–223.

Miki S, Iwano M, Miki Y, et al. Interleukin-6 (IL-6) functions as an in vitro autocrine growth factor in renal cell carcinomas. FEBS Lett. 1989;250:607–610.

Miles SA, Rezai AR, Salazar-Gonzalez JF, et al. AIDS Kaposi's sarcoma-derived cells produce and respond to interleukin-6. Proc Natl Acad Sci USA. 1990;87:4068–4072.

Miles SA, Martínez-Maza O, Rezai A, et al. Oncostatin-M as a potent mitogen for AIDS-Kaposi sarcoma derived cells. Science. 1992, in press.

Mitsuyasu RT. AIDS-related Kaposi's sarcoma: a review of its pathogenesis and treatment. Blood Rev. 1988;2:222–231.

Mitsuyasu RT, Groopman JE. Biology and therapy of Kaposi's sarcoma. Semin Oncol. 1984;11:53–59.

Mitsuyasu TT, Colman MF, Sun NCJ. Simultaneous occurrence of Hodgkin's disease and Kaposi's sarcoma in a patient with the acquired immune deficiency syndrome. Am J Med. 1986;80:954–958.

Mizuma H, Litwin S, Zolla-Pazner S. B cell activation in HIV infection: relationship of spontaneous immunoglobulin secretion to various immunologic parameters. Clin Exp Immunol. 1988;71:410–416.

Modlin RL, Hofman FM, Meyer PR, et al. Altered distribution of B and T lymphocytes in lymph nodes from homosexual men with Kaposi's sarcoma. Lancet. 1983;2:768–771.

Moore RD, Kessler H, Richman DD, Flexner C, Chaisson RE. Non-Hodgkin's lymphoma in patients with advanced HIV infection treated with zidovudine. JAMA. 1991;265:2208–2211.

Moskowitz LB, Hensley GT, Gould EW, Weiss SD. Frequency and anatomic distribution of lymphadenopathic Kaposi's sarcoma in the acquired immunodeficiency syndrome: an autopsy series. Hum Pathol. 1985;16:447–456.

Motro B, Itin A, Sachs L, Keshet E. Pattern of interleukin 6 gene expression in vivo suggests a role for this cytokine in angiogenesis. Proc Natl Acad Sci USA. 1990;87:3092–3096.

Murray HW, Welte K, Jacobs JL, Rubin BY, Mettelsmann R, Roberts RB. Production of an in vitro response to interleukin 2 in the acquired immunodeficiency syndrome. J Clin Invest. 1985;76:1959–1964.

Nakajima K, Martínez-Maza O, Hirano T, et al. Induction of IL-6 (B cell stimulatory factor 2/IFN-β_2) production by HIV. J Immunol. 1989a;142:531–536.

Nakajima K, Martínez-Maza O, Hirano T, et al. HIV-induced B cell stimulatory factor 2/interleukin-6 (BSF2/IL6) production. Ann NY Acad Sci. 1989b;557:521–524.

Nakamura S, Salahuddin SZ, Biberfeld P, et al. Kaposi's sarcoma cells: long-term culture with growth factor from retrovirus-infected $CD4^+$ T cells. Science. 1988;242:426–430.

Niedt GW, Schinella RA. Acquired immunodeficiency syndrome: clinicopathologic study of 56 autopsies. Arch Pathol Lab Med. 1985;109:727–734.

Pahwa S, Pahwa R, Saxinger C, Gallo RC, Good RA. Influence of the human T-lymphotropic virus/lymphadenopathy-associated virus on functions of human lymphocytes: evidence for immunosuppressive effects and polyclonal B cell activation by banded viral preparations. Proc Natl Acad Sci USA. 1985;82:8198–8202.

Pahwa S, Pahwa R, Good RA, Gallo RC, Saxinger C. Stimulatory and inhibitory influences of human immunodeficiency virus on normal human B lymphocytes. Proc Natl Acad Sci USA. 1986;83:9124–9128.

Palacios R, Martínez-Maza O. IFN-γ mediated suppression of Epstein-Barr virus induced activation of B lymphocytes by OKT4$^+$ T lymphocytes. In: Oppenheim JJ, Cohen S, eds. Interleukins, lymphokines and cytokines. New York, NY: Academic Press; 1983:375–380.

Pelicci PG, Knowles DM, Arlin Z, et al. Multiple monoclonal B cell expansions and c-*myc* oncogene rearrangements in AIDS-related lymphoproliferative disorders. Implications for lymphomagenesis. J Exp Med. 1986;164:2049–2060.

Pluda JM, Yarchoan R, Jaffe ES, et al. Development of non-Hodgkin lymphoma in a cohort of patients with severe human immunodeficiency virus (HIV) infection on long-term antiretroviral therapy. Ann Intern Med. 1990;113:276–282.

Podor TJ, Jirik FR, Loskutoff DJ, Carson DA, Lotz M. Human endothelial cells produce IL-6: lack of responses to exogenous IL-6. Ann NY Acad Sci. 1989;557:374–385.

Poli G, Bressler P, Kinter A, et al. Interleukin 6 induces human immunodeficiency virus expression in infected monocytic cells alone and in synergy with tumor necrosis factor α by transcriptional and post-transcriptional mechanisms. J Exp Med. 1990;172:151–158.

Prince HE, Kermani-Arab V, Fahey JL. Depressed interleukin 2 receptor expression in acquired immune deficiency and lymphadenopathy syndromes. J Immunol. 1984;133:1313–1317.

Rautonen J, Rautonen N, Martin NL, et al. Serum interleukin-6 concentrations are elevated and associated with elevated tumor necrosis factor-alpha and immunoglobulin-G and immunoglobulin-A concentrations in children with HIV infection. AIDS. 1991;5:1319–1325.

Rezai AR, Breen EC, Martínez-Maza O. HIV induces IL-6 production by THP-1, a human monocyte cell line. 1992, in preparation.

Rezai A, Martínez-Maza O, Gaynor R, Magpantay L, Kishimoto T, Miles S. HIV *tat* increases IL-6 production by and proliferation of AIDS-KS derived cells. 1992, submitted for publication.

Riggs S, Hagemeister FB. Immunodeficiency states: a predisposition to lymphoma. In: Fuller LM, Hagemeister FB, Sullivan MP, Velasquez WS, eds. Hodgkin's disease and non-Hodgkin's lymphomas in adults and children. New York, NY: Raven Press; 1988:451–478.

Roederer M, Staal FJT, Raju PA, Ela SW, Herzenberg LA, Herzenberg LA. Cytokine-stimulated human immunodeficiency virus replication is inhibited by *N*-acetyl-*L*-cysteine. Proc Natl Acad Sci USA. 1990;87:4884–4888.

Rosenberg ZF, Fauci AS. Immunopathogenic mechanisms of HIV infection: cytokine induction of HIV expression. Immunol Today. 1990;11:176–180.

Rutgers JL, Wieczorek R, Bonetti F, et al. The expression of endothelial cell surface antigens by AIDS-associated Kaposi's sarcoma: evidence for a vascular endothelial cell origin. Am J Pathol. 1986;122:493–499.

Safai B, Good RA. Kaposi's sarcoma: a review and recent developments. Clin Bull. 1980; 10:62–69.

Safai B, Lynfield R, Lowenthal DA, Ziner B. Cancer associated with HIV infection. Anticancer Res. 1987;7:1055–1068.

Salahuddin SZ, Nakamura S, Biberfeld P, et al. Angiogenic properties of Kaposi's sarcoma–derived cells after long-term culture in vitro. Science. 1988;242:430–433.

Salazar-Gonzalez JF, Moody DJ, Giorgi J, Martínez-Maza O, Mitsuyasu R, Fahey JL. Reduced lymphocyte ecto-5′-nucleotidase activity and enhanced OKT10 and HLA-DR antigen expression in the acquired immune deficiency syndrome: evidence of immaturity in CD8 (T-suppressor/cytotoxic) lymphocytes. J Immunol. 1985;135:1778–1785.

Sanchez MA, Ames ED, Erhardt A, Auer G. Analysis of DNA distribution in Kaposi's sarcoma in patients with and without acquired immunodeficiency disease. Lab Invest. 1985;52:57.

Schnittman SM, Lane HC, Higgins SE, Folks T, Fauci AS. Direct polyclonal activation of human B lymphocytes by the acquired immune deficiency syndrome virus. Science. 1986;233:1084–1086.

Schüpbach J. The etiology of AIDS and its relevance for AIDS-related neoplasias. Recent Results Cancer Res. 1988;112:6–16.

Scully PA, Steinman HK, Kennedy C, Trueblood K, Frisman DM, Voland JR. AIDS-related Kaposi's sarcoma displays differential expression of endothelial surface antigens. Am J Pathol. 1988;130:244–251.

Sehgal PB, May LT, Tamm I, Vilcek J. Human β_2-interferon and B cell differentiation factor BSF-2 are identical. Science. 1987;236:731–732.

Sirianni MC, Tagliaferri F, Aiuti F. Pathogenesis of the natural killer cell deficiency in AIDS. Immunol Today. 1990;11:81–82.

Subar M, Neri A, Inghirami G, Knowles DM, Dalla-Favera R. Frequent c-*myc* oncogene activation and infrequent presence of Epstein-Barr virus genome in AIDS-associated lymphoma. Blood. 1988;72:667–671.

Tabibzadeh SS, Santhanam U, Sehgal P, May LT. Cytokine-induced production of IFN-β_2/IL-6 by freshly explanted human endometrial stromal cells: modulation by estradiol-17b. J Immunol. 1989;142:3134–3139.

Taylor J, Afrasiabi R, Fahey JL, Korns E, Weaver M, Mitsuyasu R. Prognostically significant classification of immune changes in AIDS with Kaposi's sarcoma. Blood. 1986;67:666–671.

Tsokos GC. Defective regulation of Epstein-Barr virus infection in patients with AIDS. New Engl J Med. 1986;315:761–762.

Vogel J, Hinrichs SH, Reynolds RK, Luciw P, Jay G. The HIV tat gene induces dermal lesions resembling Kaposi's sarcoma in transgenic mice. Nature. 1988;335:606–611.

Volberding PA. Kaposi's sarcoma in AIDS. In: Levy JA, ed. AIDS pathogenesis and treatment. New York, NY: Marcel Dekker; 1989:345–358.

Volberding PA, Lagakos SW, Koch MA, et al. Zidovudine in asymptomatic human immunodeficiency virus infection. A controlled trial in persons with fewer than 500 CD4-positive cells per cubic millimeter. New Engl J Med. 1990;322:941–949.

Walker CM, Moody DJ, Stites DP, Levy JA. $CD8^+$ lymphocytes can control HIV infection in vitro by suppressing virus replication. Science. 1986;234:1563–1566.

Whittle HC, Brown J, Marsh K, et al. T cell control of Epstein-Barr virus-infected cells is lost during *P. falciparum* malaria. Nature. 1984;312:449–450.

Wijnveen A-C, Persson H, Bjorck S, Blohme I. Disseminated Kaposi's sarcoma—full regression after withdrawal of immunosuppressive therapy: report of a case. Transplant Proc. 1987;19:3735–3736.

Wright SC, Jewett A, Mitsuyasu R, Bonavida B. Spontaneous cytotoxicity and tumor necrosis factor production by peripheral blood monocytes from AIDS patients. J Immunol. 1988; 141:99–104.

Yamasaki K, Taga T, Hirata Y, et al. Cloning and expression of human interleukin-6 (BSF-2/ IFNβ_2) receptor. Science. 1988;241:825–828.

Yarchoan R, Redfield RR, Broder S. Mechanisms of B cell activation in patients with acquired immunodeficiency syndrome and related disorders. J Clin Invest. 1986;78:439–447.

Ziegler JL. Pathogenesis of AIDS-associated Kaposi's sarcoma. Lymphology. 21:1988;15–18.

Ziegler JL, Levy JA. Acquired immunodeficiency syndrome and cancer. Adv Viral Oncol. 1985;5:239–255.

Ziegler JL, Beckstead JA, Volberding PA, et al. Non-Hodgkin's lymphoma in 90 homosexual men. Relation to generalized lymphadenopathy and the acquired immunodeficiency syndrome. New Engl J Med. 1984;311:565–570.

PART **TWO**

BIOLOGICAL THERAPY

TYPES OF BIOLOGICAL THERAPY

In this section of the book we will analyze the actions of several types of biomodulator, beginning with monoclonal antibodies (mAb). Since there has been a great deal of work with monoclonal antibodies in the past 10 years, we will begin by discussing several aspects of those studies. Various types of biological therapy have shown some degree of effectiveness. We will discuss each type in detail. As elsewhere, our aim will be to indicate future directions more than to simply summarize the status of each approach.

To put subsequent chapters on the clinical applications of immunotherapy into perspective, we will outline a classification that is recognized by many investigators. Not all of the broader group of biomodulators fall into these headings. Moreover, a biomodulator with several actions may be grouped into more than one category. Still, we hope that this framework will be helpful when considering combinations of agents of different types.

1 *Active:* Stimulation of the host's intrinsic antitumor immunity.

a *Nonspecific:* Use of microbial or chemical immunomodulators ("adjuvants"). Activates macrophages, natural killer (NK) cells, and other nonspecific effectors. Activates T cells secondarily through macrophages.

Included here are the immunological "adjuvants" such as bacillus Calmette-Guérin (BCG) and its derivatives (such as muramyl dipeptide [MDP], related mycobacteria, or mycobacterial structures), pertussis toxin, pyran, poly A: poly C, endotoxin (especially detoxified endotoxin or monophosphoryl lipid A), and interferons α and β. These substances were often used singly to try to treat cancers in the 1970s, but are most useful as adjuncts to specific immunogens.

b *Specific:* Use of tumor cells or tumor-associated antigens (TAA), sometimes altered by haptens, viruses, or treatment with enzymes. Activates specific effector cells such as cytolytic T cells and antibody-armed macrophages.

Whole tumor cells (irradiated) and mechanically disrupted or virally lysed tumor cells fall into this category, as well as tumor extracts or supernates of in vitro tumor cultures.

2 *Adoptive:* Transfer of immunological cells or informational molecules (e.g., lymphokines).

Adoptive transfer of lymphoid cells was originally performed from one inbred mouse to another, but this is equivalent to autologous reinfusion of cells in a specific human being. We have arbitrarily broadened the category to include the administration of informational molecules such as interleukins even without coadministration of lymphocytes.

3 *Restorative:* Repletion of deficient immunological subpopulations such as T cells; inhibition of suppressor influences (suppressor T cells or suppressor macrophages) to accomplish the same end, indirectly.

The administration of thymic hormones or levamisole can directly accomplish such a repletion. Administration of low doses of cyclophosphamide or of type-2 histamine antagonists inhibits suppressor T cells, whereas antagonists of prostaglandin synthesis exemplify inhibitors of suppressor macrophage activity.

4 *Passive:* Transfer of antibodies or short-lived antitumor "factors." Antibodies, especially monoclonal antibodies, as carriers for killer molecules (i.e., immunoconjugates), are also included here.

Antibodies may be used by themselves, as an adjunct to substances that activate cells with receptors for the Fc portion of antibodies or as carriers for killer molecules such as radionuclides, toxins, or chemotherapeutic agents. Besides antibodies, such things as tumor necrosis factor (TNF) might be included as an example of a short-lived "factor" that accomplishes its purpose and then is cleared.

5 *Cytomodulatory:* We suggest this new category to denote a major immunological activity, particularly of the interferons and tumor necrosis factor-α (TNF-α) upregulation of TAA accessory molecules and major histocompatibility (MHC) antigens on the surface of the tumor cells. This action may be crucial to the success of other forms of immunotherapy that require the expression of those antigens. Agents within this category, like that of nonspecific active immunotherapy, may be mainly adjuncts to others, but are nonetheless important. Biochemical modulation of the cell is another activity covered by this proposed new category, perhaps with immunological consequences if the synthesis of TAA is modified or if the susceptibility of the cell to immune lysis by T cells or antibodies is increased.

These categories do not cover all aspects of biomodulators, as we mentioned in the foreword, but may provide a glossary sufficient for the more classical forms of immunotherapy. While several agents such as the interferons and retinoids have effects that fall in several different categories simultaneously, one may still attempt to achieve an effect mainly in one of the areas.

CHAPTER **10**

MONOCLONAL ANTIBODIES IN THERAPY, ALONE OR CONJUGATED WITH DRUGS

William C. Biddle
Kenneth A. Foon

The need for improved specificity in cancer chemotherapy is apparent. Monoclonal antibodies (mAb) offer the possibility of selective delivery of antineoplastic agents to the tumor site, thereby reducing systemic exposure and toxicity to normal tissue components. This approach uses the monoclonal antibody as a vehicle to transport the cytotoxic agent specifically to target tumor cells expressing the appropriate tumor-associated antigen (TAA). The idea of attaching cytotoxic agents to molecules specific for tumor cells was first postulated by Paul Ehrlich in 1906. This mode of therapy was, until recently, limited by the amount of specific heteroantisera that could be produced. In a relatively short period of time, the hybridoma technology (Köhler and Milstein, 1975, 1976) has led to an ever increasing number of unique monoclonal antibodies directed to a large variety of TAA.

Monoclonal antibodies have been shown to have clinical utility in the histologic assessment and classification of malignant diseases particularly for leukemias and lymphomas (Foon and Todd, 1986; Foon and Gale, 1987). Monoclonal antibodies raised against tumor markers such as α-fetoprotein, carcinoembryonic antigen, and CA-125, among others, have applicability in screening procedures and in monitoring clinical disease states (Bagshaw, 1983; Fritsche, 1986; Crowther et al., 1989). Monoclonal antibodies alone or monoclonal antibodies conjugated to various radioisotopes, toxins, or drugs may have potential therapeutic applications (Foon, 1989; Pimm, 1988; Dillman, 1989; Pietersz, 1990; Glassy and Dillman, 1988). The focus of this chapter is the clinical applicability of unconjugated monoclonal antibodies and monoclonal antibodies coupled to chemotherapeutic drugs.

UNLABELED MONOCLONAL ANTIBODIES—CLINICAL TRIALS

Studies using monoclonal antibodies as passive immunotherapy have helped define a number of critical factors necessary for successful monoclonal antibody therapy (Table 10-1). Although reductions in tumor loads were observed in some cases, these were for the most part transient (Dillman et al., 1982a, 1982b, 1984; Ritz et al., 1981; Oldham et al., 1984; Sears et al., 1982, 1984, 1985; Foon et al., 1984; Press et al., 1987; Harris and Mastrangelo, 1989). The isotype of a particular monoclonal antibody may be an important criterion for its selection as a therapeutic tool. Some of the most impressive clinical responses to date with unlabeled antibodies have been observed in melanoma patients treated with a monoclonal antibody (R24, IgG3) that both activates human complement and is effective in antibody-dependent cellular cytotoxicity (Vadhan-Raj et al., 1988). Activation of immune effector mechanisms, complement mediated lysis, or direct antiproliferative actions by monoclonal antibody alone, however, appears insufficient in generating an effective, sustained eradication of tumor cells.

One novel therapeutic approach involves the use of monoclonal anti-idiotype antibodies in B-cell malignancies. Unlike the aforementioned antibodies, in which the antigen is a TAA, anti-idiotype antibodies are directed against a tumor-specific antigen (TSA), which is the idiotype of the cell surface immunoglobulin present on the malignant B cells. Since B-cell lymphomas and leukemias are clonal, all of the malignant cells should express the same idiotype. Each patient's lymphoma idiotype is therefore unique, and anti-idiotype antibodies must be "tailor-made" for each patient.

The largest experience with anti-idiotype therapy is that of Miller et al. (1982). Their initial report of this therapy was in a patient with a rapidly progressive lymphoma resistant to chemotherapy and interferon. Following eight continuous 6-hour IV infusions spaced over the period of 1 month, the patient entered a complete clinical remission that was sustained for 6 years without further treatment (Levy R, personal communication). The mechanism responsible for this is not clear. Because the antitumor response continued long after the period of passive antibody administration, evidence of an anti–anti-idiotype antibody response by the patient was investigated; none was detected. It remains possible that indirect mechanisms may be involved. The immune system is regulated by networks of interactions between idiotypes and anti-idiotypes (Jerne, 1974, 1984). The anti-idiotype could have triggered these interactions, leading to an antiproliferative response against the tumor.

These investigators treated 10 additional patients with individually tailored anti-idiotype antibodies of different subclasses (Meeker et al., 1985a). Some were treated with multiple antibodies with different isotype or epitope specificity. Tumor responses were reported in 50% of patients. No complete responses were observed and most lasted for less than 6 months. Problems included antiglobulin responses and free idiotype antibody in the serum, which blocked the murine antibody and led to fever, anthralgias, dyspnea, and headaches. A more serious problem was emergence of idiotype variants within tumors during treatment (Meeker et al., 1985b). These investigators are currently generating monoclonal anti-idiotype antibodies that identify public or "shared idiotypes" (Brown et al., 1989). Shared anti-idiotype antibodies react with the tumor cells from more than one patient. Panels of "shared idiotype" antibodies would lead to a much broader application of this novel approach to B-leukemia/lymphoma therapy.

It must be taken into account that most patients in these initial trials were poor candidates either due to the debilitating nature of their disease or because, as a consequence of previous treatment regimens, they were unable to mount adequate antitumor responses. Strategies to improve host effector cell mechanisms and increase the interactions of monoclonal antibodies with these cells will be required to improve these results (discussed in subsequent sections). However, these initial clinical studies are encouraging in that monoclonal antibody treatment did result in effective localization with tolerable toxicities (reviewed in Dillman, 1989; Dillman and Royston, 1984; Foon, 1989; Oldham, 1987; Harris and Mastrangelo, 1989).

Strategies to Improve Host Immune Response with Unconjugated Monoclonal Antibodies

The limited therapeutic efficacy observed in prior passive serotherapy studies using unconjugated monoclonal antibodies appears to be at least partially attributable to inadequate involvement of host immune effector cells with the tumor. With the possible exception of monoclonal antibodies raised against receptors required for cell proliferation, such as epidermal growth factor (Sato et al., 1983; Masui et al., 1984), transferrin (Taetle and Honeysett, 1987; Sauvage et al., 1987; Trowbridge, 1983), somatomedin (Arteaga and Osborne, 1989), and IL-2 (Waldmann et al., 1985; Waldmann, 1986) or class II molecules (Vaickus et al., 1989), direct effects on tumor cell growth cannot usually be obtained. A recent report, however, has demonstrated that monoclonal antibodies can be directly cytotoxic to tumor cells by induction of apoptotic lysis (Trauth et al., 1989) responsible for cell death. The clinical utility of many of these monoclonal antibodies is debatable due to (1) the large systemic pool of normal cells expressing these receptors and (2) the question of whether or not a substantial sustained antiproliferative response can be obtained. Partial clinical responses have been obtained, however, in two patients with adult T-cell leukemia following administration of anti-CD25 (IL-2 receptor) antibody (Waldmann et al., 1985).

To be most effective, unconjugated monoclonal antibodies need to initiate a potent immune response against the tumor. Monoclonal antibodies can indeed elicit tumor cell lysis by either complement-mediated or antibody-dependent cell-mediated cytotoxicity (ADCC) mechanisms. Both of these antitumor mechanisms, however, require an intact monoclonal antibody, which is attributed to the necessity of having an intact Fc portion of the immunoglobulin for interaction with either effector cell Fc receptor sites or complement proteins. The monoclonal antibody subclass is an additional constraint because (1) murine IgG3 monoclonal antibodies are most effective at complement-mediated lysis with other isotypes less, or not, effective and (2) IgG3 and IgG2a mouse antibodies are the most potent at initiating ADCC due to their interaction with

TABLE 10-1
HUMAN CLINICAL TRIALS USING UNLABELED MURINE MONOCLONAL ANTIBODIES

Disease	Antibody/class	No. of patients	Toxicity	Effect	Reference
cALL	Anti-J5/IgG2a (anti-CD10)	4	Fever	Transient reduction in circulating cells	Ritz et al., 1981
T-ALL	Anti-Leu-1/IgG2a (anti-CD5), 12E7/IgG1, 4H9/IgG2a	8	Coagulopathy	Transient reduction in circulating cells	Levy and Miller, 1983
AML	PM/81/IgM, AML-2-23/IgG2b, PMN 29/IgM	3	Fever, arthralgia, myalgia	Transient reduction in circulating cells	Ball et al., 1983
ATL	Anti-Tac (anti-CD25)	2	None	1 partial response	Waldmann et al., 1985
B-CLL	T101/IgG2a (anti-CD5)	18	Dyspnea, fever, hypotension, malaise, urticaria	Transient reduction in circulating cells	Bertram et al., 1986; Foon et al., 1984; Dillman et al., 1982b, 1984

B-CLL	Anti-idiotype/IgG1 and IgG2b	1	Fever, urticaria	Transient reduction in circulating cells	Giardinia et al., 1985
CTCL	T101/IgG2a, anti-Leu-1/IgG2a (anti-CD5)	30	Dyspnea, urticaria, fever, hypotension	10 minor responses	Miller et al., 1983; Bertram et al., 1986; Dillman et al., 1984
B-lymphoma	1F5/IgG2a (anti-CD20)	4	Fever, myelosuppression	1 partial response	Press et al., 1987
B-lymphoma	Anti-idiotype/IgG1, IgG2a, or Ig2b	11	Fever, chills, nausea, vomiting, headache, diarrhea, transient dyspnea	1 complete and 5 partial responses	Miller et al., 1982; Meeker et al., 1985
B-lymphoma	Lym-1/IgG2a	10	Fever, urticaria	3 minor responses	Hu et al., 1989
Gastrointestinal	17-1A/IgG2a	20	Urticaria, bronchospasm, mild hypotension	Limited responses	Sears et al., 1984
Melanoma	9.2.27/IgG2a	20	Fever, serum sickness	None	Schroff et al., 1987; Oldham et al., 1984
Melanoma	R24/IgG3	21	Urticaria, pruritis, fever, wheezing	4 partial responses	Vadhan-Raj et al., 1988

Alphabetical listing of abbreviations: ATL, adult T-cell leukemia/lymphoma; AML, acute myelogenous leukemia; B-CLL, B-chronic lymphocytic leukemia; cALL, common acute lymphoblastic leukemia; CTCL, cutaneous T-cell lymphoma.

appropriate Fc gamma receptors. The Fc gamma receptors type I, II, and III are differentially expressed on human monocytes, lymphocytes, and granulocytes, and their relative number and affinity for monoclonal antibodies is an important consideration for effector cell "triggering" in ADCC (Gergely and Sarmay, 1989; Fanger et al., 1989). To amplify the host immune response in this regard will require the recruitment of large numbers of immunocompetent cells that can then interact with monoclonal antibodies to mount an effective ADCC response.

Several possibilities for addressing this issue have been proposed and include the use of human monoclonal antibodies, human/mouse chimeric monoclonal antibodies, and various cytokines to upregulate host antitumor response. Human monoclonal antibodies obviously are the best candidates for increasing the potency of ADCC because they would have the highest avidity for immune effector cells in an allogeneic system. However, problems in obtaining an appropriate lymphocyte source, low cell-fusion yields, and the stability of resulting clones that generally secrete low amounts of monoclonal antibodies (the majority of which are IgM) have severely limited their development and use (for review, Glassy and Dillman, 1988). Although intralesional therapy of malignant melanoma with human monoclonal antibodies has shown responses (Irie and Morton, 1986), systemic therapy with human monoclonal antibodies has not been reported.

Another approach to circumvent the poor responses observed with murine monoclonal antibodies is to create human/mouse chimeric monoclonal antibodies. These genetically engineered monoclonal antibodies consist of a monoclonal antibody composed of the murine Fab portion responsible for antigen binding and the constant region of human immunoglobulin. Successful creation of such chimeric monoclonal antibodies has been described (Sun et al., 1987; Liu et al., 1987a, 1987b; Shaw et al., 1987). Chimeric monoclonal antibodies constructed through the use of the murine V region genome of mAb CO17-1A and either the $\gamma 1$, $\gamma 2$, $\gamma 3$, or $\gamma 4$ human C domains were recently tested for their ability to participate in human ADCC against colorectal carcinoma cells (Steplewski et al., 1988). Chimeric IgG1 mAb and, to a lesser extent, IgG2, IgG3, and IgG4 were capable of mediating ADCC together with either human monocytes, macrophages, lymphocytes, or granulocytes. A chimeric IgG1-κ 17-1A mAb was recently administered to 10 patients with metastatic colon cancer (LoBuglio et al., 1989) to evaluate pharmacokinetics and immunogenicity. This chimeric form of 17-1A mAb was less immunogenic, with only one patient developing an antibody response, which was directed only against the murine variable region of the chimera. In addition, the chimera had a sixfold longer circulation time than its murine counterpart. Another chimeric mAb (CAMPATH-1) has been shown to be effective in the treatment of otherwise refractory B-cell lymphoma patients (Hale et al., 1988).

Combination therapy of monoclonal antibodies with cytokines such as interleukin-2 (IL-2), interferons, or colony-stimulating factors (CSF) might further increase the antitumor effect. Interleukin-2 can activate human killer cells (Grimm et al., 1983; Lotze et al., 1980, 1981) and has been shown to enhance monoclonal antibody–mediated ADCC by human effector cells in vitro (Biddle et al., 1990a; Morgan et al., 1989; Masucci et al., 1989; Munn and Cheung, 1987). The in vivo relevance of combination therapy of recombinant IL-2 and anti–B-cell monoclonal antibodies was recently demonstrated. The antitumor effect of an anti-CD19 IgG2a mAb and the Lym-1 IgG2a mAb (Gill et al., 1989; Vuist et al., 1989) was potentiated by recombinant IL-2 in these studies and was attributed to increased ADCC.

Interferon-gamma (IFN-γ) has similarly been reported to augment human granulocyte ADCC with murine monoclonal antibody (Vaickus et al., 1990) and chimeric monoclonal antibody (Steplewski et al., 1988) and may be attributed to upregulation of Fc gamma receptors on these cells. Interleukin-2 and interferon have been shown to synergistically enhance the effect of anti-idiotype antibodies in a transplantable murine B-cell lymphoma (Berinstein and Levy, 1987; Basham et al., 1986). Human monocytes/macrophages are reported to have increased effector function and potentiation of ADCC following exposure to macrophage CSF (Mufson et al., 1989), GM-CSF (Kushner and Cheung, 1989), or IFN-γ (Shen et al., 1986b; Weiner et al., 1988a).

Although these in vitro results are promising, they have not, as yet, been translated into successful clinical regimens. Weiner et al. (1986, 1988b) and Douillard et al. (1986) have used IFN-γ in combination with the CO17-1A mAb for the treatment of colorectal carcinoma. No responses were noted in these studies. Ex vivo treatment of peripheral blood mononuclear cells with IFN-γ and/or CO17-1A prior to reinfusion has similarly resulted in a poor response rate (Frödin et al., 1988; Douillard et al., 1986; Verrill et al., 1986). Proper dosaging and scheduling of both monoclonal antibodies and cytokines to obtain and sustain high circulating levels and allow adequate time for effector-cell recruitment appear necessary for this form of therapy.

Anti-Idiotype Vaccines

Another novel approach for increasing the host immune response to tumor is the use of anti-idiotype vaccines. Tumor-associated antigens are often a part of "self" and evoke a very poor immune response in the tumor-bearing host because of T cell–mediated suppression (Haubeck and Kolsch, 1982; Howle and McBride, 1982) and tolerance to the antigen (McBride and Howle, 1986). According to the idiotypic network hypothesis (Jerne, 1974), certain anti-idiotype antibodies express three-dimensional shapes that resemble the structure of external antigens. These "internal" antigens are stereochemical copies of nominal antigens, which produce specific immune responses similar to responses induced by nominal antigen and can also compete with normal antigens in binding assays. The anti-idiotype hybridoma route of making surrogate antigens could alleviate the problems of making large amounts of purified TAA for immunotherapy. If a tumor-specific hybridoma (Ab1) is available, then a second antihybridoma (anti-idiotypic hybridoma Ab2) can be made and selected for the structure that represents the tumor antigen. This Ab2β mAb can then be used as a vaccine and may improve the host immune response and result in generation of TSA (Ab3) by presenting the "antigen" in a dissimilar form. This technique may overcome immunogenicity and tolerance problems often associated with normal TAA.

The experimental evidence that idiotypes or anti-idiotypes mimic antigens and produce antitumor immunity is quite strong (Bona and Köhler, 1984; Kennedy et al., 1987; Köhler, 1985). Treatment of mice with anti-idiotype that appears to mimic tumor antigen structures has been reported to induce antitumor immunity in human tumor model systems (Nepon et al., 1985; Gorczynski et al., 1984), and specific Ab3 responses have also been observed in animals immunized with anti-idiotype antibodies (Herlyn et al., 1986; Bhattacharya-Chatterjee et al., 1987, 1988).

In one clinical trial (Herlyn et al., 1988), patients with colorectal carcinoma were immunized with goat anti-idiotypic antibodies to murine mAb CO17-1A (Ab1). All patients developed Ab3 with binding specificities to the tumor cells similar to that obtained with Ab1. Clinical responses were noted in 10% of the treated patients. In another trial, monoclonal anti-idiotypic antibodies were used to immunize patients with disseminated melanoma (Mittelman et al., 1988). Seven of 15 patients developed specific Ab3 responses and three patients showed tumor reductions. Clinical trials are currently ongoing to further evaluate the viability of anti-idiotype vaccines as a therapeutic modality.

Use of Monoclonal Antibodies in Transplantation Procedures

Various chemotherapeutic or radiation treatments can require the use of "marrow rescue" to optimize therapy. Also, some patients with hematopoietic malignancy can respond to standard first-line therapy, with the absence of clinically detectable disease; however, nondurable remissions often occur. Undetectable "spared" tumor cells in the bone marrow can result in the reappearance of occult disease, which then can be refractory to further therapy. Monoclonal antibodies, together with complement or various monoclonal antibody conjugates themselves, could potentially be useful in detecting and eradicating these tumor cells, provided that the monoclonal antibody or its conjugates do not react with the normal pleuripotent hematopoietic stem-cell population. In addition, other limitations associated with in vivo monoclonal antibody use are of no concern. Such an approach has been utilized in the treatment of non-Hodgkin's lymphoma and acute lymphoblastic leukemia (ALL) (Takvorian et al., 1987; Ramsay et al., 1985; Ritz et al., 1982). Encouragingly, these initial studies have demonstrated that successful marrow reconstitution can be obtained, the therapy is well tolerated, and the majority of patients can undergo disease remission. However, in the ALL patient groups studied, the remission rate and durability of remission were not dissimilar to that which can be obtained with allogeneic transplant procedures. The results for non-Hodgkin's lymphoma are more promising, with greater than 50% of patients remaining in remission for a median duration of 22 months. Controlled trials will be required to determine if these results can be attributed to monoclonal antibody treatment.

Allogeneic transplantation procedures have the advantage that marrow truly devoid of tumor cells is transfused to the patient, and reputed graft-versus-leukemia effects can be obtained. The major obstacle in the use of allogeneic marrow source, however, is the ultimate development of graft-versus-host disease. Depletion of T cells responsible for these effects has been successful in prevention of this, but has led to higher incidences of graft rejection and recurrent leukemia (Waldmann et al., 1984; Mitsuyasu et al., 1986; Martin et al., 1985). A more selective ablation of specific T-cell subsets or addition of specific factors necessary for graft establishment appears necessary to optimize this procedure.

MONOCLONAL ANTIBODY–DRUG CONJUGATES

Representative members of virtually every class of chemotherapeutic agents have been successfully conjugated to monoclonal antibodies specific for a vast array of tumors (Table 10-2). Some of the special problems associated with mAb–drug conjugates and

TABLE 10-2
CHEMOTHERAPEUTIC AGENTS THAT HAVE BEEN SUCCESSFULLY CONJUGATED TO MONOCLONAL ANTIBODIES

Classification	Agent
Antitumor antibiotics	Doxorubicin (adriamycin) Daunorubicin (daunomycin) Idarubicin Bleomycin Mitomycin C
Antimetabolites	Methotrexate Cytosine arabinoside 5-fluorouridine Aminopterin
Alkylating agents	Melphalan Chlorambucil
Plant alkaloids	Vindesine Vinblastine derivatives Etoposide
Synthetics	*Cis*-platinum
Photosensitizing agents	Hematoporphyrin Hematoporphyrin derivative 5-10-15-20 tetracarboxyphenylporphine Chlorin e_6
Radiosensitizing agents	Misonidazole
Miscellaneous agents	Neocarzinostatin

TABLE 10-3
PROBLEMS ASSOCIATED WITH MONOCLONAL ANTIBODY–DRUG CONJUGATES

Chemical linkage should not impair drug activity or mAb immunoreactivity
Number of accessible epitopes on tumor cells
Delivery of adequate amount of mAb–drug conjugates
Large-scale production
In vitro and in vivo stability
Noncovalent association of drug to mAb and polymerization problems
Alterations in mAb biodistribution and pharmacokinetics
Internalization of conjugate
In vivo toxicity
Broad-spectrum drug resistance

strategies for improving their use are shown in Tables 10-3 and 10-4. These drugs have mainly been coupled to monoclonal antibodies by covalent linkage, although non-covalent complexes have been studied. Doxorubicin noncovalently associated to mAb T101 has been shown to be more efficacious than covalently attached drug (Dillman et al., 1986). However, studies using other monoclonal antibodies have reported different results (Matsui et al., 1988; Yang and Reisfeld, 1988). Noncovalent linkage of drug does have the advantage that specific chemical reactions need not be devised so as not to impair drug activity following conjugation. Covalent coupling necessitates that drugs be complexed so that (1) pharmacologically active sites on the drug are not compromised, (2) the monoclonal antibody–drug complex is stable in the circulation, and (3) the linkage permits dissociation of free active drug following conjugate binding and internalization by tumor cells.

Chemotherapeutic agents have been attached to monoclonal antibody using a number of chemical modification techniques. However, the maximum number of drug molecules coupled directly to monoclonal antibody has been limited to approximately 5 to 10 molecules without subsequent impairment of antibody-binding activity to target antigen. The use of intermediate carriers has been shown to increase the amount of drugs that can be effectively bound to monoclonal antibody.

Optimal strategies for chemical coupling of drug to monoclonal antibody must be technically straightforward, reproducible, and allow for high incorporation of drug

TABLE 10-4
STRATEGIES FOR IMPROVING MONOCLONAL ANTIBODY–DRUG DELIVERY SYSTEM

Intermediate carriers
More potent drug analogues
Novel chemistry procedures
Chemically reversible linkages (e.g., *cis*-aconitic acid)
Enzymatic conversion of pro-drugs to active drugs by mAb–enzyme conjugates
Cytokines to increase cell-surface antigen level
Vasoactive substances may increase vascular permeability

without interference of drug or antibody activity. In addition, they should allow for scale-up procedures required for clinical implementation. Some of the more common chemical coupling procedures are detailed elsewhere (Ghose et al., 1983; Sezaki and Hashida, 1984; Sela and Hurwitz, 1987; Pietersz, 1990). Maximal recovery of homogeneous chemically characterized and highly active products will be necessary and underscores the need for limiting any noncovalent associations of drug and monoclonal antibody. Homopolymerization of monoclonal antibodies with resultant high molecular weight species can result in insoluble aggregated material, which can severely reduce yields. Soluble high molecular weight species should be removed to prevent nonspecific in vivo trafficking and removal by the reticuloendothelial system, which can increase toxicity to the host.

Most importantly, the cytocidal agent must be delivered to sensitive tumor target cells in a form that is fully active or that can be activated in situ. This criterion necessitates that the drug be either active when attached to monoclonal antibody or can be metabolized to an active form by intracellular mechanisms. Compounding this problem is the fact that monoclonal antibody–drug conjugates should be chemically stable with little or no release of free drug during systemic traversation in the bloodstream. Although the relative toxicities and maximal obtainable dosages are known for presently used chemotherapeutic agents, monoclonal antibody–drug conjugates should be reevaluated for possible adverse cross-reactivity and toxicities prior to embarking on clinical studies.

More potential analogues of presently available chemotherapeutic agents need also be reevaluated for their clinical usefulness when conjugated to monoclonal antibodies. Due to their increased potency, these agents may offset the reductions in drug pharmacologic activity normally associated with covalent attachment of drug to monoclonal antibody. Site-directed therapy of these mAb–drug conjugates may therefore prove more effective than with conventional drugs. Three potent drug analogues, idarubicin, melphalan, and aminopterin, have all been shown to be more effective both in vitro and in vivo than their respective counterparts doxorubicin, chlorambucil, and methotrexate, when conjugated to monoclonal antibodies (Kanellos et al., 1987; Pietersz et al., 1988d).

Antitumor Antibiotics

The anthracyclines doxorubicin (adriamycin) and daunorubicin (daunomycin) have been covalently coupled to monoclonal antibody either directly or through the use of intermediate drug carriers. Hurwitz et al. (1975) and Levy et al. (1975) were the first to demonstrate direct conjugation of doxorubicin (DXR) and daunorubicin (DNR) to antibody. Conjugation of drugs to monoclonal antibody was accomplished in these early studies via (1) a Schiff base linkage between drug and protein following periodate oxidation of the anthracycline amino sugar that was subsequently reduced by sodium borohydride, (2) glutaraldehyde cross-linking of amino groups on drugs and protein, or (3) by carbodiimide resulting in amino sugar coupling to protein carboxylic acid groups. These procedures resulted in 2 to 10 moles of drug per mole of immunoglobulin. Carbodiimide treatment resulted in complete ablation of antibody activity. Glutaraldehyde linkage resulted in 50% of the product being in aggregated forms. Periodate oxidation was determined to be the method of choice, and compromises in molar substitution levels were necessary to generate a conjugate that displayed both significant binding activity and pharmacologic activity. Subsequent reports by Hurwitz et al. (1976) demonstrated that DNR substituted $F(ab')_2$ antilymphoma antibody was as effective as free DNR in vitro. Although other reports by this group indicated that this technique resulted in active conjugates with good antitumor activity in vitro and in vivo (Hurwitz et al., 1978a, 1978b, 1979, 1983a, 1983b) and cellular uptake and nuclear accumulation of drugs could be demonstrated (Hurwitz et al., 1978a, 1978b), this coupling strategy has not found widespread utility.

A number of other methods for direct covalent attachment of anthracyclines to antibody have been described. In contrast to the original published report by Hurwitz et al. (1975) direct attachment of DNR to antiserum specific for mouse α-fetoprotein via glutaraldehyde cross-linking of amino groups was shown to result in a conjugate more active than free drug (Belles-Isles and Pagé, 1980). Pagé et al. (1981, 1984) further demonstrated the validity of this technique and were able to generate anti-carcinoembryonic antigen (CEA)–DNR conjugates that were more effective than free drug both in vitro and in vivo. Other studies indicate, however, that problems with polymerization when using this technique may severely limit its clinical ability (Arnon and Sela, 1982; Hermentin and Seiler, 1988).

Doxorubicin, daunorubicin, and mitomycin C have been coupled to antibody by a cyanogen bromide method; however, the appreciable losses in both drug and antibody activity observed with molar substitution ratios of only 1–2:1 may also preclude its use (Suzuki et al., 1981).

Direct linkage of DNR to immunoglobulin via the methyl ketone side chain of the drug has been reported to maintain its pharmacologic activity (Zunino, 1981). A subsequent study (Gallego et al., 1984) using 14-bromo-DNR coupled to mAb 791T/36 resulted in a conjugate that was selectively cytotoxic to osteogenic sarcoma cells in vitro. In an extension of these studies, it was further demonstrated that this particular conjugate could effectively localize to xenogeneic human tumors in athymic nude mice (Pimm et al., 1988a). The biodistribution profile of this conjugate appeared similar to unconjugated monoclonal antibody, although less accumulation in the tumor was noted. The conjugate did remain stable and accumulation of drug in the tumor was 100 times greater than that observed following administration of free drug. Toxicity studies further indicated that 791T/36–DNR was at least five times less toxic than free drug with a LD_{50} value greater than 80 mg/kg compared to 14 mg/kg for free DNR. Increased hepatic clearance of the conjugate was observed, however, and should be a consideration for clinical studies.

Comparing a number of different chemical coupling procedures, Gallego et al. (1984) reported that direct attachment of DNR to monoclonal antibody using a *cis*-aconityl linkage resulted in the greatest selective cytotoxicity. This *cis*-aconitic acid spacer was previously demonstrated to result in a pH-sensitive linkage by which DNR can be effectively released following internalization and sequestration in the lysosomal compartment of cells (Shen and Ryser, 1981). To date, this linkage system appears one of the most promising. Selective depletion of murine T cells by an anti-Thy 1.2 IgM Ab coupled to DNR by this linkage has been reported (Diener et al., 1986). Additional studies by this group have shown that this conjugate was effective in prevention of graft-versus-host disease in mice who were repopulated with a T cell–depleted alloreactive bone marrow/spleen mixture (Diener et al., 1988). This purging of alloreactive T cells did not affect hematopoietic stem cells, and similar techniques may have clinical application.

Doxorubicin covalently coupled to the antimelanoma mAb 9.2.27 by *cis*-aconitic anhydride has been shown to result in conjugates with molar ratios of drug:monoclonal antibody ranging from 2–10:1, with immunoreactivity being retained and which were two times more potent than free drug in killing tumor cells in vitro (Yang and Reisfeld, 1988). Nuclear accumulation of DXR was observed following in vitro treatment of melanoma cells in vitro. The kinetics for this accumulation were slower, however, than observed with free drug, indicating the need for lysosomal processing and resultant release of free drug. Biodistribution studies indicated that this conjugate delivered at least four times more DXR to the tumor (3.7% injected dose/gram tumor) as compared to free drug. Marked antitumor responses and increased survival time were observed. Most interestingly, these conjugate-mediated antitumor effects were accomplished with a tumor that was resistant to treatment with free DXR.

Daunorubicin was conjugated to the T101 mAb via *cis*-aconitate by a somewhat different approach (Dillman et al., 1988a, 1988b). Higher molar ratios of 25:1 were obtained by generating active amino groups on mAb carbohydrate prior to conjugation with DNR via an active ester intermediate of *cis*-aconitate. Functional activities of both drug and antibody were retained and therapeutic efficacy was demonstrated in vivo. Interestingly, a synergistic antitumor effect between an antimelanoma mAb (CL207) *cis*-aconitate–DNR conjugate and IFN-γ has also been reported (Matsui et al., 1988).

Three different derivatives of DXR, including iodoacetyl-DXR, succinyl DXR, and maleimidophenylbutyl-DXR, have been conjugated to monoclonal antibody (Pietersz et al., 1988a). These derivatives were prepared by modifying the amino group of the sugar moiety on DXR. Results of these studies indicated that only iodoacetyl DXR was active after coupling, and only 2.5% of free-drug activity was retained. The severe losses in drug activity following attachment of these derivatives can be attributed to adverse effects on the amino sugar that appears to be necessary for optimal drug activity.

Idarubicin (IDA), a more potent therapeutic analogue of DNR, has been extensively studied as a potential candidate agent for monoclonal antibody delivery (Pietersz et al., 1988b, 1988d; Smyth et al., 1988b). Covalent attachment of 14-bromo-IDA was accomplished using methodologies similar to those previously described by Zunino et al. (1981) and Gallego et al. (1984). Although some loss of IDA activity occurred upon conjugation, antibody reactivities were retained. These conjugates were effective in vivo against murine thymoma and human colon tumor models (Pietersz et al., 1988b, 1988d). Elimination of T-cell subsets in vivo and immunosuppression of tumor graft rejection with anti-Ly 2.1, anti-L3T4, or anti-Thy-1 IDA conjugates have also been demonstrated by this group (Smyth et al., 1988b).

Antimetabolites

Although the active ester approach has been most widely used for the direct conjugation of methotrexate (MTX) to antibody, other strategies, including the use of carbodiimide (Shen et al., 1986a; Hurwitz, 1983; Kulkarni et al., 1981) or disulfide linkages (Umemoto et al., 1989), have been reported. The mechanism of action of these conjugates may be dependent upon the nature of this linkage (Endo et al., 1988). It also appears that many of these conjugates exert their cytocidal effects following internalization and subsequent degradation in lysosomal compartments (Shen et al., 1986a; Uadia et al., 1985; Smyth et al., 1987b; Shen and Ryser, 1984; Endo, 1987a, 1987b, 1987c, 1987d; Singh et al., 1989).

Initial studies showing the feasibility of conjugating MTX by an active ester derivative were reported by two independent groups (Kulkarni et al., 1981, 1985; Kanellos et al., 1985). Other investigators have subsequently reported that in vivo therapeutic effects could be obtained in tumor xenograft systems using a number of mAb–MTX conjugates (Shawler et al., 1988; Baldwin et al., 1987; Deguchi et al., 1986). Effective localization of a mAb 791T/36–MTX conjugate into human osteogenic sarcoma xenografted tumors has been demonstrated with 20 times more accumulation of drug into the tumor than could be obtained by administration of free drug (Pimm et al., 1987, 1988b).

Aminopterin (AMN), a folic acid antagonist similar in structure and function but more potent than MTX, has recently been studied (Kanellos et al., 1987). Methotrexate or AMN was coupled to monoclonal antibody at similar molar substitution ratios and their in vitro and in vivo activity compared. The mAb–AMN conjugate was demonstrated to be the more potent conjugate in vitro and in vivo, and in addition, its therapeutic efficacy in vivo was superior to either free AMN or MTX.

Vinca Alkaloids

Initial studies demonstrating that antibody–vindesine conjugates could be successfully prepared and were selectively cytotoxic against a number of malignant target cells were reported in the early 1980s (Rowland et al., 1981, 1983; Johnson et al., 1981; Embleton et al., 1983). Ford et al. (1987) further showed that the in vitro efficacy of anti-CEA–vindesine conjugates directly correlated with the level of CEA expression when tested against a panel of malignant cell lines. Similar effects were observed by these investigators in vivo with these anti-CEA–vindesine conjugates, indicating the importance of tumor cell antigen expression for successful therapy (Casson et al., 1987).

Also of importance was the finding that this conjugate was not effective against CEA-expressing xenografts that were resistant to free drug. Successful localization, antitumor activity, and decreased toxicity in vivo with other anti-CEA–vindesine conjugates have been reported (Rowland et al., 1986; Casson et al., 1987).

The vinca-derivative desacetyl-vinblastine (DAVLB) was shown by Rowland et al. (1985) to be effective against a number of different tumor xenografts in athymic nude mice. Another derivative, desacetyl-vinblastine-hydrazide (DAVLB-HZ), appears to be more potent than DAVLB when conjugated to monoclonal antibody (Johnson et al., 1987). However, both of these derivatives were effective antitumor agents in vivo when coupled to monoclonal antibody, and fewer toxicities than with free drug were demonstrated in rodents and primates (Johnson et al., 1987, 1988; Johnson and Laguzza, 1987). Due to their respective differences in oncolytic potency and toxicity, it is unclear which analogue may provide a superior therapeutic index for clinical application.

Other Agents

The alklyating agents melphalan, chlorambucil, and trenimon (Ghose et al., 1982) have also been studied, but to a lesser extent than other drugs. Chlorambucil (CBL) has been shown to have specific in vitro cytotoxicity when noncovalently bound to anti-idiotype antibody (Tung et al., 1983) or covalently attached to anti-CEA monoclonal antibody by an isocyanate derivative (Bernier et al., 1983). Recently, Smyth et al. (1986) have covalently coupled an active ester derivative of CBL to antibody without impairing drug or antibody activity. In fact, this study is one of the first to demonstrate greater in vitro activity of drug when coupled to antibody. Similarly, enhanced therapeutic effects were observed in vivo using this conjugate.

Using a different approach, an inactive melphalan analog, N-acetyl melphalan was directly conjugated to either intact or $F(ab')_2$ mAb fragments (Smyth et al., 1987a, 1987c). Conjugation of this analogue resulted in restoration of its alkylating ability. N-acetyl melphalan due to acetylation is unable to be actively transported across cell membranes. However, when coupled to monoclonal antibody, it can be actively endocytosed after binding of monoclonal antibody to TAA. This conjugate was reported to have considerable cytotoxic activity in vitro and antitumor activity in vivo.

Another strategy for using pro-drugs has been devised by Senter et al. (1988). Their approach was to attach the enzyme alkaline phosphatase to monoclonal antibody, which could then deliver these enzymes to the tumor surface where they are then capable of converting etoposide phosphate to its active form. Using a two-step approach, mAb-enzyme is first directed to the tumor followed by administration of the relatively noncytotoxic pro-drug. The pro-drug can then be activated extracellularly and would be capable of diffusing into nearby cells. Antigenic heterogeneity and the nonmodulating nature of some TAA could perhaps be circumvented using this type of approach. In fact, potent antitumor effects were observed with this conjugate in human colon tumor xenografts.

The antitumor agent neocarcinostatin (NCS) is another example of how a pro-drug can be coupled to antibody and subsequently activated. Neocarcinostatin is composed of an inert apoprotein containing a biologically active chromophore (Edo et al., 1980; Koide et al., 1980). This chromophore can be released from the protein and can adversely affect DNA molecules (Povirk et al., 1981; Jung and Köhnlein, 1981). After separating the chromophore from the apoprotein, the protein can be coupled to monoclonal antibody (Lüders et al., 1985; Jung et al., 1981; Takahashi et al., 1988). The chromophore is then reassociated, with resultant restoration of biological activity. An anticolon mAb–NCS conjugate has recently undergone clinical trial (see Clinical Studies below).

Other agents that have been directly coupled to monoclonal antibody but have received little study include *cis*-platinum, 5-fluorouridine (Hurwitz, 1983), and the radiation sensitizer misonidazole (Borlinghaus et al., 1987).

Indirect Conjugates

In an attempt to increase the potency of mAb–drug conjugates, a number of investigators have coupled drugs indirectly to monoclonal antibodies via the use of intermediate carriers. This method of coupling chemotherapeutic agents may prove most efficacious in that sufficient cytotoxic quantities of drugs may be introduced into tumor cells, especially those exhibiting limited expression of TAA. Intermediate carriers such as dextran and its substituted derivatives, albumin, and polyglutamic acid have all proven useful.

The first demonstration of successful indirect conjugation of DNR to antibody was through the use of a dextran intermediate (Hurwitz et al., 1978a, 1978b; Bernstein, 1978; Arnon, 1982). In these experiments, DNR and antibody were coupled to periodate oxidized-polyaldehyde dextran by a Schiff base linkage, which was subsequently reduced by sodium borohydride treatment. Antitumor efficacy was demonstrated in these initial studies; however, suboptimal tumor model systems were used to evaluate conjugate effectiveness.

Daunorubicin covalently linked via dextran to polyclonal or monoclonal antibody specific for α-fetoprotein was subsequently proven to be more effective than either free drug, nonspecific conjugates, or a noncovalent mixture of DNR and antibody against rat hepatomas in vivo (Tsukada et al., 1982, 1983, 1987). Similarly, monoclonal antibodies against human hepatocellular carcinoma antigens have shown effectiveness when conjugated to DXR (Shouval et al., 1988). An anti-idiotype antibody–DNR conjugate directed against a lymphoma cell-surface IgM was also shown to be effective in vivo (Hurwitz et al., 1983a). Pimm et al. (1982) were the first to demonstrate effective localization of a DXR–dextran mAb conjugate in vivo. In addition, this conjugate containing approximately 20 moles DXR per mole of antibody was significantly more effective than free drug or appropriate controls in reducing tumor size and extending survival time in rats bearing subcutaneous tumors.

Recent reports have further demonstrated the therapeutic efficacy of anthracycline–dextran mAb conjugates against established human tumor xenografts in athymic nude mice. An antiprostatic acid, DXR–mAb conjugate, although less effective than free drug in vitro, showed equivalent or greater antitumor activity in vivo (Deguchi et al., 1987). Similar findings were reported by Biddle et al. (1989), using monoclonal antibodies directed against acute lymphoblastic leukemia. A combination of mAb–DNR conjugates was shown to retard the growth of leukemia xenografts and, in addition, was significantly less toxic than free DNR. Yu et al. (1988b) demonstrated that mAb F36/22-dextran-DNR conjugates were effective against human ovarian carcinoma cells in vivo and that their antitumor effects could be enhanced by verapamil. Similar findings were reported by this group using an anti–human bladder cancer mAb (Yu et al., 1988a). Our group has also recently completed studies with a mAb F36/22 dextran–DNR conjugate and significant antitumor efficacy against subcutaneous human breast carcinoma tumors following intravenous administration was observed with less systemic toxicity as compared to free drug (unpublished).

Dillman et al. (1986) have reported somewhat different findings using a DXR–dextran T101 mAb conjugate. Although this conjugate displayed some antitumor effects, it was inferior to a noncovalent mixture of T101 and DXR. In other tumor model systems, however, this finding has not been reproduced (Yu et al., 1988; Yang and Reisfeld, 1988; Matsui, 1988) and, in one study, noncovalent mixtures were as acutely toxic as free anthracycline (Ohkawa et al., 1986a). Although physicochemical differences of these conjugates or experimental differences may account for these findings, further studies will be necessary to resolve this issue.

Other carriers that have been used successfully to couple anthracyclines to antibody include carboxymethyl dextran hydrazide (Hurwitz et al., 1983b) and poly-L-glutamic acid (Kato et al., 1984; Tsukada et al., 1985). *Cis*-platinum, cytosine arabinoside, 5-fluorouridine, bleomycin, and MTX have also been covalently attached to monoclonal antibody via polyaldehyde dextran or dextran derivatives, with retention of both antibody and drug activity (Schechter et al., 1987; Hurwitz et al., 1985; Shih et al., 1988; Manabe et al., 1983).

Human serum albumin (HSA) and bovine serum albumin (BSA) have been used extensively as drug carriers because they can be heavily substituted due to the availability of a large number of reactive lysine residues. Mitomycin C has been successfully coupled to antibody via serum albumin (Umemoto, 1984; Ohkawa et al., 1986b; Takahashi et al., 1987). A releasable bond was used, which resulted in retention of drug activity. The single free thiol group of albumin was used to couple the complex to antibody and resulted in molar ratios of drug:monoclonal antibody of 30:1. The HSA carrier conjugates have also been constructed with DNR, resulting in conjugates with more drug substitution than can be obtained by direct coupling procedures (Pimm et al., 1988a; Ognumuyiwa et al., 1987; Baldwin, 1987). Conjugates coupled through ester linkages appear to be rapidly removed from the circulation by hepatic clearance and may be related to the overall net negative charge of these complexes (Monsigny et al., 1980). Conjugates created by using a 14-bromo-DNR derivative do not display this aberrant charge, and improved biodistribution profiles were obtained (Pimm et al., 1988a; Ognumuyiwa et al., 1987).

The mAb–HSA–MTX conjugates have been widely studied and this linkage has proven to be efficacious in a number of model systems (Endo et al., 1987b, 1987c; Garnett et al., 1983; Garnett and Baldwin, 1986a; Pietersz et al., 1988c). In most of these studies, the active ester of MTX was used to conjugate the drug to albumin, whereas various strategies were utilized to link this complex to antibody. Endocytosis followed by lysosomal processing and release of active drug from these conjugates may account for their cytotoxicity (Endo et al., 1987a, 1987b, 1987c, 1987d; Garnett et al., 1985; Embleton and Garnett, 1985). The antihuman osteosarcoma mAb 791T/36 has been the most thoroughly evaluated mAb–MTX conjugate to date (Baldwin and Byers, 1987; Garnett and Baldwin, 1986a; Garnett et al., 1983; Embleton and Garnett, 1985; Pimm et al., 1987). These conjugates have proven to be very effective cytotoxic agents in vitro and, in some cases, have shown to be superior to free drug. In a series of studies (Embleton and Garnett, 1985), this indirect conjugate had superior in vivo therapeutic activity compared to either a directly linked MTX conjugate or free drug. In addition, treatment with this conjugate resulted in no evidence of host toxicity, whereas a comparable dose of MTX showed considerable toxicity. Plasma pharmacokinetic patterns in mice indicate that this conjugate is cleared more rapidly than unconjugated monoclonal antibody or directly labeled MTX–mAb 791T/36 conjugate. However, it was cleared less rapidly than free MTX, with liver and spleen being the major sites of accumulation. Possibly, the overall net negative charge of this complex may account for these findings and is similar to what has been reported elsewhere (Pimm et al., 1988b; Ognumuyiwa et al., 1987). Although no evidence for antitumor efficacy of these conjugates was reported, the directly labeled MTX conjugate appears superior from a pharmacology standpoint, and clinical evaluations have been initiated (see Clinical Studies below).

Photoactive Conjugates

Photochemotherapy presents a unique strategy for the treatment of malignant disease. Activation of light-absorbing chemicals by an exogenous penetrating light source that emits the proper absorption wavelength spectrum can result in photodestruction of cells incorporating these agents. Porphyrin, psoralen, and chlorin derivatives, as well as various dyes, have been studied in this regard. The advantage of these photosensitizing agents is that they are innocuous and present little toxocological consequence unless "excited" by light. The resultant formation of cytotoxic reactive oxygen species that irreversibly oxidize an as yet unclarified essential metabolic or structural component(s) is the generally accepted mechanism for cell destruction by many of these agents (Dougherty, 1986).

Photodynamic therapy relies on the fact that, although tumor cells, in general, do not selectively incorporate these compounds, disparate accretion rates between normal and neoplastic cells result in significant retention and accumulation of the drug in the tumor. Confined illumination of the tumor site can be accomplished by (1) laser light transferred through fiberoptics via endoscopy for deep lesions or (2) light banks for the treatment of peripheral cutaneous disease or for extracorporeal (ex vivo) therapy. The active component of hematoporphyrin derivative (HPD), dihematoporphyrin ether (Photofrin II) (Quadralogic Technologies [QLT] Phototherapeutics, Inc., Vancouver, British Columbia, Canada), used in photodynamic therapy clinical trials to date, has been shown to generate impressive response rates in advanced lung, bladder, esophageal, skin, and head and neck cancers (Dougherty, 1989). Extracorporeal phototherapy of disseminated cutaneous T-cell lymphoma with 8-methoxypsoralen resulted in 27 responses of 37 treated patients with otherwise resistant disease (Edelson et al., 1987). Photocutaneous toxicity, access to tumors containing appreciable levels of compound with sufficient penetrating light dosages, and photodestruction of surrounding normal tissue appear to be the major problems confronting this form of therapy.

A dual selective advantage may be obtained by conjugating photoactive drugs to monoclonal antibodies, in that both successful targeting and illumination are requirements for cell kill. This may allow the use of monoclonal antibodies that do not have the desired restricted specificity necessary for other types of immunoconjugates (i.e., toxins, radioisotopes, chemotherapeutic drugs). Antigen internalization appears not to be required for destruction, in that light-initiated formation of singlet oxygen results in actively diffusable molecules that may then permeate the target cell. An additional benefit of this form of therapy may be that adjacent tumor cells devoid of antigen may also be susceptible to attack by these molecules.

The feasibility of using photoactive immunoconjugates to destroy neoplastic cells was first demonstrated by Mew et al. (1983). Hematoporphyrin (HP) coupled to monoclonal antibody by a carbodiimide procedure resulted in an immunoconjugate that was cytocidal in vitro and could suppress the growth of a murine myosarcoma tumor in vivo. A subsequent study by this group (Mew et al., 1985) used a monoclonal antibody against an acute nonlymphocytic leukemia antigen (CAMAL-1), which when conjugated to HP, displayed a selective light-activated cell kill in vitro that correlated with antigen expression. Selective in vitro photodestruction of human T-cell leukemia was further demonstrated when the photosensitizer chlorin e_6 was coupled to anti-Leu-1 mAb via an intermediate dextran carrier (Oseroff et al., 1986). Phototoxicity was both conjugate- and light dose–dependent, with approximately 10^{10} molecules of singlet oxygen required for cell kill. This conjugate (molar ratio of chlorin e_6:Leu-1 of 21:1) appeared to elicit a potent cell kill with 200 to 1000 times less photosensitizer than normally required for HP cytotoxicity. Free uncoupled chlorin e_6 displayed no cytotoxicity even at dosages 100 times higher than the conjugate.

In other studies, a monoclonal antibody (B16G) linked to HPD (molar ratio of 1:50) was an effective form of murine suppressor T-cell deletion therapy in vivo (Steele et al., 1988). Studies by our group using the non-lipophilic porphyrin 5-10-15-20 tetracarboxyphenylporphine directly conjugated to an antivariant class II HLA-DR mAb (Lym-1) has shown similar findings (Biddle et al., 1990b). Immunoreactivity and immunospecificity of this conjugate were comparable to native Lym-1, and selective photodestruction of malignant leukemia and lymphoma cell lines was observed. Of particular importance, the Lym-1 antigen does not readily internalize (Epstein et al., 1987), yet a significant cell kill could be obtained, suggesting that cytotoxic reactive oxygen species can elicit a potent cell kill regardless of the extent of mAb–antigen complex endocytosis.

The mAb–porphyrin conjugates may also be useful for delivery of certain radioisotopes, in that naturally occurring porphyrins are known to complex a variety of metals including iron, magnesium, and copper. Recently, the successful preparation of stable copper-67 porphyrin-antibody conjugates (Roberts et al., 1987; Mercer-Smith et al., 1988) and ^{111}indium–porphyrin-antibody conjugates (Foster et al., 1985) has been demonstrated. Although still early, this development may lead to other novel chelation strategies for delivery of radionuclide by this approach.

Monoclonal Antibody–Drug Uptake and Role in Tumor Cell Resistance

One of the most important reasons for failure of conventional chemotherapeutic modalities in the treatment of cancer is directly attributed to tumor-cell resistance to the cytotoxic agent (Harrap et al., 1971; Kaye and Merry, 1985; Moscow and Cowan, 1987). Inherently resistant individuals are generally refractory to chemotherapy and therefore their prognosis is poor. Development of acquired drug resistance is also often encountered following first-line therapeutic modalities, resulting from the ultimate emergence of genetically altered drug-resistant malignant clones. Development of resistance is probably multifactorial and stems from the genetic instability of tumor cells. The underlying mechanism(s) of resistance appears to be related to either decreased uptake of the drugs, increased drug efflux, and/or altered sensitivity to drug action through somatic mutations. Alterations of active pathways in the cell membrane, including calcium channel transport (Nair et al., 1986; Kaye and Merry, 1985), gene amplifications (Fojo et al., 1987; Jongsma et al., 1987), and development of cell-surface glycoproteins (Hamada et al., 1986, 1987; Danks et al., 1985), have been demonstrated in association with drug resistance of tumor cells.

Monoclonal antibody–drug conjugates perhaps can circumvent resistance at the level of the cell membrane via binding to target antigen and subsequently being internalized by endocytic mechanisms (Garnett and Baldwin, 1988b; Matzku et al., 1986; Shen and Ryser, 1984; Shen et al., 1986a), which is a distinctly dissimilar mode of entry than for free drugs. The rapid efflux of drugs often associated with resistance may also be compromised due to covalent attachment of drug to immunoglobulin. Methotrexate linked to immunoglobulin has been shown to be more effective in inhibiting tumor growth than free MTX (Uadia et al., 1983, 1984, 1985), and this has been attributed to increased intracellular accumulation resulting from decreased efflux of MTX. Active catabolites of this conjugate have been shown to contain amino acid residues (Uadia et al., 1988) that may be responsible for the favorable prolonged retention.

Release of free drug need not always be a prerequisite for drug activity, and complexed drug has been shown capable of inducing cytotoxic effects (Tritton and Yee, 1982; Wingard et al., 1985; Tokes et al., 1982; Rogers et al., 1983). If, indeed, release is necessary for cytotoxic activity, it appears plausible that the kinetics of release and the accumulation of free drug would be less rapid than with free-drug uptake. This gradual release may prevent the initiation of active homeostatic mechanisms that normally result in rapid drug efflux from a cellular compartment. Rapid internalization of a mAb–vinblastine conjugate has indeed been demonstrated not to be a requirement for effective cytotoxicity (Starling et al., 1988). It also has been observed that a conjugate consisting of antihepatoma antibodies coupled to the alkylating agent trenimon could be cytotoxic to target cells without internalization (Ghose et al., 1982). Monoclonal antibody–drug conjugates may also act on cellular compartments or impair intracellular metabolic pathways in a dissimilar fashion to free drug, due to differences in subcellular trafficking or physicochemical differences in molecular structure.

The acquired broad-spectrum resistance of tumors to cytotoxic agents often observed following chemotherapy may be reduced by using cocktails of monoclonal antibodies conjugated to optimal panels of drugs. In at least one study, treatment with a mAb–MTX conjugate designed to allow the "escape" of viable osteogenic sarcoma cell clones failed to show emergence of tumor-cell variants that differed from parental cells either in antigenicity or in susceptibility to MTX (Embleton et al., 1984). Monoclonal antibody–drug and toxin cocktails have proven to be more effective than single-agent conjugates in vitro (Embleton, 1987) and in vivo (Pietersz et al., 1988d; Hara et al., 1988; Ceriani et al., 1987). Although these concepts are appealing, few data exist on this potential application of monoclonal antibody–drug conjugates. However, one study using newly established colorectal cell lines resistant to MTX demonstrated that these cells were sensitive to destruction by a mAb (791T/36)–drug conjugate (Durrant et al., 1987). The implications of a successful impact of monoclonal antibody–drug conjugate on tumor-cell resistance warrant testing.

Clinical Studies

Although preclinical data using a vast array of polyclonal and monoclonal antibodies coupled to chemotherapeutic agents via various chemical-linkage strategies are readily available, clinical studies to date are limited. Early studies by Ghose et al. (1972, 1977) using CBL-bound antimelanoma immunoglobulins failed to demonstrate significant antitumor effects in patients with disseminated disease. Localization and toxicity of a vindesine–anti-CEA sheep immunoglobulin conjugate in patients with refractory disseminated colorectal or ovarian carcinoma were evaluated in a subsequent study by Ford et al. (1983). Radiolocalization of this iodine-131 (^{131}I)-labeled conjugate that equated with clinical disease state was demonstrated in five of eight patients by external photoscanning. Although no alterations in circulating CEA levels were observed with a radiolocalizing dose of this conjugate, escalating doses of this conjugate resulted in transient declines of CEA level from pretreatment levels. Although no clinical responses were noted, the maximum dose administered was less than the conventionally used therapeutic dose of vindesine. No obvious hypersensitivities or toxicities could be directly attributed to radiolocalizing or escalated doses of conjugate, although some liver dysfunction was reported.

Biodistribution patterns of an mAb (791/T6)–MTX conjugate in patients with colorectal cancer (Ballantyne et al., 1988) were shown to be similar to those previously observed using unconjugated ^{131}I-labeled monoclonal antibody (Armitage et al., 1984). Successful tumor localization images were observed in four of six patients' primary sigmoid cancer lesions and two of six with rectal cancer lesions. Free ^{131}I accumulation in the bladder obscured the remainder. There was visualization of hepatic metastasis in three of five patients, with negative patients having secondary foci less than 2 centimeters in size. Tumor:nontumor uptake ratios ranged from less than 2.0 to 8.0 (mean 3.0), with necrotic tumors exhibiting approximately 50% to 60% less accumulation of conjugate. Therefore, it appears that the relatively avascular necrotic areas of tumors may impede conjugate penetration and limit its effectiveness in advanced disease states. Encouraging, however, is that this conjugate remained stable in vivo, showed a biphasic pharmacokinetic clearance profile similar to unconjugated mAb 791/T6, and tumor:nontumor uptake ratios of greater than 2:1 could be demonstrated in 86% of actively growing tumors. These studies indicate that, at least with this monoclonal antibody conjugate, physicochemical alteration in macromolecular structure did not appear to alter pharmacokinetics nor impede localization to tumors.

Daunorubicin and CBL conjugated to allogeneic antibody have been shown to be an effective regimen in a preliminary study of children with stage II, III, and IV neuroblastoma (Melino et al., 1985). Treatment was continued for up to 1 year with 1 mg DNR/kg and/or 0.5 mg CBL/kg, one to two times per week, with cumulative dosages of 35 to 50 mg/kg DNR obtained. Complete clinical responses were observed in three of three stage II and III patients, with no evidence of disease and posttreatment survival times ranging from 32 to 46 months. Partial responses were noted in three of four persons with stage IV disease. Catecholamine reduction was observed in all patients and toxicity was limited to minor bone marrow depression. Although this study has shown impressive response rates and is encouraging, a more detailed control study is necessary to fully evaluate the future clinical utility of this treatment.

A phase I dose escalation study of MTX coupled to monoclonal antibody directed against colon cancer has recently been reported (Pietersz et al., 1988d). Patients with metastatic, histologically confirmed colorectal cancer received up to 100 mg of mAb and 4 mg of MTX in conjugated form. No objective clinical responses were observed using these suboptimal dosages of MTX, although plateau levels of CEA were obtained and disease state appeared to remain stable during treatment (3–10 months). Development of antimouse antibodies was observed in all patients treated (four of four) by 3 months following the initiation of therapy. With the exception of mild nausea in one patient, no deleterious side effects resulting from treatment were noted.

Monoclonal antibody A7 directed against human colon cancer has been shown to be an effective regimen in preclinical models when conjugated to either mitomycin C or NCS (Takahashi et al., 1988). In a subsequent clinical trial by this group, 41 patients with colorectal cancer were treated with A7–NCS. Due to difficulties in obtaining adequate amounts of conjugate, A7–mitomycin C was not used (Ogawa, 1982; Takahashi et al., 1988). Patients received dosages ranging from 15 to 90 mg of mAb and 1000 to 6000 units of NCS, the majority of intra-arterial administration. Studies on resected tumor specimens showed localization of the A7–NCS conjugate with significant accumulation of drug. Favorable clinical responses were observed in four of eight patients with liver metastasis, with up to 67% reductions in tumor burden observed in a CT scan. Follow-up studies on 31 patients with primary carcinoma of the colon and rectum, which were resected surgically, who were given A7–NCS, are being performed. No serious side effects of treatment were noted. Fever greater than 38°C was common (20 patients), whereas leukocytosis, focal pain in the tumor area, and slight hypotension were observed in only a small number of patients.

Immunoconjugates DXR–mAb have been used in the treatment of a variety of human malignancies (Oldham et al., 1988). Of 23 patients enrolled in this study with disseminated disease refractory to other conventional therapies, 5 partial responses were observed. The major limiting factor in treatment was the variable dissociation of active DXR from the conjugate, resulting in hematopoietic depression. Tumor-cell antigenic phenotype was shown to vary in several patients over time. Results from the study further support the idea that monoclonal antibody cocktails may prove most efficacious in combating tumor diversity and underscore the need for fully characterized stable drug immunoconjugates for targeted therapy.

CRITICAL ISSUES FOR MONOCLONAL ANTIBODY–BASED THERAPY

Some of the critical issues that need to be considered for successful monoclonal antibody–based treatment are described in Table 10-5.

TABLE 10-5
CRITICAL ISSUES FOR MONOCLONAL ANTIBODY CLINICAL USE

Cross-reactivity of mAb with normal histotypes
Development of antiglobulin or anti-hapten (drug) response
Accessibility and permeability of tumor to mAb (vascular architecture of tumor)
Antigenic heterogeneity of tumor cell population
Antigen modulation (internalization, secretion of antigen)
Ability of mAb to mediate human effector-cell function or complement activity
Affinity or avidity of mAb for tumor cell

Monoclonal Antibody Cross-Reactivity with Normal Tissue

Monoclonal antibodies should be as tumor-specific as possible to minimize injury to normal tissues. Most monoclonal antibodies react with some normal tissue(s). This stems from the fact that monoclonal antibodies are directed against tumor-associated, not tumor-specific, antigens. However, quantitative differences in expression of these antigens can exist between certain normal and neoplastic tissues. The extent and site(s) of this cross-reactivity are of paramount importance in addressing whether or how a particular monoclonal antibody may be used. In fact, physicochemical alterations in monoclonal antibodies after coupling to drugs may dictate that they be reevaluated to ensure that no changes in nonspecific reactivity occur. This is especially important because monoclonal antibody–drug conjugates can exert potent direct cytotoxic effects in contrast to unconjugated monoclonal antibodies, which require activation of the complement cascade or mediate immune effector-cell cytotoxicity. Direct cytotoxicity of monoclonal antibody conjugates can therefore alleviate the necessity of using monoclonal antibodies of a particular isotype, in contrast to passive serotherapy studies, which have shown greater efficacy of mAb of the Ig2a or Ig3 subclass. The use of $F(Ab')_2$, FAb fragments, or intact mAbs of the murine IgG1 isotype may be useful in reducing nonspecific binding of conjugates to cells via Fc receptor recognition sites.

Heterogeneity of Tumors and Tumor Cells

Tumor heterogeneity has long been recognized as a major obstacle to cancer treatment resulting from differences in tissue architecture, vascularization patterns, and microenvironment, as well as genotypic, phenotypic, and physiologic variability (for review, Heppner and Miller, 1989). These, as well as the immunotherapeutic consequences of varying amounts of TAA expression in tumors, must be considered.

Tumor-Cell Antigen Expression Tumor cells devoid, or expressing low levels, of antigen may escape destruction. Reduction of antigen levels has been observed on cultured cells following repeated passage and has resulted in concomitant decreases in sensitivity to passive immunotherapy in experimental models (Hand et al., 1983; Capone et al., 1984). The number of antigenic determinants per cell and the extent of tumor positivity for TAA will, similarly, be an important consideration for therapy by drug immunoconjugates. It is likely, therefore, that successful treatment will require the use of monoclonal antibody "cocktails" specific for distinct TAA and also for different epitopes on the same TAA, to reduce the impact of tumor-cell diversity. Unlike radioimmunoconjugates that can kill adjacent non–antigen-bearing cells through radiation crossfire, monoclonal antibody–toxin or monoclonal antibody–drug conjugates require cell-surface antigen presentation for binding and, in most cases, appear to require internalization to elicit a cytocidal effect. Toxins require only one internalized molecule to induce a lethal "hit" (Yamaizumi et al., 1978), whereas chemotherapeutic drugs require relatively large molar amounts. It has been reported that cytotoxicity of human breast cells in culture required 10 to 20 $\times$ 10^6 molecules of DXR per cell (Trouet and Tolles, 1984).

Several strategies have been utilized to counteract the problem of antigenic heterogeneity. Interferons have been shown to upregulate the level of TAA and histocompatibility antigen expression on human tumor cells both in vivo and in vitro (Greiner, 1986; Greiner et al., 1985, 1987; Anichini et al., 1986; Guadagni et al., 1988; Marley et al., 1989; Schlom et al., 1990). Tumor necrosis factor (TNF) and transforming growth factor-β also have been reported to upregulate cell-surface antigen expression (Walker-Jones, 1989; Marley et al., 1989). Although not all TAA or class II molecules are susceptible to upregulation via cytokine treatment, monoclonal antibody directed against those that are susceptible should be more thoroughly investigated. Interferon treatment has also resulted in increased localization and accumulation of radiolabeled monoclonal antibodies in vivo (Rowlinson et al., 1986; Greiner et al., 1987). Synergistic antitumor effects between IFN-γ and an antimelanoma monoclonal antibody conjugated to DNR, which recognizes a 96-kDa cell-surface molecule susceptible to IFN-γ upregulation, have been reported (Matsui et al., 1988). More efficient endocytosis (Webb et al., 1983) and increased cytotoxicity (Embleton, 1987) have been shown to occur following administration of various panels of monoclonal antibody or monoclonal antibody–drug conjugates.

Tumor-Cell Antigen Modulation The phenotypic expression level of a particular TAA is not the only consideration for the use of monoclonal antibody–directed therapy. Also of concern is the ultimate intracellular or extracellular fate of the antigen. The ability of the TAA to modulate (i.e., be internalized or shed from the cell membrane) can dictate which type of therapeutic approach (if any) should be taken. Antigenic modulation has been observed in vivo following administration of monoclonal antibody or monoclonal antibody conjugates (Dillman et al., 1986; Foon et al., 1984).

When using monoclonal antibodies in a passive immunotherapy mode to interact with human immune effector-cell populations, a nonmodulating antigen is preferable to allow for adequate immune effector-cell:tumor interactions. Due to the high emission path length of most beta particle–emitting radionuclides, radioimmunotherapeutic approaches, with the exception of alpha-emitting isotopes, do not require internalization to elicit a cytotoxic event. Most chemotherapeutic agents, however, act either by intercalation between DNA base pairs or through perturbance of intracellular metabolism. Internalization of antigen following monoclonal antibody binding, therefore, appears to be necessary for most monoclonal antibody–drug conjugates. However, the rate of internalization may be of little consequence. When mAb–vinblastine conjugates were compared, no difference in ultimate in vivo cytotoxicity was observed, even though they recognized either rapid or slow internalizing molecules (Starling et al., 1988). Binding to cell-surface antigen without internalization may be sufficient to elicit a cell kill in some cases. For example, anthracyclines can exert cytocidal effects on the cell membrane (Tritton and Yee, 1982; Wingard et al., 1985; Tokes et al., 1982; Rogers et al., 1983).

Neutralization of monoclonal antibody or monoclonal antibody–drug conjugates by circulating antigen may impair effective localization and result in formation of immune complexes. Resultant "end organ" accumulation in hepatic, renal, reticuloendothelial, or other sites may limit the number of monoclonal antibodies that can be considered for therapy (Halpern and Dillman, 1987). However, effective localization despite high levels of circulating antigen has been reported in several studies (Ishii et al., 1983; Warenius et al., 1981). Alternatively, the use of saturating amounts of cold monoclonal antibody, appropriate scheduling, and/or plasmapheresis may be required to alleviate this problem.

Tumor Accessibility The atypical vascular architecture and physiologic differences found in most tumors can impede effective penetration and localization of monoclonal antibodies. Avascular areas, arteriovenous shunts, decreased cross-sectional area, and decreased flexibility can all inhibit perfusion through the endothelial lining. The more acidic microenvironment and high protease activity associated with necrotic areas could adversely affect stability and result in increased catabolic breakdown of monoclonal antibody–drug conjugates.

The use of vasoactive substances may allow greater tumor accessibility by monoclonal antibody. The β-adrenergic blocking agents propranolol, pindolol, and oxyprenolol have been shown to increase the localization of an iodine-125 (^{125}I)-labeled Ly 2.1 mAb in murine thymomas (Pietersz et al., 1988d). In addition, an IDA–Ly 2.1 mAb conjugate was shown by these investigators to have increased therapeutic efficacy in vivo when administered in conjunction with these agents. The increased efficacy was attributed to enhanced blood flow through the tumor vasculature resulting in greater accumulation of conjugate in the tumor bed. Similarly, TNF has been shown to increase the antitumor effects of a mAb–melphalan conjugate (Smyth et al., 1988a). Although TNF can be directly cytocidal to tumor cells, it also affects the vascular compartments, which may account for this enhanced antitumor response (Stolphen et al., 1986; Sato et al., 1986; Creasy et al., 1987; MacPherson and North, 1986).

The use of monoclonal antibody fragments is thought to increase tumor accessibility due to their smaller molecular size, more rapid diffusion rate through the vasculature, and noninteraction with Fc receptors. However, the rapid pharmacokinetic clearance, lower affinity, and lower amount of drug that can be attached to fragments without impairing immunoreactivity may be restrictive. A mathematical modeling analysis that addresses these and other issues of monoclonal antibody treatment and ultimate tumor distribution has recently been described (Fujimori et al., 1989). A $F(Ab')_2$–melphalan conjugate that was less immunogenic and exhibited greater tumor permeability than intact monoclonal antibody conjugate has shown similar antitumor effects, indicating that the increased diffusion rate of these molecules is offset by their rapid in vivo clearance rate (Pietersz et al., 1988d; Smyth et al., 1987c).

Host Immune Response

Neutralization of monoclonal antibody or immunoconjugates because of host immunological recognition may also prove limiting. Host antiglobulin response can vary depending on tumor type, treatment dosage, scheduling, and degree of immunosuppression. Hypogammaglobulinemic chronic lymphocytic leukemia (CLL) patients rarely develop antiglobulins (Foon et al., 1984; Dillman et al., 1984). The majority of patients with solid tumors and cutaneous T-cell lymphomas have shown antiglobulin responses (Schroff et al., 1985; Schroff and Stevenson, 1985).

The use of monoclonal antibody fragments (Carrasquillo et al., 1984), tolerating dosages of specific monoclonal antibody (Schroff et al., 1987; Sears et al., 1984), administration of nonspecific antibody together with the specific monoclonal antibody, or proper dosaging and scheduling may reduce specific antiglobulin response. Immunosuppressive agents such as cyclophosphamide or cyclosporine may prove useful (Khazaeli et al., 1988). Human or chimeric antibodies (Liu et al., 1987a, 1987b; Shaw et al., 1987; LoBuglio et al., 1989) are less immunogenic than xenogeneic monoclonal antibodies. Allotypic or idiotypic responses, however, could still be expected. The use of monoclonal antibody–drug conjugates may also result in host antibody raised against the haptenic drug portion of the complex. If immunologic intermediate carriers are used to couple drugs to monoclonal antibody, they likewise could initiate an immune response.

SUMMARY

Taken together, several general observations can be made from these studies. Successful utilization of unconjugated monoclonal antibodies for systemic treatment will probably require the use of recombinant cytokines to enhance host immune effector-cell mechanisms. Recruitment of large numbers of these cells to the tumor, together with sufficient amounts of monoclonal antibody capable of mediating cytotoxic actions, would appear necessary for optimal antitumor responses. Major problems such as the host immune response and tumor heterogeneity need to be overcome. Some alternative strategies have been discussed herein and other new approaches may prove useful in developing monoclonal antibodies as a true clinical treatment modality.

Preclinical studies of monoclonal antibody–drug conjugates are encouraging. It has been demonstrated that drugs can be covalently coupled to monoclonal antibody albeit some losses in antibody binding activity and drug pharmacological activity can be expected. For the most part, these conjugates appear to be selective in their actions with greater therapeutic efficacy than free drug. Several studies have demonstrated that these conjugates can be effectively internalized by tumor cells expressing specific TAA. Preliminary information in xenogeneic tumor model systems suggests that these conjugates can localize to tumors in vivo with delivery of adequate amounts of drug necessary for significant reduction in tumor burdens and increased survival time. In addition, several of these conjugates have proven to be less toxic than their respective free drug when directly compared in these animal model systems. However, to date, it is not abundantly clear from all these studies which type of conjugation procedure or which monoclonal antibodies will be most appropriate for future drug immunotherapy. Phase I and II clinical trials will be required to address the problems inherent in this form of therapeutic modality and to delineate the future role of monoclonal antibody–drug conjugates may have as an alternative form of cancer therapy.

REFERENCES

Anichini A, Mortarini R, Fossati G, Parmiani G. Phenotypic profile of clones from early cultures of human metastatic melanomas and its modulation by recombinant interferon. Int J Cancer. 1986;38:505–511.

Armitage NC, Perkins AC, Pimm MV, Farrands PA, Baldwin RW, Hardcastle HD. The localization of an anti-tumor monoclonal antibody (791T36) in gastrointestinal tumours. Br J Surg. 1984;71:407–412.

Arnon R, Sela M. In vitro and in vivo efficacy of conjugates of daunomycin with anti-tumor antibodies. Immunol Rev. 1982;62:5–27.

Arteaga CL, Osborne CK. Growth inhibition of human breast cancer cells in vitro with an antibody against the type I somatomedin receptor. Cancer Res. 1989;49:6237–6241.

Bagshawe KD. Tumor markers—where do we go from here? Br J Cancer. 1983;48:167–175.

Baldwin RW. Comparative biodistribution of daunomycin-HSA-monoclonal antibody conjugates with different linkages. Br J Cancer. 1987;56:186.

Baldwin RW, Byers VS. Monoclonal antibodies in drug targeting. In: Den Otterm W, Ruitenberg EJ, eds. Tumor immunology—mechanisms, diagnosis, therapy. New York, NY: Elsevier Science, 1987:251–264.

Baldwin RW, Embleton MJ, Garnett MC, Pimm MV. Conjugates of monoclonal antibody 791T/36 with methotrexate in cancer therapy. NCI Monogr. 1987;3:95–99.

Ball ED, Bernier GM, Cornwell GG, McIntyre OR, O'Donnell JF, Fanger MW. Monoclonal antibodies to myeloid differentiation antigens: in vivo studies of three patients with acute myelogenous leukemia. Blood. 1983;62:1203–1210.

Ballantyne KC, Perkins AC, Pimm MV, et al. Biodistribution of a monoclonal antibody-methotrexate conjugate (791T.36-MTX) in patients with colorectal cancer. Int J Cancer. 1988; 2:103–108.

Basham TY, Kaminski M, Kitamura K, Levy R, Merigan T. Synergistic antitumor effect of interferon and anti-idiotype monoclonal antibody in murine lymphoma. J Immunol. 1986; 137:3019–3024.

Belles-Isles M, Page M. In vitro activity of daunomycin-anti-alphafaetoprotein conjugate on mouse hepatoma cells. Br J Cancer. 1980;41:841–842.

Berinstein N, Levy R. Treatment of a murine B-cell lymphoma with monoclonal antibodies and IL-2. J Immunol. 1987;139:972–976.

Bernier LG, Page M, Dumas L, Gauthier C, Gaudreault R, Joly LP. Monoclonal anti-CEA antibodies for targeting chlorambucil to human colon carcinoma cells in vitro. Prot Biol Fluids. 1983;31:787–790.

Bernstein A, Hurwitz E, Maron R, Arnon R, Sela M, Wilckek M. Higher antitumor efficacy of daunomycin when linked to dextran: in vivo and in vitro studies. J Natl Cancer Inst. 1978;60:379–384.

Bertram JH, Gill PS, Levine AM, et al. Monoclonal antibody T101 in T cell malignancies: a clinical pharmacokinetic and immunologic correlation. Blood. 1986;68:752–761.

Bhattacharya-Chatterjee M, Price MW, Seon BK, Kohler H. Idiotype vaccines against human T-cell acute lymphoblastic leukemia. I. Generation and characterization of biologically active monoclonal antiidiotopes. J Immunol. 1987;139:1354–1360.

Bhattacharya-Chatterjee M, Chatterjee SK, Vasile S, Seon BK, Kohler H. Idiotype vaccines against human T-cell leukemia. II. Generation and characterization of a monoclonal idiotype cascade (Ab1, Ab2, and Ab3). J Immunol. 1988;141:1298–1403.

Biddle WC, Hauta Y, Seon BK, Henderson ES, Sarcione EJ. In vitro and in vivo cytotoxic activity of anti-human leukemia monoclonal antibodies SN5c and SN6 daunorubicin conjugates. Leukemia Res. 1989;13(8):699–707.

Biddle WC, Pancook J, Goldrosen M, Han T, Foon KA, Vaickus L. Antibody-dependent, cell-mediated cytotoxicity by an anti–class II murine monoclonal antibody: effects of recombinant interleukin-2 on human effector cell lysis of human B-cell tumors. Cancer Res. 1990a; 50:2991–2996.

Biddle WC, Musser DA, Goldrosen MH, Foon KA. Selective destruction of malignant human B cells by a photoimmunotherapeutic approach in vitro. Proc Am Assoc Cancer Res. 1990b;31(No. 1740):293.

Bona CA, Köhler H. Anti-idiotypic antibodies and internal images. In: Venter JC, Fraser CM, Lindstrom J, eds. Probes for receptor structure and function, vol. 4. New York, NY: Alan R. Liss; 1984:141–150.

Borlinghaus KP, Fitzpatrick DA, Heindel ND, et al. Radiosensitizer conjugation to the carcinoma 19–9 monoclonal antibody. Cancer Res. 1987;47:4071–4075.

Brown SL, Miller RA, Levy R. Anti-idiotype antibody therapy of B-cell lymphoma. Semin Oncol. 1989;16(No. 3):199–210.

Capone PM, Papsidero LD, Chu TM. Relationship between antigen density and immunotherapeutic response elicited by monoclonal antibodies against solid tumors. J Natl Cancer Inst. 1984;72(No. 3):673–677.

Carrasquillo JA, Krohn KA, Beaumier PL. Diagnosis and therapy of solid tumors with radiolabeled antibodies and immune fragments. Cancer Treat Rep. 1984;68:317–327.

Casson AG, Ford CHJ, Marsden CH, Hallant ME, Bartlett SE. Efficacy and selectivity of vindesine monoclonal anti-carcinoembryonic antigen antibody conjugates on human tumor cell lines grown as xenografts in nude mice. NCI Monogr. 1987;3:117–124.

Ceriani RL, Blank EW, Petersons JA. Experimental immunotherapy of human breast carcinomas implanted in nude mice with a mixture of monoclonal antibodies against human milk fat globule components. Cancer Res. 1987;47:532–540.

Creasy AA, Doyle LV, Reynolds MT, Jung T, Lin LS, Vitt CR. Biological effects of recombinant human tumor necrosis factor and its novel muteins on tumor and normal cell units. Cancer Res. 1987;47:145–149.

Crowther ME, Britton KE, Granowska M, Shepherd JH. Monoclonal antibodies and their usefulness in epithelial ovarian cancer. A review. Br J Obstet Gynecol. 1989;96:516–521.

Danks MK, Metzger DW, Ashmund RA, Beck WT. Monoclonal antibodies to glycoproteins of vinca alkaloid-resistant human leukemic cells. Cancer Res. 1985;45:3220–3224.

Deguchi T, Chu TM, Leong SS, Horoszewicz JS, Lee C-L. Effect of methotrexate-monoclonal anti-prostatic acid phosphatase antibody conjugate on human prostate tumor. Cancer Res. 1986;46:3751–3755.

Deguchi T, Chu TM, Leong SS, Horoszewicz JS, Lee C-L. Potential therapeutic effect of adriamycin monoclonal anti-prostatic acid phosphatase antibody conjugate on human prostate tumor. J Urol. 1987;137:353–358.

Diener E, Diner UE, Sinha A, Xie S, Vergidis R. Specific immunosuppression by immunotoxins containing daunomycin. Science. 1986;231:148–150.

Diener E, Xie S, Yu L, Longenecker BM, Sinha AA. Experimental application of target specific immunoconjugates containing daunomycin as the cytocidal component. In: Rodwell JD, ed. Antibody-mediated delivery systems. New York, NY: Marcel Dekker, 1988.

Dillman RO, Royston I. Applications of monoclonal antibodies in cancer therapy. Br Med Bull. 1984;40:240–246.

Dillman RO, Shawler DL, Johnson DR, Meyer DL, Koziol JA, Frincke JM. Preclinical trials with combinations and conjugates of T101 monoclonal antibody and doxorubicin. Cancer Res. 1982a;46:4886–4891.

Dillman RO, Shawler DL, Sobel RE, et al. Murine monoclonal antibody therapy in two patients with chronic lymphocytic leukemia. Blood. 1982b;59:1036–1045.

Dillman RW, Shawler DL, Dillman JB, Royston I. Therapy of chronic lymphocytic leukemia and cutaneous T-cell lymphoma with T101 monoclonal antibody. J Clin Oncol. 1984;2:881–891.

Dillman RO, Shawler DL, Johnson DE, Meyer DL, Koziol JA, Frincke JM. Preclinical trials with combinations and conjugates of T101 monoclonal antibody and doxorubicin. Cancer Res. 1986;46:4886–4891.

Dillman RO, Johnson DE, Shawler DL, Koziol JA. Superiority of an acid-labile daunorubicin–monoclonal antibody immunoconjugate compared to free drug. Cancer Res. 1988a;48:6097–6102.

Dillman RO, Johnson DE, Shawler DL. Comparisons of drug and toxin immunoconjugates. Antibody Immunoconjugates Radiopharmaceuticals. 1988b;1:65–77.

Dillman RO. Monoclonal antibodies for treating cancer. Ann Intern Med. 1989;111:592–603.

Dougherty TJ. Photosensitization of malignant tumors. Sem Surg Oncol. 1986;2:24–37.

Dougherty TJ. Photodynamic therapy: status and potential. Oncology. 1989;3:67–73.

Douillard JY, Lehur PA, Vignoud J, et al. Monoclonal antibodies specific immunotherapy of gastrointestinal tumor. Hybridoma. 1986;5:139–149.

Durrant LG, Garnett MC, Gallego J, et al. Sensitivity of newly established colorectal cell lines to cytotoxic drugs and monoclonal antibody drug conjugates. Br J Cancer. 1987;56:722–726.

Edelson R, Berger C, Gasparro F, et al. Treatment of cutaneous T-cell lymphoma by extracorporeal photochemotherapy. N Engl J Med. 1987;316:297–303.

Edo K, Katamine S, Kitame S, Ishida N. Napthalenecarboxylic acid from neocarzinostatin (NCS). J Antibiot. 1980;33:347–351.

Ehrlich P. Collected studies on immunology, Vol. 11. New York, NY: John Wiley and Sons; 1906:442–447.

Embleton MJ, Rowland GF, Simmonds RG, Jacobs E, Marsden CH, Baldwin RW. Selective cytotoxicity against human tumour cells by a vindesine-monoclonal antibody conjugate. Br J Cancer. 1983;47:43–49.

Embleton MJ, Garnett MC, Jacobs E, Baldwin RW. Antigenicity and drug susceptibility of human osteogenic sarcoma cells "escaping" a cytotoxic methotrexate-albumin-monoclonal antibody conjugate. Br J Cancer. 1984;49:559–565.

Embleton MJ, Garnett MC. Antibody targeting of anti-cancer agents. In: Monoclonal antibodies for cancer detection and therapy. London: Academic Press; 1985:317–344.

Embleton MJ. Cytotoxic action of combinations of drug-antibody conjugates against human tumour cells. Med Sci Res. 1987;15:1107–1108.

Endo N, Takeda Y, Kishida K, et al. Target-selective cytotoxicity of methotrexate conjugated with monoclonal anti-mm46 antibody. Cancer Immunol Immunother. 1987a;25:1–6.

Endo N, Kato Y, Takeda Y, et al. Drug/antibody conjugates. In vitro cytotoxicity of a human serum albumin-mediated conjugate of methotrexate with anti-mm46 monoclonal antibody. Acta Pediatr Jpn. 1987b;29:566–568.

Endo N, Kato Y, Takeda Y, Saito M, et al. Drug/antibody conjugates. In vitro cytotoxicity of a human serum albumin-mediated conjugate of methotrexate with anti-mm46 monoclonal antibody. Cancer Res. 1987c;47:1076–1080.

Endo N, Kato Y, Takeda Y, et al. In vitro cytotoxicity of a human serum albumin-mediated conjugate of methotrexate with anti-mm46 monoclonal antibody. Cancer Res. 1987d;47: 1076–1080.

Endo N, Takeda Y, Umemoto N, et al. Nature of linkage and mode of action of methotrexate conjugated with antitumor antibodies: implications for future preparation of conjugates. Cancer Res. 1988;48:3330–3335.

Epstein AL, Marder RJ, Winter JN, et al. Two new monoclonal antibodies, Lym-1 and Lym-2, reactive with human B-lymphocytes and derived tumors, with immunodiagnostic and immunotherapeutic potential. Cancer Res. 1987;47:830–840.

Fanger MW, Shen L, Graziano RF, Guyre PM. Cytotoxicity mediated by human Fc receptors for IgG. Immunol Today. 1989;10:92–99.

Fojo A, Cornwell M, Cardarelli C, et al. Molecular biology of drug resistance. Br Cancer Res Treat. 1987;9:5–16.

Foon KA. Biological response modifiers: the new immunotherapy. Cancer Res. 1989;49:1621–1639.

Foon KA, Todd RF. Immunologic classification of leukemia and lymphoma. Blood. 1986;68:1–31.

Foon KA, Gale RP. Immunologic classification of lymphoma and lymphoid leukemia. Blood Rev. 1987;1:77–88.

Foon KA, Schroff RW, Bunn PA, et al. Effects of monoclonal antibody therapy in patients with chronic lymphocytic leukemia. Blood. 1984;64:1085–1094.

Ford CHJ, Newman CE, Johnson JR, et al. Localization and toxicity study of a vindesine-anti-CEA conjugate in patients with advanced cancer. Br J Cancer. 1983;47:35–42.

Ford CHJ, Bartlett SE, Casson AH, Marsden CH, Gallant ME. Efficacy and specificity of vindesine monoclonal anti-carcinoembryonic antigen conjugate with nine human cancer cell lines. NCI Monogr. 1987;3:107–116.

Foster N, Woon DV, Kaltovich F, Emrich J, Ljungquist C. Delineation of a transplanted malignant melanoma with Indium-111-labeled porphyrin. J Nucl Med. 1985;26:756–760.

Fritsche HA. Some new and prospective tumor markers; their nature and clinical status. Lab Management. 1986;25–34.

Frödin JE, Harmenberg U, Biberfeld P, et al. Clinical effects of monoclonal antibodies (MAb 17-1A) in patients with metastatic colorectal carcinomas. Hybridoma. 1988;7:309–321.

Fujimori K, Corvell DG, Fletcher JE, Weinstein JN. Modeling analysis of the global and microscopic distribution of immunoglobulin G, $F(Ab')_2$ and FAB in tumors. Cancer Res. 1989;49:5656–5663.

Gallego J, Price MR, Baldwin RW. Preparation of four daunomycin-monoclonal antibody 791T/36 conjugates with anti-tumour activity. Int J Cancer. 1984;33:737–744.

Garnett MC, Baldwin RW. An improved synthesis of a methotrexate-albumin-791T/36 monoclonal antibody conjugate cytotoxic to human osteogenic sarcoma cell lines. Cancer Res. 1986a;46:2407–2412.

Garnett MC, Baldwin RW. Endocytosis of a monoclonal antibody recognizing a cell surface glycoprotein antigen visualized using fluorescent conjugates. Eur J Cell Biol. 1986b;41:214–221.

Garnett MC, Embleton MJ, Jacobs E, Baldwin RW. Preparation and properties of a drug-carrier-antibody conjugate showing selective antibody-directed cytotoxicity in vitro. Int J Cancer. 1983;31:661–670.

Garnett MC, Embleton MJ, Jacobs E, Baldwin RW. Studies on the mechanism of action of an antibody-targeted drug-carrier conjugate. Anti-Cancer Drug Design. 1985;1:3–12.

Gergely J, Sarmay G. IgG-Fc-receptors: ligand binding and lysis induction. Immunol Lett. 1989;20:1–4.

Ghose T, Norvell ST, Guclu A, Cameron D, Bodurtha A, MacDonald AS. Immunochemotherapy of cancer with chlorambucil-carrying antibody. Br Med J. 1972;3:495–499.

Ghose T, Norvell ST, Guclu A, Bodurtha A, Tai J, MacDonald AS. Immunochemotherapy of malignant melanoma with chlorambucil-bound anti-melanoma globulins: preliminary results in patients with disseminated disease. J Natl Cancer Inst. 1977;58:845–852.

Ghose T, Guclu A, Raman RR, Huntley Blair A. Inhibition of a mouse hepatoma by the alkylating agent trenimon linked to immunoglobulins. Cancer Immunol. Immunother. 1982;13: 185–189.

Ghose TI, Blair AH, Kulkarni PN. Preparation of antibody-linked to cytotoxic agents. Meth Enzymol. 1983;93:280–333.

Giardinia SL, Schroff RW, Kipps T, et al. Generation of monoclonal antiidiotype antibodies to human B-cell derived leukemias and lymphomas. J Immunol. 1985;135:653–658.

Gill I, Agah R, Hu E, Mazumder A. Synergistic antitumor effects of interleukin-2 and the monoclonal Lym-1 against human Burkitt lymphoma cells in vitro and in vivo. Cancer Res. 1989;49:5377–5379.

Glassy MC, Dillman RO. Molecular biotherapy with human monoclonal antibodies. Mol Biother. 1988;1:7–13.

Gorczynski RM, Kennedy M, Polidoulis I, Price GB. Altered tumor growth in vivo after immunization of mice with antitumor antibodies. Cancer Res. 1984;44:3291–3298.

Greiner JW. Modulation of antigen expression in human tumor cell populations. Cancer Invest. 1986;4:239–256.

Greiner JW, Tobi M, Fisher PB, Langer JA, Pestka S. Differential responsiveness of cloned mammary carcinoma cell populations to the human recombinant leukocyte interferon enhancement of tumor antigen expression. Int J Cancer. 1985;36:159–166.

Greiner JW, Guadagni F, Doguchi P, Pestka S, Colcher P, Fisher B, et al. Recombinant interferon enhances monoclonal antibody-targeting of carcinoma lesions in vivo. Science. 1987; 235:895–898.

Grimm EA, Robb RJ, Roth JA, et al. Lymphokine-activated killer cell phenomenon. III. Evidence that IL-2 is sufficient for direct activation of peripheral blood lymphocytes into lymphokine-activated killer cells. J Exp Med. 1983;158:1356–1361.

Guadagni F, Schlom J, Pothen S, Pestka S, Greiner JW. Parameters involved in the enhancement of monoclonal antibody targeting in vivo with recombinant interferon. Cancer Immunol Immunother. 1988;26:222–230.

Hale G, Clark MR, Marcus R, et al. Remission induction in non-Hodgkin's lymphoma with reshaped human monoclonal antibody. CAMPATH-1H. Lancet. 1988;1394–1398.

Halpern SE, Dillman RO. Problems associated with radioimmunodetection and possibilities for future solutions. J Biol Resp Mod. 1987;6:235–262.

Hamada H, Tsuruo T. Functional role for the 170 to 180 kDa glycoprotein specific to drug-resistant tumor cells as revealed by monoclonal antibodies. Proc Natl Acad Sci USA. 1986;83:7785–7789.

Hamada H, Hagiwara K-I, Nakajima T, Tsuruo T. Phosphorylation of the Mr 170,000 to 180,000 glycoprotein specific to multidrug-resistant tumor cells: effects of verapamil, trifluoperazine, and phorbol esters. Cancer Res. 1987;47:2860–2865.

Hand PH, Ruti M, Colcher D, Schlom J. Definition of antigenic heterogeneity and modulation among human mammary carcinoma cell populations using monoclonal antibodies to tumor-associated antigens. Cancer Res. 1983;43:728–735.

Hara H, Luo Y, Haruta Y, Seon BK. Efficient transplantation of human non-T-leukemia cells into nude mice and induction of complete regression of the transplanted distinct tumors by ricin A-chain conjugates of monoclonal antibodies SN5 and SN6. Cancer Res. 1988;48: 4673–4680.

Harrap KR, Hill BT, Furness ME, Hart LI. Sites of action of amethopterin intrinsic and acquired drug resistance. Ann NY Acad Sci. 1971;186:312–324.

Harris DT, Mastrangelo MJ. Serotherapy of cancer. Semin Oncol. 1989;16:180–198.

Haubeck HD, Kolsch E. Tumor-specific T suppressor cells induced at early stage of tumorigenesis act on the induction phase of cytotoxic T cells. Immunology. 1982;47:503–519.

Heppner GH, Miller BE. Therapeutic implications of tumor heterogeneity. Semin Oncol. 1989;16:9–15.

Herlyn D, Ross AH, Koprowski H. Anti-idiotypic antibodies bear the internal image of a human tumor antigen. Science (Washington D.C.). 1986;232:100–102.

Herlyn D, Wettendorff M, Iliopoulos D, Schmoll E, Schedel I, Koprowski H. Immunotherapy of colorectal cancer with anti-idiotypic antibodies. Proc Am Assoc Cancer Res. 1988;2: 408.

Hermentin P, Seiler FR. Investigations with monoclonal antibody drug (anthracycline) conjugates. Behring Inst Mitt. 1988;82:197–215.

Howle SM, McBride WH. Tumor specific T helper activity can be abrogated by two distinct suppressor cell mechanisms. Eur J Immunol. 1982;12:671–675.

Hu E, Epstein AL, Naeve GS, et al. A phase 1a clinical trial of Lym-1 monoclonal antibody serotherapy in patients with refractory B-cell malignancies. Hematol Oncol. 1989;7:155–166.

Hurwitz E, Levy R, Maron R, Wilchek M, Arnon R, Sela M. The covalent binding of daunomycin and adriamycin to antibodies with retention of both drug and antibody activities. Cancer Res. 1975;35:1175–1181.

Hurwitz E, Maron R, Arnon R, Sela M. Fab dimers of antitumor immunoglobulins as covalent carriers of daunomycin. Cancer Biochem Biophys. 1976;1:197–202.

Hurwitz E, Maron R, Bernstein A, Wilchek M, Sela M, Arnon R. The effect in vivo of chemotherapeutic drug-antibody conjugates in two murine experimental tumor systems. Int J Cancer. 1978a;21:747–755.

Hurwitz E, Maron R, Arnon R, Wilchek M, Sela M. Daunomycin-immunoglobulin conjugates, uptake and activity in vitro. Eur J Cancer. 1978b;44:1213–1220.

Hurwitz E, Schechter B, Arnon R, Sela M. Binding of anti-tumor immunoglobulins and their daunomycin conjugates to the tumor and its metastases. In vitro and in vivo studies with Lewis lung carcinoma. Int J Cancer. 1979;24:461–470.

Hurwitz E. Specific and nonspecific macromolecule-drug conjugates for the improvement of cancer chemotherapy. Biopolymers. 1983;22:557–567.

Hurwitz E, Kashi R, Burowsky D, Arnon R, Haimovich H. Site-directed chemotherapy with a drug bound to anti-idiotypic antibody to a lymphoma cell surface IgM. Int J Cancer. 1983a;31:745–748.

Hurwitz E, Arnon R, Sahar E, Donon Y. A conjugate of adriamycin and monoclonal antibodies to the THY-1 antigen inhibits human neuroblastoma cells in vitro. Ann NY Acad Sci. 1983b;83:125–136.

Hurwitz E, Kashi R, Arnon R, Wilchek M, Sela M. The covalent linking of two nucleotide analogues to antibodies. J Med Chem. 1985;28(No. 1):137–140.

Irie RF, Morton DL. Regression of cutaneous metastatic melanoma by intralesional injection with human monoclonal antibody to ganglioside GD2. Proc Natl Acad Sci USA. 1986; 83:8694–8698.

Ishii N, Nakata K, Munehisa T, Koji T, Nishi S, Hirai H. Radioimmunodetection of cancer-using radiolabelled antibodies to alpha fetoprotein. Prot Biol Fluids. 1983;321:305–308.

Jerne NK. Towards a network therapy of the immune system. Ann Immunol (Paris). 1974; 125c:373–389.

Jerne NK. Idiotypic networks and other preconceived ideas. Immunol Rev. 1984;79:5.

Johnson DA, Laguzza BC. Antitumor xenograft activity with a conjugate of a vinca derivative and the squamous carcinoma reactive monoclonal antibody PFI/D. Cancer Res. 1987;47: 3118–3122.

Johnson DA, Zimmermann JL, Laguzza BC, Etole JN. In vivo antitumor activity demonstrated with squamous carcinoma reactive monoclonal antibody-vinca immunoconjugates. Cancer Immunol Immunother. 1988;27:241–245.

Johnson JR, Ford CHJ, Newman CE, Woodhouse CS, Rowland GF, Simmonds RG. A vindesine-anti-CEA conjugate cytotoxic for human cancer cells in vitro. Br J Cancer. 1981;44: 472–475.

Johnson IS, Spearman ME, Todd GC, Zimmerman JL, Bumol TF. Monoclonal antibody drug conjugates for site-directed cancer chemotherapy: preclinical pharmacology and toxicology studies. Cancer Treat Rev. 1987;14:193–196.

Jongsma APM, Spengler BA, Van de Blick AM, Borst P, Biedler JL. Chromosomal localization of three genes co-amplified in the multidrug resistant CHRC5 Chinese hamster ovary cell line. Cancer Res. 1987;47:2875–2878.

Jung G, Kohnlein W, Lupers G. Biologic activity of the antitumor protein neocarzinostatin coupled to a monoclonal antibody by N-succinimidyl 3-(2-pyridyldithio) propionate. Biochem Biophys Res Commun. 1981;101:599–606.

Jung G, Kohnlein W. Neocarzinostatin: controlled release of chromophore and its interaction with DNA. Biochem Biophys Res Commun. 1981;98:176–183.

Kanellos J, Pietersz GA, McKenzie IFC. Studies of methotrexate-monoclonal antibody conjugates for immunotherapy. J Natl Cancer Inst. 1985;75(No. 2):319–329.

Kanellos J, Pietersz GA, Cunningham Z, McKenzie IFC. Anti-tumour activity of aminopterin-monoclonal antibody conjugates; in vitro and in vivo comparison with methotrexate-monoclonal antibody conjugates. Immunol Cell Biol. 1987;65(Pt. 6):483–493.

Kato Y, Umemoto N, Kayama Y, Fukushima H, Takeda Y, Hara T, et al. A novel method of conjugation of daunomycin with antibody with a poly-L-glutamic acid derivative as intermediate drug carrier. An anti-alpha-fetoprotein antibody-daunomycin conjugate. J Med Chem. 1984;27:1602–1607.

Kaye S, Merry S. Tumour cell resistance to anthracyclines—a review. Cancer Chemother Pharmacol. 1985;14:96–103.

Kennedy RC, Zhou E-M, Lanford RE, Chanh TC, Bona CA. Possible role of anti-idiotypic antibodies in the induction of tumor immunity. J Clin Invest. 1987;80:1217–1224.

Khazaeli M, Lo Buglio AF, Wheeler R, Haynes A, Miscchak R, Spitler LE. The effects of immunosuppressive regimens on human immune response to murine monoclonal anti-melanoma antibody-ricin A chain. Proc Am Soc Clin Oncol. 1988;29:418.

Köhler G, Milstein C. Continuous cultures of fused cells secreting antibody of predefined specificity. Nature. 1975;256:495–497.

Köhler G, Milstein D. Derivation of specific antibody-producing tissue culture and tumor lines by cell fusion. Eur J Immunol. 1976;6:511–519.

Köhler H. The immune network revisited. In: Köhler H, Urgain J, Cazenave P, eds. Idiotypes in biology and medicine. New York, NY: Academic Press; 1985;13–28.

Koide Y, Ishii, Hasuda K, et al. Isolation of non-protein compound and a protein-component from neocarzinostatin (NCS) and their biological activities. J Antibiot. 1980;33:342–346.

Kulkarni PN, Blair AH, Ghose TI. Covalent binding of methotrexate to immunoglobulins and the effect of antibody-linked drug on tumor growth in vivo. Cancer Res. 1981;41:2700–2706.

Kulkarni PN, Blair AH, Ghose T, Mammen M. Conjugation of methotrexate to IgG antibodies and their $F(ab)_2$ fragments and the effects of conjugated methotrexate on tumor growth in vivo. Cancer Immunol Immunother. 1985;19:211–214.

Kushner BH, Cheung N-K. GM-CSF enhances 3F8 monoclonal antibody-dependent cellular cytotoxicity against human melanoma and neuroblastoma. Blood. 1989;73:1936–1941.

Levy R, Hurwitz E, Maron R, Arnon R, Sela M. The specific cytotoxic effects of daunomycin conjugated to antitumor antibodies. Cancer Res. 1975;35:1182–1186.

Levy R, Miller RA. Tumor therapy with monoclonal antibodies. Fed Proc. 1983;42:2650–2656.

Liu AY, Robinson RR, Hellstrom KE, Murray ED Jr, Chang CP, Hellstrom I. Chimeric mouse-human IgG1 antibody that can mediate lysis of cancer cells. Proc Natl Acad Sci USA. 1987a;84:3439–3443.

Liu AY, Robinson RR, Murray ED Jr, Ledbetter JA, Hellstrom KE. Production of a mouse human chimeric monoclonal antibody to CD20 with potent Fc-dependent biologic activity. J Immunol. 1987b;139:3521–3526.

LoBuglio AF, Wheeler RH, Trang J, et al. Mouse/human chimeric monoclonal antibody in man: kinetics and immune response. Proc Natl Acad Sci USA. 1989;86:4220–4224.

Lotze MT, Grimm EA, Mazumder A. The in vivo distribution of autologous human and murine lymphoid cells grown in T cell growth factor (TCGF): implications for the adoptive immunotherapy of tumors. J Immunol. 1980;125:1487–1493.

Lotze MT, Grimm EA, Mazumder A. Lysis of fresh and cultured autologous tumor by human lymphocytes cultured in T-cell growth factor (TCGF). Cancer Res. 1981;41:4420–4425.

Lüders G, Köhnlein W, Sorg C, Bruggen J. Selective toxicity of neocarzinostatin-monoclonal antibody conjugates to the antigen-bearing human melanoma cell line in vitro. Cancer Immunol. Immunother. 1985;20:85–90.

MacPherson GG, North RJ. Endotoxin-mediated necrosis and regression of established tumors in the mouse. A correlative study of quantitative changes in blood flow and ultrastructural morphology. Cancer Immunol Immunother. 1986;21:209–216.

Manabe Y, Tsubota T, Haruta Y, et al. Production of a monoclonal antibody–bleomycin conjugate utilizing dextran T-40 and the antigen-targeting cytotoxicity of the conjugate. Biochem Biophys Res Commun. 1983;115:1009–1014.

Marley GM, Doyle LA, Ordonez JV, Sisk A, Hussain A, Chiu-Yen R-W. Potentiation of interferon induction of class I major histocompatibility complex antigen expression by human tumor necrosis factor in small cell lung cancer cell lines. Cancer Res. 1989;49:6232–6236.

Martin PJ, Hansen JA, Buckner DC, et al. Effects of in vitro depletion of cells in HLA-identical allogeneic marrow grafts. Blood. 1985;66:664–672.

Masucci G, Wersall P, Nielson J, Kierlulff-Nielson H, Wigzell H, Mellstedt H. Lymphokine activated killer (LAK) cells in antibody-dependent cellular cytotoxicity (ADCC) using MAb 17-1A: a combination of potential usefulness in tumor therapy. Hybridoma. 1989;8:507–516.

Masui H, Kawamoto T, Sato J-D, Wolf B, Sato G, Mendelsohn J. Growth inhibition of human tumor cells in athymic mice by anti-epidermal growth factor receptor monoclonal antibodies. Cancer Res. 1984;44:1002–1007.

Matsui M, Nakanishi T, Nogucki T, Ferrone S. Synergistic in vitro and in vivo anti-tumor effect of daunomycin-anti-96-kDa melanoma-associated antigen monoclonal antibody CL207 conjugate and recombinant IFN-gamma. J Immunol. 1988;141:1410–1417.

Matzku S, Brocker E-B, Bruggen J, Dippold WC, Tilgen W. Modes of binding and internalization of monoclonal antibodies to human melanoma cell lines. Cancer Res. 1986;46:3848–3854.

McBride WH, Howle SM. Induction of tolerance to a murine fibrosarcoma in two zones of dosage—the involvement of suppressor cells. Br J Cancer. 1986;53:707–711.

Meeker TC, Lowder J, Maloney DG, et al. The generation of monoclonal anti-idiotype therapy for B cell malignancy. Blood. 1985a;65:1349–1363.

Meeker T, Lowder J, Cleary ML. Emergence of idiotype variants during treatment of B-cell lymphoma with anti-idiotype antibodies. N Engl J Med. 1985b;312:1658–1665.

Melino G, Hobbs JR, Radford M, et al. Drug targeting for seven neuroblastoma patients using human polyclonal antibodies. Prot Biol Fluid. 1985;32:413–416.

Mercer-Smith JA, Roberts JC, Figard SD, Lavallee DK. The development of copper-67-labeled porphyrin-antibody conjugates. In: Rodwell JD, ed. Antibody-mediated delivery systems. New York, NY: Marcel Dekker; 1988:317–352.

Mew D, Wat C-H, Towers GHN, Levy JG. Photoimmunotherapy: treatment of animal tumors with tumor-specific monoclonal antibody-hematoporphyrin conjugates. J Immunol. 1983;130 (No. 3):1473–1477.

Mew D, Lum V, Wat C-K, et al. Ability of specific monoclonal antibodies and conventional antisera conjugated to hematoporphyrin to label and kill selected cell lines subsequent to light activation. Cancer Res. 1985;45:4380–4386.

Miller RA, Maloney BG, Warnke R, Levy R. Treatment of a B cell lymphoma with monoclonal anti-idiotype antibody. N Engl J Med. 1982;306:517–522.

Miller RA, Oseroff AR, Stratte PT, Levy R. Monoclonal antibody therapeutic trials in seven patients with T cell lymphoma. Blood. 1983;62:988–995.

Mitsuyasu RT, Champlin RE, Gale RP, et al. Treatment of donor bone marrow with monoclonal anti–T-cell antibody and complement for the prevention of graft-versus-host disease. A prospective randomized, double-blind trial. Ann Intern Med. 1986;105:20–26.

Mittelman A, Kageshita T, Kusama K, Kim JW, Arlin Z, Ferrone SA. A clinical trial of murine anti-idiotype monoclonal antibodies to high molecular weight melanoma associated antigens. Proc Am Soc Clin Oncol. 1988;7:248.

Monsigny M, Kieda C, Roche AC, Delmoiete F. Preparation and biological properties of a covalent antitumor drug-arm-carrier (DAC conjugate). FEBS Lett. 1980;119:181–186.

Morgan AC, Sullivan W, Graves S, Woodhouse CS. Murine monoclonal IgG3 to human colorectal tumor associated antigens: enhancement of antibody-dependent cell-mediated cytotoxicity by interleukin-2. Cancer Res. 1989;49:2773–2776.

Moscow JW, Cowan KH. Multidrug resistance. J Natl Cancer Inst. 1988;80:14–20.

Mufson RA, Aghajanian J, Wong G, Woodhouse C, Morgan AC. Recombinant human macrophage colony stimulating factor enhances the activity of human macrophages in antibody-dependent cell-mediated cytotoxicity. Cell Immunol. 1989;119:182–192.

Munn DH, Cheung N-K. Interleukin-2 enhancement of monoclonal antibody-mediated cellular cytotoxicity against human melanoma. Cancer Res. 1987;47:6600–6605.

Nair S, Samy TSA, Krishan A. Calcium, calmodulin, and protein content of adriamycin-resistant and sensitive murine leukemic cells. Cancer Res. 1986;46:229–232.

Nepon GT, Nelson KA, Holbeck SL, Hellstrom I, Hellstrom KE. Induction of immunity to a human tumor marker by in vivo administration of anti-idiotypic antibodies in mice. Proc Natl Acad Sci USA. 1985;81:2864–2867.

Ogawa M. An overview of mitomycin C study in Japan. In: Ogawa M, ed. Mitomycin C. New York, NY: Excerpta Medica; 1982;41–50.

Ognumuyiwa Y, Clegg JA, Pimm MV, Price MR, Baldwin RW. Comparative biodistribution of daunomycin-HSA-monoclonal antibody conjugates with different linkages. Br J Cancer. 1987;56:186.

Ohkawa K, Hibi N, Tsukada Y. Evaluation of a conjugate of purified antibodies against human AFP-dextran-daunorubicin to human APT-producing yolk sac tumor cell lines. Cancer Immunol Immunother. 1986a;22:81–86.

Ohkawa K, Tsukada Y, Hibi N, Umemoto N, Hara T. Selective in vitro and in vivo growth inhibition against human yolk sac tumor cell lines by purified antibody against human alphafetoprotein conjugated with mitomycin C via human serum albumin. Cancer Immunol Immunother. 1986b;23:81–86.

Oldham RK, Foon KA, Morgan AC, et al. Monoclonal antibody therapy of malignant melanoma: in vivo localization in cutaneous metastasis after intravenous administration. J Clin Oncol. 1984;2:1235–1244.

Oldham RK. Monoclonal antibodies: does sufficient selectivity to cancer cells exist for therapeutic application? J Biol Resp Mod. 1987;6:227–234.

Oldham RK, Lewis M, Orr DW, et al. Adriamycin custom tailored immunoconjugate in the treatment of human malignancies. Mol Biother. 1988;1:103–113.

Oseroff AR, Ohuoha D, Hasan T, Bommer JC, Yarmush ML. Antibody-targeted photolysis: selective photodestruction of human T-cell leukemia cells using monoclonal antibody-chlorin E_6 conjugates. Proc Natl Acad Sci USA. 1986;83:8744–8748.

Pagé M, Emond JP, Gauthier C, Dufour C, Innes L. Drug targeting with monoclonal antibodies. Prot Biol Fluids. 1981;29:933–936.

Pagé M, Delorme F, Lafontaine F, Dumas L. Chemotherapy with daunorubicin-anti-CEA conjugates in human colon adenocarcinoma grafted in nude mice. Semin Oncol. 1984;11 (No. 4):56–58.

Pietersz GA, Smyth MJ, McKenzie IFC. The use of anthracycline-antibody complexes for specific antitumor activity. In: Rodwell JD, ed. Antibody-mediated delivery systems. New York, NY: Marcel Dekker; 1988a:25–53.

Pietersz GA, Smyth MJ, McKenzie IFC. Immunochemotherapy of a murine thymoma with the use of idarubicin monoclonal antibody conjugates. Cancer Res. 1988b;48:926–931.

Pietersz GA, Cunningham Z, McKenzie IFC. Specific in vitro anti-tumor activity of methotrexate monoclonal antibody conjugates prepared using human serum albumin as an intermediary. Immunol Cell Biol. 1988c;66(Pt. 1):43–49.

Pietersz GA, Smyth MJ, Kanellos J, Cunningham Z, Sacks NPM, McKenzie IFC. Preclinical and clinical studies with a variety of immunoconjugates. Antibody Immunoconjugates Radiopharmaceuticals. 1988d;1(No. 1):79–103.

Pietersz GA. The linkage of cytotoxic drugs to monoclonal antibodies for the treatment of cancer. Bioconjugate Chem. 1990;1:89–95.

Pimm MV, Jones JA, Price MR, Middle JG, Embleton MJ, Baldwin RW. Tumour localization of monoclonal antibody against a rat mammary carcinoma and suppression of tumour growth with adriamycin-antibody conjugates. Cancer Immunol Immunother. 1982;12:125–134.

Pimm MV, Clegg JA, Caten JE, et al. Biodistribution of methotrexate-monoclonal antibody conjugates and complexes: experimental and clinical studies. Cancer Treat Rev. 1987;14: 411–420.

Pimm MV. Drug-monoclonal antibody conjugates for cancer therapy: potentials and limitations. Crit Rev Ther Drug Carrier Systems. 1988;5:189–227.

Pimm MV, Paul MA, Ogumiryiwa Y, Baldwin RW. Biodistribution and tumour localization of a daunomycin-monoclonal antibody conjugate in nude mice with human tumour xenografts. Cancer Immunol Immunother. 1988a;27:267–271.

Pimm MV, Clegg JA, Garnett MC, Baldwin RW. Biodistribution and tumour localization of a methotrexate monoclonal antibody 791T/36 conjugate in nude mice with human tumour xenografts. Int J Cancer. 1988b;41:886–891.

Povirk LF, Datta Gupta N, Warf BC, Goldberg TH. Neocarzinostatin chromophore binds to deoxyribonucleic acid by intercalation. Biochemistry. 1981;20:4007–4014.

Press OW, Appelbaum F, Ledbetter JA, et al. Monoclonal antibody IF5 (anti-CD20) serotherapy of human B-cell lymphomas. Blood. 1987;69:584–591.

Ramsay N, Le Bien T, Nesbit M, et al. Autologous bone marrow transplantation for patients with acute lymphoblastic leukemia after in vivo treatment with monoclonal antibodies BA-1, BA-2, and BA-3 plus complement. Blood. 1985;66:508–513.

Ritz J, Pesando JM, Sallan SE, et al. Serotherapy of acute lymphoblastic leukemia with monoclonal antibody. Blood. 1981;58:141–152.

Ritz J, Bast RC, Clavell LA, et al. Autologous bone marrow transplantation in CALLA-positive acute lymphoblastic leukemia after in vivo treatment with J5 monoclonal antibody and complement. Lancet. 1982;2:60–63.

Roberts JC, Figard SD, Mercer-Smith JA, Svitra Z, Anderson WL, Lavallee DK. Preparation and characterization of copper-67 porphyrin-antibody conjugates. J Immunol Meth. 1987; 105:153–164.

Rogers KE, Carr BI, Tokes ZA. Cell surface-mediated cytotoxicity of polymer bound adriamycin against drug resistant hepatocytes. Cancer Res. 1983;43:2741–2748.

Rowland GF, Simmonds RG, Corvalan JRF, et al. The potential use of monoclonal antibodies in drug targeting. Prot Biol Fluids. 1981;29:921–926.

Rowland GF, Simmonds RG, Corvalan JRF, et al. Monoclonal antibodies for targeted therapy with vindesine. Prot Biol Fluids Proc Colloq. 1983;30:375–379.

Rowland GF, Axton CA, Baldwin RW, et al. Antitumor properties of vindesine-monoclonal antibody conjugates. Cancer Immunol Immunother. 1985;19:1–7.

Rowland GF, Simmonds RG, Gore VA, Marsden CH, Smith W. Drug localization and growth inhibition studies of vindesine-monoclonal anti-CEA conjugates in human tumour xenograft. Cancer Immunol Immunother. 1986;21:183–187.

Rowlinson G, Balkwill F, Snook D, Hooker G, Epenetos AA. Enhancement of gamma-interferon of in vivo tumor radiolocalization by a monoclonal antibody against HLA-DR antigen. Cancer Res. 1986;46:6413.

Sato JD, Kawamoto T, Le AD, Mendelsohn J, Polikoff J, Sato GH. Biological effects in vitro of monoclonal antibodies to human epidermal growth factor receptors. Mol Biol Med. 1983;1:511–529.

Sato N, Goto T, Haranama K, et al. Actions of tumor necrosis factor on cultured vascular endothelial cells morphologic modulation, growth inhibition and cytotoxicity. J Natl Cancer Inst. 1986;76:1113–1121.

Sauvage CA, Mendelsohn JC, Lesley JF, Trowbridge IS. Effects of monoclonal antibodies that block transferrin receptor function on the in vivo growth of a syngeneic murine leukemia. Cancer Res. 1987;47:747–753.

Schechter B, Pauzner R, Arnon R, Haimovich J, Wilchek M. Selective cytotoxicity against tumor cells by cisplatin complexed to antitumor antibodies via carboxymethyl dextran. Cancer Immunol Immunother. 1987;25:225–230.

Schlom JC, Horan-Hand P, Greiner JW, et al. Innovations that influence the pharmacology of monoclonal antibody guided tumor targeting. Cancer Res. 1990;50:8205–8275.

Schroff RW, Stevenson HC. Human immune responses to murine monoclonal antibodies. In: Foon KA, Morgan AC, eds. Monoclonal antibody therapy of human cancer. The Hague: Martinus Nijhoff; 1985:121–138.

Schroff RW, Foon KA, Beatty SM, Oldham RK, Morgan AC. Human anti-murine immunoglobulin responses in patients receiving monoclonal antibody therapy. Cancer Res. 1985; 45:779–885.

Schroff RW, Morgan AC, Woodhouse CS, et al. Monoclonal antibody therapy in malignant melanoma: factors effecting in vivo localization. J Biol Resp Mod. 1987;6:457–472.

Sears HF, Atkinson B, Mattis J. Phase I clinical trial of monoclonal antibody in treatment of gastrointestinal tumors. Lancet. 1982;1:762–765.

Sears HG, Herlyn D, Steplewski Z, Koprowski H. Effects of monoclonal antibody immunotherapy in patients with gastrointestinal adenocarcinoma. J Biol Resp Mod. 1984;3:138–150.

Sears HF, Herlyn D, Steplewski Z, Koprowski H. Phase II clinical trial of a murine monoclonal antibody cytotoxic for gastrointestinal adenocarcinoma. Cancer Res. 1985;45:5910–5913.

Sela M, Hurwitz E. Conjugates of antibodies with cytotoxic drugs. In: Vogel CW, ed. Immunoconjugates, antibody conjugates in radioimaging and therapy of cancer; New York, NY: Oxford University Press; 1987:189–216.

Senter PD, Saulnier MG, Schreiber GJ, et al. Anti-tumor effects of antibody-alkaline phosphatase conjugates in combination with etoposide phosphate. Proc Natl Acad Sci USA. 1988;85:4842–4846.

Sezaki H, Hashida M. Macromolecule drug conjugates in targeted cancer chemotherapy. Crit Rev Ther Drug Carrier Systems. 1984;1:1–38.

Shaw DR, Khazaeli MB, Sun LK, et al. Characterization of a mouse/human chimeric monoclonal antibody (17-1A) to a colon cancer tumor associated antigen. J Immunol. 1987;138: 4534–4538.

Shawler DL, Johnson DE, Sweet MD, et al. Preclinical trials using an immunoconjugate of

T101 and methotrexate in an athymic mouse/human T-cell tumor model. J Biol Resp Mod. 1988;7:608–618.

Shen L, Guyre PM, Ball ED, Fanser MW. Glucocorticoid enhances γ-interferon effects on human monocyte antigen expression and ADCC. Clin Exp Immunol. 1986b;65:387–395.

Shen W-C, Ryser HJ-P. Cis-aconityl space between daunomycin and macromolecular carriers: a model of pH sensitive linkage releasing drug from a lysomotropic conjugate. Biochem Biophys Res Commun. 1981;102:1048–1054.

Shen W-C, Ryser HJ-P. Selective killing of Fc-receptor-bearing tumor cells through endocytosis of a drug-carrying immune complex. Proc Natl Acad Sci USA. 1984;81:1445–1447.

Shen W-C, Ballou B, Ryser HJ-P, Hakala TR. Targeting internalization and cytotoxicity of methotrexate-monoclonal anti-stage specific embryonic antigen-1 antibody conjugates in cultured F-9 teratocarcinoma cells. Cancer Res. 1986a;46:3912–3916.

Shih LB, Sharkey RM, Primus FJ, Goldenberg DM. Site-specific linkage of methotrexate to monoclonal antibodies using an intermediate carrier. Int J Cancer. 1988;41:832–839.

Shouval D, Adler R, Wands JR, Hurwitz E, Isselbacher KJ, Sela M. Doxorubicin conjugate of monoclonal antibodies to hepato-associated antigens. Proc Natl Acad Sci. 1988;85:8276–8280.

Singh M, Kralovec J, Mezei M, Ghose T. Inhibition of human renal cancer by methotrexate linked to a monoclonal antibody. J Urol. 1989;141:428–431.

Smyth MJ, Pietersz GA, Classon BJ, McKenzie IFC. Specific targeting of chlorambucil to tumors with the use of monoclonal antibodies. J Natl Cancer Inst. 1986;76(No. 3):503–510.

Smyth MJ, Pietersz GA, McKenzie IFC. Selective enhancement of antitumor activity of N-acetyl melphalan upon conjugation to monoclonal antibodies. Cancer Res. 1987a;47:62–69.

Smyth MJ, Pietersz GA, McKenzie IFC. The mode of action of methotrexate-monoclonal antibody conjugates. Immunol Cell Biol. 1987b;65(Pt. 2):189–200.

Smyth MJ, Pietersz GA, McKenzie IFC. The in vitro and in vivo anti-tumour activity of N-ACMEL-$(Fab')_2$ conjugate. Br J Cancer. 1987c;55:7–11.

Smyth MJ, Pietersz GA, McKenzie IFC. Increased antitumor effect of immunoconjugates and tumor necrosis factor in vivo. Cancer Res. 1988a;48:3607–3612.

Smyth MJ, Pietersz GA, McKenzie IFC. Immunosuppression of graft rejection with idarubicin-monoclonal antibody conjugates by elimination of T-cell subsets in vivo. Transplantation. 1988b;46:126–131.

Starling JJ, Hinson NA, Marder P, Maciak RS, Laguzza BC. Rapid internalization of antigen-immunoconjugate complexes is not required for anti-tumor activity of monoclonal antibody-drug conjugates. Antibody Immunoconjugates Radiopharmaceuticals. 1988;1(No. 4):311–323.

Steele JK, Liu D, Stammers AT, Deal H, Whitney S, Levy JG. Suppressor deletion therapy. In: Rodwell JD, ed. Antibody-mediated delivery systems. New York, NY: Marcel Dekker; 1988:8–39.

Steplewski Z, Sun LK, Shearman CW, Ghrayeb J, Daddona P, Koprowski H. Biological activity of human-mouse IgG1, IgG2, IgG3, and IgG4 chimeric monoclonal antibodies with antitumor specificity. Proc Natl Acad Sci USA. 1988;85:4852–4856.

Stolphen AH, Guinan EC, Fiers W, Pobet JS. Recombinant tumor necrosis factor and immune interferon act singly and in combination to recognize human vascular endothelial cell monolayers. Am J Pathol. 1986;123:16–24.

Sun LK, Curtis P, Rakowicz-Szulczynska E, et al. Chimeric antibody with human constant regions and mouse variable regions directed against carcinoma-associated 17-1A. Proc Natl Acad Sci USA. 1987;84:214–218.

Suzuki T, Sato D, Goto K, Katsunada Y, Unno K, Takahashi T. The preparation of mitomycin C, adriamycin and daunomycin covalently bound to antibodies as improved cancer chemotherapeutic agents. Chem Pharm Bull. 1981;29(No. 3):844–848.

Taetle R, Honeysett JM. Effects of monoclonal anti-transferrin antibodies on in vitro growth of human solid tumor cells. Cancer Res. 1987;47:2040–2044.

Takahashi Y, Mai M, Umemoto N, Kato Y, Hara T, Tsukada Y. Conjugates of mitomycin with anti-alpha-fetoprotein antibody: antitumor effect against alpha-fetoprotein-producing human gastric carcinoma implanted in nude mice. NCI Monogr. 1987;3:101–105.

Takahashi T, Yamaguchi T, Kitamura K, et al. Clinical application of monoclonal antibody-drug conjugates for immunotargeting chemotherapy of colorectal carcinoma. Cancer. 1988;61: 881–888.

Takvorian T, Canellos GP, Ritz J, et al. Prolonged disease-free survival after autologous bone marrow transplantation in patients with non-Hodgkin's lymphoma with a poor prognosis. N Engl J Med. 1987;316:1499–1505.

Tokes ZA, Rogers KE, Rembaum A. Synthesis of adriamycin coupled polyglutaraldehyde microspheres and evaluation of their cytostatic activity. Proc Natl Acad Sci USA. 1982;79: 2026–2030.

Trauth BC, Klas C, Peters AMJ, et al. Monoclonal antibody mediated tumor regression by induction of apoptosis. Science. 1989;245:301–304.

Tritton TR, Yee G. The anticancer agent adriamycin can be actively cytotoxic without entering cells. Science. 1982;217:248–250.

Trouet A, Tolles G. Targeting of daunorubicin by association with DNA or proteins: a review. Semin Oncol. 1984;11:64.

Trowbridge IS. Therapeutic potential of monoclonal antibodies that block biological function. In: Boss BD, Langmann R, Trowbridge I, Dulbecco R, eds. Monoclonal antibodies and cancer. New York, NY: Academic Press; 1983:53–61.

Tsukada Y, Hurwitz E, Kashi R, et al. Chemotherapy by intravenous administration of conjugates of daunomycin with monoclonal and conventional anti-rat alpha-fetoprotein antibodies. Proc Natl Acad Sci USA. 1982;79:7896–7899.

Tsukada Y, Hurwitz E, Kashi R, et al. Effect of a conjugate of daunomycin and purified polyclonal or monoclonal antibodies to rat alpha-fetoprotein on the growth of alpha-fetoprotein and producing tumor cells. Ann NY Acad Sci. 1983;83:262–269.

Tsukada Y, Ohkawa K, Hibi N. Suppression of human alpha-fetoprotein-producing hepatocellular carcinoma growth in nude mice by an anti alpha-fetoprotein antibody-daunorubicin conjugate with a poly-L-glutamic acid derivative as intermediate drug carrier. Br J Cancer. 1985;52:111–116.

Tsukada Y, Okhawa K, Hibi N. Therapeutic effect of treatment with polyclonal or monoclonal antibodies to alpha-fetoprotein that have been conjugated to daunomycin via dextran bridge: studies with alpha-fetoprotein-producing rat hepatoma tumor model. Cancer Res. 1987; 47:4293-4295.

Tung E, Goust JM, Chen WY, Kang SS, Wang IY, Wang AC. Cytotoxic effect of anti-idiotype antibody-chlorambucil conjugates against human lymphoblastoid cells. Immunology. 1983;50: 57–64.

Uadia P, Blair AH, Ghose T. Uptake of methotrexate linked to an anti-EL4-lymphoma antibody by EL4 cells. Cancer Immunol Immunother. 1983;16:127–129.

Uadia P, Blair AH, Ghose T. Tumor and tissue distribution of a methotrexate-anti-EL4 immunoglobulin conjugate in EL4 lymphoma-bearing mice. Cancer Res. 1984;44:4263–4266.

Uadia P, Blair AH, Ghose T, Ferrone S. Uptake of methotrexate linked to polyclonal and monoclonal antimelanoma antibodies by a human melanoma cell line. J Natl Cancer Inst. 1985;74:29–35.

Uadia PO, Blair AH, Ghose T. Hydrolysis of methotrexate-immunoglobulin conjugates by liver homogenates and characterization of catabolites. Cancer Chemother Pharmacol. 1988;22: 175–177.

Umemoto N, Kato Y, Takeda Y. Conjugates of mitomycin C with the immunoglobulin M monomer fragment of a monoclonal anti-mm46 immunoglobulin M antibody with or without serum albumin as intermediary. J Appl Biochem. 1984;6:297–307.

Umemoto N, Kato Y, Hara T. Cytotoxicities of two disulfide-bond-linked conjugates of methotrexate with monoclonal anti-mm46 antibody. Cancer Immunol Immunother. 1989;28:9–16.

Vadhan-Raj S, Cordon-Cardo C, Carswell E, et al. Phase I trial of a mouse monoclonal antibody against CD3 ganglioside in patients with melanoma: induction of inflammatory response at tumor sites. J Clin Oncol. 1988;6:1636–1648.

Vaickus L, Jones VE, Morton CC, Whitford K, Bacon RN. Antiproliferative mechanism of anti-class II monoclonal antibodies. Cell Immunol. 1989;119:445–458.

Vaickus L, Biddle W, Cemerlic D, Foon K. Interferon-gamma augments Lym-1-dependent, granulocyte-mediated tumor cell lysis. Blood. 1990;75:2408–2416.

Verrill H, Goldberg M, Rosenbaum R, et al. Clinical trial of Wistar Institute 17-1A monoclonal antibody in patients with advanced gastrointestinal adenocarcinoma: a preliminary report. Hybridoma. 1986;5:175–183.

Vuist WMJ, Buitenen FV, deRie A, Hekman P, Rumke P, Mebef CJM. Potentiation by interleukin-2 of Burkitt's lymphoma therapy with anti-pan B (anti-CD19) monoclonal antibodies in a mouse xenotransplantation model. Cancer Res. 1989;49:3783–3788.

Waldmann H, Polliak A, Hale G, et al. Elimination of graft-versus-host disease by in vitro depletion of alloreactive lymphocytes with a monoclonal rat anti-human lymphocyte antibody (CAMPATH-1). Lancet. 1984;2:483–486.

Waldmann TA, Longo DL, Leonard WJ, et al. Interleukin-2 receptor (Tac antigen) expression in HTLV-1 associated adult T-cell leukemia. Cancer Res. 1985;45:4559–4562.

Waldmann TA. The structure, function and expression of interleukin-2 receptors on normal and malignant lymphocytes. Science. 1986;232:727–732.

Walker-Jones D, Valverius EM, Stampter MK, Lippman ME, Dickson RB. Stimulation of epithelial membrane antigen expression by transforming growth factor-β in normal and oncogene-transformed human mammary epithelial cells. Cancer Res. 1989;49:6407–6411.

Warenius HM, Golfe G, Bleeher NM, Milstein C. Attempted targeting of a monoclonal antibody in a human tumour xenograft system. Br J Cancer. 1981;17(No. 9):1009–1015.

Webb KS, Paulson DF, Parks SF, Tuck FL, Walther PJ, Ware JL. Characterization of prostate-tissue-directed monoclonal antibody, α-Pro 13. Cancer Immunol Immunother. 1984;17: 7–17.

Weiner LM, Steplewski Z, Koprowski H, Sears HF, Litwin S, Comis RL. Biological effects of γ-interferon pie-treatment followed by monoclonal antibody 17-1A administered in patients with gastrointestinal carcinoma. Hybridoma. 1986;5:65–77.

Weiner LM, Steplewski Z, Koprowski H, Litwin S, Comis RL. Divergent dose-related effects of γ-interferon on in vitro antibody-dependent-cellular-cytotoxicity by numan peripheral blood monocytes. Cancer Res. 1988a;48:1042–1046.

Weiner LM, Moldofsky PJ, Gatenby RA, et al. Antibody delivery and effector-cell activation in a phase II trial of recombinant γ-interferon and the murine monoclonal antibody CO17-1A in advanced colorectal carcinoma. Cancer Res. 1988b;48:2568–2573.

Wingard LB Jr, Tritton JR, Egler KA. Cell surface effects of adriamycin and carminomycin immobilized on cross-linked polyvinyl alcohol. Cancer Res. 1985;45:3529–3536.

Yamaizumi M, Mekada E, Uchida T, Okada Y. One molecule of diphtheria toxin fragment A introduced into a cell can kill the cell. Cell. 1978;15:255.

Yang HM, Reisfeld RA. Doxorubicin conjugated with a monoclonal antibody directed to a human melanoma-associated proteoglycan suppresses the growth of established tumor xenografts in nude mice. Proc Natl Acad Sci USA. 1988;85:1189–1193.

Yu D-S, Chu TM, Yeh M-Y, Chang S-Y, Ma C-P, Han SH. Antitumor activity of doxorubicin-monoclonal antibody conjugate on human bladder cancer. J Urology. 1988a;140:415–421.

Yu D-S, Kawinski E, Chu TM. Effect of verapamil on antitumor activity of adriamycin-monoclonal antibody conjugate against intraperitoneal human ovarian cancer xenograft. J Tumor Marker Oncol. 1988b;3(No. 2):237–249.

Zunino F, Gambetta R, Vigevani A, Penco S, Geroni C, Di Marco A. Biologic activity of daunorubicin linked to proteins via the methylketone side chain. Tumori. 1981;67:521–524.

CHAPTER 11

IMMUNOTOXINS IN CANCER TREATMENT

Robert W. Baldwin
Vera S. Byers

Monoclonal antibodies (mAb) have been produced that react with a significant spectrum of human malignant cells (Boyer et al., 1988). These include antibodies reacting with solid cancers of epithelial origin such as colorectal, breast, lung, and ovarian cancers, as well as antibodies recognizing "neoantigens" on malignant melanoma and bone and soft-tissue sarcomas. Antibodies reacting with antigens on leukemias and lymphomas have also been produced, which mainly recognize epitopes associated with the CD cluster markers. While the antigens recognized by these monoclonal antibodies are not tumor-specific, they are expressed at the tumor cell surface in high enough concentration, compared with their level of expression on normal tissues, to be considered for targeting therapeutic agents. In this approach to cancer treatment, the choice of cytotoxic agent is a compromise between the desire to employ highly cytotoxic agents so that tumor-cell kill is effective and the need to minimize side effects of the immunoconjugate through interactions with target antigen expressed on normal tissues. Drug resistance associated with many chemotherapeutic agents also needs to be taken into account. From these considerations, the antibody delivery of toxin molecules has been advocated and there are a number of immunotoxins derived by conjugating plant and bacterial toxins at the stage of clinical assessment (Byers and Baldwin, 1991; Vitetta and Thorpe, 1991; Wawrzyczak, 1991).

DESIGN OF IMMUNOTOXINS

Ricin

Ricin, isolated from the seeds of *Ricinus communis* plant, has been extensively used for immunotoxin synthesis (Baldwin et al., 1988; Blakey et al., 1988b; Baldwin and Byers, 1990; Vitetta and Thorpe, 1991). This toxin in its mature form is composed of two polypeptide chains, A and B, of approximately comparable size (30 kDa), each of which has a distinct role in target-cell toxicity. In the normal course of events, the toxin binds through a site on the B chain to galactose-containing cell receptors. The B chain also plays a role, still not well defined, in transporting the A chain into the cytoplasm of the cell (Olsnes and Sandvig, 1988; Richardson et al., 1988). Following entry into the cytoplasm, through a series of endosome vesicles and trafficking through the Golgi network, the A chain inhibits protein synthesis by catalytically inactivating the 60S ribosomal subunit (May et al., 1989). This is achieved by an *N*-glycosidic cleavage, which releases a specific adenine base from the sugar phosphate of 28S RNA (Endo et al., 1987; Endo and Tsurugi, 1987).

Immunotoxins have been constructed by conjugation of whole ricin to antibody. This can be effected by introducing a free thiol group into the antibody and reacting the derivatized antibody with toxin having an introduced alkylating function (Blakey et al., 1988b). This interaction results in toxin–antibody binding through a thioether linkage. Although this linkage is stable to reduction, conjugates retain the natural disulfide bond linking the A and B chains, thus allowing intracellular cleavage and release of A chain to effect inhibition of cell protein synthesis. Variables affecting ricin–antibody conjugate efficacy have been studied with respect to the number of conjugated ricin molecules and the use of spacer molecules in conjugate design. Direct linkage of ricin to antibody may produce steric interference with the B chain. This led to the construction of an immunotoxin in which ricin was coupled to immunoglobulin through a 29-residue flexible peptide spacer arm and this resulted in an almost 10-fold increase in potency (Marsh and Neville, 1988).

Immunotoxins constructed with intact ricin are highly cytotoxic, since they retain the multiple functions of the B chain, thus augmenting cell binding and internalization of the A chains. But they lack target-cell specificity, since the B chain binds nonspecifically to galactose residues on the surface of cells. Various maneuvers have been utilized in order to prevent this B-chain binding such as in vitro incubation of target cells and immunotoxin in the presence of excess concentrations of galactose or lactose. This is not a feasible approach in vivo and methods have been devised for constructing conjugates to block the B-chain galactose binding site. Monoclonal antibody anti-Thy 1.1 bound to ricin through a short linker was unable to bind to galactose, probably through antibody causing steric hindrance of the B-chain binding site (Thorpe et al., 1984). This approach was also adopted in the construction of a thioether-linked ricin–antibody immunotoxin and fractionation into "blocked" and "nonblocked" components (Brusa et al., 1989). The blocked immunotoxin was most effective when used to treat human colorectal carcinoma xenografts by intraperitoneal injection and was less toxic than the unblocked product.

Ricin A Chain

Immunotoxins constructed with ricin A chain (RTA) have increased target cell specificity, although this is achieved at the expense of cytotoxic potential compared to whole ricin. In this approach, the A- and B-chain polypeptides of ricin are separated following reductive cleavage of the disulfide bond joining the two chains of the toxin and the RTA conjugated to antibody. This is achieved by linking RTA to antibody by means of a reducible disulfide bond so that the RTA can be released intracellularly. This is accomplished by modifying antibody with a heterobifunctional reagent to introduce an activated disulfide group, and by reacting it with reduced RTA. A thiol–disulfide exchange reaction results, leaving the A chain attached to antibody by a disulfide linkage (Fig. 11-1).

Many immunotoxins have been constructed using the heterobifunctional reagent *N*-succinimidyl-3-(2-pyridyldithio)propionate (SPDP) following its introduction for protein–protein conjugation (Carlsson et al., 1978). The choice of linker between antibody and RTA is a compromise, since it must be sufficiently stable to preserve intact immunotoxin in the circulation, while readily undergoing cleavage intracellularly, thus releasing the RTA moiety (Vitetta and Thorpe, 1991). In this respect, some immunotoxins constructed using SPDP as the bifunctional coupling agent have proven to be unstable in vivo and other coupling agents have been introduced. These include 2-iminothiolane and 4-succinimidyloxycarbonyl-α methyl-α(2 pyridyldithio) toluene (SMPT). Coupling of SMPT introduces a sterically hindered disulfide linkage in which a methyl group and a benzene ring protect the disulfide bond from reduction and thus increase immunotoxin stability (Thorpe et al., 1987). Other heterobifunctional cross-

FIGURE 11-1
Linkages introduced between antibody and ricin A chain.

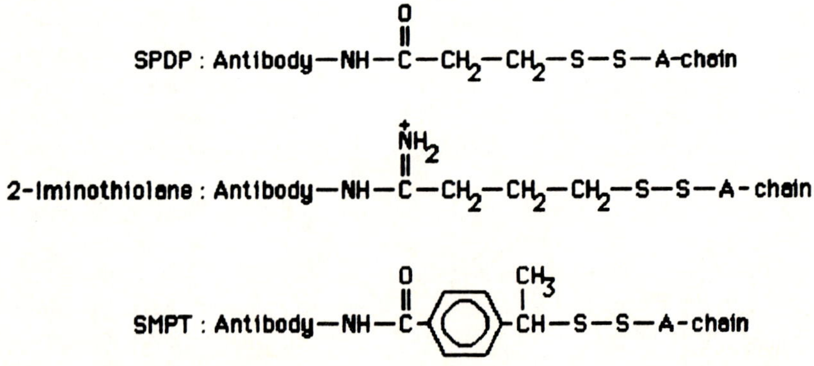

linking agents introduced for immunotoxin construction have maleiimide as the protein reactive group. These include m-maleimidobenzoyl-*N*-hydroxysuccinimide ester (Myers et al., 1989) and the acetone ketal bis(maleimidoethoxy)propane (BMEP), which is readily cleaved at the pH of acidified cellular vesicles (p4-6), but is stable at pH in the range pH7-8 (Srinivasachar and Neville, 1989).

Ribosome-Inhibiting Proteins

Ribosome-inhibiting proteins occur naturally in several plant species, probably as a defense against predators in evolutionary terms. Some, like ricin, are produced as two-chain toxins, whereas others occur as single-chain products akin to RTA. These potential candidates for construction of immunotoxins include trichosanthin, trichokirin, gelonin, saporin, mormordin, and pokeweed antiviral protein (Yeung et al., 1988).

Of particular interest is trichosanthin, which is isolated from the root tuber *Trichosantes kirilowii,* a Cucurbitaceae used in traditional Chinese medicine as an abortifactant and for the treatment of choriocarcinoma. This basic single-chain protein consisting of 234 amino acid residues has been sequenced and a molecular model derived from X-ray structure analysis. These analyses indicate a very striking degree of homology between RTA and trichosanthin, suggesting that they may originate from a common ancestor (Zhang and Wang, 1986). Unlike RTA, trichosanthin is not glycosylated, making it an attractive candidate for construction of immunoconjugates. As discussed later, the in vivo fate of RTA immunotoxins is very heavily influenced by associated mannose-containing oligosaccharides because of their uptake by mannose receptors on hepatic Kupffer's cells. The ribosome-inactivating activity of trichosanthin has been demonstrated in rabbit reticulocyte lysate assay (Yeung et al., 1988). Furthermore, this protein was reported to inhibit replication of human immunodeficiency virus (HIV) in both T lymphoblastoid cells and mitogen-activated peripheral blood mononuclear cells (McGrath et al., 1989), activities that have led to its use in phase I trials in acquired immunodeficiency syndrome (AIDS) patients (Byers et al., 1990).

Immunotoxins constructed with trichosanthin are being developed and the properties of an immunoconjugate constructed with a related ribosome-inhibiting protein (RIP), trichokirin, have been described (Casellas et al., 1988). Trichokirin is extracted from the seeds rather than the root of *Trichosanthes kirilowii* Maximowicz. It is strongly basic but, unlike trichosanthin, is glycosylated. The immunotoxin constructed by conjugation of trichokirin to an antibody directed against the murine Thy 1.2 antigen was highly cytotoxic for leukemia cells expressing the Th 1.2 antigen.

Pseudomonas Exotoxin

Pseudomonas exotoxin (PE) is a bacterial protein (MW 66KD) consisting of three domains (FitzGerald and Pastan, 1989). Domain 1 (also termed 1a) at the *N* terminus mediates binding, domain 2 is required for cellular translocation, and domain 3 at the

C terminus has adenosine diphosphate (ADP)-ribosylation activity. Removal of domain 1a (amino acid residues 1-252) yields a residual protein (PE40) that retains both translocating and ADP-ribosylating activity. Protein PE40 lacks cell-binding activity and so has been used to construct immunotoxins. In one approach, PE was treated with 2-iminothiolane to block lysine residues, including lysine-57 in the binding domain, which is important for PE binding. This treatment also introduced sulfhydryl groups into the modified PE and these were used to link to antibody by a disulfide exchange reaction (Pirker et al., 1985). In an alternative approach, recombinant forms of PE have been synthesized by deleting DNA coding for cell binding and used to construct immunotoxins (Kondo et al., 1988). This has subsequently led to the construction of recombinant immunotoxins consisting of antibody–toxin fusion protein. As an example of this approach, a recombinant product has been produced containing the variable region of the anti-Tac monoclonal antibody recognizing the p55 subunit of interleukin-2 (IL-2) receptor joined through a peptide linkage to PE40 (Chaudhary et al., 1989).

Immunotoxins constructed by conjugation of PE to murine monoclonal antibodies, particularly antiovarian cancer antibody OVB3, have been used to treat xenografts of ovarian and colorectal carcinomas (Willingham et al., 1987; FitzGerald et al., 1987; Pearson et al., 1989) and mesothelioma (Griffin et al., 1987). These studies demonstrated the therapeutic efficacy of PE immunotoxins given intraperitoneally to treat intraperitoneal tumors and the effects with colon tumors being enhanced when combined with cyclophosphamide. Drawing from these experiences, a clinical trial has been initiated treating ovarian cancer with immunotoxin PE-OVB3.

IMMUNOTOXIN THERAPY: HUMAN TUMOR XENOGRAFTS

Immunotoxins have been constructed with monoclonal antibodies reacting with several types of solid cancer, including colorectal, breast, and ovarian cancer, malignant melanoma, and bone and soft tissue sarcomas. These immunotoxins have been constructed mainly with ricin or RTA and PE. They display specific in vitro cytotoxicity for tumor cells and studies have progressed to in vivo evaluation against human tumor xenografts in athymic mice. Two general approaches have been adopted in these studies. First, immunotoxins have been administered systemically and their effectiveness assessed against tumor xenografts at distant sites. This essentially provides a model for systemic treatment of solid cancers such as recurrent local disease or less satisfactorily for metastatic disease and requires the immunotoxin to have good pharmacokinetic properties. The second approach involves injection of immunotoxin directly into the site of the tumor xenografts (intracavity therapy) and this has been used particularly as a model for therapy of peritoneal tumor deposits.

The site-specific delivery of immunotoxins requires adequate blood survival following systemic administration. But RTA immunotoxins have proven to be rapidly eliminated from the circulation with preferential localization in liver (Byers et al., 1987a; Bourrie et al., 1986; Fulton et al., 1988). This is due to the recognition of mannose-containing oligosaccharide sidechains of RTA by specific cell-surface receptors on nonparenchymal hepatic (Kupffer's) cells (Blakey et al., 1988a). Several strategies have been adopted to modify hepatic uptake including the use of RTA subfractions with reduced oligosaccharide content or by chemically modifying the mannose and fucose residues of the A chain (Thorpe et al., 1988; Vitetta and Thorpe, 1991). In the latter approach, so-called deglycosylated RTA is produced by modifying the carbohydrate component of ricin by oxidation with metaperiodate-cyanoborohydride mixtures prior to separation of the ricin A and B chains for antibody conjugation. This markedly improves the pharmacokinetics of the immunotoxin, although the product is still cleared from the circulation more rapidly than unconjugated antibody. Immunotoxins have also been constructed with recombinant ricin A chain (rRA), which is nonglycosylated (O'Hare et al., 1990; Bjorn et al., 1985). The influence of the oligosaccharide in this type of immunoconjugate is illustrated in experiments comparing the blood survival of RTA and rRA when complexed with an anti-RTA monoclonal antibody that binds both toxin species (Pimm et al., 1990). Both RTA and rRA in free form are rapidly eliminated from the circulation by clearance through the kidneys. When complexed with anti-RTA monoclonal antibody, RTA complexes were taken up by the liver, but rRA complexes showed much lower clearance, resulting in a fivefold increase in blood survival.

A third approach for limiting RTA immunotoxin uptake in liver is to administer the conjugate with mannose-containing agents, which will preferentially block mannose receptors on Kupffer's cells (Byers et al., 1987a). One such agent was a conjugate of mannose and lysine (Man_3Ly_2) designed specifically for hepatic targeting of drugs (Ponpipom et al., 1981). When this compound was administered with RTA immunotoxin, there was a marked reduction in liver uptake of immunotoxin and a concomitant increase in blood survival. These observations indicate the desirability of utilizing toxin moieties deficient in mannose-containing oligosaccharides such as recombinant RTA and naturally occurring nonglycosylated A chain RIP, for example, trichosanthin (Yeung et al., 1988). Hepatic clearance by recognition of mannose-containing residues is not the only factor to be taken into account, since other features still to be defined contribute to the rapid elimination of immunotoxin from the circulation.

The blood survival of immunotoxin is further influenced by the stability of the linkage between toxin molecule and antibody. This has already been commented upon since some immunoconjugates constructed using SPDP as the heterobifunctional agent are readily degraded in serum and this becomes an important issue when blood survival is increased by blocking hepatic uptake. For example, in one series of studies, immunotoxins constructed using deglycosylated RTA and a new coupling agent (SMPT) that produces a more stable bond between RTA and antibody showed improved antitumor activity (Thorpe et al., 1987).

Even with these reservations, immunotoxins have been constructed that are efficacious in suppressing growth of human tumor xenografts. These include RTA immunotoxins constructed with mAb 791T/36 reacting with a cell-surface glycoprotein gp72 on colorectal cancer (Byers et al., 1987b) and with antibody reacting with a large molecular weight (220-kDa, 500-kDa) melanoma-associated antigen. An RTA conjugate with anti–common acute lymphoblastic leukemia antigen (CALLA) antibody also suppressed growth of xenografts of NALM-6 (a pre-B-ALL cell line) cells (Hara et al., 1988).

Intracavity immunotherapy has advantages over systemic treatment in that immunotoxin can be delivered more effectively to the tumor site. This approach has been explored largely for the treatment of peritoneal tumor growths. In particular, an immunotoxin constructed by conjugating PE to the antiovarian cancer mAb OVb3 was effective for intracavity therapy of xenografts of ovarian (Willingham et al., 1987) and colon (Pearson et al., 1989) tumors.

CLINICAL STUDIES

Following on from what are now quite extensive preclinical studies, phase I clinical trials have been conducted with RTA immunotoxins in colorectal cancer (Byers et al., 1989) and malignant melanoma (Spitler et al., 1987) and with recombinant RTA containing immunotoxin in breast cancer (Weiner et al., 1989). The overall objectives of the studies were to establish the safety of immunotoxins when given systemically to patients with metastatic disease and to determine maximum tolerated doses. Related issues addressed included the pharmacokinetics of immunotoxins in relation to their in vivo stability and tumor penetration and the influence of antibody responses to RTA and mouse immunoglobulin. The trials also provided initial evidence of therapeutic responses.

A second approach is evaluating immunotoxins when administered systemically for the elimination of target cells where at least a proportion are present in the circulation (Byers and Baldwin, 1991a, 1991b; Vitetta and Thorpe, 1991). This has been successfully employed in the use of an RTA immunotoxin constructed with an anti–T-cell antigen (CD5) monoclonal antibody in the treatment of acute and chronic graft versus host disease in patients receiving bone marrow transplantation (Kernan et al., 1988; Byers et al., 1990). This is leading to trials with immunotoxins constructed with a range of antibodies reacting with B- and T-cell antigens (CD4, CD5, CD7, CD19, CD22) in the treatment of lymphoid malignancies (Vitetta et al., 1990; Vitetta and Thorpe, 1991) and for the clinical management of bone marrow–transplanted patients (Byers et al., 1990).

Immunotoxin 791T/36–RTA in Colorectal Cancer

Patients with metastatic colorectal carcinoma were entered into a dose-escalation study with immunotoxin 791T/36–RTA (Byers et al., 1989). The antibody component recognizes a tumor cell membrane glycoprotein (gp72) that, by flow-cytometry analysis of tumor cells derived by disaggregation of surgical specimens, is expressed on colorectal cancer cells with 2 to 8 $\times$ 10^5 copies expressed per cell (Durrant et al., 1985, 1989b). This antibody labeled with iodine 131 (^{131}I) and indium 111 (^{111}In) has been used extensively for gamma camera imaging of primary and metastatic colorectal cancers (Armitage et al., 1984, 1985; Perkins and Pimm, 1991). Radioisotope counting of normal and malignant colonic tissue derived from surgically resected specimens indicated tumor:normal tissue ratios ranging up to 10:1 (Armitage et al., 1984), indicating preferential localization of antibody in tumor. In the phase I study, patients with metastatic colorectal cancer received immunotoxin 791T/36–RTA in doses ranging from 0.02 to 0.2 mg/kg/day in 1-hour infusions for a 5-day course. The side effects included a composite of reversible signs and symptoms, including decreased serum albumin levels with mild weight gain, mild fever, and flulike effects, which seem to be generic to RTA immunotoxins (Byers et al., 1989; Spitler et al., 1987). Two other side effects, reversible proteinuria and mental status changes, were also observed in patients treated with immunotoxin 791T/36–RTA. Proteinuria probably occurs as a consequence of anti-immunotoxin antibody responses. The changes in mental status were originally considered to be characteristic of the immunotoxin, since they were not observed in melanoma studies (Spitler et al., 1987). But neurological toxicity has been observed in breast cancer patients treated with another immunotoxin (Weiner et al., 1989). Neurotoxic effects may be related to the affinity of RIP for neural cells (Wiley et al., 1990; Foxwell et al., 1985). For example, the RIP trichosanthin, which has a high degree of structural homology with RTA, has been reported to be neurotoxic in a clinical trial in HIV-infected patients (Byers et al., 1990). The neurotoxic effects observed in immunotoxin-treated patients may therefore reflect localization of residual RTA following their in vivo cleavage.

Patients produced IgG and IgM antibodies to the murine immunoglobulin mAb 791T/36 (IgG2b isotype) and to the RTA moiety of the immunotoxin (Byers et al., 1989; Durrant et al., 1989a). Dissection of the human antimouse antibody (HAMA) responses revealed that the strongest response was to the idiotypic determinant of mAb 791T/36. Anti-idiotypic antibody was produced extremely rapidly following immunotoxin treatment, and in several patients, significant levels of antibody persisted throughout the period of observation (Fig. 11-2). High levels of IgM and IgG anti-RTA antibodies were also produced in patients following immunotoxin treatment. In many patients, anti-RTA antibodies became detectable within 5 to 10 days following completion of immunotoxin treatment (days 1 to 5) with, in one patient, a peak serum titer of 316,000.

The humoral immune response to murine immunoglobulin is undesirable with respect to immunotoxin treatment, since it results in rapid elimination of product from the circulation. Antibodies to both the constant and variable sites on mAb 791T/36 alter the biodistribution and pharmacokinetics of mAb 791T/36. This has been investigated in experimental systems showing that the blood survival of ^{125}I-labeled mAb 791T/36 as well as normal mouse IgG2b was markedly reduced with an associated liver uptake in rats producing anti-791T/36 antibody (Pimm et al., 1988). The influence of antibodies reacting with the combining site of mAb 791T/36 has been demonstrated using mice immunized with the immunotoxin (Pimm et al., 1989). In this case, the biodistribution of mAb 791T/36, but not normal mouse IgG2b, was modified by anti–combining site antibodies (Fig. 11-3).

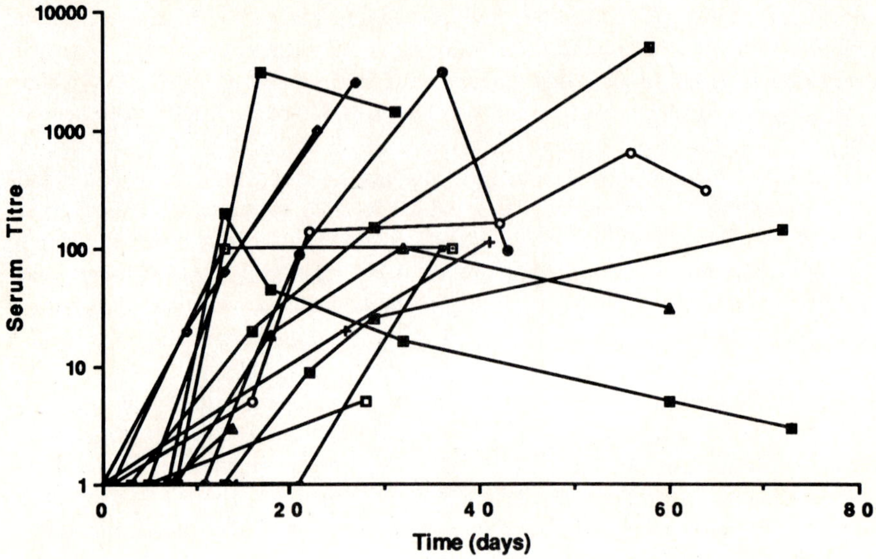

FIGURE 11-2
Anti-idiotypic antibodies in colorectal cancer patients with immunotoxin 791T/36–RTA. Serum from patients treated with 791T/36–RTA assayed for anticombining site (idiotypic) antibodies by determining the capacity to block binding of fluorescein-labeled mAb 791T/36 (FITC-791T/36) to gp72 antigen on tumor 791T cells (Durrant et al., 1989a). Serum titer expressed as the serum dilution producing 50% inhibition of FITC-791T/36 binding.

Although this was a phase I dose-escalation study, some evidence of therapeutic responses was obtained. Of 16 patients with hepatic metastases, 2 had objective evidence by abdominal computerized tomography (CT) scan of decreasing size in large metastases and disappearance of smaller lesions. These responses were seen at 3 months without additional intervening therapy, and similar delayed responses were seen in the melanoma study (Spitler et al., 1987). Fixed supraclavicular node metastases in 3 patients responded to immunotoxin treatment being reduced in size or becoming nondetectable. However, these patients also had liver metastases that increased in size or number. These observations, while encouraging, could not be classified as clinical responses by accepted criteria.

XOMAZYME Mel in Malignant Melanoma

Patients with metastatic malignant melanoma (stage IV) have been treated in two phase I/phase II trials with an immunotoxin constructed by conjugation of RTA to a monoclonal antibody (IgG2a) that reacts with melanoma-associated antigens (Mol. wt. 220 kDa and 500 kDa) (Spitler et al., 1987). Doses up to 0.5 mg/kg/day for 5 days were

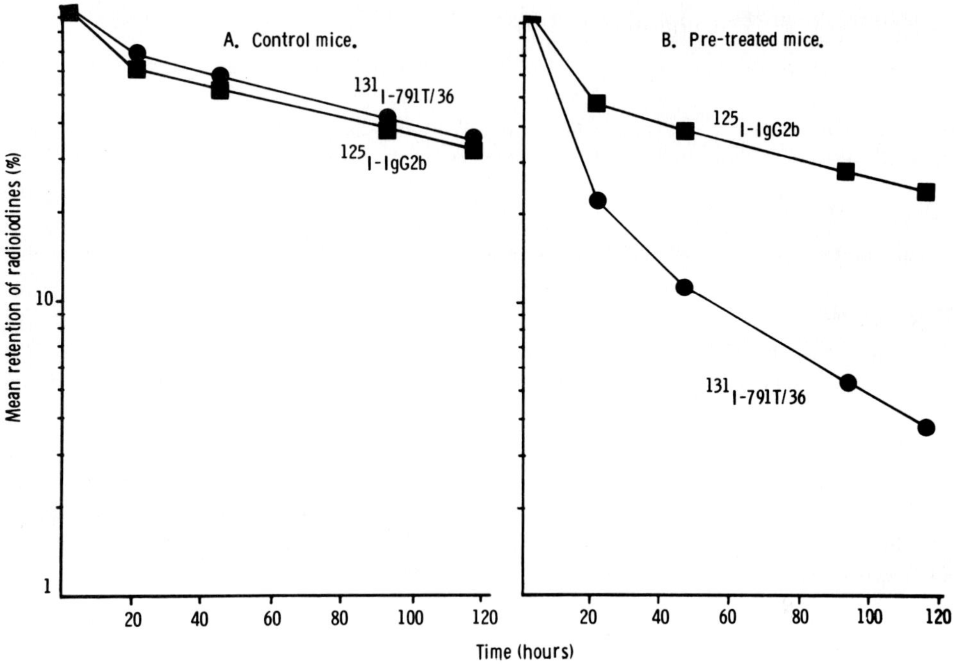

FIGURE 11-3
Influence of anti-idiotypic antibody on the rate of catabolism of radiolabeled mAb 791T/36 (Pimm et al., 1989). Whole body retention of ^{131}I-791T/36 mAb and ^{125}I-control IgG2b in BALB/c mice producing anti-791T/36 idiotypic antibody following treatment with 791T/36–RTA compared to control mice (Pimm et al., 1989).

tolerated, the major dose-limiting effect being transient decrease in serum albumin levels. This was associated with weight gain and edema in some patients. All patients generated an immune response to the immunotoxin, and antibodies to the murine IgG2a immunoglobulin (HAMA) and RTA were demonstrated (LoBuglio et al., 1988b). Clinical responses were observed in a number of patients, but these could not be categorized in terms of objective responses by currently defined criteria. Of the 65 patients treated with immunotoxin, a degree of response was observed in 23 patients (Byers and Baldwin, 1991a). These included 1 patient having a complete response with disappearance of a pulmonary metastasis and 5 patients having mixed responses defined as a 50% or greater reduction in size of one or more metastases, while concurrently one or more lesions increased in size or new lesions appeared. The duration of tumor regressions ranged from 2 to 13 months and 5 patients had ongoing stabilization of pulmonary metastases from 2 to 6 months. A particular feature noted in these evaluations was that tumors continued to regress for prolonged periods following a single course of immunotoxin treatment and without additional therapy.

Immunotoxin 260-F_9-RA in Breast Cancer

An immunotoxin has been constructed by conjugation of rRA to a monoclonal antibody (260 F_9) reacting with a 55-kDa antigen expressed on about 50% of breast cancer cells (Bjorn et al., 1985). Four patients with metastatic breast cancer have been treated with this immunotoxin by daily intravenous injection for up to 8 days (Weiner et al., 1989). The trial was then suspended in the light of neurological toxicity in patients treated under another protocol with continuous infusions of immunotoxin (Gould et al., 1989). Analysis of the patients treated by intravenous injection of immunotoxin demonstrated significant toxicity revealed as a symptom complex consisting of hypoalbuminemia, weight gain, edema, and dyspnea. It was suggested that this capillary-leak syndrome resulted from delivery of immunotoxin to nonmalignant cells. In this respect, it was shown that the immunotoxin bound to human monocytes, the proposed mechanism being interaction through Fc receptors.

In keeping with trials with other immunotoxins, patients developed anti-immunoconjugate antibodies including anti-idiotypic antibodies in at least one patient and anti-RTA antibodies. Although this study was curtailed because of toxicities in the related continuous infusion trial, the findings with four patients suggested that the toxicity syndrome was seen at doses of immunotoxin insufficient to deliver adequate levels of immunotoxin to tumors.

Immunotoxin H65–RTA in the Treatment of Graft-versus-Host Disease Arising Following Bone Marrow Transplantation

The lymphocyte maturation antigen CD5 found on almost all mature human T lymphocytes as well as on a subpopulation of B cells implicated in autoantibody formation. An RTA immunotoxin has been constructed by conjugating RTA to mAb H65, reacting with this antigen. The immunotoxin reacts with over 95% of human T lymphocytes and is cytotoxic to them in vitro at concentrations of about 1 ng/mL (Byers, 1990). A phase I/II trial was designed to treat patients with steroid-resistant graft-versus-host (GVH) disease to study safety and efficacy of this drug (Kernan et al., 1988; Byers et al., 1988; Byers and Baldwin, 1991a, 1991b). Graft-versus-host disease is a complication of bone marrow transplantation (BMT), which is caused by the mature T lymphocytes in the donor transplant reacting against antigens on host cells. The disease affects skin, gastrointestinal tract, and liver, and in its most severe form can result in complete desquamation of the skin, massive bloody diarrhea with fluid and electrolyte disturbances, and loss of liver function. This life-threatening disease has limited the use of BMT, which can be curative for leukemia and lymphoma. The initial study defined the side effects as being constitutional symptoms such as fatigue, myalgias, and hypoalbuminemia with weight gain. These side effects are the same as have been seen with other RTA immunotoxins and were dose-limiting. Thirty-four patients were given the immunotoxin as 1-hour infusions daily for 14 days. These patients had failed to respond to the only available therapy for this disease, namely steroids. Thirty-two patients could be evaluated for improvement or resolution of disease. Complete or partial responses were seen in 16 patients, with skin disease being most responsive (73%), and gastrointestinal tract (45%) and liver (28%) responding at lower incidences. Survival in responding patients was significantly prolonged at all times compared to those with no response. Treatment was associated with a rapid decrease in peripheral blood T lymphocytes, which persisted for longer than 1 month after therapy (Byers et al., 1990).

A second study treated 17 patients with GVH disease receiving H65–RTA as initial therapy. Responses were noted in about 50% of patients, and this second study differed from the first study in that all patients who responded had complete responses. Of those who responded, about half relapsed, but they were easily controlled on steroids, which now provide an effective second-line therapy (Byers and Baldwin, 1991a).

The BMT technique is well suited for prophylactic therapy, since there is a 15- to 25-day period after the transplant before GVH disease is expected to begin. Relatively low-risk donor–recipient pairs are HLA-matched siblings, in which the recipient is less than 20 years of age; in these populations, the incidence of GVH disease is about 50%. Higher-risk patients are those older than 30 years of age or those receiving transplants from donors who are related, but partially HLA-mismatched, or HLA-matched, but unrelated (and thus mismatched at minor HLS loci). Clinical trials are ongoing in all three of these high-risk populations, in which H65–RTA is given shortly after transplantation through day 10 post-BMT, in an attempt to reduce incidence of severe GVH disease. The first study, in which patients received BMT from partially matched related donors starting 7 to 10 days post-BMT, is complete. Those patients with one and two antigen mismatches fared significantly better than controls, with severe GVH disease developing in 4 of 21 patients receiving immunotoxin, compared to 9 of 12 in controls. Similar results are being seen in other high-risk populations, and it is anticipated that this agent will allow expansion of the procedure to other high-risk patients (Henslee-Downey et al., in preparation).

Immunotoxin H65–RTA in T-Cell Leukemia/Lymphoma

Since the CD5 antigen is also expressed on leukemias and lymphomas, immunotoxin H65–RTA can also serve as an antitumor agent. Immunotoxin H65–RTA has been given to 14 patients with cutaneous T-cell lymphoma (CTCL) and Sézary syndrome with encouraging results. Eleven patients were treated with doses from 0.2 to 0.5 mg/kg/day for 10 days, and the side effects were the same as those seen in the patients with GVH disease and in those patients treated with other RTA immunotoxins. However, two of three patients at the highest dose developed dyspnea at rest, without pulmonary edema, establishing the maximum tolerated dose. Three patients showed a partial response by day 35, one of whom had a greater than 80% reduction in Sézary cells after the first course, with complete clearance after the second cycle. Another attained a complete response after a second cycle. Although antimouse antibodies developed in most patients, this did not preclude induction of responses (LeMaistre et al., 1990). An ongoing study treating patients with chronic lymphocytic leukemia has also reported encouraging results with several patients showing complete resolution of lymphoadenopathy (LeMaistre et al., 1991).

Additional ongoing studies are aimed at treating autoimmune diseases such as rheumatoid arthritis and diabetes with H65–RTA (Byers and Baldwin, 1991a). In the first of these studies, 16 patients with severe rheumatoid arthritis refractory to conventional immunosuppressive agents were treated with a 5-day course of escalating doses of the immunotoxin. The drug was well tolerated with the same side effects as those noted in other studies, and significant improvement was seen in the joint scores of 7 of 16 patients. In 3 of these patients, this improvement has persisted for over 1 year, and clinical studies are in progress evaluating patients earlier in the disease process. Because of their success in autoimmune diseases such as GVH disease, these antilymphocyte immunotoxins are proving to be the most successful types of targeted therapy to date, and their use in cancers is continuing to be explored.

Anti-CD22 Monoclonal Antibody–Ricin A Chain Immunotoxins in B-Cell Lymphoma

The CD22 antigen is a B cell–restricted, two-chain glycoprotein (130 kDa and 140 kDa) that during B-cell ontogeny is first expressed in the cytoplasm at the pre–B-cell stage. The marker then is expressed on the cell surface of B cells and is also expressed on some B-cell tumors. Immunotoxins have been constructed for the treatment of B-cell lymphoma by conjugation of chemically deglycosylated RTA (dgA) to a murine antibody (RFB4) reacting with CD22 antigen (Shen et al., 1988). Two variants of the immunotoxin have been constructed for clinical study (Vitetta et al., 1991). One contains CD22 antibody conjugated to dgA through a hindered disulfide bond; this product being 10- to 20-fold more toxic than whole ricin for cells of a B lymphoblastoid cell line. The other immunotoxin was prepared by linking Fab fragments of the anti-CD22 antibody through a cystine bridge to dgA. This immunotoxin is twofold more potent than ricin (Vitetta et al., 1991). The immunotoxins are in clinical trial with patients with B-cell lymphomas. Side effects include a vascular-leak syndrome with decreases in serum albumin levels similar to those observed in immunotoxin trials in patients with solid cancers. The generation of low-titer antibody responses to the immunotoxin has been observed in only 4 of 14 patients. This is probably partly due to the patients being immunosuppressed and also because the immunotoxin is directed against a B-lymphocyte antigen. The trials are still ongoing, but transient partial or mixed responses (more than 50% reduction in tumor mass) have been reported in 60% of patients treated with either anti-CD22–dgA or Fab anti-CD22–dgA (Vitetta et al., 1991).

Anti-CD19 Antibody–"Blocked-Ricin" Immunotoxin in Human B-Cell Malignancies

Antigen CD19 is a B-cell glycoprotein (95 kDa) restricted in its expression to normal and neoplastic B cells. An immunotoxin has been constructed by conjugation of a murine anti-CD19 mAb B4, which reacts with greater than 99% of B-cell malignancies (Nadler et al., 1983) to "blocked" whole ricin (Nadler, unpublished finding). Blocked ricin has the carbohydrate binding sites of the ricin B chain blocked by reaction with an affinity reagent and this is then conjugated to antibody. The objective of constructing immunotoxin in this manner is to eliminate the target-cell binding of the ricin B chain, but to retain its function for internalizing the cytotoxic A chain. Thus, the blocked immunotoxin was highly cytotoxic for CD19 antigen positive cell line (Burkitt's cells), and while toxicity was reduced by treating target cells with unconjugated B4 antibody, galactose had no effect. Following preclinical studies in mice and monkeys, which identified hepatocellular injury as the major toxicity, a phase I clinical trial has been initiated in 25 patients with CD19 antigen positive B-cell malignancies (23 patients with non-Hodgkin's lymphoma, 1 with acute lymphoblastic leukemia [ALL], and 1 with chronic lymphocytic leukemia [CLL] [reviewed in Vitetta and Thorpe, 1991]). The majority of the patients had disease resistant to salvage therapy and about one third had failed BMT. Almost all patients had bulky tumor masses with infiltration of lymphoid organs and bone marrow.

Immunotoxin was administered daily for 5 days by infusion at doses up to 60 μg/kg/day. Pharmacokinetic studies indicated peak serum levels were achieved at the completion of infusion (1 hour) and thereafter rapidly decreased. For example, at a dose of 50 μg/kg blood levels of immunotoxin in the range 10^{-9} M were achieved for less than 4 hours. Hepatotoxicity manifested as elevations in SGOT/SGPT in the range 10 times normal was a major side effect and defined maximum tolerated dose (50 μg/kg/day, for 5 days). At this dose, decreased serum albumin levels (25%) were noted in most patients.

Tumor responses were determined by bone marrow biopsies, X-ray, and CT and gallium scans. One complete response (disappearance of cervical and mediastinal adenopathy) has been noted in one patient (greater than 10 months). Partial remissions in two patients with extensive bone marrow replacement have been noted, and seven patients had transient or mixed responses.

Immunotoxin treatment produced a 40% to 70% decrease in circulating $CD19^{+}$ cells (B cells or tumor cells) and a complete inhibition of peripheral blood B-cell immunoglobulin synthesis. B-cell function recovered 2 to 10 days following treatment. Even with these profound effects on peripheral B cells, patients made antibody responses to the mouse monoclonal antibody and ricin.

A second phase I trial has been initiated, the aim being to maintain significant levels of immunotoxin for longer periods of time. This is being achieved by administering immunotoxin as a bolus infusion (20 μg/kg over 1 hour) followed by a constant daily infusion (10 to 50 μg/kg for 7 days). These are ongoing trials, and at the time of reporting (8 patients), 2 patients have had partial remissions and 1 a complete remission.

HUMORAL IMMUNE RESPONSES TO IMMUNOTOXINS

The generation in patients of antibody responses to murine monoclonal antibody and toxin components of immunotoxins is a particularly important side effect. Most of the clinical trials with ricin or RTA immunotoxins have reported that patients produce HAMA and anti-RTA antibodies (Spitler et al., 1987; Byers et al., 1989; Weiner et al., 1989; Vitetta et al., 1991).

The actual extent of HAMA will depend in some part on the underlying disease as well as any concomitant immunosuppression. For example, patients receiving an immunotoxin containing an anti-CD5 lymphocyte monoclonal antibody conjugated to RTA, who have GVH disease and therefore are suppressed both exogenously and endogenously, produced little HAMA (Byers et al., 1990). Also, HAMA responses occurred infrequently in lymphoma patients treated with an immunotoxin constructed with an anti B-lymphocyte antibody (Vitetta et al., 1991). Overall, the HAMA responses elicited by immunotoxins are similar to those produced following treatment of patients with unconjugated monoclonal antibodies. For example, most patients treated with murine anticolorectal cancer mAb 17-1A generated HAMA responses with peak levels occurring 15 to 22 days after infusion (Khazaeli et al., 1988). Comparably, all colorectal patients treated with immunotoxin 791T/36–RTA generated IgM and IgG antibodies recognizing mouse immunoglobulin with peak responses 7 to 22 days after initiation of therapy (Durrant et al., 1989a).

Immunologically mediated side effects are not common responses in patients producing HAMA when retreated with monoclonal antibody. This is exemplified by the trial of mAb 17-1A in colorectal cancer patients where no significant toxicity was ascribed to immunological reactions even when patients received multiple infusions (400 mg) of antibody (LoBuglio et al., 1988a). But HAMA responses do lead to altered pharmacokinetics of the injected monoclonal antibody or immunotoxin, and also lead to tissue deposition of immune complexes (Perkins et al., 1988). This may not be a significant problem when unconjugated antibodies are administered. Thus, the overall pharmacokinetics of mAb 17-1A was not significantly altered in patients producing HAMA, since in this study the large dose of antibody administered obscured the effect of the HAMA response (Khazaeli et al., 1988). The effects of HAMA responses are more significant with immunotoxins, since the amounts administered are considerably less (generally below 200 μg/kg/day) and deposition of immune complexes may result in tissue accumulation of toxin components producing toxicity.

APPROACHES TO ABROGATION OF ANTIBODY RESPONSES TO IMMUNOTOXINS

Major approaches in attempting to control immune responses to immunotoxins include immunosuppression of patients and/or construction of less immunogenic immunoconjugates. Concomitant treatment with azathoprine and prednisone to produce generalized immunosuppression has been reported to blunt HAMA responses in melanoma patients treated with immunotoxin (LoBuglio et al., 1988b). Significant inhibition of the primary HAMA response to unconjugated monoclonal antibody has also been achieved with cyclosporin A pretreatment (Lederman et al., 1988). The problems with such regimens is the overall nonspecific immunosuppression, and the toxicity of the drugs given an adjunct therapy with immunotoxin. An alternative approach being investigated is to suppress specific antibody responses to immunoconjugate components. Theoretically, immunotoxins themselves should exert a cytotoxic effect against antigen-processing cells. For example antigen-processing B lymphocytes expressing receptors for mouse immunoglobulin should react with immunotoxin. This should lead to endocytosis of the immunotoxin and intracellular release of the toxin moiety, and result in cytotoxicity. The HAMA response seen with immunotoxins indicates that this process is not effective. But immunoconjugates have been constructed that have the ability to abrogate antibody responses to murine immunoglobulins (Durrant et al., 1989c). These conjugates contain monoclonal antibody conjugated to *cis*-aconityl daunomycin and, in model animal studies, have proven to suppress antibody responses to the mouse monoclonal antibody.

Construction of Humanized Monoclonal Antibodies

Methods are being devised by which the variable region of the murine monoclonal antibody may be engineered onto a human constant region (Orlandi et al., 1989). A chimeric antibody composed of the variable regions of murine mAb 17-1A (IgG2a-κ), which recognizes a glycoprotein present on human colorectal cells, has been coupled with the constant region of human IgG (Shaw et al., 1987, 1988). This chimeric mAb 17-1A has the same reactivity against colon tumor cells as the native antibody, and both have identical capacity to inhibit radiolabeled native 17.1A binding to tumor cells (Shaw et al., 1987). Native 17-1A has been used extensively in clinical trials in colorectal cancer patients and it elicits a very pronounced HAMA response (LoBuglio et al., 1988a; Khazaeli et al., 1988). In contrast, antibody responses have not been uniformly detected in patients receiving multiple treatments with the chimeric mAb 17-1A, and the pharmacokinetics of the chimeric mAb 17-1A was not modified, which is additional evidence of lack of an antibody response (LoBuglio et al., 1989). This result was unexpected since this construct still has the whole of the variable region as murine-derived and since the idiotypic component of the immune response forms a prominent proportion of the HAMA response. Several groups, therefore, are in the process of "humanizing" murine monoclonal antibodies, using various techniques such as the chimeric antibody constructed from rat antibody CAMPATH I by introducing only the six hypervariable regions from the heavy- and light-chain domains into a human IgG1 molecule (Riechmann et al., 1988). This chimera was as effective as the native monoclonal antibody in complement-mediated lysis of B-cell lymphocytic leukemia cells. However, a chimeric antibody composed of the V regions of the murine mAb B72-3 and the constant regions of human immunoglobulin γ4 heavy and K light chain is immunogenic in human subjects (Khazaeli et al., 1991). Seven of twelve colon cancer patients who were administered this antibody had an antibody response, primarily directed to the murine V regions.

Since antibodies to binding domain of a monoclonal antibody have been found to markedly modify its pharmacokinetics (Pimm et al., 1989), it is considered necessary to produce more human-like "reshaped" products. In one approach termed CDR-grafting or reshaping (Riechmann et al., 1988), the complementary determining regions (CDR) of a murine monoclonal antibody are transplanted onto the corresponding regions in a human immunoglobulin. The CDR (three in monoclonal antibody heavy chains and three in light chains) are manipulated by genetic engineering by cloning murine heavy and light chain variable (V) region gene segments and transferred to corresponding human V regions by site-directed mutagenesis. Human constant region gene segments of the desired isotype are added and the "reshaped" heavy and light chain genes are co-expressed in mammalian cells to produce soluble humanized antibody.

A humanized antilymphocyte monoclonal antibody (CAMPATH-1 H) has been used to treat two patients with non-Hodgkin's lymphoma without the production of an antibody response (Hale et al., 1988). Also a genetically reshaped human IgG1 monoclonal antibody (Hu2PLAP) reacting with human placental alkaline phosphatase has been used for immunoscintigraphy of ovarian carcinoma patients (Hird et al., 1991). None of the patients developed antibodies reacting with this antibody preparation. Although experience is still limited, genetically reshaped antibodies may be satisfactory for immunoconjugate design. The problem of antibody responses to the targeted molecule, especially toxin proteins, still remains. Thus, some patients receiving human mAb Hu2PLAP conjugated to a chelating agent for ^{111}Ind labeling produced antibodies to the chelate group (a macrocyclic compound).

IDIOTYPIC INTERACTIONS AND TUMOR THERAPY

There is a growing awareness of the potential of anti-idiotypic antibodies as vaccines in the treatment of infectious diseases (Geha, 1986). This approach to immunotherapy is based upon the concept that an antibody (Ab2) directed against the combining site of an antibody (Ab1) can itself function as a surrogate antigen, thus producing an immune response against the original antigen (Köhler et al., 1989; see Chapter 8). The concept of using anti-idiotypic antibody to manipulate immune responses has been extended to tumor immunotherapy (Nepom and Hellström, 1987; see Chapter 8). Antitumor, cell-mediated and humoral immune responses induced by anti-idiotypic antibodies have been demonstrated against mouse (Chen et al., 1989) and rat (Dunn et al., 1987) tumor-associated antigens. This has led to the view that idiotypic manipulation may be effective therapy of human cancer, and anti-idiotypic antibodies have been produced against antibodies reacting with human TAA (Herlyn et al., 1987; Viale et al., 1987; Steinitz et al., 1988; Monestier et al., 1989; Kusama et al., 1989; Barth et al., 1989; Austin et al., 1989). Treatment of colorectal cancer patients with goat anti-idiotypic antibodies to the murine mAb 17-1A demonstrated the production of anti-[anti-idiotypic] antibodies, this being reported to be associated with a clinical response (Herlyn et al., 1987). Furthermore, patients treated with mAb 17-1A produce autologous anti-[anti-idiotypic] antibodies binding to tumor cells (Wettendorff et al., 1989). A human monoclonal anti-idiotypic antibody (105AD7) that reacts with the binding site of mAb 791T/36, a mouse monoclonal antibody to a colorectal cancer antigen, has been developed (Austin et al., 1989). A phase I clinical trial treating patients with advanced colorectal cancer with a vaccine containing anti-idiotypic mAb 105AD7 in aluminum hydroxide gel has been carried out (Robins et al., 1991). The major objective of this study was to demonstrate that vaccine treatment generated a T-lymphocyte response and this was shown both by lymphocyte proliferative responses and production of elevated interleukin-2 levels in serum of treated patients.

In this context, the possibility has been considered that in immunotoxin treatment the induction of anti-idiotypic antibodies to the immunoglobulin component of the immunoconjugate leads to activation of the idiotypic network, which indirectly contributes to the therapeutic response (Spitler et al., 1987; Byers et al., 1989). This is supported by the finding that colorectal cancer patients treated with immunotoxin 791T/36–RTA generate very pronounced levels of anti-idiotypic antibody to immunoglobulin 791T/36 (Byers et al., 1989; Durrant et al., 1989a). Furthermore, immunotoxin-treated patients produce antibodies reacting with tumor-associated antigens (Durrant et al., 1989a). The clinical significance of the antibody responses in patients treated with immunotoxin 791T/36-RTA remains to be elucidated. Interestingly, however, patients treated both with this immunotoxin (Byers et al., 1989) and with an antimelanoma immunotoxin (Spitler et al., 1987) showed clinical responses continuing long after completion of the course of treatment.

CONCLUSIONS

Clinical trials with several types of immunotoxin have highlighted factors that need to be addressed for improving therapeutic efficacy. These include modifications in immunoconjugate design so as to enable adequate amounts of toxin molecules to be delivered to solid cancers in relation to overall side effects arising from normal tissue localization. Target antigen expression on tumor cells has to be taken into account if therapy is to be efficacious, particularly against solid cancers. Downregulation of antibody responses to immunotoxin components is important in order to allow the design of retreatment schedules. This has to take into account the intriguing finding that anti-idiotypic antibody may actually potentiate immunotoxin efficacy through stimulation of antitumor immune responses in patients.

Delivery of immunotoxins to target tissues is dependent upon a number of factors that govern blood survival and integrity of the immunoconjugate, its ability to extravasate and to localize and bind to cell-surface antigens. Ricin A chain and "blocked" ricin immunotoxins are rapidly removed from the circulation by hepatic nonparenchymal and parenchymal cells (Blakey et al., 1988b). The blood survival of immunoconjugates can be considerably improved by modifying the carbohydrate component of the ricin to reduce or eliminate recognition of mannose residues. This has led to the construction of immunoconjugates with so-called deglycosylated RTA for clinical studies (Till et al., 1989; Vitetta et al., 1990, 1991; Vitetta and Thorpe, 1991). Overall, however, these immunoconjugates are still cleared from blood more rapidly than the parent antibody. This is a common experience with several types of immunoconjugates, including daunorubicin (DNR) and methotrexate (MTX)–human serum albumin-antibody conjugates (Pimm et al., 1987), and may reflect conformational changes induced by antibody conjugation. Further refinements in antibody conjugation procedures are desirable and it is anticipated that this will also encompass the utilization of antibody fragments, which may have a greater facility to penetrate target tissues. The ultimate aim is to reduce the overall size of the antibody recognition site, and one of the most important advances here is the synthesis of single-domain antibodies (d Ab) (Ward et al., 1989). In this approach, genomic DNA from immune splenic lymphocytes is amplified by the polymerase chain reaction, with primers designed to react with rearranged VH genes. The amplified DNA is cloned into plasmids transfected into *Escherichia coli* leading to the synthesis of single domain antibodies.

Classically, it is held that cytotoxic drugs need to react with essentially all cells in a tumor to elicit a significant therapeutic response. Thus, antibody targeting of toxins has to take into account the frequency of target antigen expression. Immunotoxin H65–RTA binding to pan T-lymphocyte CD5 marker and RFB4–RTA binding to the CD22 marker on B lymphocytes recognize antigens expressed on essentially all target cells (Byers et al., 1990; Byers, 1990; Shen et al., 1988). But the frequency of antigen-positive cells in solid cancers is generally more variable. This is illustrated by flow cytometric screening studies of a panel of monoclonal antibodies binding to colorectal and ovarian tumor cells derived by collagenase disaggregation of tumor tissues (Durrant et al., 1989b). For example, colorectal cancer cells binding an anti-CEA monoclonal antibody and ovarian cancer cells binding antiepithelial membrane antigen antibody ranged from 90% to less than 5% of the tumor cell populations. Immunophenotyping of tumors will be necessary, therefore, to allow combinations of monoclonal antibodies to be selected that will overcome the effect of intertumor variation in antigen expression.

Finally, procedures are evolving that significantly reduce the impact of patient antibody responses to immunotoxin components. These include the construction of chimeric and humanized monoclonal antibodies that do not provoke significant HAMA responses (LoBuglio et al., 1989; Hird et al., 1991), and toxin molecules are being produced that are only weakly immunogenic, if at all. Added to this experience is showing that retreatment with RTA immunotoxins can be given safely in the presence of anti-immunotoxin antibodies, thus permitting the design of multicycle therapy.

REFERENCES

Armitage NC, Perkins AC, Pimm MV, Farrands PA, Baldwin RW, Hardcastle JD. The localisation of an antitumour monoclonal antibody (791T/36) in gastrointestinal tumours. Br J Surg. 1984;71:407–409.

Armitage NC, Perkins AC, Pimm MV, Wastie ML, Baldwin RW, Hardcastle JD. Imaging of primary and metastatic colorectal cancer using an ^{111}In-labelled antitumour monoclonal antibody (791T/36). Nucl Med Comm. 1985;6:623–631.

Austin EB, Robins RA, Durrant LG, Price MR, Baldwin RW. Human monoclonal anti-idiotypic antibody to the tumour-associated antibody 791T/36. Immunology. 1989;67:525–530.

Baldwin RW, Byers VS, Mann RD, eds. Monoclonal antibodies and immunoconjugates in cancer treatment. Carnforth, U.K.: Parthenon Publishing; 1990.

Baldwin RW, Byers VS, Pimm MV. Monoclonal antibodies and immunoconjugates for cancer treatment. In: Pinedo HM, Longo DL, Chabner BA, eds. Cancer chemotherapy and biological response modifiers, Annual 10. New York, NY: Elsevier Science; 1988:397–415.

Barth A, Waibel R, Stahel RA. Monoclonal anti-idiotypic antibody mimicking a tumor-associated sialoglycoprotein antigen induces humoral immune response against human small-cell lung carcinoma. Int J Cancer. 1989;43:896–900.

Bjorn MJ, Ring D, Frankel A. Evaluation of monoclonal antibodies for the development of breast cancer immunotoxins. Cancer Res. 1985;45:1214–1221.

Blakey DC, Skilleter DN, Price RJ, Thorpe PE. Uptake of native and deglycosylated ricin A-chain immunotoxins by mouse liver parenchymal and nonparenchymal cells in vitro and in vivo. Biochim Biophys Acta. 1988a;968:172–178.

Blakey DC, Wawrzynczak EJ, Wallace PM, Thorpe PE. Antibody toxin conjugates: a perspective. Prog Allergy. 1988b;45:50–90.

Bourrie BJP, Casellas P, Blythman HE, Jansen FK. Study of the plasma clearance of antibody–ricin-A-chain immunotoxins. Eur J Biochem. 1986;155:1–10.

Boyer CM, Lidor Y, Lottich SC, Bast RC Jr. Antigenic cell surface markers in human solid tumors. Antibody Immunoconjugates Radiopharmaceuticals. 1988;1:105–162.

Brusa P, Pietribiasi F, Bussolati G, et al. Blocked and not blocked whole-ricin-antibody immunotoxins: intraperitoneal therapy of human tumour xenografted in nude mice. Cancer Immunol Immunother. 1989;29:185–192.

Byers VS. Anti-pan T-lymphocyte immunotoxin for therapy of autoimmune diseases: preclinical and clinical development. In: Baldwin RW, Byers VS, eds. Monoclonal antibodies and immunoconjugates in cancer treatment. Nashville, Tenn.: Parthenon Press; 1990:47–59.

Byers VS, Pimm MV, Pawluczyk IZA, et al. Biodistribution of ricin toxin A chain-monoclonal antibody 791T/36 immunotoxin and influence of hepatic blocking agents. Cancer Res. 1987a;47:5277–5283.

Byers VS, Pimm MV, Scannon PJ, Pawluczyk I, Baldwin RW. Inhibition of growth of human tumor xenografts in athymic mice treated with ricin toxin A chain–monoclonal antibody 791T/36 conjugates. Cancer Res. 1987b;47:5042–5046.

Byers VS, Rodvien R, Grant K, et al. Phase I study of monoclonal antibody–ricin A chain immunotoxin XomaZyme-791 in patients with metastatic colon cancer. Cancer Res. 1989; 49:6153–6160.

Byers VS, Henslee PJ, Kernan NA, et al. Use of an anti-pan T lymphocyte ricin A chain immunotoxin in steroid resistant acute graft vs. host disease. Blood. 1990;75:1426–1432.

Byers VS, Baldwin RW. Rationale for clinical use of immunotoxins in cancer and autoimmune disease. In: Lord JM, ed. Seminars in cell biology. Philadelphia, Pa: W.B. Saunders; 1991a:59–70.

Byers VS, Baldwin RW. Immunotoxins in haematological oncology. In: Newland A, Burnett A, Keating A, Armitage J, eds. Haematological oncology. Cambridge: Cambridge Medical Reviews; 1991b:49–62.

Carlsson J, Drevin H, Axen R. Protein thiolation and reversible protein–protein conjugation. *N*-succinimidyl 3-(2 pyridyldithio)propionate, a new heterobifunctional agent. Biochem J. 1978;173:723–737.

Casellas P, Dussossoy D, Falasca AI, et al. Trichokirin, a ribosome-inactivating protein from the seeds of *Trichosanthes kirilowii* Maximowicz. Eur J Biochem. 1988;176:581–588.

Chaudhary VK, Queen C, Junghans RP, Waldmann TA, FitzGerald DJ, Pastan I. A recombinant immunotoxin consisting of two antibody variable domains fused to *Pseudomonas* exotoxin. Nature. 1989;339:394–397.

Chen J-J, Saeki Y, Shi L, Köhler H. Tumor idiotype vaccines: VI. Synergistic anti-tumor effects with combined "internal image" anti–idiotypes and chemotherapy. J Immunol. 1989;143: 1053–1057.

Dunn PL, Johnson CA, Styles JM, Pease SS, Dean CJ. Vaccination with syngeneic monoclonal anti-idiotype protects against a tumour challenge. Immunology. 1987;60:181–186.

Durrant LG, Robins RA, Armitage NC, Brown A, Baldwin RW. Association of antigen expression and DNA ploidy in human colorectal tumors. Cancer Res. 1985;46:3543–3549.

Durrant LG, Byers VS, Scannon PJ, et al. Humoral immune responses to XMMCO-791-RTA immunotoxin in colorectal cancer patients. Clin Exp Immunol. 1989a;75:258–264.

Durrant LG, Robins RA, Baldwin RW. Flow cytometric screening of monoclonal antibodies for drug or toxin targeting to human cancer. J Natl Cancer Inst. 1989b;81:688–696.

Durrant LG, Robins RA, Marksman RA, Garnett MC, Ogunmuyiwa Y, Baldwin RW. Abrogation of antibody responses in rats to murine monoclonal antibody 791T/36 by treatment with daunomycin–cis-aconityl-791T/36 conjugates. Cancer Immunol Immunother. 1989c;28: 37–42.

Endo Y, Tsurugi K. RNA *N*-glycosidase activity of ricin A chain. J Biol Chem. 1987;262:8128–8130.

Endo Y, Mitsui K, Motizuki M, Tsurugi K. The mechanism of action of ricin and related toxic lectins on eukaryotic ribosomes. The site and the characteristics of the modification in 28S ribosomal RNA caused by the toxins. J Biol Chem. 1987;262:5908–5912.

FitzGerald DJ, Bjorn MJ, Ferris RJ, et al. Antitumor activity of an immunotoxin in a nude mouse model of human ovarian cancer. Cancer Res. 1987;47:1407–1410.

FitzGerald D, Pastan I. Targeted toxin therapy for the treatment of cancer. J Natl Cancer Inst. 1989;81:1455–1463.

Foxwell BMJ, Detre SI, Donovan TA, Thorpe PE. The use of anti-ricin antibodies to protect mice intoxicated with ricin. Toxicology. 1985;34:79–88.

Fulton RJ, Tucker TF, Vitetta ES, Uhr JW. Pharmacokinetics of tumor-reactive immunotoxins in tumor-bearing mice: effect of antibody valency and deglycosylation of the ricin A chain on clearance and tumor localization. Cancer Res. 1988;48:2618–2625.

Geha RS. Idiotypic interactions in the treatment of human diseases. Adv Immunol. 1986; 39:255–297.

Gould BJ, Borowitz MJ, Groves ES, et al. Phase I study of an anti-breast cancer immunotoxin by continuous infusion: report of a targeted toxic effect not predicted by animal studies. J Natl Cancer Inst. 1989;81:775–781.

Griffin TW, Richardson C, Houston LL, LePage D, Bogden A, Raso V. Antitumor activity of intraperitoneal immunotoxins in a nude mouse model of human malignant mesothelioma. Cancer Res. 1987;47:4266–4270.

Hale G, Clark MR, Marcus R, et al. Remission induction in non-Hodgkin lymphoma with reshaped human monoclonal antibody CAMPATH-1H. Lancet. 1988;2:1394–1399.

Hara H, Luo Y, Haruta Y, Seon BK. Efficient transplantation of human non–T-leukemia cells into nude mice and induction of complete regression of the transplanted distinct tumors by ricin A-chain conjugates of monoclonal antibodies SN5 and SN6. Cancer Res. 1988; 48:4673–4680.

Herlyn D, Wettendorff M, Schmoll E, et al. Anti-idiotype immunization of cancer patients: modulation of the immune response. Proc Natl Acad Sci USA. 1987;84:8055–8059.

Hird V, Verhoeyen M, Badley RA, et al. Tumour localisation with a radioactively labelled reshaped human monoclonal antibody. Br J Cancer. 1991;64:911–914.

Kernan NA, Byers VS, Scannon PJ, et al. Treatment of steroid-resistant acutegraft-vs-host disease by in vivo administration of an anti–T-cell ricin A chain immunotoxin. JAMA. 1988; 259:3154–3157.

Kondo T, FitzGerald D, Chaudhary VK, Adhya S, Pastan I. Activity of immunotoxins constructed with modified *Pseudomonas* exotoxin A lacking the cell recognition domain. J Biol Chem. 1988;263:9470–9475.

Khazaeli MB, Saleh MS, Wheeler RH, et al. Phase I trial of multiple large doses of murine monoclonal antibody CO17-1A. II. Pharmacokinetics and immune response. J Natl Cancer Inst. 1988;80:937–942.

Khazaeli MB, Saleh MN, Liu TP, et al. Pharmacokinetics and immune response of ^{131}-chimeric mouse/human B72.3 (human $\gamma 4$) monoclonal antibody in humans. Cancer Res. 1991;51: 5461–5466.

Köhler H, Kiber-Emmons T, Srinivasan S, et al. Short analytical review: revised immune network concepts. Clin Immunol Immunopath. 1989;52:104–116.

Kusama M, Kageshita T, Chen ZJ, Ferrone S. Characterization of syngeneic antiidiotypic monoclonal antibodies to murine anti-human high molecular weight melanoma-associated antigen monoclonal antibodies. J Immunol. 1989;143:3844–3852.

Lederman JA, Begent RHJ, Bagshawe KD, et al. Repeated antitumour antibody therapy in man with suppression of the host response by cyclosporin A. Br J Cancer. 1988;58:654–657.

LeMaistre CF, Frankel A, Kornfeld S, Rosen S, Scannon P, Byers VS. Phase I/II study of a pan T cell immunotoxin (IT) in cutaneous T cell lymphoma (CTCL). Blood. 1990;(suppl):161a. Abstract.

LeMaistre CF, Deissoeroth A, Fogel B, et al. Phase I trial of H65–RTA in patients with chronic lymphocytic leukemia. Blood. 1991; in press.

LoBuglio AF, Saleh MN, Lee J, et al. Phase I trial of multiple large doses of murine monoclonal antibody CO17-1A. I. Clinical aspects. J Natl Cancer Inst. 1988a;80:932–936.

LoBuglio AF, Khazaeli MB, Lee J, et al. Pharmacokinetics and immune response to Xomazyme-Mel in melanoma patients. Antibody Immunoconjugates Radiopharmaceuticals. 1988b; 1:305–310.

LoBuglio AF, Wheeler RH, Trang J, et al. Mouse/human chimeric monoclonal antibody in man: kinetics and immune response. Proc Natl Acad Sci USA. 1989;86:4220–4224.

Marsh JW, Neville DM Jr. A flexible peptide spacer increases the efficacy of holoricin anti–T cell immunotoxins. J Immunol. 1988;140:3674–3678.

May MJ, Hartley MR, Roberts LM, Krieg PA, Osborn RW, Lord JM. Ribosome inactivation by ricin A chain: a sensitive method to assess the activity of wild-type and mutant polypeptides. EMBO J. 1989;8:301–308.

McGrath MS, Hwang KM, Caldwell SE, et al. GLQ223: an inhibitor of human immunodeficiency virus replication in acutely and chronically infected cells of lymphocyte and mononuclear phagocyte lineage. Proc Natl Acad Sci USA. 1989;86:2844–2848.

Monestier M, Debbas ME, Goldenberg DM. Syngeneic anti-idiotype monoclonal antibodies to murine anticarcinoembryonic antigen monoclonal antibodies. Cancer Res. 1989;49:123–126.

Myers DE, Uckun FM, Swaim SE, Vallera DA. The effects of aromatic and aliphatic maleimide crosslinkers on anti-CD5 ricin immunotoxins. J Immunol Methods. 1989;121:129–142.

Nadler LM, Anderson KC, Marti G, et al. B4, a human B lymphocyte–associated antigen expressed on normal, mitogen-activated, and malignant B lymphocytes. J Immunol. 1983; 131:244–250.

Nepom GT, Hellström KE. Anti-idiotypic antibodies and the induction of specific tumor immunity. Cancer Metastasis Rev. 1987;6:489–502.

O'Hare M, Brown AN, Hussain K, et al. Cytotoxicity of a recombinant ricin A chain fusion protein containing a proteolytical cleavable spacer sequence. FEBS. 1990;273:200–204.

Olsnes S, Sandvig K. How protein toxins enter and kill cells. In: Frankel AE, ed. Immunotoxins. Norwell, Mass.: Kluwer Academic Publishers; 1988:39–72.

Orlandi R, Gussow DH, Jones PT, Winter G. Cloning immunoglobulin variable domains for expression by the polymerase chain reaction. Proc Natl Acad Sci USA. 1989;86:3833–3837.

Pearson JW, FitzGerald DJP, Willingham MC, Wiltrout RH, Pastan I, Longo DL. Chemoimmunotoxin therapy against a human colon tumor (HT-29) xenografted into nude mice. Cancer Res. 1989;49:3562–3567.

Perkins AC, Pimm MV, Powell MC. The implications of patient antibody responses for the clinical usefulness of immunoscintigraphy. Nucl Med Comm. 1988;9:273–282.

Perkins AC, Pimm MV. Immunoscintigraphy: practical aspects and clinical applications. New York, NY: Wiley-Liss; 1991:208.

Pimm MV, Clegg JA, Caten JE, et al. Biodistribution of methotrexate–monoclonal antibody conjugates and complexes: experimental and clinical studies. Cancer Treat Rev. 1987;14: 411–420.

Pimm MV, Perkins AC, Durrant LG, Baldwin RW. A rat model for imaging the effect of anti-mouse antibody responses on the biodistribution of radiolabelled mouse monoclonal antibodies. Eur J Nucl Med. 1988;14:507–511.

Pimm MV, Durrant LG, Baldwin RW. The influence of syngeneic anti-idiotypic antibody on the biodistribution of an anti-tumour monoclonal antibody in BALB/c mice. Int J Cancer. 1989;43:147–151.

Pimm MV, Gunn B, Lord JM, Baldwin RW. The influence of anti-ricin toxin A monoclonal antibodies on the pharmacokinetics of ricin toxin A chain and recombinant ricin A chain in mice. Cancer Immunol Immunother. 1990;32:235–240.

Pirker R, FitzGerald DJP, Hamilton TC, Ozols RF, Willingham MC, Pastan I. Anti-transferrin receptor antibody linked to *Pseudomonas* exotoxin as a model immunotoxin in human ovarian carcinoma cell lines. Cancer Res. 1985;45:751–757.

Ponpipom MM, Bugianesi RL, Robbins JC, Doebber TW, Shen TY. Cell-specific ligands for selective drug delivery to tissues and organs. J Med Chem. 1981;24:1388–1395.

Richardson PT, Gilmartin P, Colman A, Roberts LM, Lord JM. Expression of functional ricin B chain in *xenopus* oocytes. Biotechnology. 1988;6:565–570.

Riechmann L, Clark M, Waldmann H, Winter G. Reshaping human antibodies for therapy. Nature. 1988;332:323–327.

Robins RA, Denton GWL, Hardcastle JD, Austin EB, Baldwin RW, Durrant LG. Antitumour immune response and interleukin 2 production induced in colorectal cancer patients by immunization with human monoclonal anti-idiotypic antibody. Cancer Res. 1991;51:5425-5429.

Shaw DR, Khazaeli MB, Sun LK, et al. Characterization of a mouse/human chimeric monoclonal antibody (17-1A) to a colon cancer tumor-associated antigen. J Immunol. 1987; 138:4534–4538.

Shaw DR, Khazaeli MB, LoBuglio AF. Mouse/human chimeric antibodies to a tumor-associated antigen: biologic activity of the four human IgG subclasses. J Natl Cancer Inst. 1988; 80:1553–1559.

Shen G-L, La J-L, Ghetie M-A, et al. Evaluation of four CD22 antibodies as ricin A chain–containing immunotoxins for the in vivo therapy of human B-cell leukaemias and lymphomas. Int J Cancer. 1988;42:792–797.

Spitler LE, Del Rio M, Kentigan A, et al. Therapy of patients with malignant melanoma using a monoclonal antimelanoma antibody–ricin A chain immunotoxin. Cancer Res. 1987;47: 1717–1723.

Srinivasachar K, Neville DM Jr. New protein cross-linking reagents that are cleaved by mild acid. Biochemistry. 1989;28:2501–2509.

Steinitz M, Tamir S, Frödin J-E, Lefvert A-K, Mellstedt H. Human monoclonal anti-idiotypic antibodies. I. Establishment of immortalized cell lines from a tumor patient treated with mouse monoclonal antibodies. J Immunol. 1988;141:3516–3522.

Thorpe PE, Ross WCJ, Brown ANF, et al. Blockade of the galactose-binding sites of ricin by its linkage to antibody. Eur J Biochem. 1984;140:63–71.

Thorpe PE, Wallace PM, Knowles PP, et al. New coupling agents for the synthesis of immunotoxins containing a hindered disulfide bond with improved stability in vivo. Cancer Res. 1987;47:5924–5931.

Thorpe PE, Wallace PM, Knowles PP, et al. Improved antitumor effects of immunotoxins prepared with deglycosylated ricin A-chain and hindered disulfide linkages. Cancer Res. 1988;48:6396–6403.

Till MA, Zolla-Pazner S, Gorny MK, Patton JS, Uhr JW, Vitetta ES. Human immunodeficiency virus-infected T cells and monocytes are killed by monoclonal human anti-gp41 antibodies coupled to ricin A chain. Proc Natl Acad Sci USA. 1989;86:1987–1991.

Viale G, Grassi F, Pelagi M, et al. Anti-human tumor antibodies induced in mice and rabbits by "internal image" anti-idiotypic monoclonal immunoglobulins. J Immunol. 1987;139:4250–4255.

Vitetta ES, Thorpe PE. Immunotoxins containing ricin or its A chain. In: Lord JM, ed. Seminars in cell biology. Philadelphia, Pa: W.B. Saunders; 1991:47–58.

Vitetta ES, Till MA, Ghetie V, et al. Immunoconjugates containing ricin A chain can kill lines of HIV-infected T cells and monocytes. In: Baldwin RW, Byers VS, eds. Monoclonal antibodies and immunoconjugates in cancer treatment. Nashville, Tenn.: Parthenon Press; 1990:771.

Vitetta ES, Stone M, Amolt P, et al. Phase I immunotoxin trial in patients with B-cell lymphoma. Cancer Res. 1991;51:4052–4058.

Ward ES, Güssow D, Griffiths AD, Jones PT, Winter G. Binding activities of a repertoire of single immunoglobulin variable domains secreted from *Escherichia coli*. Nature. 1989;341: 544–546.

Wawrzyczak EJ. Systemic immunotoxin therapy of cancer: advances and prospects. Br J Cancer. 1991;64:624–630.

Weiner LM, O'Dwyer J, Kitson J, et al. Phase I evaluation of an anti-breast carcinoma monoclonal antibody 260F9-recombinant ricin A chain immunoconjugate. Cancer Res. 1989;49: 4062–4067.

Wettendorff M, Iliopoulos D, Tempero M, et al. Idiotypic cascades in cancer patients treated with monoclonal antibody CO17-1A. Proc Natl Acad Sci USA. 1989;86:3787–3791.

Wiley RG, Stirpe F, Thorpe PE, Oeltmann TN. Neuronotoxic effects of monoclonal anti-Thy 1 antibody (OX7) coupled to the ribosome inactivating protein, saporin, as studied by suicide transport experiments in the rat. Brain Res. 1989;505:44–54.

Willingham MC, FitzGerald DJ, Pastan I. *Pseudomonas* exotoxin coupled to a monoclonal antibody against ovarian cancer inhibits the growth of human ovarian cancer cells in a mouse model. Proc Natl Acad Sci USA. 1987;84:2474–2478.

Yeung HW, Li WW, Feng Z, Barbieri L, Stirpe F. Trichosanthin, α-momorcharin and β-momorcharin: identity of abortifacient and ribosome-inactivating proteins. Int J Peptide Protein Res. 1988;31:265–268.

Zhang L, Wang J. Homology of trichosanthin and ricin A chain. Nature. 1986;321:477–478.

CHAPTER 12

IMAGING AND THERAPY OF CANCER WITH SPECIFICALLY TARGETED RADIONUCLIDES

Paul G. Abrams
Alan R. Fritzberg
Darrell J. Salk

Current diagnostic staging procedures are organ and/or regionally directed. None routinely scan the entire body for metastatic tumor. Current cancer therapy is either unavoidably local (surgery, radiation therapy) or indiscriminately systemic (chemotherapy).

Targeted radionuclides may overcome these diagnostic and therapeutic limitations. The current focus on antibody targeting represents the culmination of nearly a century of theory, practice, and development of Paul Ehrlich's "magic bullet" proposition (Ehrlich, 1956). Current genetic engineering and protein synthesis techniques have produced other targeting molecules whose clinical application should be apparent in the near future.

Diagnostic radionuclides are gamma emitters. The most widely used are technetium 99m (^{99m}Tc), indium 111 (^{111}In), iodine 123 (^{123}I), and iodine 131 (^{131}I). After attachment to a targeting molecule, they can be injected and total body imaging performed using standard gamma cameras. Computerized tomography (CT) or magnetic resonance imaging (MRI) may then be directed to suspicious areas, if necessary, to confirm the presence of disease.

Therapeutic radionuclides may be alpha, beta, or even Auger electron emitters. Examples of beta emitters include ^{131}I, rhenium 188 (^{188}Re), copper 67 (^{67}Cu), and yttrium 90 (^{90}Y). Astatine 211 (^{211}At) and bismuth 212 (^{212}Bi) (either itself or as a degradation product of lead 212 [^{212}Pb], a beta emitter) are two alpha emitters considered suitable for targeted therapy applications. Iodine 125 is an example of a long half-life Auger electron emitter. Once linked to antibody, these radioconjugates can deliver lethal radiation to nests of tumor cells wherever they may have lodged in the body. Of interest is that, unlike all the other diagnostic techniques, successful diagnostic imaging with targeting molecules have direct, predictive implications for patient selection, internal radiation dose estimates, and treatment outcome of targeted therapy.

CHOICE OF RADIONUCLIDE

Diagnostic

The gamma-emitting radionuclides suitable for use as imaging agents have high-abundance gamma rays, preferably with energies between 100 and 200 keV for which current gamma cameras are most efficient. Their physical half-life should be matched to the kinetics of tumor localization and background clearance, but should not be so long as to remain in tissues long after images are obtained.

Technetium 99m has long been the radionuclide of choice for most nuclear medicine procedures. Its 140-keV gamma ray and high photon flux provide excellent image resolution and single photon emission computerized tomography (SPECT) capabilities. Its lack of particulate radiation provides a wide margin of safety, but its short half-life (T1/2) of 6 hours limits carriers to those with rapid kinetics of tumor localization and background clearance. It is inexpensive, generator-produced, and routinely available.

Iodine 123 has better physical qualities than ^{99m}Tc for antibody imaging due to its 13-hour half-life. It is, however, extremely expensive and not routinely available. By contrast, ^{131}I is inexpensive and readily available, but has too long a half-life and its gamma rays are too energetic (364 keV) for optimal imaging. Both are also compromised by dehalogenation in vivo when standard techniques of radiolabeling are employed.

Indium 111 has two gamma ray energies (173 and 247 keV). The basic challenge has been to engineer a chelate that slows the kinetics of transchelation of ^{111}In to transferrin. Indium 111-transferrin traffics to liver and, in some cases, to spleen and marrow, thus compromising imaging in these organs. Indium 111 is also moderately expensive and, up to now, has not been routinely available in nuclear medicine departments.

In summary, each radionuclide considered for antibody imaging has some positive quality. Technetium 99m and ^{123}I have optimal physical properties for image resolution and safety. Further considerations include the availability of appropriate chemistries to link them stably to proteins, their metabolic fate as elements, and practical issues such as ease of use, cost, and experience in nuclear medicine departments.

Therapy

The lure of targeted radiotherapy to treat cancer arises from the established efficacy of external beam treatment in achieving local control in large numbers of malignancies, but its well-known litany of failure outside the radiation port. Targeted radiotherapy can, at least theoretically, be used systemically to treat metastatic disease with little toxicity to normal organs.

There is now an abundance of radionuclides with a variety of physical properties to choose from for antibody labeling. The choice of the appropriate radionuclide is much more complex than for imaging, because issues of absorbed dose to tumor compared to total body exposure, innocent bystander toxicity (e.g., bone marrow), and tumor architecture must be added to considerations of availability, cost, chelation chemistry, and safety to medical personnel.

Humm (1986) has provided a useful classification and analysis of the therapeutic radionuclides that are summarized in Table 12-1.

Alpha emitters depend on a reasonably homogeneous distribution in the tumor because of their short range (50–90 μm). If this also markedly decreases innocent bystander toxicity, then alpha-emitter conjugates may be used as drugs in multiple doses, killing nests of cells with each dose. They have a high linear-energy transfer (LET) of approximately 80 keV/μm; a single alpha particle traversing a 10-μm nucleus deposits 800 keV, 400 times greater than a single beta particle. Alpha-particle therapy may kill cells independent of their state of hypoxia and may demonstrate no "shoulder" on the radiation sensitivity curve.

The most promising alpha emitters for therapeutic application are ^{211}At (T1/2, 7.2 hours) and ^{212}Bi (T1/2, 60.6 minutes). Astatine 211 is a halogen, produced in a cyclotron and conjugated to proteins in a manner similar to ^{131}I. Technology is now available to conjugate ^{211}At stably to antibodies. Its short half-life and cyclotron requirement will limit its use to regional cancer centers.

Bismuth 212 is a product of the beta decay of ^{212}Pb (T1/2, 10.6 hours). Lead 212 is potentially generator-produced in high specific activity. Chelators for lead that can withstand the 2-eV beta recoil that occurs with its transmutation to ^{212}Bi could be applied as "in situ generators." Lead 212 is eluted from a generator, chelated to antibody, injected and accumulated at the tumor site; in situ ^{212}Pb would then transmute via beta decay to ^{212}Bi, that would then emit alpha particles (T1/2, 60.6 minutes). The peak ^{212}Bi alpha activity would occur at 3.8 hours. Although previously considered too short a time for tumor localization, recent studies with ^{99m}Tc-labeled fragments (Eary et al., 1986) suggest that this may be compatible with a reasonable therapeutic index between tumor and normal organs.

Sources of alpha particles applicable to the targeted antibody approach are limited, because the elements that decay with alpha emissions usually produce unstable daugh-

TABLE 12-1
CLASSIFICATION OF THERAPEUTIC RADIONUCLIDES

1. Alpha emitters;
2. Low-range beta emitters (mean range ≤ 200 μm);
3. Medium-range beta emitters (200 μm ≤ mean range ≤ 1 mm);
4. High-range beta emitters (mean range ≥ 1 mm);
5. Electron capture and/or internal conversion.

ters that escape from the tumor site following rupture of the radionuclide–antibody bond. Beta sources are more plentiful, permitting both clinicians and chemists the choice of appropriate characteristics for particular tumor.

The low-range ($\leq$200 μm) beta sources are phosphorus 33 (^{33}P), tin 121 (^{121}Sn), lutetium 177 (^{177}Lu), osmium 191 (^{191}Os), and gold 199 (^{199}Au). Because of their short range, they require relatively uniform distribution throughout the tumor. Of these, ^{199}Au can be produced carrier-free from platinum 198 (^{198}Pt), has Auger electrons that increase local energy deposition, and a gamma ray (159 keV) that is suitable for simultaneous imaging.

The medium range (between 200 μm and 1 mm) beta sources include, as examples, scandium 47 (^{47}Sc), ^{67}Cu, arsenic 77 (^{77}As), ^{105}Rh, palladium 109 (^{109}Pd), silver 111 (^{111}Ag), ^{131}I, praseodymium 143, (^{143}Ps), ytterbium 161 (^{161}Yb), and rhenium 186 (^{186}Re). The most widely used, of course, is ^{131}I, which has been successfully employed for decades to treat Graves' disease and thyroid cancer, as well as in early studies of antibody-directed therapy. It is, however, not the ideal choice on the basis of its physical properties: its gamma ray escapes from most tumor masses and yet accounts for a substantial fraction of the total body dose. Rhenium 186 is now being used in several phase I clinical trials.

The long-range beta particles ($\geq$1 mm) include ^{32}P, ^{90}Y, and ^{188}Re. The latter can be generator produced. Yttrium 90 is currently the subject of intense preclinical and clinical antibody-targeted therapy research.

Electron-capture and internal-conversion radionuclides result from the creation of an inner-shell electron vacancy that causes a cascading of electron transitions with the release of X-rays and Auger electrons. These short-range energies require proximity to target DNA to be effective and, therefore, must be internalized into tumor cells.

Considering the physical characteristics described, the actual choice of therapeutic radionuclides for antibody labeling is quite complex. Generally, the longer particle length radionuclides are preferred in tumors that have heterogeneous distribution of antibody and consist of large numbers of "packed" tumor cells. In this situation, the salutary effects of "cross fire" compensate for the increased toxicity to normal tissues. Importantly, it is not necessary to target every cell with antibody.

In cases of homogeneous distribution of labeled antibody or loosely packed or linear growth of tumor cells, most particles emitted from antibody bound to tumor cell surfaces will miss the tumor cell and "hit" surrounding normal cells. Humm (1986) suggests that shorter particle length radionuclides would be preferred to decrease toxicity because the dose advantage to tumor cells becomes inexploitably small for alpha particles and medium- and long-range beta particles. Electron capture or internal conversion decaying radionuclides may deliver the best tumor:nontumor absorbed dose ratios providing the antibody–nuclide conjugate is internalized.

More detailed discussion of the physical properties of these elements and their impact on strategic decisions for antibody labeling is beyond the scope of this chapter. The reader is referred to several reviews on the subject (Humm, 1986; Jungermar et al., 1984; O'Brien, 1983; Wessels and Rogers, 1984).

CHOICE OF ANTIBODY

The application of antibodies as targeting vehicles was catapulted into the modern era by the Nobel Prize winning discovery by Köhler and Milstein that myeloma cells could incorporate DNA from programmed and stimulated B lymphocytes so that the resulting hybrid (hybridoma) produced, secreted, and immortalized the monoclonal antibodies derived from the normal, immunized B lymphocyte (Köhler and Milstein, 1975). The earlier radiolocalization studies performed with polyclonal antibodies had suggested that more highly purified antibodies were required to transform this interesting science into clinically useful agents.

It was not until the late 1970s to early 1980s that sufficient clinical-grade monoclonal antibodies to tumor-associated antigens (TAA) became available. This has made possible repeated studies with highly purified single antibodies with exquisite specificity and insignificant lot-to-lot variation. Finally, it has permitted careful selection from a host of antibodies directed to a particular tumor and the identification of those with the best binding and localization potential and low cross-reactivity.

In this section, we will briefly review the considerations that ought to be addressed in choosing an antibody for development as delivery vehicle for the radionuclide. At this time, there is no clear answer as to which qualities are essential or even the most critical.

Specificity

Specificity is usually assessed by immunohistochemistry studies on frozen sections of normal and cancerous human tissues. All murine antibodies to TAA surveyed to date display some normal tissue cross-reactivity. Nonetheless, sufficient quantitative differences in specific binding of antibody to tumor and normal tissues have been achieved to effect qualitative resolution of small tumors and to widen the therapeutic index between tumor and normal cells compared to untargeted chemotherapy.

Specificity must be interpreted with a view toward its impact on selective localization. These issues include relative accessibility and quantity of antigen in normal organs compared to tumor and antigen heterogeneity in tumors. Generally, antibodies with less cross-reactivity and those directed to relatively dense and homogeneous cell-surface antigens will be the best candidates. Specific localization in tumor sites has been demonstrated, however, using antibody to secreted or intracellular antigens and, in some cases, to antigens with extensive normal tissue expression as assessed in vitro.

Nonspecific Binding

Different antibody or antibody subclasses bind less avidly to human reticuloendothelial system (RES) cells. Fc receptors appear to account for only one of these interactions. The better antibody will display less binding in vivo.

Affinity

Monoclonal antibodies can be selected with adequate affinities (10^{-8} mol/L or greater) to bind antigen at the tumor site. Monovalent fragments formed by enzymatic digestion of whole antibody usually display decreased affinity compared to whole, bivalent antibody. Genetically engineered fragments, however, appear to retain the affinity of the parent molecule. Generally the higher affinity antibodies ($\geq 10^{-10}$ mol/L) would be expected to have improved kinetics of uptake and greater stability and will likely produce monovalent fragments with slower dissociation. These higher-affinity antibodies are more likely to complex with circulating antigen and will also exhibit improved binding to low levels of antigen in normal tissues.

Antigen

In addition to expression, accessibility, and heterogeneity, antigen modulation may be critical for some applications. Once internalized, the rate of metabolism and fate of the metabolites may be important. Generally, stable cell-surface antigens that slowly internalize offer the best target for imaging and therapy with most radionuclides. A more rapidly internalized complex is best for Auger electron emitters. Antigen density above 10^5 sites/cells appears to predict for better localization.

Molecular Species

Several studies have been reported comparing whole antibody, $F(ab')_2$, and Fab fragments (150,000, 100,000, and 50,000 Mol. wt., respectively). Through Fc receptors and other mechanisms, whole Ig binds nonspecifically in the RES, although there are strategies to prevent this. At doses above 10 mg, its half-life is approximately 24 to 30 hours. $F(ab')_2$ has an intermediate half-life of approximately 10 to 12 hours and may cleave to F(ab′). F(ab′) and Fab have half-lives of approximately 90 minutes and tend to accumulate in the kidney. Genetically engineered targeting molecules (GETM) can be designed to provide optimal characteristics of size, percolation into tumor, and kinetics. Choice of the appropriate molecular form depends on an appreciation of these kinetics, the relative rates of uptake into tumor and clearance, and the standard pharmacokinetic "[concentration × time]" required to get enough antibody into the tumor. Because Fab is monovalent, it has lower affinity, so that its "off rate" may be faster than that of bivalent species. This may be important in therapeutic applications. Choice of antibody form must be coordinated with its intended use and the particular radionuclide employed.

GENETICALLY ENGINEERED TARGETING MOLECULES

The past few years have witnessed the predicted marriage between monoclonal antibody technology and recombinant DNA. The pace at which this union has been consummated, however, has already surpassed the expectations of even the most starry-eyed optimist. This technology has provided an alternative to efforts to develop human antibodies de novo, the problems and prospects of which have been reviewed (Abrams et al., 1986). These molecules can be engineered to display a varied array of properties.

Chimeras are produced by substituting the human constant region (heavy and light chain) for the murine constant region, retaining the murine-binding domains that impart specificity. These GETM are approximately two thirds "human" and one third "murine," and demonstrate markedly reduced immunogenicity (LoBuglio et al., 1989).

Replacing all murine sequences with human sequences, except for the complement determining regions (CDR) that impart specificity, yields GETM that are more than 90% human.

Novel constructs include rearrangements or elimination of domains to retain or enhance certain properties (e.g., complement fixation) without requiring the full 150,000-Mol. wt. antibody. They also include CDR mutations to enhance affinity and the production of GETM in bacteria. Most recently, a technique to produce and screen an entire library of random recombinants of heavy and light regions had been described (Huse et al., 1989). The GETM can be constructed with virtually any property or for any use.

The full clinical implications of these new molecules will not be realized for many years. Even now, however, evidence suggests that some chimeras markedly reduce the immunogenicity. Improved complement fixation may enhance effector function and, perhaps, specific delivery to target cells by provoking a local inflammatory response. Genetically engineered targeting molecules from bacteria will dramatically reduce the cost, and increase the batch-to-batch homogeneity, of these products.

PRETARGETING AND HAPTEN CHELATES

One of the major problems associated with antibody tumor targeting is the tension between the requirement for increased serum half-life (area under the curve) to improve delivery and its negative impact on signal-to-noise ratios (imaging) and innocent bystander toxicity (therapy).

The antibody supplies the "targeting principle" and the radiolabel, the "signal" or "cytotoxic principle." Only the radiolabel is compromised by longer serum half-life. Thus, one solution is to administer the antibody and the radiolabel separately. Goodwin et al. (1988) pioneered the use of prelocalizing an unlabeled antihapten antibody in tumors and then administering a labeled hapten that clears the bloodstream rapidly. Stickney et al. (1989) have reported the first human clinical trials using a bifunctional antibody: one arm that binds a carcinoembryonic antigen (CEA) and another that binds an ^{111}In-labeled hapten.

IMPORTANT PARAMETERS IN ANALYZING TARGETED RADIONUCLIDE STUDIES

The first parameter that must be assessed is the labeled reagent itself. Knowledge of its specific activity and the percentage of protein bound counts is critical in interpreting the biodistribution of the radioactivity. High-performance liquid chromatography (HPLC) can analyze and, if necessary, separate the different molecular weights of the radioactive components in the preparation. Verification of the absence of aggregates is critical, for injected aggregates have altered biodistribution and are more immunogenic than monomers. Thin-layer chromatography is used to assess the percentage of protein-bound counts.

Analysis of the labeled material for binding to the target should be performed and compared to an established standard. Competition experiments with cold antibody can provide an indication of relative affinities. We, and others, have shown that antibodies can now be labeled to very high specific activities without compromising immunoreactivity or affinity.

Second, the vagaries of the tumor system used must be assessed. In animal studies using nude mouse/human tumor xenograft models, degree of vascularization, antigen heterogeneity, and necrosis may significantly influence localization. A 1-cm (1-g) tumor constitutes 5% of the total mass of mouse; in a human, it is approximately 0.0014%. Tumor bulk (size of single tumors) and its relative vascularity are important both in animal studies and in human applications.

Third, bioavailability of the labeled reagent for the tumor should be assessed following injection. Because uptake in tumor sites appears to depend in part on standard pharmacokinetics, that is, serum concentration over time or the area under the curve, it is important to measure blood disappearance curves, urine excretion, whole body retention, presence of circulating antigen, and antigen modulation on cells. Serum should be monitored for antibody and radioactivity independently. There are now stable labeling systems that show a serum disappearance parallel to the antibody (Schroff et al., 1990).

Finally, biopsies of tumor and other organs should be obtained in animal studies to determine the percentage of the injected dose per gram (%ID/g) that localized. This provides assessment of the relative localization of the labeled molecule corrected for the size of the organ (%ID/g). Administration of a matched, nonspecific molecule along with the specific antibody and then comparing the %ID/g for specific and nonspecific antibodies in each organ provide an indication of the contribution specificity to localization.

For obvious reasons this level of analysis is not possible in humans. Region of interest (ROI) data obtained by gamma camera imaging corrected for organ size based upon computer modeling are a surrogate for actual counting and weighing of normal organs, except blood and, occasionally, tumors. A pixel (picture element) group is chosen over an organ and counted in comparison to a "standard" part of the body to determine relative uptake. Comparison to a phantom with a known source placed a defined distance from the camera improves accuracy of this technique. Determination of tumor size by CT scan volumetrics and computer merging of images will improve accuracy further. Biopsies of tumor and blood sampling should be performed where possible to analyze the %ID/g accurately and determine tumor:blood ratios.

ANTIGLOBULINS

Development of host antimurine antiglobulin could result in the formation of immune complexes with subsequent immune complex–mediated tissue damage, alterations in the rate of clearance and normal organ distribution of injected monoclonal antibodies, or inhibition of the localization of the monoclonal antibody to tumor cells (blocking antibody) upon subsequent administration of antibody.

Clinical studies that have been performed with murine monoclonal antibodies suggest that a variety of factors may influence elevation of human antimouse antibody (HAMA) titers. Patients with different diseases respond differently to the same murine antibody (Schroff et al., 1985b). For example, patients with chronic lymphocytic leukemia (CLL) treated with the T101 murine monoclonal antibody had a very low incidence of HAMA, whereas patients with cutaneous T-cell lymphoma (CTCL) routinely developed elevated HAMA to the same monoclonal antibody administered at similar doses. This is most likely due to the underlying disease, since CLL patients often have hypogammaglobulinemia. On the other hand, 70% of melanoma patients developing HAMA means that nearly one third do not. Melanoma patients appear to be immunologically intact. In general, both $F(ab')_2$ and Fab fragments have been demonstrated to be immunogenic in man (Carrasquillo et al., 1987).

The specificity of the HAMA response must be analyzed to determine subsequent dosing strategies. In most cases, the antiglobulins cross-react with most, or all, murine immunoglobulin classes. Schroff and co-workers (1985a) demonstrated that cross-reactive antiglobulin responses were largely IgG, had a rapid onset within 2 weeks of immunization, and thus appeared to represent a secondary immune reaction with elevation of levels of preexisting cross-reactive antiglobulins. In some cases, however, a component of the patient's antiglobulin response appears to be specific for the administered antibody (anti-idiotypic). An anti-idiotypic response represents a primary immune response (assuming that the individual has never before encountered this particular antigen).

We have tested a ^{99m}Tc-Fab fragment (NR-LU-10 Fab) in patients with small-cell lung cancer (Abrams et al., 1990a). Among 56 patients in a phase III clinical trial analyzed for HAMA, only 2 patients developed marginally increased and transient HAMA elevations and only 1 ($<$2%) had evidence of significant increase, but this elevation also appeared to be returning toward normal. More than 60 patients have received subsequent injections without evidence of side effects, altered biodistribution, or pharmacokinetics of the labeled Fab. There was also no increased rate of HAMA following the second injection. The influence of antibody (some may be more immunogenic than others), patient population, and chemotherapy is currently undergoing analysis.

The advent of humanized novel constructs (see earlier section) appears in some cases to ameliorate the problem of immunogenicity. LoBuglio et al. (1989) administered a chimera of 17-1A antibody and found a low incidence of anti-idiotype. Antibodies to B72.3 chimera, however, appear in preliminary reports to be of greater incidence. Ledermann et al. (1988) reported a marked decrease in HAMA using cyclosporin A concomitantly with the antibody. It appears, therefore, that the HAMA problem will become a phenomenon of historical interest only. Perhaps some degree of transient immunosuppression, along with use of GETM, will definitively solve this problem.

IN VIVO APPLICATIONS

Historical Overview

In 1948, Pressman and Keighly demonstrated that ^{133}I-labeled anti–rat kidney antibodies localized preferentially in rat kidneys following intravenous injection (Pressman and Keighly, 1948). Pressman (1957) also pioneered the use of radiolabeled antibodies for tumor localization. He showed, in 1957, that ^{131}I-labeled specific antisera localized preferentially into rat sarcomas when compared to ^{125}I-labeled nonimmune serum. Since the specific antiserum itself contained a large fraction of nonspecific antibody, it was not surprising that the ratio of specific:nonspecific antibody localization was only 2:1. In the 1960s and 1970s Bale and co-workers demonstrated that labeled antibodies to fibrin, which is often deposited in rapidly growing tumors, localized in rat, dog, and human tumors (65% of 141 patients) (Bale et al., 1980; Spar et al., 1969). Human studies using ^{131}I anti-CEA antiserum were performed in the early 1970s, revealing uptake in metastatic tumors by external gamma camera scanning (Hoffer and Gottschalk, 1974).

Therapeutic attempts using labeled monoclonal antibodies were also pursued in this period. In 1956, Vial and Callahan reported Beierwaltes' case of a dramatic, complete response in a patient with widely metastatic malignant melanoma treated with ^{131}I-antibodies raised against his own tumor (Vial and Callahan, 1956). McCardle et al. (1966) reported tumor regression in one of two patients treated with ^{131}I-labeled antibodies to human fibrinogen. In 1974, Ghose and Gulcu reported inhibition and complete suppression of the murine EL4 lymphoma with a ^{131}I-labeled anti-EL4 antibody (Ghose and Gulcu, 1974). All noted that delivery of more ^{131}I to tumor by the use of more specific antibody would be required to improve results. In 1974, Chao and colleagues demonstrated the use of affinity chromatography to improve the specificity of the injected antibody preparation and the selective localization of radiolabeled Fab fragments (Chao et al., 1974).

The advent of monoclonal antibodies in 1975 (Köhler and Milstein, 1975) with their promise of improved specificity for tumor cells, unlimited availability, and lack of lot-to-lot variation suggested that the solution to the deficiencies of the antibody preparation had arrived. As we will see, advances in labeling technology and genetic engineering were also required.

Monoclonal Antibodies: Imaging Studies

Iodine-Labeled Antibodies The first studies of radiolabeled monoclonal antibodies used ^{125}I or ^{131}I as the radionuclide because they are easily incorporated into tyrosyl residues by one of several procedures (Ballou et al., 1979; Ghose and Gulcu, 1974). Ballou et al. (1979) reported the first example of a radiolabeled monoclonal antibody directed at a tumor antigen in vivo. They showed localization of an IgM anti-SSEA-1 antibody in human teratocarcinoma xenografts. Houston et al. (1980) demonstrated a high level of localization into target tissues of the murine monoclonal antibody against the murine Thy 1.1 antigen present on AKR/J SL2 lymphoma. In 1981, Moshakis et al. described selective localization in a human germ cell tumor nude mouse xenograft of an ^{131}I-labeled murine monoclonal antibody (Moshakis et al., 1981). These studies established the feasibility of injecting radiolabeled monoclonal antibodies intravenously and achieving localization of the radiolabel at the site of tumor.

The same year (1981) saw what was probably the first use of radiolabeled monoclonal antibodies in humans. Mach et al. (1981) successfully imaged tumors using antibodies to CEA. Farrands et al. (1982) reported successful imaging of colorectal carcinomas using ^{131}I-labeled 791T/36 antibody raised originally against osteogenic sarcoma. Prior to background subtraction, however, the tumor:nontumor ratios were unimpressive, the highest (2:1) compared to normal colon. Epenetos et al. (1982) reported a series of patients with breast, ovarian, and colon carcinoma whose tumors imaged following the injection of ^{123}I-labeled HMFG-1 and HMFG-2 antibodies to the human milk-fat globule. Samples of the patient's tumors were prescreened for the presence of antigen. Of note is that no background subtraction was required for image interpretation and there was no loss of immunoreactivity of the antibody following iodination.*

Larson's group from the University of Washington performed the first systematic human studies of ^{131}I-labeled monoclonal antibodies in melanoma. Using Fab fragments, they found approximately 60% of known sites detectable by scanning, although more than 90% of the patients had at least one site detected. Tumors less than 1.5 cm and those with poor antigen expression accounted for all of the negative findings when appropriately labeled reagents were employed. Without excising a tumor sample, they

*The uptake in tumors was reported to range between 0.26% and 3.5% of the injected dose, the latter in malignant ascites. These values were not corrected for the weight of the tissue (i.e., percentage of the injected dose per gram) so that relative targeting could not be assessed. This demonstrates the difficulty in comparing studies where the data are not comparably analyzed. See earlier discussion in this chapter.

estimated 0.04% ID/g was in the tumor compared to 0.29% ID/g in liver. Human antimurine antibodies detected in several patients were presumably directed at the previously administered subclass. Switching to another subclass permitted subsequent successful imaging without toxicity. Finally, they also noted significant deiodination of the protein in vivo as there were substantial counts in the thyroid gland, a bioassay for the phenomenon (Carrasquillo et al., 1984; Larson et al., 1983).

There have been numerous other studies using iodinated antibodies for diagnosis of metastatic cancer. No attempt was made here to be exhaustive. Deiodination that occurs most vigorously in the liver for whole antibody, and in kidney for fragments, actually improved the apparent specific localization.

Wilbur et al. (1986) have described a new method that prevents dehalogenation. This stability has been demonstrated in nude mice using iodine-, bromine-, and astatine-labeled antibodies and in humans using ^{131}I-labeled antibody. Because toxicity from the radiolabeled antibody at therapy doses occurs during the period of conjugate circulation through normal organs, the period of "free" cytotoxicity to tumors (cytotoxicity with no further normal organ toxicity) is 4 to 8 days (^{131}I has a T1/2 of 8 days). Vigorous dehalogenation at the tumor site compromises therapeutic efficacy and increases potential toxicity.

Indium 111-Labeled Antibodies Fairweather et al. compared ^{111}In-labeled to conventionally labeled ^{131}I anti-CEA antibodies in patients with gastrointestinal malignancies. Indium 111 antibody detected greater than 50% more of the known lesions than ^{131}I antibody when compared in the same patient and produced better signal:noise ratios, showing the lesions with greater certainty (Jungermar et al., 1984). This indicated that choice of radionuclide could be critical.

There have been many studies reported with ^{111}In-labeled antibodies (Murray et al., 1985, 1987), all using diethylenetriaminepentaacetic acid (DTPA) as the metal chelator. Lesions as small as 1.5 cm × 1.5 cm have been detected in subcutaneous sites (Carrasquillo et al., 1987). Subcutaneous, lymph node, and pulmonary lesions were seen at 72 to 144 hours following injection. Problems encountered include the substantial RES (liver, spleen, and marrow) uptake of the ^{111}In-labeled antibody, a pattern that parallels the distribution of ^{111}In-transferrin, except for spleen. This not only compromises imaging of lesions in liver (and spleen), but also suggests that therapy doses using ^{90}Y may be limited by marrow and hepatic toxicity and the contribution by the liver to whole body radiation.

Several improvements in ^{111}In labeling are on the horizon. First, Carrasquillo et al. (1985) have shown excellent imaging of CTCL patients. The antibody was known to bound to circulating cells and the antigen–antibody complex modulated internally, apparently trapping the ^{111}In. The authors speculated that cells with internalized complex trafficked to lymph nodes and skin, enhancing the apparent localization. Concentrations of 0.01% to 0.03% ID/g were achieved in diseased nodes; this is approximately 1 log greater than described in other systems. Rodwell et al. (1986) have reported that linking the chelate to oxidized carbohydrate decreases RES uptake in animal studies of the labeled antibody. At this time, however, patient studies do not appear to corroborate that observation.

More recently, Rosselli et al. (1989) have proposed a new chelating system for ^{111}In and tested it in animal studies in which a marked reduction in RES localization was observed. Confirmation of this observation in human clinical trials is eagerly awaited.

Bifunctional Antibodies Stickney et al. (1989) have demonstrated successful tumor imaging and reduced RES uptake with the bifunctional antibody (BFA) system described earlier. $F(ab')_2$ fragments of anti-CEA antibody and anti–^{111}In-benzyl EDTA bleomycin were chemically linked using the homobifunctional, noncleavable bis-(maleimido) methyl ether (BMEE). Doses between 5 and 40 mg of the BFA were administered 24 to 120 hours prior to the labeled hapten.

Although this was only a phase I study with small patient and lesion numbers, two observations seem justified. Reticuloendothelial system accumulation was markedly decreased compared to identical studies by the same group with ^{111}In-DTPA anti-CEA antibody, and hepatic metastases were detected as "hot" spots rather than the "cold" spots previously described. In addition, a high percentage of known lesions was identified.

Several factors may, however, temper enthusiasm for this approach. The procedure is somewhat cumbersome, requiring preinjection of BFA, waiting 96 hours for localization and clearance, injecting the labeled hapten, and then imaging 72 hours later for a total of 1 week from initial injection until results are finally obtained. Whether or not this is viewed as a problem in the practice of medicine remains to be tested. On the other hand, this technique appears worth further study since high tumor:normal tissue ratios can be achieved with more rapid clearance from the total body, providing a potential advantage in therapeutic applications. If this advantage is indeed realized, the practical problems will seem trivial.

Technetium 99m-Labeled Antibodies Technetium 99m has many of the more desirable qualities for imaging applications: excellent image resolution, ready availability, low cost, safety, standard camera settings, and SPECT applications. Because of its short half-life, it was long considered incompatible with tumor localization and sufficient background clearance to image tumors. In addition, as a transition metal with a +7 oxidation state, it tends to be unstable in most chelate systems.

Fritzberg et al. (1988) have applied a diamide-dithiolate (N_2S_2) chelate to labeling antibody with ^{99m}Tc; initially, pertechnetate (TcO_4^-) (+7 oxidation state) is reduced and complexed by an exchangeable chelating agent. The ^{99m}Tc is then transferred into the stable N_2S_2 chelate at the +5 oxidation level. Another method involves reduction of disulfides to provide intrinsic sites for direct chelation of ^{99m}Tc. We have shown that this procedure, followed by lyophilization, allows for the retention of these intrinsic sites and rapid binding of ^{99m}Tc to the mercapto-proteins. The ^{99m}Tc-N_2S_2 preformed chelate method of labeling is depicted in Figure 12-1.

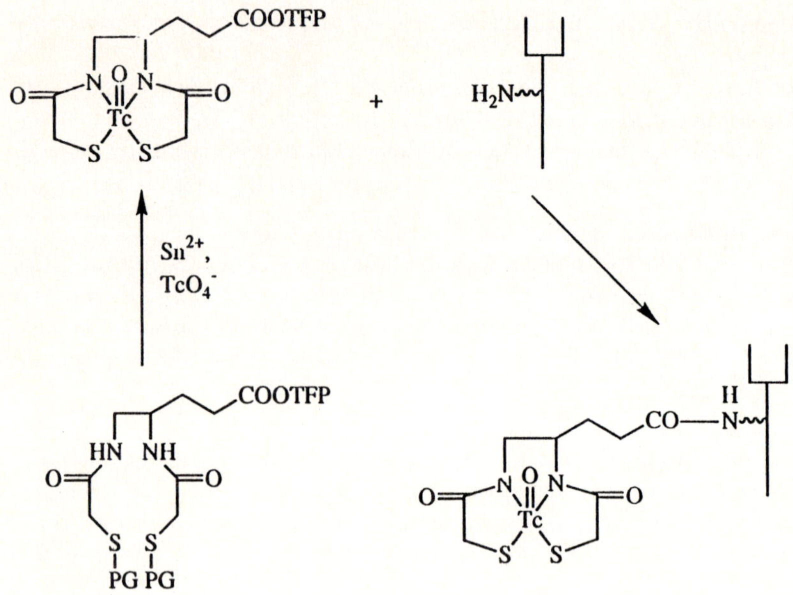

PG = protecting group
TFP = 2,3,5,6-tetrafluorophenyl

FIGURE 12-1
Preformed chelate strategy of protein labeling. The N_xS_y ligand is reacted with reduced TcO_4^- that has been weakly chelated to gluconate. The sulfur-protecting groups dissociate from the ligand as the ^{99m}Tc is chelated. The tetrafluorophenyl active ester remains intact during the chelation process. It is then used to bind to lysine amino groups in polypeptide molecules.

Salk et al. (1988) reported the results of the first, formal phase III trial of a labeled monoclonal antibody for imaging tumors. The study was conducted using a ^{99m}Tc-N_2S_2–labeled (NR-ML-05) Fab directed at the 250-kDa melanoma-associated antigen. Cold, whole NR-ML-05 was preinjected to block nontumor, cross-reactive antigen in marrow, spleen, and liver. Such blockade was shown to be epitope-specific by failure of another anti-250-kDa antibody to prevent deposition of labeled NR-ML-05 Fab into these organs.

Several observations can be made from this study. First, the procedure is safe. Allergic reactions were observed in only 2% of the patients, all of whom had histories of general atopy. No patient could not complete the study nor suffered any sequelae. Elevation of HAMA titers, however, occurred frequently (over 70%).

Second, antibody imaging detects an equal number, but noncongruent set of lesions compared to conventional diagnostic imaging techniques. This observation appears to be unrelated to antigen distribution and more related to site and size of the tumor. Other differences in individual tumors are similar to those described for nude mouse xenografts. The lowest detection rates, for example, appear to be in lung; putative pulmonary lesions, however, have a high false-positive rate with other diagnostic procedures (about 30% in a surgical series), so only a surgical study can determine the true sensitivity of the procedure in this organ.

Third, in a small, but definite, subset of patients, the detection of lesions by antibody imaging made a difference in patient care despite the prior evaluation of the patient with standard techniques. This included improved delineation of the extent of locoregional tumors (either altering or canceling a scheduled surgical procedure), discovery of unsuspected distant metastases (altering or canceling a scheduled surgical procedure), and discovery of unsuspected distant metastases (altering therapy).

Fourth, detection rates were highest for lesions in liver and bone.

Finally, as a single test that can evaluate all anatomical regions simultaneously, antibody imaging, after standard physical examination and chest X-ray, is highly accurate (97%) for establishing a patient's stage of disease; stage determines prognosis.

A second phase III trial using ^{99m}Tc-NR-LU-10 Fab in patients with previously untreated, newly diagnosed small cell lung cancer (SCLC) has been completed (Abrams et al., 1990a). The results differ slightly from those described for melanoma, with a few critical exceptions. The incidence of HAMA was less than 6% of patients and transient in all but 2%. Over 60 second injections have been administered without evidence of altered pharmacokinetics, biodistribution, or toxicity.

Antibody imaging alone was shown to be nearly as accurate as a large standard battery of conventional tests (chest X-ray, CT-abdomen, bone scan, CT-head) in distinguishing limited and extensive SCLC disease. This distinction is critical for making correct therapeutic decisions. The positive predictive value of antibody imaging for establishing a diagnosis of extensive disease is over 95%.

Detection rates for hepatic and osseous metastases were lower than in melanoma, but bone marrow metastases were also occasionally detected by the imaging procedure. SPECT imaging improved the detection of primary pulmonary lesions and mediastinal metastases. SPECT imaging was not part of the melanoma study.

A phase II study in non-SCLC has recently been reported (Friedman et al., 1990). The ^{99m}Tc-NR-LU-10 Fab was slightly better than CT in staging the mediastinum; the two tests together were 100% accurate as judged by surgical staging.

ROLE OF TARGETED RADIONUCLIDE IMAGING IN CANCER TREATMENT

In general, the role of targeted radionuclide imaging (TRI) in cancer patients is becoming better defined. The original vision of reproducibly detecting smaller lesions earlier in a patient's course of illness has not been realized. Complicating factors include variable vascular access to tumor nodules and the resulting differences in signal:noise ratios, the short physical half-life of the best imaging radionuclides, and physical limitations on resolution imposed by current gamma camera imaging technology. Similar problems were encountered in preclinical animal models. The prospect of hot spot cancer imaging with specifically targeted ^{99m}Tc may well prompt a new generation of hardware.

Nonetheless, pivotal phase III studies have now established a different role for TRI in managing patients with cancer. By detecting disease outside regions routinely assessed by conventional techniques, it can improve the definition of patients with truly localized disease; results of local therapies such as surgery and external beam radiation can therefore be improved by excluding patients upstaged by TRI. Alternatively, more extensive local procedures may be undertaken.

Because TRI provides a total body scan, it can be used as a general metastatic survey to stage patients with one test and, if necessary, to direct other tests to suspicious areas. As with all diagnostic techniques, its role will vary from tumor type to tumor type and from stage to stage.

Because of the specificity of targeting and the very low false-positive rates that occurred in our imaging studies, the imaging procedure has a high positive predictive value. Not only does this allow therapeutic decisions to be made on the basis of positive results, but it also suggests a role in corroborating the nature of questionable lesions detected by other tests. Because its negative predictive value is not sufficiently high (i.e., perhaps up to 15% to 20% false-negatives), negative results cannot by themselves be used as a determinant of the absence of metastatic disease when critical therapeutic decisions hang in the balance.

TARGETED RADIOTHERAPY (TRT)

Application of radionuclides for targeted therapy of cancer raises many more basic and clinical issues. Whereas imaging radionuclides generate very little "local" energy, therapeutic radionuclides can cause radiolysis of the protein and/or the chelate system attaching it to the protein. "Innocent bystander" toxicity of circulating radioactivity must be successfully ameliorated. High doses of radioactivity must be handled by medical personnel. For these, and other, reasons, there is less experience with TRT than with imaging applications of antibodies.

Historically, Beierwaltes' 1952 case of curing metastatic melanoma with ^{131}I-labeled polyclonal antiserum raised to the patient's own tumor was the first indication that this approach was feasible. Beierwaltes himself, however, was unsuccessful in treating 13 more patients with the same strategy (Beierwaltes, 1986). Order and coworkers (1982) showed that ^{131}I-anti-ferritin *polyclonal* antiserum could produce regressions of bulky hepatomas. Four of 24 patients had partial responses (PR) and none had complete response (CR). Patients received as much as 150 mCi in a single dose with acceptable hematologic toxicity. For reasons that remain obscure, however, monoclonal antiferritin did not work (Order et al., 1986). Subsequent studies combined cytotoxic agents (5-FU and adriamycin) and external beam radiation with lower doses (50 mCi in divided doses) of TRT and achieved an overall response rate of 48% (7% CR; 41% PR). Yttrium 90 has now been substituted for ^{131}I, with 1 CR and 1 PR in 8 patients (Order et al., 1986). The dose-limiting toxicity was the bone marrow, but marrow transplantation was not required. These responses in hepatoma patients are quite remarkable. A randomized, controlled trial will be necessary to determine the role of the labeled antibody in achieving these results.

Badger et al. (1985) performed a series of elegant experiments in mice using ^{131}I–anti-Thy 1.1 in the AKR/J SL2 lymphoma system. They studied factors that would influence the localization of labeled antibody, including tumor size, quantity, and subclass of administered antibody, specific activity, and host anti-Thy 1.1 immune response. They found that uptake into tumor was maximum at 24 hours with a mean of 6.5% ID/g. The half-life for residence in the tumor was 104 hours. A control, subclass-matched, irrelevant antibody cleared more slowly from the blood than anti-Thy 1.1, a phenomenon noted by Larson in patient studies (Larson et al., 1983). However, when another irrelevant antibody was substituted, its clearance was identical to Thy 1.1. This indicates that subclass is not the only factor that influences antibody clearance.

Tumor uptake of radiolabel varied widely and was inconsistently associated with tumor size. Specific antibody:irrelevant antibody ratios were more consistent, suggesting vascularity and vascular permeability were important factors. The presence of an immune response to the administered antibody did not affect localization of a large dose of labeled antibody.

Human studies of the impact of mass of antibody administered have been inconsistent. This is perhaps, at least in part, due to marked differences in antigen "sink" in both tumor and normal tissue. Oldham has shown increased saturation of antigen sites in melanoma with increasing doses of unlabeled antibody (Oldham et al., 1984), but there was no indication that the *percentage* of the ID/g increased (Oldham et al., 1984; Abrams et al., 1985) because this issue cannot be addressed with unlabeled antibody. Indeed, Badger and his co-workers (1985) found no difference in the percentage of the ID/g up to 400 mg, after which the number actually decreased, although the major decreases occurred at doses greater than 1000 μg.

Based on biodistribution and avidity studies, Badger's group determined they could label 1 μg of antibody with 24 μCi ^{131}I without deleterious effects to the antibody molecules. Fifteen hundred microcuries was the maximum tolerated dose (MTD) to mice with bone marrow the target organ of toxicity. Based upon dosimetry from biodistribution trials, a mean of 3300 cGy, with a wide variance could be delivered to a tumor at the expense of 290 cGy to marrow.

Cheung et al. (1986) have achieved complete regressions of 0.45 to 2 cm^3 human neuroblastoma nude mouse xenografts by administering 0.5 to 1 mCi ^{131}I-labeled anti-GD_2 monoclonal antibody. The critical determinant of response was the actual delivered dose to tumor with complete responses achieved only with greater than 4100 rads. Recurrent tumors showed no loss of GD_2 antigen and no evidence of relative radioresistance.

We have demonstrated (Beaumier et al., submitted) antibody-specific regressions and occasional cures of palpable small-cell lung cancer xenografts using ^{186}Re-labeled NR-LU-10 when the delivered dose to the tumor was 2800 rads or greater. Interestingly, standard chemotherapy that produces regressions in about 90% of patients could not effect partial responses in this model even with excessively high doses. The xenograft was derived from the tumor of a patient who had received no prior chemotherapy. There was a correlation between tumor size and therapeutic efficacy; 17-mm^3 (barely palpable) tumors underwent complete regressions and frequently did not recur. By contrast 107-mm^3 tumors demonstrated substantial tumor regressions, but often recurred. Both of these effects, however, were shown to be specific as the same millicurie dose of irrelevant antibody failed to produce regressions. The results with small tumors suggest a role for TRT in the adjuvant setting.

Human Studies

There is now emerging an increasing body of abstracts and literature of phase I human clinical trials using radiolabeled monoclonal antibodies. The pioneers in this field are Order et al. (1986). Although they found monoclonal antiferritin inferior to polyclonal antisera in treating hepatoma, they have noted ^{90}Y-labeled antiferritin to be better than ^{131}I-antiferritin. Larson et al. (1983) performed the first phase I therapeutic study of a labeled fragment in patients. Despite good localization in selected melanoma patients of ^{131}I-labeled Fab, with calculated (but not measured) doses of 3800 to 8500 rads to tumor, the antitumor effects were few and modest. The first critical organ of toxicity was bone marrow.

Iodine 131 Some of the most impressive results of TRT to date have been achieved, not surprisingly, in lymphoma. Using marrow ablative doses, Press et al. (1990) have achieved complete responses in at least 8/9 cases. Of potential significance to understanding radiobiological effects, patients who recurred have tolerated a standard marrow transplant (high-dose chemotherapy, total body irradiation [TBI], and marrow infusion). This suggests the calculated doses from TRT to critical organs such as lung, kidney, and liver may be overestimating the true biological effects as if they were the same from doses delivered by external beam. More time and more patients will be required to determine whether this speculation is a valid extrapolation from the data.

DeNardo et al. (1990) have employed fractionated doses in more than 20 non-Hodgkin's lymphoma patients with 30 to 60 mCi ^{131}I-labeled Lym-1 antibody every 2 to 6 weeks. The total dose administered, however, was high, 300 to 750 mCi. Two patients had complete responses and all but 1 of the remaining patients had partial responses. Toxicity was mostly allergic in nature; 2 patients experienced transient thrombocytopenia. Fevers and chills were observed in 20% to 25% of the patients.

Epenetos et al. (1982) treated several patients with intraperitoneal ^{131}I-labeled antiovarian (HMFG2) antibody and saw some suggestion of antitumor effect. Several other groups, including our own, are studying the same approach using ^{131}I-, ^{90}Y-, or ^{186}Re-labeled antibodies. Small residual disease appears to be amenable to this therapeutic approach. Peritoneal lavage following antibody localization may reduce peritoneal toxicity if this becomes a problem, but that procedure does not uniformly recover most or all of the infused agent.

Yttrium 90 Yttrium 90 has a more energetic beta particle than ^{131}I (2.2 vs. 0.6 MeV). As mentioned, Order et al. (1986) have shown improved results with ^{90}Y-labeled antiferritin than with the ^{131}I-labeled molecule. Most attempts to use ^{90}Y, however, have been limited by marrow toxicity secondary to transchelation of the radionuclide and hepatic uptake. The use of DOTA type compounds may slow the kinetics of transchelation sufficiently to overcome some of the marrow toxicity that has occurred at doses of 15 mCi/m^2 in most studies. The application of the bifunctional approach is also eagerly awaited.

Rhenium 186 Studies Rhenium has two different beta-emitting isotopes that are linked to antibody with the same N_xS_y preformed chelate system described for ^{99m}Tc. For any given "expense" of total body radiation dose, ^{186}Re and ^{90}Y provide 20% to 30% greater absorbed dose to tumor than ^{131}I or ^{188}Re. A 100-mCi dose of ^{186}Re exposes medical personnel to one fifth the radiation of 100-mCi dose of ^{131}I and less than a typical 30-mCi dose of ^{99m}Tc. Because ^{186}Re has an imageable gamma, it has an advantage over ^{90}Y for dosimetry calculations.

We have now conducted three phase I dose-escalation clinical trials using single doses of ^{186}Re-labeled antibodies (Abrams et al., 1990b). The F(ab′)$_2$ of an anti-CEA variant murine monoclonal antibody has been labeled with up to 300 mCi (total dose) and administered to patients with refractory tumors with evidence of dose-limiting bone marrow toxicity at the highest dose. To qualify for the study, patients were first imaged with ^{99m}Tc-labeled antibody. The pharmacokinetics, metabolism, and clearance of ^{99m}Tc- and ^{186}Re-labeled F(ab′)$_2$ appeared nearly identical. Doses to tumor ranged from 1 to 17 rads/mCi. Images from a patient selected by ^{99m}Tc-antibody and then treated with ^{186}Re-antibody F(ab′)$_2$ fragments are shown in Figure 12-2. Two significant PR in a patient who had end-stage colon cancer refractory to standard treatment were observed at the 150-mCi level (Schroff et al., 1990). In this study we noted that recalculation of the administered dose (in mCi) on the basis of body surface area provided a better prediction of dose to marrow. The MTD in this study was 150 to 200 mCi/m^2 depending upon the intensity of prior therapy with marrow toxic agents.

The second study employed the whole NR-LU-10 antibody that had been studied extensively as a ^{99m}Tc Fab in a phase III study in patients with small-cell lung cancer. Patients qualified for the ^{186}Re-NR-LU-10 study if their tumors imaged with ^{99m}Tc-NR-LU-10 Fab; because of the different molecular species used for imaging (Fab) and therapy (whole), dosimetry comparisons were not relevant. Doses up to 90 mCi/m^2 ^{186}Re-labeled were administered without dose-limiting toxicity. At 120 mCi/m^2 bone marrow toxicity, primarily thrombocytopenia, emerged as dose-limiting. No responses were achieved in a diverse patient population. Dose escalation with autologous marrow support is the next step in this phase I study. If responses are achieved, hematopoietic

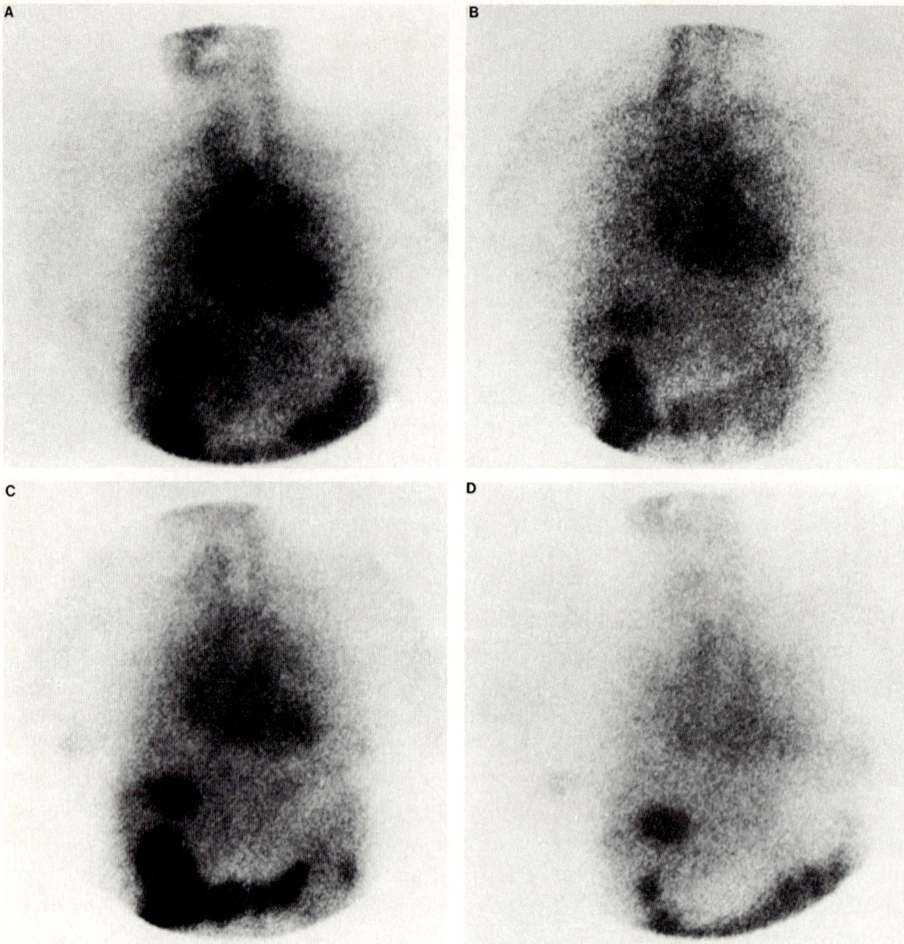

FIGURE 12-2
^{99m}Tc-NR-CO-02 F(ab′)$_2$ and ^{186}Re-NR-CO-02 F(ab′)$_2$ in the same patient in a phase I study. A patient with colorectal carcinoma metastatic to liver receives 30 mCi ^{99m}Tc-NR-CO-02 F(ab′)$_2$ week 1. Twenty hours after injection, an imaging study is performed. (A) Note blood pool (8–12 hr T1/2 of F[ab′]$_2$) not observed in images with Fabs. Density in liver represents tumor. The labeled metabolite is partially excreted in the intestine. One week later the patient receives the same F(ab′)$_2$ preparation with 50 mCi ^{186}Re substituted for ^{99m}Tc. Images are taken at 24 hours (B), 48 hours (C), and 72 hours (D). Note progressive clearing of blood pool and intestinal excretion, and persistence of radioactivity in the hepatic metastasis. The calculated dose to the tumor was 850 rads. Note excellent images obtained using the 9% abundant, 137-keV gamma ray of ^{186}Re.

growth factors may be able to replace the requirement for autologous marrow reinfusion.

The third study involves intraperitoneal ^{186}Re-NR-LU-10 in patients with ovarian cancer. No dose-limiting toxicity has been observed in doses up to 120 mCi/m^2. The MTD has been determined to be 150 mCi/m^2, approximately 10 times that achieved with similarly administered ^{90}Y-labeled antibodies. Five of the first 13 patients showed surgical or laparoscopic evidence of response to a single dose.

FUTURE INVESTIGATIONS

There are several problems that have compromised the application of TRT in cancer therapy. The first was inadequately specific and pure targeting vehicles; monoclonal antibody technology was a major step forward in solving that problem.

The second problem, identified when monoclonals were shown not to solve all the problems, was inadequate chelation of radionuclides. These chemical and biochemical problems have been solved for rhenium; ^{186}Re can be stably and irreversibly linked to antibody using a bifunctional chelate system without affecting immunoreactivity or causing aggregate formation even at high doses. The biodistribution, clearance, and pharmacokinetics appear reasonably identical to trace-labeled, no-carrier-added ^{99m}Tc conjugates. The stability and preserved immunoreactivity of both the ^{186}Re- and ^{99m}Tc-labeling systems are qualitatively different from prior methods.

The major remaining problem compromising TRT is inadequate delivery to tumor. Targeted radiotherapy has the advantage over drug and toxin conjugates of not requiring antibody targeting of every cell; rather, nontargeted cells can be killed by cross fire. On the other hand, improving delivery by increasing serum half-life also increases "innocent bystander" toxicity from circulating radioactivity. The relative advantages of TRT compared to drug and toxin conjugates are summarized in Table 12-2.

There are ongoing studies to increase uptake selectively to tumor. Human antibodies with intact effector mechanisms seem to improve the %ID/g into tumor. The availability of these humanized molecules provides the opportunity for demonstrating the impact of this phenomenon in large patient studies over the next 2 years. A 5- to 10-

TABLE 12-2
COMPARISON OF TRT TO OTHER IMMUNOCONJUGATES

TRT		Drug/toxin conjugates
No	Need to target "every" cell	Yes
Yes	Innocent bystander toxicity	No
Low	Immunogenicity	High (toxins)
Yes	Available agents to ameliorate toxicity	No
No (?)	Unique mechanism of cytoxicity	Yes

fold improvement in selective delivery would transform TRT overnight from a curiosity with potential into a major weapon in the arsenal against cancer. Imaging would then have the additional role of selecting patients for therapy.

Short of such a breakthrough, TRT has several intermediate applications. Wessels has proposed the extra 1500 to 2000 rads that can be delivered today by safe doses of ^{186}Re-labeled antibody as a boost to conventional radiation therapy (XRT). Such an increment could have a dramatic effect on local control for XRT doses that are just "off the shoulder" of the radiation response curve.

The intraperitoneal approach in ovarian cancer provides another application in which tolerable doses of TRT have already demonstrated patient benefit.

With human antibodies, multiple doses may be administered, with or without mild immunosuppressive treatment, to patients with diseases other than lymphoma, delivering a greater total dose to tumor. In addition, tumor cells may be recruited from G_0 into the cell cycle where they are more sensitive to radiation. Scheduling of doses may then become a critical parameter in successful treatment. Cloned hematopoietic growth factors (G-CSF, GM-CSF, IL-3) have already facilitated the use of higher doses of chemotherapy than were previously tolerable. Unfortunately, the bone marrow is only one target for the ravages of chemotherapy. Toxicities to kidney, lung, eighth nerve, peripheral nerve, intestine, and heart are not only common but often occur at doses that are not very much higher, if at all, than those causing unacceptable hematopoietic toxicity.

Indications from our studies (Abrams et al., 1990b; Schroff et al., 1990) and those of Press et al. (1990) suggest that the second critical organ of toxicity (kidney, intestine, or liver) requires perhaps up to a 10-fold greater dose than the marrow can tolerate before clinical toxicity due to TRT occurs. This may be secondary to intrinsic repair mechanisms in these slowly replicating cells. Thus, hematopoietic growth factors could have a more profound effect on the TRT dose range that can be administered than for chemotherapy and may largely abrogate TRT toxicity. Radioprotectors such as WR-2721, IL-1, and others may also enhance the marrow recovery rate by preventing stem-cell toxicity.

Finally, the use of alpha emitters should not go unmentioned. Their high LET and short particle lengths suggest that they could be both safer and more efficacious than beta-emitter therapy. Multiple doses would allow targeting of different nests of tumor cells with each dose, thereby overcoming the problem of short particle length of the alpha emitters. The chemistry of ^{211}At coupling has progressed to the point where clinical trials can be contemplated, but a well-controlled phase I clinical trial has not yet begun.

We are now at the threshold of a major revolution in the treatment of cancer: effective, targeted therapy. Tumor regressions have been achieved by several different groups in refractory lymphoma, hepatoma, ovarian, and colorectal cancers. In most cases, the toxicities associated with these treatments have been mild or nonexistent. Technologies exist to link appropriate radionuclides to targeting agents, to design these carriers to fit any purpose, and to facilitate multiple dosing. These improved carriers will be able to deliver an increased percentage of the injected dose to tumors that should induce regressions at tolerable doses. Either alternatively, or additionally, the hematopoietic growth factors and the radioprotectors will almost assuredly increase the dose intensity of RIT that can be safely administered to patients. These strategies merely await the resources, and the commitment, to learn how to apply them most advantageously.

REFERENCES

Abrams PG, Morgan AC, Schroff RW, et al. Localization and biodistribution studies of a monoclonal antibody in patients with melanoma. In: Reisfeld, Sell, eds. Monoclonal antibodies and cancer therapy. New York, NY: Alan R. Liss; 1985:233–236.

Abrams P, Fer M, Faubion C, et al. A new procedure for staging small cell lung cancer (SCLC): gamma camera imaging using technetium-99m labeled monoclonal antibody Fab. Proc Am Soc Clin Oncol. 1990a;9:232.

Abrams P, Fer M, Schroff R, et al. Radioimmunotherapy with ^{186}Re-labeled antibodies. Ant Immunoconjugates Radiopharmacol. 1990b;3:39.

Abrams PG, Rossio JR, Stevenson HC, Foon KA. Optimal strategies for developing human monoclonal antibodies. Meth Enzymology. 1986;121:107–119.

Badger CC, Krohn KA, Peterson AV, Shulman H, Bernstein ID. Experimental radiotherapy of murine lymphoma with ^{131}I-labeled anti–thy 1.1 monoclonal antibody. Cancer Res. 1985; 45:1536–1544.

Bale WF, Centeras MA, Goody ED. Factors influencing localization of antibodies in tumors. Cancer Res. 1980;40:2965–2972.

Ballou B, Levine G, Hakala RR, et al. Tumor localization detected with radioactively labeled monoclonal antibody and external scintigraphy. Science. 1979;206:844–847.

Beaumier PL, Venkatesan P, Vanderheyden JL, et al. Rhenium-186 radioimmunotherapy of small cell lung carcinoma xenografts in nude mice (submitted).

Beierwaltes WH. Radioimmunotherapy of cancer: historical perspectives and prospects for the future. Text of talk delivered at NATO Conference on "Radiolabeled monoclonal antibodies for imaging and therapy: potential, problems, and prospects." Barga, Italy; 1986.

Carrasquillo JA, Krohn KA, Beaumier PL, et al. Diagnosis and therapy of solid tumors with radiolabeled antibodies and immune fragments. Cancer Treat Rep. 1984;68:317–327.

Carrasquillo JA, Bunn PA Jr, Keenan AM, et al. Radioimmunodetection of cutaneous T-cell lymphoma with ^{111}In-labeled T101 monoclonal antibody. New Engl J Med. 1985;315:673–679.

Carrasquillo JA, Abrams PG, Schroff RW, et al. Effect of ^{111}In-9.2.27 monoclonal antibody dose on the imaging of metastatic melanoma. J Nucl Med. 1987;29:130–133.

Chao HF, Peiper SC, Philpott GW, Parker CW, Asch RD. Selective uptake of specifically purified antibodies to carcinoembryonic antigen of human adenocarcinoma. Res Comm Chem Pathol and Pharmacol. 1974;9:746–761.

Cheung N-K, Landmeier B, et al. Complete tumor ablation with ^{131}I-labeled disialoganglioside GD2-specific monoclonal antibody against human neuroblastoma xenografted in nude mice. J Natl Cancer Inst. 1986;77:739–745.

DeNardo GL, DeNardo SJ, O'Grady LF, et al. Radiation treatment of B-cell malignancies with immunoconjugate. Frontiers Radiation Ther Oncol. 1990;24:194–201.

Eary JF, Schroff RW, Kasina S, et al. Clin Nucl Med. 1986;9. Abstract.

Ehrlich P. The relationship existing between chemical constitution, distribution and pharmacologic action. In: Himmelweight F, Marquardt M, Sir Henry Dale, eds. The collected papers of Paul Ehrlich, vol. I. New York, NY: Pergamon Press, 1956:596–618.

Epenetos AA, Mather S, Granowska M, et al. Targeting of iodine-123-labeled tumor-associated monoclonal antibodies to ovarian, breast and gastrointestinal tumors. Lancet. 1982;2:999–1004.

Farrands PA, Pimm NW, Embleton MJ, et al. Radioimmunodetection of human colorectal cancers by an antitumor monoclonal antibody. Lancet. 1982;2:397–400.

Friedman S, Sullivan K, Salk D, et al. Staging nonsmall cell lung cancer using technetium-99m-labeled monoclonal antibodies. Hematol Oncol Clin N Am. 1990;4:1069–1078.

Fritzberg AR, Abrams PG, Beaumier PL, et al. Specific and stable labeling of antibodies with ^{99m}Tc using a diamide dithiolate chelating agent. Proc Natl Acad Sci (USA). 1988;85:4025–4029.

Ghose T, Gulcu A. Cure of a mouse lymphoma with radio-iodinated antibody. Eur J Cancer. 1974;10:787–791.

Goodwin DA, Meares CF, McCall MJ, et al. Pretargeted immunoscintigraphy of murine tumors with indium-111-labeled bifunctional haptens. J Nucl Med. 1988;29:266–234.

Hoffer PB, Gottschalk A. Tumor scanning agents. Semin Nucl Med. 1974;4:305–316.

Houston LL, Nowinski RC, Bernstein ID. Specific in vivo localization of monoclonal antibodies directed against the Thy 1.1 antigen. J Immunol. 1980;125:837–843.

Huse WD, Sastry L, Iverson SA, et al. Generation of a large combinatorial library of the immunoglobulin repertoire in phage. Science. 1989;246:1275–1281.

Humm JL. Dosimetric aspects of radiolabeled antibodies for tumor therapy. J Nucl Med. 1986;27:1014–1017.

Jungermar JA, Kin-Hung PYu, Zanelli CI. Radiation absorbed dose estimates at the cellular level for some electron-emitting radionuclides for radioimmunotherapy. Int J Appl Radiation Isotopes. 1984;35:883–888.

Köhler G, Milstein C. Continuous cultures of fused cells secreting antibody of pre-defined specificity. Nature. 1975;256:495–497.

Larson SM, Carrasquillo JA, Krohn KA, et al. Localization of ^{131}I-labeled p97 specific Fab fragments in human melanomas as a basis for radiotherapy. J Clin Invest. 1983;72:2101–2114.

Ledermann JA, et al. Br J Cancer. 1988;58:654.

LoBuglio AF, et al. Clinical experience with chimeric antibodies. Fourth International Conference on Monoclonal Antibody Immunoconjugates for Cancer. March 30, 1989. Abstract.

McCardle RJ, Harper PV, Spar IL, et al. Studies with iodine-131-labeled antibody for diagnosis and therapy of tumors. J Nucl Med. 1966;7:873–844.

Mach JP, Bucheggar F, Forni M, et al. Use of radiolabeled monoclonal anti-CEA antibodies for detection of human carcinomas by external photoscanning and tomoscintigraphy. Immunol Today. 1981;2:239–249.

Moshakis V, McIllhinney RAJ, Raghavan D. Localization of human tumor xenografts after IV administration of radiolabeled monoclonal antibodies. Br J Cancer. 1981;44:91–99.

Murray JL, Rosenblum MG, Sobol RE, et al. Radioimmunoimaging in malignant melanoma with ^{111}In-labeled monoclonal antibody 96.5. Cancer Res. 1985;45:2376–2381.

Murray JL, Rosenblum MG, Lamki L, et al. Clinical parameters related to optimal tumor localization of indium-111-labeled mouse antimelanoma monoclonal antibody ZME-018. J Nucl Med. 1987;28:25–33.

O'Brien HA, Jr. Overview of radionuclides useful for radioimaging/radioimmunotherapy and current status of preparing radiolabeled antibodies. In: Burchiel SW, Rhodes BA, eds. Radioimaging and radioimmunotherapy. New York, NY: Elsevier Science; 1983:161–169.

Oldham RK, Foon KA, Morgan AC, et al. Monoclonal antibody therapy of malignant melanoma: in vivo localization in cutaneous metastases after intravenous administration. J Clin Oncol. 1984;2:1235.

Order SE, Klein JL, Leichner PK, Warham MD, Ettinger DS, Seigelman SS. Advances in iodine-131 labeled antiferritin immunoglobulin cancer therapy. Cancer Biol. 1982;34:264–267.

Order SE, Klein JL, Leichner PK. Radiation therapy of hepatoma with I-131 and Y-90 labeled antiferritin antibodies. International Conference of Monoclonal Antibody Immunoconjugates for Cancer. 1986;1:27–28.

Press OW, Eary JF, Badger CC. High-dose radioimmunotherapy of B-cell lymphomas. Frontiers Radiation Ther Oncol. 1990;24:204–213.

Pressman D. Radiolabeled antibodies. Ann NY Acad Sci. 1957;69:644–650.

Pressman D, Keighley G. The zone of activity of antibodies as determined by the use of radioactive tracers: the zone of activity of nephrotoxic antikidney serum. J Immunol. 1948; 59:141–146.

Rodwell JD, Alvarez VL, Lee C, et al. Site-specific covalent modification of monoclonal antibodies: In vitro and in vivo evaluations. Proc Natl Acad Sci USA. 1986;83:2632–2636.

Roselli M, Schlom J, Gansow OA, et al. Comparative biodistribution of yttrium- and indium-labeled monoclonal antibody B72.3 in athymic mice bearing human colon carcinoma xenografts. J Nucl Med. 1989;30:672–682.

Salk D, et al. Technetium-labeled monoclonal antibodies for imaging metastatic melanoma: results of a multicenter clinical study. Semin Oncol. 1988;15:608–618.

Schroff RW, Foon KA, Beatty SM, Oldham RK, Morgan AC. Human anti-murine immunoglobulin responses in patients receiving monoclonal antibody therapy. Cancer Res. 1985a; 45:879–885.

Schroff RW, Stevenson HC. Human immune responses to murine monoclonal antibodies. In: Foon KA, Morgan AC, eds. Monoclonal antibody therapy of human cancer. Hingham, Mass: Martinus Nijhoff Publishing; 1985b:121–138.

Schroff RW, Weiden PL, Appelbaum J, et al. Rhenium-186 labeled antibody in patients with cancer: report of a pilot phase I study. Ant Immunoconjugates Radiopharmacol. 1990;3:99–111.

Spar IL, Bale WF, Manach D. ^{131}I-labeled antibodies to human fibrinogen: diagnostic studies and therapeutic trials. Cancer. 1969;78:731–759.

Stickney DR, Slater JB, Kirk GA, et al. Bifunctional antibody: ZCE/CHA ^{111}indium BLEDTA-IV clinical imaging in colorectal carcinoma. Ant Immunoconjugates Radiopharmacol. 1989; 2:1–13.

Vial AB, Callahan W. Univ Mich Med Bull. 1956;20:284–286.

Wessels BW, Rogers RD. Radionuclide selection and model absorbed dose calculations for radiolabeled tumor associated antibodies. Med Phys. 1984;11:638–645.

Wilbur DS, Jones DS, Fritzberg AR, Morgan AC, Jr. Radioiodination of monoclonal antibodies. Labeling with *para*-iodophenyl (PIP) derivatives for in vivo stability of the radioiodination. J Nucl Med. 1986;27:959. (Abstract).

CHAPTER **13**

VACCINIA VIRAL LYSATES IN TREATMENT OF MELANOMA

Peter Hersey

There is much clinical and histopathological evidence that suggests melanoma incites an immune response that may influence the clinical course of tumor growth. Hence, many primary melanomas have areas of regression (McGovern, 1982), and this is associated with histopathological evidence of lymphoid infiltration, particularly by T lymphocytes (Hersey et al., 1985; McGovern, 1982). Other clinical phenomena such as long latent periods to recurrence and spontaneous stabilization or (rarely) remission of metastatic disease are also generally held to reflect immune responses to the tumor.

This evidence has provided the incentive for a number of clinical studies of immunotherapy over the past two decades (Hersey and Balch, 1984; Hersey, 1989). The most extensive of these were trials of nonspecific active immunotherapy that appeared to show minimal benefit from this approach (Hersey and Balch, 1984). Nevertheless, there was evidence of benefit in certain patient subgroups such as the improved survival of patients in the WHO trial of adjuvant therapy who converted from skin test negative to positive during immunotherapy with *Mycobacterium bovis* strain bacillus Calmette-Guérin (BCG).

Interest in the use of viral lysates for immunotherapy dates from studies on viral oncolysis in animal tumor models, in which it was observed that animals surviving viral oncolysis were often strongly immune to subsequent transplants of syngeneic tumors (Koprowski et al., 1957; Lindenmann and Klein, 1967). Subsequent studies in animal models defined many of the characteristics of this response and established that the immunity was T cell–dependent and specific for the tumor cells used in the vaccines (Austin and Boone, 1979). The appeal of this therapeutic approach suggested from these studies in animal models is the possible induction of strong, long-lasting immunity against tumor cells by injection of viral lysates.

Initial results from phase I/II studies in human cancer also appear promising. These include studies by Cassel et al. (1983, 1986) on the treatment of melanoma patients with Newcastle disease virus (NDV)-induced lysates of melanoma cells and those on influenza viral-induced lysates in treatment of vulval, cervical, and ovarian cancer (Freedman et al., 1980, 1983) and patients with melanoma (Sinkovics et al., 1981). Wallack et al. (1981, 1986) carried out phase I/II studies with vaccinia viral lysates in patients with melanoma and confirmed the safety of this approach. This chapter reviews the scientific basis of the viral lysate approach, our experience with vaccinia viral lysates in treatment of patients with melanoma, and analysis of the immune response induced in the patients. The main questions and areas for future research are discussed.

VIRAL LYSATES IN IMMUNOTHERAPY—THEORETICAL CONSIDERATIONS

Several basic principles concerning the mode of action of viral lysates in immunotherapy have been established from studies in experimental animal models (Austin and Boone, 1979; Lindenmann, 1974; Lindenmann and Klein, 1967). First, in most models, injection of virus alone, tumor cells alone, or tumor cells admixed with ultraviolet light (UV)-inactivated virus did not induce immunity against tumor transplants, that is, integration of viral antigens into the host cell membrane appeared necessary to produce an effective vaccine. Similarly, immunization with viral-induced lysates of normal cells was not protective (Austin and Boone, 1979). These experiments indicated that the virus did not act as an adjuvant, such as complete Freund's adjuvant. They also suggested that the effects were not induced by release of interferon or other nonspecific mediators, since these were released after viral infection alone or after injection of viral lysates of normal cells.

Second, it was necessary for the tumor cell in the vaccine to have antigens recognized by T cells, that is, animals made tolerant to the viral antigens were not protected by the lysates (Austin and Boone, 1974). Also, vaccines made from virus infection of tumor-cell variants that did not express antigens recognized by cytotoxic T lymphocytes (CTL) did not induce immunity against tumors (Schirrmacher, 1987). It appeared from these studies that it was necessary for both viral- and tumor-associated antigens (TAA) to be expressed on the tumor cell membranes.

Why Vaccinia Virus?

Vaccinia virus (VV) may be particularly favorable for induction of T-cell responses in that the virus is known to be strongly immunogenic and to induce lifelong immunity.

Some of the antigens recognized by the immune system (in mice) are shown in Table 13-1. Viral antigens were shown to distribute in the cell membrane during entry of the virus into the cell (Chang and Metz, 1976). Additional new antigens appeared on the cell surface during the early phase of viral replication (Mallon et al., 1985; Wilton et al., 1986). Some VV antigens such as the hemagglutinin appear to be physically associated with major histocompatibility complex (MHC) antigens on the cell membrane and this may present a more immunogenic complex to T cells (Dales and Oldstone, 1982). This ability to associate with MHC antigens does not appear to be a general property of viral antigens, because those of the vesicular stomatitis virus (VSV) did not appear to associate with host-cell MHC antigens (Wise, 1977). This may account for the ineffectiveness of VSV to induce immunity in some studies (Livingston et al., 1985a).

The most plausible hypothesis to account for the mode of action of viral lysates is that the viral antigens act as helper determinants for B cells or CTL that recognize TAA. This idea was supported by evidence of increased antibody and CTL responses to tumor cells when mice were immunized with VV-infected tumor cells (Fujiwara et al., 1984). Similarly, the number of CTL precursors against tumor cells was increased in mice immunized with NDV-infected tumor cells (Schirrmacher, 1987). Studies on helper activity in model systems demonstrated increased CTL and antibody production against the hapten TNP when this was coupled to VV-infected target cells compared to noninfected target cells (Fujiwara et al., 1984; Shimizu et al., 1984). This (proposed) mode of action of viral-infected tumor cells in induction of immunity to tumors is shown in Figure 13-1. It demonstrates that the VV antigens expressed on MHC antigens of antigen-presenting cells (APC) stimulate helper T-cell activity and that the latter release lymphokines such as interleukin 2 (IL-2) and interleukin 4 (IL-4) that stimulate, in a paracrine fashion, CTL activity and immunoglobulin (Ig) production by B cells against adjacent TAA on the APC. This model is similar to that proposed for T-cell and Ig responses to proteins of the hepatitis B virus (Milich, 1988). In the case of B-cell responses it is more likely that B cells act as APC and that the VV helper determinants are expressed on MHC class II D related (DR) antigens after ingestion of the VV TAA complex (Howard, 1985).

A second possibility indicated in Figure 13-1 is that VV infection of melanoma cells may induce new antigens on the cell membrane or increase the concentration of TAA recognized by T cells. It is well established that certain viruses may either inhibit the expression of certain cell-surface antigens, such as the suppression of MHC antigens by type 12 adenovirus (Bernards et al., 1983), or result in expression of new antigens, such as certain class I-like MHC antigens by several RNA and DNA oncogenic viruses (Brickwell et al., 1983) or various heat-shock or stress proteins (Polla, 1988). Once T cells are generated against these antigens, they may then be able to recognize them on the VV-uninfected melanoma cells of the host. Figure 13-1 also incorporates the possibility that some CTL do not need help and appear to respond directly to antigens (Widmer and Bach, 1981).

TABLE 13-1
VACCINIA VIRUS–ASSOCIATED ANTIGENS DETECTED IN INFECTED CELLS

	Mol. wt. of antigens in SDS-PAGE gels																
Virion-derived			65						41	35–37	32–34					20	14–16
Cell membrane 120 min.*			65			58	48–50	42		36–37†	34	32†	29				14–16
Serologically defined	94	70		62‡	60			42	40	35‡				28‡	25		

*Antigens detected in cell membranes 120 minutes post infection with VV (Mallon et al., 1985).
†Possible target antigens for CTL (Mallon et al., 1985).
‡Major responses are underlined in table (Wilton et al., 1986).

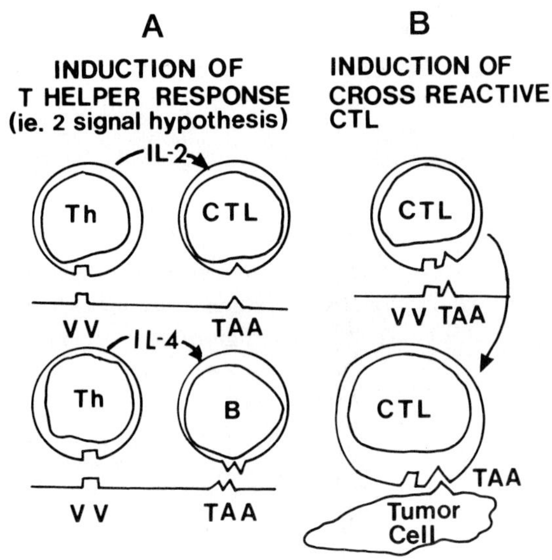

FIGURE 13-1
(A) Diagrammatic representation of how helper T cells that recognize VV on MHC class II antigens of APC (e.g., Langerhans cells in skin or dendritic cells in lymph nodes) may provide help to CTL or B cells that recognize adjacent TAA on APC. In the case of antibody responses, it is more likely that the B cells act as APC (see text). (B) The second possibility is that VV infection may increase the expression of TAA, which are recognized directly by CTL. These latter are expanded and then interact with similar determinants on the melanoma cells of the host (see text).

EFFECT OF THERAPY WITH VACCINIA MELANOMA CELL LYSATES ON SURVIVAL OF MELANOMA PATIENTS FOLLOWING SURGICAL REMOVAL OF LYMPH NODE METASTASES

Prognosis in Stage II Melanoma

The detection of metastases from melanoma in regional lymph nodes is associated with a poor prognosis. As shown in Table 13-2, overall survival rates at 5 years range from 23% to 42% (Lindenmann, 1974; Livingston et al., 1985a, 1985b, 1987; McGovern,

TABLE 13-2
PERCENTAGE OF PATIENTS FREE OF RECURRENCES AND SURVIVING 2 YEARS AFTER SURGICAL TREATMENT FOR STAGE II MELANOMA*

	% Recurrence-free + S.E.		% Survival + S.E.		
Study	Number of patients	2 years	Number of patients	2 years	5 years
Hilal et al., 1981	47	44 ± 18	47	58 ± 14	
Hill et al., 1981	84	46 ± 10	84	45 ± 10	
Camacho et al., 1981					
DNCB +ve	120	44 ± 10	147	57 ± 8	30 ± 4
DNCB −ve	28	28 ± 16	35	43 ± 16	
Veronesi et al., 1982	185	38 ± 8	185	55 ± 8	30 ± 3
Bukowski et al., 1983			36	54 ± 16	
Balch et al., 1985a			280 (<50 yrs)	60 ± 6	42 ± 3
			168 (>50 yrs)	55 ± 8	23 ± 3
Cascinelli et al., 1984			255	50 ± 2	33 ± 2

*Estimates made from figures and by calculation of S.E. from formula $(p(1-p)/n)^{1/2}$.

1982; Mallon et al., 1985; Mehra et al., 1984; Milich, 1988). Prognosis in stage II melanoma is determined predominantly by the number of lymph nodes found to contain metastases, and many of the clinical and pathological features of primary melanoma that influence prognosis in stage I melanoma lose their significance in patients with lymph node disease, for example, thickness of the primary melanoma appears to be of only marginal significance, except perhaps in patients with microscopically detected lymph node metastases (Roses et al., 1985). Ulceration of the primary melanoma, however, still appears to be associated with adverse prognosis in patients with lymph node disease (Balch et al., 1985a). In view of the adverse prognosis and the relatively well-defined prognostic criteria in melanoma patients with lymph node metastases, phase II studies were commenced in late 1982 to determine whether vaccination with vaccinia-induced melanoma cell lysates (VMCL) may influence their survival.

Clinical Studies with VMCL

Production of the vaccine is described in detail elsewhere and was similar to that described by Wallack (1981). Only one melanoma cell line was used. This was established from a primary melanoma of a 43-year-old woman in 1972. The MHC phenotype was A2,3.B7,35. DR2,4. VV was added at 2.5-pock–forming units per melanoma cell and the resulting lysate collected at 24 hours. Low-speed (400 g) centrifugation was used to remove nuclei and other large particulate material, and the vaccine was prepared from a high-speed (38,000 g) centrifugation of the supernatant. Electron microscopic appearance of the vaccine is shown elsewhere (Hersey et al., 1986). Each vaccine contained lysate from the equivalent of 5×10^6 melanoma cells in the original culture (100–200 μg protein). It was shown to contain MHC class I and II antigens and most of the melanoma-associated antigens defined by immune monoclonal antibodies. Analysis of the vaccine by thin-layer chromatography by Cheresh (Immunology Unit, Scripps Research Institute, La Jolla, CA) confirmed the presence of the ganglioside GD_3 and the absence of GD_2 from the vaccine.

The vaccines were given intradermally at one site rotating around each limb with successive injections. They were given every 2 weeks for 4 injections, then every 3 weeks for 6 injections, and then monthly for 18 injections (total of 2 years).

The results of the initial study on 96 patients are presented in detail elsewhere (Hersey et al., 1987). A more recent analysis of the survival of these patients is shown in Figure 13-2. The control groups referred to are (1) historical controls (151 patients) treated at the Sydney Melanoma Unit from September 1978 to December 1981 and (2) concurrent controls (55 patients) who had lymph node metastases during the period of the trial, but who were not treated with the vaccine. (The main reason for their exclu-

FIGURE 13-2
Survival of patients with stage II melanoma treated with VMCL □——□ compared with the historical control ●——● and concurrent nonrandomized ▼——▼ groups. The number of patients at risk is indicated below the abscissa.

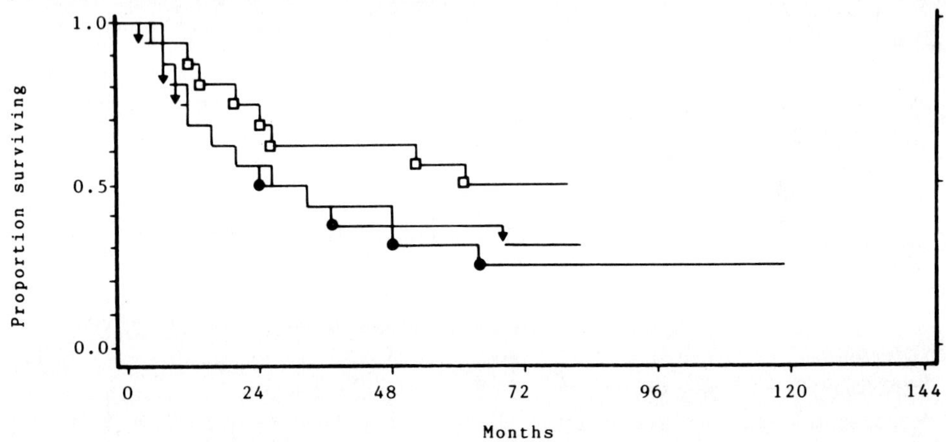

Number at risk

80	59	45	8	0	0	0
151	84	58	46	32	1	0
55	32	24	7	0	0	0

sion was [inadvertent] nonreferral to the Immunotherapy Clinic by intern staff at the time of discharge of the patient.) Although the study was not randomized, the groups of patients were well matched for age, sex, and thickness and ulceration of the primary melanoma. Surgical treatment of all patients in the study was carried out by the same surgeons (Professors Milton and McCarthy) according to a well-defined protocol that included elective lymph node dissections for primary melanoma >1.5 mm in thickness and incontinuity dissections when feasible (Balch et al., 1985b). Referral patterns, investigative procedures, and follow-up of the patients did not change over the period of the study.

As shown in Figure 13-2 and summarized in Table 13-3, the survival of the VMCL-treated group was significantly longer than both the historical and concurrent control groups. This was mainly evident in the patients with lymph node metastases detected more than 2 months after removal of the primary (delayed metastases), but was also evident in those with metastases detected at the time of treatment of the primary (synchronous metastases).

Side effects of the injections were mainly related to the primary response to VV in the vaccine. Previous immunity to vaccinia did not appear to influence the results. Vitiligo developed during the vaccination program in approximately 10 patients about the hairline, neck, shoulders, and arms. The extent of the vitiligo was marked in two patients and necessitated special precautions to avoid skin damage on sun exposure.

Influence of Low-Dose Cyclophosphamide on Treatment with VMCL

Studies on leukocyte-dependent antibody (LDA) activity in some of the patients treated with VMCL alone indicated that titers of antibody activity decreased with repeated vaccinations (Hersey et al., 1986). These findings, as well as the depression of natural killer (NK)-cell activity noted in some patients early in treatment, were consistent with the hypothesis that the injections may have increased suppressor-cell activity in the patients. In view of this, the effects of low-dose cyclophosphamide were examined in a second group of 102 patients treated with VMCL.

The rationale for the use of cyclophosphamide came from previous experimental studies showing that immune responses were increased in animals by pretreatment with cyclophosphamide, for example, Greenberg and Cheever (1984) and Dye and North (1984) were able to transfer immunity to established tumors in mice only when the mice had been pretreated with cyclophosphamide to remove suppressor cells in the recipients. Pretreatment of animals with cyclophosphamide was shown to increase syngeneic antibody responses to a tumor-cell vaccine (Livingston et al., 1985b), and studies in human subjects indicated that cyclophosphamide in low doses had selective effects on $CD8^+$ cytotoxic suppressor T cells in the circulation (Bast et al., 1983; Berd and Mastrangelo, 1987). Similarly, studies in humans showed that delayed skin test and antibody responses to keyhole-limpet hemocyanin (KLH) were increased in cancer

TABLE 13-3
SUMMARY OF MEDIAN AND 75% SURVIVAL OF TREATED AND HISTORICAL CONTROL GROUPS

	Number dead	Total number	Survival (months) Median	75%	χ^2	P*
All patients						
VMCL + cyclo	29	102	—†	22.3	5.01	.025
VMCL	33	80	—	23.7	12.2	.0025
Historical controls	106	151	32	12		
Synchronous nodal metastases						
VMCL + cyclo	9	36	—	21	0.3	.52
VMCL	10	31	61.4	52	4.1	.043
Historical controls	40	71	50	19		
Delayed nodal metastases						
VMCL + cyclo	20	66	37	22.3	8.65	.003
VMCL	23	49	60.4	17.1	9.7	.002
Historical controls	66	80	19.5	10		

*Comparisons made with historical control group in each case.
†Indicates median survival not reached.

patients (8 with malignant melanoma) given low-dose IV cyclophosphamide (300 mg/m^2) (Berd et al., 1984, 1986). Subsequent studies showed that delayed type hypersensitivity (DTH) responses were increased against melanoma antigens in 11 of 23 patients given low-dose cyclophosphamide before treatment with melanoma cell vaccine (Berd and Mastrangelo, 1987, 1988). Livingston et al. (1987) reported that pretreatment with cyclophosphamide of 20 patients with melanoma did not increase their DTH responses to dinitrochlorobenzene (DNCB) and recall antigens or serological responses to pneumococcal influenzal or melanoma antigens. However, in patients shown to have increased suppressor activity by several in vitro assays of suppressor-cell activity, there was a significant reduction from 1 to 4 weeks after pretreatment with cyclophosphamide.

The protocol used in our studies on patients with melanoma was to give four doses of cyclophosphamide orally at 300 mg/m^2 over the first 3 months of the VMCL treatment. The first dose of cyclophosphamide was given at the time of the second injection of the vaccine, after immunity to vaccinia had been established, since it was considered that the immunosuppressive effects of cyclophosphamide may have resulted in dissemination of the VV in nonimmune subjects.

Analysis of the effect of this treatment is shown in Figure 13-3 and summarized in Table 13-3. Although the follow-up on these patients is relatively short, there was no suggestion from the univariate analysis that survival was improved by addition of cyclophosphamide. Similarly, the multivariate analysis did not indicate any benefit from the addition of cyclophosphamide. As shown in Table 13-3 and Figure 13-3, the im-

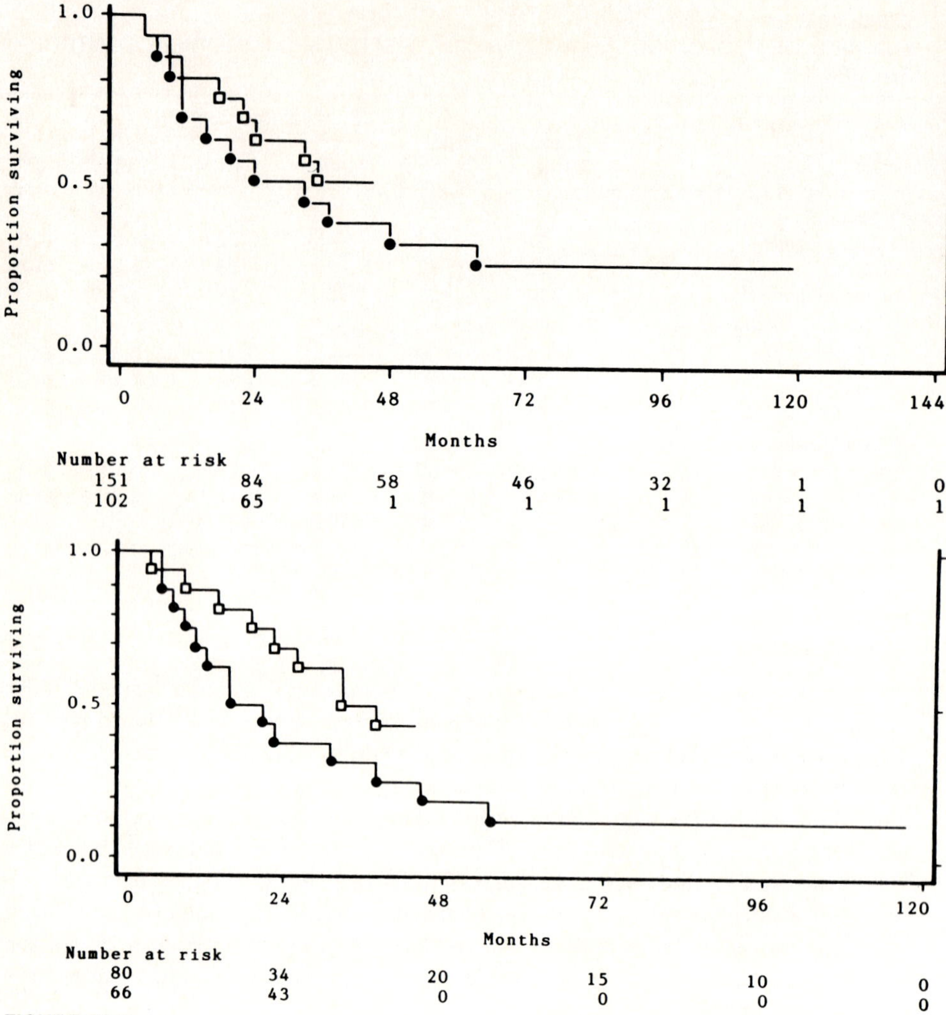

FIGURE 13-3
Delayed nodal metastases. Survival of patients treated with VMCL + low-dose cyclophosphamide □——□ compared to historical controls ●——●. The upper figure indicates survival of all patients, whereas the lower figure is a comparison of survival of treated and control patients with delayed metastases.

proved survival of patients treated with VMCL plus cyclophosphamide appeared to be confined to those with delayed metastases. Patients with synchronous nodal metastases did not appear to benefit from VMCL when combined with low-dose cyclophosphamide. It is possible, therefore, that low-dose cyclophosphamide had an adverse effect on the response to the vaccine in this patient group, perhaps because effects on helper T cells outweighed effects on suppressor T cells. Whether a different protocol of administration may have resulted in improved survival is not known.

Influence of the Number of Involved Lymph Nodes on Survival

As shown in Table 13-4, treatment with VMCL appeared to prolong survival in patients with one and three or more lymph nodes involved, whereas improved survival of patients with delayed metastases (Table 13-4) only appeared evident in those with metastases in one lymph node. The number of patients in these subgroups, however, were small, and these conclusions need to be substantiated in studies on larger patient numbers. They may indicate that treatment with VMCL was most effective in patients with small tumor burdens. Previous multivariate analysis of the influence of size of the lymph nodes on survival, however, revealed that the size of lymph nodes did not influence survival (Hersey et al., 1987).

TABLE 13-4
SUMMARY OF SURVIVAL ACCORDING TO NUMBER OF LYMPH NODES INVOLVED

			Survival (months)			
Group	**No.**	**% Alive**	**Median**	**75%**	χ^2	***P***
All patients						
One lymph node						
Control	57	42	53	15		
VMCL	32	78	—*	53	4.4	.035
VMCL + cyclo	64	81	—	—	2.4	.12
Two lymph nodes						
Control	26	35	49	20		
VMCL	21	52	—	24	.17	.68
VMCL + cyclo	17	59	25	19	.699	.403
Two lymph nodes						
Control	65	17	18	9		
VMCL	24	42	60	15	4.1	.043
VMCL + cyclo	18	44	26	12	.145	.703
Patients with delayed nodal metastases						
One lymph node						
Control	29	24	23	12		
VMCL	19	68	—	22	4.54	.033
VMCL + cyclo	39	79	—	—	4.9	.027
Two lymph nodes						
Control	12	17	19	12		
VMCL	14	50	—	17	1.8	.175
VMCL + cyclo	13	62	25	19	.25	.617
Two lymph nodes						
Control	38	13	16	7		
VMCL	15	31	25	11	1.64	.20
VMCL + cyclo	11	36	25	15	.186	.666

*Indicates median survival not reached.

Summary of Clinical Studies

The current information from these clinical studies suggests that intradermal injection of VMCL in the postoperative period may significantly improve survival of patients with lymph node metastases, especially in those with only one lymph node involved. There was no evidence that concomitant administration of low-dose cyclophosphamide further improved survival. In numerical terms (and assuming the present improvement in survival continues with longer follow-up of the patients), a salvage rate of 15 to 20 patients per 100 treated could be expected.

It is unlikely that the results reflect changes in the surgical management, investigation, or postoperative follow-up of the patients or differences in known prognostic factors. It also appears unlikely that the results merely reflect selection of control groups that have poor survival (reportedly a common error in historical controls [Sacks et al., 1982]), since the survival of the historical and concurrent control groups in the present study were similar to each other and comparable, or superior, to those reported for patients with stage II melanoma from a number of institutions, as shown in Table 13-2. Hence, although it cannot be excluded that the improved survival may reflect unidentified diagnostic factors, these have not been identified.

IMMUNOLOGICAL EFFECTS OF TREATMENT WITH VMCL

Serological Responses

In previous studies using assays of LDA, it was shown that immunization of melanoma patients with VMCL was associated with the rapid (i.e., within 4 weeks) development of antibody to allogeneic melanoma cells, but not to Epstein-Barr virus (EBV)-transformed B cells from the same donor as the allogeneic melanoma cells in 54% of patients (Hersey et al., 1986). However, tests carried out on IgG fractions separated from sera of patients not showing a response revealed that, in most instances, these were reactive to the melanoma cells, suggesting that circulating antigen may have neutralized the LDA activity (Hersey et al., 1986).

The nature of the antigens recognized by the antibody responses was analyzed by Western blot techniques. As shown in Figure 13-4, studies on extracts of the VMCL revealed at least 15 fractions that were identified by antibody responses. The number of fractions identified by sera from individual patients ranged from approximately 3 to 10. This variability was particularly noticeable against fractions above 50 kDa and below 40 kDa. Practically all patients responded to fractions of approximately 46 kDa and this was associated with responses to fractions of approximately 43 kDa and/or 49 kDa. Particularly strong responses were detected in approximately half the patients against fractions of 77, 85, 91, and 100 kDa, and a smaller number to fractions of approximately 34 to 36 kDa. Fractions in the Mol. wt. range of 60 to 69 were identified by antibodies in a number of sera, but were of low intensity compared to responses against the 43, 49, 46, and 77 kDa fractions.

The majority of these responses did not appear to be against antigens associated

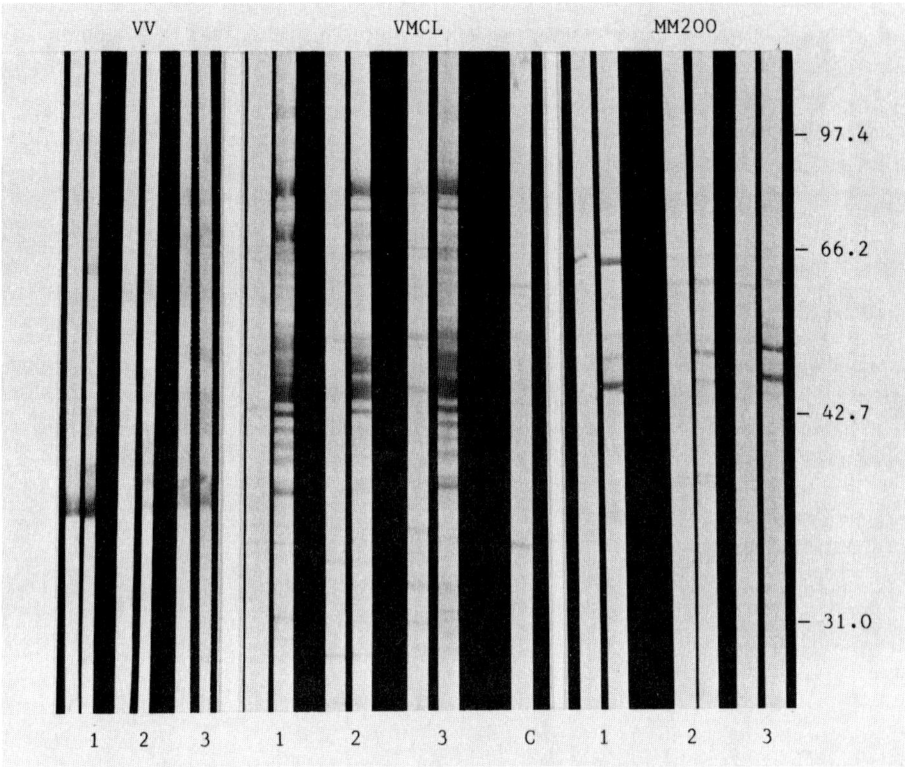

FIGURE 13-4
Western blot analysis of antibody responses of three patients treated with VMCL to extracts of vaccinia virus (VV), the vaccine (VMCL), and the allogeneic melanoma cell line MM200 used for preparation of the vaccine. C refers to sera from a control normal subject and 1, 2, and, 3 refer to three patients. Position of the standard Mol. wt. markers is indicated on the right-hand side. (See text.)

with the VV, since parallel studies on extracts of the virus showed that the fractions identified by antibody responses were located at different positions on the blot. Major responses against the virus appeared to be against fractions of approximately 27, 32, 34, 56 to 58, and 135 kDa. The 27-, 34-, and 58-kDa fractions were similar in Mol. wt. to the 28-, 35-, 60-, and 62-kDa vaccinia antigens recognized by mice, but the latter also recognized minor antigens at 25, 40, 42, 70, and 94 kDa that were not apparent in the present studies (Wilton et al., 1986).

Comparison of reactivity against extracts of VMCL and MM200 indicated that a number of fractions identified in VMCL were not identified in extracts of MM200, the main fractions identified in the latter being at 35, 38, 43, 46, and 49 kDa. The majority of patients did not appear to respond to fractions in the higher Mol. wt. range. One of the possible explanations for the disparity in responses to extracts of MM200 and VMCL is that the VMCL contained nonviral antigens induced by the virus infection. Examples of this include the 85-kDa hemagglutinin induced by VV on murine cells (Dales and Oldstone, 1982) and various members of the so-called heat shock proteins that may be induced by virus infection such as the 20-, 70- (68-, 72-, 78-kDa), and 90-kDa family (83, 90, 94, and 110 kDa) (Polla, 1988). Some of the latter appear to be immunogenic in their hosts such as the 65-kDa heat shock protein from mycobacteria (Polla, 1988) and the gp96 proteins in chemically induced murine tumors that induce individual specific tumor-rejection responses (Srivastava, 1989). The latter are homologous to human gp96 on human melanoma and other cells, but it seems uncertain whether the latter is immunogenic in humans or whether it is related to the immunogenic gp90 (Real et al., 1988).

One of the main questions is whether immunization with VMCL induced responses to the patient's (autologous) tumor. Studies on autologous extracts from six different melanomas clearly indicated that the vaccination procedure was associated with the development of antibody responses against fractions in autologous extracts that corresponded closely with those identified in VMCL. Most patients responded to the 43-, 46-, and 49-kDa fractions, but there was marked variability in response to the 35-, 39-, 77-, 85-, and 100-kDa fractions (Hersey et al., 1990). This variability in response to certain antigens in the vaccine is puzzling, because it might be expected that the same pattern of response would be seen in the patients. Comparison of responses to the vaccine and autologous melanomas suggested similar patterns of reactivity against both. This raises the possibility that the antigens in the vaccine recruited responses already initiated in response to the patient's tumor or that responses to some antigens are suppressed in certain patients. We are unable to distinguish between these possibilities at present.

Another question is whether the antibody responses have prognostic significance. We have previously reported that detection of LDA activity in serum of patients in the postoperative period was associated with a good prognosis (Hersey et al., 1983b). Bash and Wallack (1988), Jones et al. (1981), and Portoukalian et al. (1989) also reported that antibody responses to melanoma lines and gangliosides, respectively, were associated with a good prognosis. Vlock et al. (1986), however, in studies on 43 patients, found that antibody to a melanoma cell line predicted eventual disease recurrence. Generation of IgG antibody responses against melanoma does not necessarily indicate that the antibodies mediate antitumor effects. Instead, they may be markers of a helper T-cell response that may recruit other effector mechanisms against the tumor cells and hence be useful in characterization of antigens recognized by T cells. Whether responses against certain of the fractions identified on Western blots may be more prognostically significant than others is currently under investigation.

Cell-Mediated Cytotoxic Responses to the Vaccine

Studies on cell-mediated responses of peripheral blood lymphocytes (PBL) of patients were carried out on blood samples taken pretreatment and immediately prior to the next injection of VMCL, that is, cell-mediated cytotoxicity (CMC) was studied 2 weeks after the injections in the first 8 weeks, 3 weeks after the injections from 8 to 24 weeks, and 4 weeks after the injections given after 24 weeks. It is possible that CMC may have increased after each injection and then waned by the time the next blood sample was taken. This may explain why, in general, the changes in CMC were not marked, but nevertheless may be valuable in indicating lasting effects on CMC. (The term CMC is used rather than NK-cell activity, because it is possible that, in patients receiving therapy, T cells, as well as NK cells, were responsible for the cytotoxic effects.)

As reported elsewhere, in many patients, there was a decrease in CMC against an allogeneic melanoma cell and the K562 TCs (Hersey et al., 1986). However, these results may have been biased by the inclusion of a number of patients who subsequently showed clinical recurrence of their disease and who probably had significantly higher tumor load than those who have not relapsed. Tumor burden was shown in previous studies to be associated with low NK-cell activity in blood (Pross and Baines, 1976). Figure 13-5 illustrates the data on a larger sample of the patients treated with VMCL alone (31 patients) or VMCL plus low-dose cyclophosphamide (24 patients). The results can be summarized as follows: (1) A small but significant increase in CMC activity was seen at 4 weeks in patients treated with VMCL who did not develop recurrences, but there was a significant decrease in those who developed recurrences. These results would be consistent with the hypothesis that this latter group of patients had increased suppressor-cell activity that was further increased by treatment with VMCL. (2) Concomitant administration of low-dose cyclophosphamide did not appear to have significant effects on CMC in those not developing recurrent disease, but appeared to prevent depression of CMC in those who subsequently developed clinically recurrent disease compared to those treated with VMCL alone. Cessation of cyclophosphamide at 12 weeks appeared to result in a "rebound" increase in CMC. These results are consistent with the hypothesis that low-dose cyclophosphamide may have inhibited suppressor-cell activity. Table 13-5 indicates similar data from studies against the MM200 melanoma TCs.

FUTURE DIRECTIONS

The results from these studies with VMCL provide grounds for optimism that this treatment approach may improve the survival of patients with stage II melanoma. This is currently being tested in a randomized clinical trial on a national basis. Encouraging as the results may be, it is clear that a large proportion of patients with stage II melanoma treated with VMCL still develop recurrences and that further improvement in this treatment approach is needed. Focus on several main areas may help to achieve this.

Development of More Effective Vaccines

As discussed above, the main hypothesis for the efficacy of viral lysates is that the viral determinants in the membrane generate helper T-cell responses that amplify B

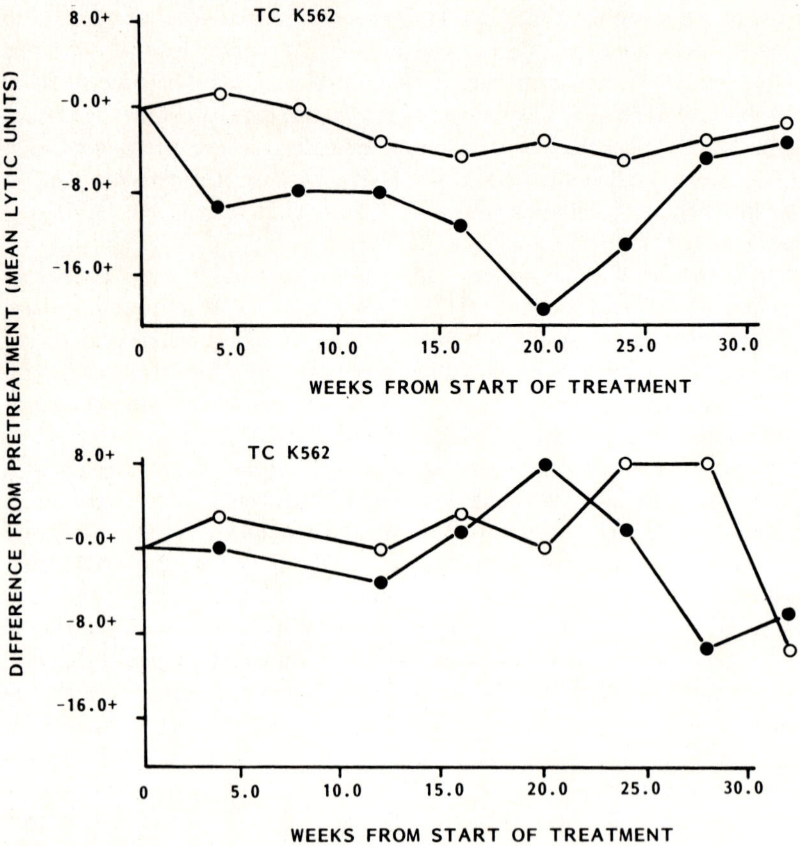

FIGURE 13-5
Cell-mediated cytotoxic (CMC) activity of blood lymphocytes from patients with stage II melanoma treated with VMCL alone (upper panel) or VMCL + low-dose cyclophosphamide (lower panel). Patients developing recurrences in the first 2 years ●——● treated with VMCL had a decrease in CMC during vaccination compared to those disease-free at 2 years ○——○. The decrease was not seen in patients who developed recurrences and who had received low-dose cyclophosphamide in the first 12 weeks of treatment with VMCL. Points shown are mean values of the change in lytic units compared with pretreatment values. Patient numbers shown at each time period are as indicated in Table 13-5.

and CTL responses to closely associated tumor-cell determinants in the cell membrane (Austin and Boone, 1979; Fujiwara et al., 1984; Shimizu et al., 1984). If this view is correct, the essential requirement of the vaccine is that it contain (1) antigens (melanoma-associated or nonmelanoma, e.g., viral antigens) recognized by helper T cells and (2) melanoma antigens recognized by CTL and B lymphocytes that cross-react with those on melanoma cells of the host. At present, information about the extent of

TABLE 13-5

EFFECTS OF TREATMENT WITH VMCL ± LOW-DOSE CYCLOPHOSPHAMIDE ON CELL-MEDIATED TOXICITY OF PATIENTS WITH STAGE II MELANOMA

	Weeks from commencement of treatment							
	0	4	8	12	16	20	24	28
VMCL Alone								
TC = MM200								
n	24	24	24	24	22	20	13	11
No rec.	15.2 ± 0.9	16.5 ± 0.8	15.3 ± 0.9	13.7 ± 0.8	13.2 ± 0.7	14 ± 0.7	14.2 ± 0.8	13.6 ± 0.9
n	7	7	7	7	6		4	5
Rec.	16.7 ± 1.8	11.8 ± 1.6	12.9 ± 0.9	13.2 ± 1.5	11.7 ± 1.4	—	10.6 ± 0.7	12.3 ± 1.2
	31	31	31	31	28	20	17	16
Total	15.5 ± 0.8	15.5 ± 0.8	14.8 ± 0.7	13.6 ± 0.7	12.8 ± 0.6	13.5 ± 0.7	13.7 ± 0.7	13.7 ± 0.9
VMCL + low-dose cyclophosphamide								
n	18	13	13	13	13	13	13	8
No rec.	13.8 ± 0.8	17.7 ± 0.6	17.4 ± 1.0	14.3 ± 0.8	15.7 ± 0.7	14.3 ± 1.1	16.7 ± 1.0	16.7 ± 1.1
n	6	5	5	5	5	5	5	3
Rec.	12.6 ± 1.7	12.5 ± 2.8	12.8 ± 2.8	12.8 ± 2.5	15.7 ± 1.8	17.6 ± 0.8	14.8 ± 0.9	13 ± 3.5
n	24	18	18	18	18	18	18	11
Total	13.5 ± 0.7	16.2 ± 1.1	16.6 ± 1.2	13.9 ± 0.9	15.7 ± 0.7	14.9 ± 1.0	16.1 ± 0.7	15.7 ± 1.3

Values shown are mean lytic units (20%/10^6 PBL) ± I.S.E. against the MM200 TC. n, number of patients studied; Rec., recurrence within 2 years of regional lymph node dissection.

cross-reactivity of serologically and T cell–defined antigens on melanoma cells is limited. As shown above, the serological response of patients treated with VMCL appear to define at least 15 different fractions on Western blots. Whether these are separate structures, proteins with variable glycosylation, or breakdown products of a more restricted number of structures is not clear. The antibodies appeared to be predominantly IgG, which suggests that the structures have been closely associated with, or contain, determinants recognized by T cells.

Certain of the fractions identified in these studies may be similar to those described previously; for example, the 32-, 49-, and 96-kDa fractions described by Savage et al. (1986), and the 22-, 38-, 43-, and 70-kDa fractions described by Fareed et al. (1988). Melanoma antigens of 66-kDa (Vlock et al., 1988), 80-kDa (Preddie et al., 1978), and 90-kDa (Real et al., 1988) as well as responses to ganglioside antigens (Cahan et al., 1982; Tai et al., 1983; Watanabe et al., 1982) have also been described.

Western blot studies to identify fractions stimulating T-cell responses suggested that there may be a more restricted number of structures on melanoma cells recognized by T cells than by antibody responses (Hersey et al., 1988). Further information about these structures should assist in the design of vaccines containing antigens that cross-react with those on melanoma cells from the majority of melanoma patients. If, as suggested by Van Waes et al. (1986), some tumor-cell variants lack antigens recognized by CTL, it is possible that specific immunotherapy will be ineffective in individuals with such variants. Clones of melanoma cells from the one tumor were shown to vary in their susceptibility to killing by cloned CTL (Anichini et al., 1986), but whether some clones are devoid of antigens recognized by other clones of CTL is unknown. It is also not known whether clones of tumor cells not recognized by CTL will nevertheless be killed by the so-called nonspecific responses mediated by activated macrophages, NK cells, and other lymphokine-activated killer (LAK) cells.

Overcoming Selective Immunosuppression Against Melanoma

There is evidence from several studies that melanoma cells may release factors that inhibit release of IL-2 (Hersey et al., 1983a) and the generation of DTH responses (Farram et al., 1982). Immunization with vaccines at sites distant to the tumor may largely circumvent this problem. It is also possible that administration of IL-2 with the vaccine may overcome the effects of such inhibitors. In addition to inhibitory factors from melanoma cells, there is good evidence for suppression of immune responses by suppressor T cells in melanoma patients (Hoon et al., 1987; Mukherji et al., 1986a, 1986b, 1987, 1989). The factors underlying their nature and mechanism of induction are, however, poorly understood. For example, it is unknown whether some melanoma antigens may have determinants that selectively induce suppressor T cells such as those described in leprosy (Mukherji et al., 1989) and for β galactosidase (Krzych et al., 1988) or whether their induction depends on the nature of antigen presentation to T cells. If our studies on NK-cell activity referred to above are any guide, immunization may increase their activity, particularly in patients with a significant tumor burden. A number of studies suggest that low-dose cyclophosphamide may reduce suppressor activity, particularly in patients with high levels of spontaneous suppressor-cell activity (Berd and Mastrangelo, 1988; Livingston et al., 1987). Cyclophosphamide is, however, relatively nonselective against lymphocyte subsets in humans, and more selective approaches for control of suppressor-cell activity are needed.

Antigen Presentation and Adjuvants

Induction of T-cell responses against most antigens is believed to require presentation of the antigen on MHC antigens compatible with those on T cells (Howard, 1985). These requirements are met in the case of VMCL by processing of the particulate material either by macrophages, dendritic cells, and B cells at the site of vaccination or in regional lymph nodes after transport of the antigen to these sites by the lymph. Coexpression of antigens from vaccinia and melanoma by the same antigen-presenting cell would presumably create conditions favorable for helper T cells responding to VV to help cytotoxic T cells and B cells with specificity to melanoma antigens coexpressed on APC of the host. Adjuvants may assist this process by creating an inflammatory focus to attract more APC and T cells to the site and by creating a depot of antigens for repeated stimulation of T cells. They may also act to orientate antigens in such a way as to facilitate recognition by B and T cells. Very little work has yet been carried out on different adjuvants in patients with melanoma, but it is of interest that use of an adjuvant composed of detoxified endotoxin or monophosphyl lipid A plus cell-wall skeletons was associated with a high remission rate in the studies of Mitchell et al. (1988). Design of trials to evaluate this and other adjuvants would appear to be a high priority in future studies.

Sanctuary Sites and Influence of Treatment on Sites of Distant Metastases

We have been impressed by the number of patients who relapse from metastases in the central nervous system (CNS). This may indicate that immune responses generated by the vaccine were not effective in the CNS. Similarly, local recurrences in scar tissue at the site of operation may indicate failure of T-cell traffic through these sites. If there were indeed sites not accessible to the immune system it might be expected that the sites of metastases may differ in the vaccine treated compared to untreated patients. Examination of this in patients treated with VMCL revealed that the relative incidence of metastases in brain and lung was similar to that in the control group. There appeared to be a marked decrease, however, in distant metastases to the skin in the treated group (Hersey, 1992). This unexpected result may have indicated that the immune response induced by the vaccine was more effective in the skin than at other body sites. Such a result would be consistent with recruitment of lymphocytes that home to the skin and raises a question as to whether immunization at certain body sites will preferentially induce immune responses in discrete regions of lymphocyte traffic.

In conclusion, active immunotherapy with melanoma vaccines is potentially an important additional treatment for melanoma that appears safe and relatively inexpensive. It seems crucial, however, that all that has been learned over the past decades about the conduct of clinical trials be applied in the evaluation of melanoma vaccines and that the power of molecular biology and cell-culture techniques be utilized to characterize and develop carefully defined vaccine products. In so doing, small gains from past studies may be used to hasten progress in this complex biological system.

ACKNOWLEDGMENTS

The work of the author described in this chapter was supported by grants from the New South Wales State Cancer Council, National Health and Medical Research Council, and the Sydney and Newcastle Melanoma Foundations.

REFERENCES

Anichini A, Fossati G, Parmiani G. Heterogeneity of clones from a human metastatic melanoma detected by autologous cytotoxic T lymphocytes. J Exp Med. 1986;163:215–220.

Austin FC, Boone CW. Virus augmentation of the antigenicity of tumor cell extracts. Adv Cancer Res. 1979;30:301–345.

Balch CM, Soong SJ, Shaw HM, Milton GW. An analysis of prognostic factors in 4000 patients with cutaneous melanoma. In: Balch CM, Milton GW, eds. Cutaneous melanoma. Philadelphia, Pa: JB Lippincott; 1985a:338–352.

Balch CM, Urist MM, Maddox WA, Milton GW, McCarthy WH. Management of regional metastatic melanoma. In: Balch CM, Milton GW, eds. Cutaneous melanoma. Clinical management and treatment results worldwide. Philadelphia, Pa: JB Lippincott; 1985b:93–130.

Bash JA, Wallack MK. Vaccinia virus oncolysates in the treatment of malignant melanoma. In: Nathanson L, ed. Malignant melanoma: biology, diagnosis and therapy. Boston, Mass: Kluwer Academic Publishers; 1988:177.

Bast RC, Reinherz EC, Maver C, Lavin P, Schlossman SF. Contrasting effects of cyclophosphamide and prednisone on phenotype of human peripheral blood leukocytes. Clin Immunol Immunopathol. 1983;28:101–114.

Berd D, Maguire HC, Mastrangelo MJ. Potentiation of human cell mediated and humoral immunity by low dose cyclophosphamide. Cancer Res. 1984;44:5439–5443.

Berd D, Maguire HC, Mastrangelo MJ. Induction of cell-mediated immunity to autologous melanoma cells and regression of metastases after treatment with a melanoma cell vaccine preceded by cyclophosphamide. Cancer Res. 1986;46:2572–2577.

Berd D, Mastrangelo MJ. Effect of low dose cyclophosphamide on the immune system of cancer patients: reduction of T suppressor function without depletion of the $CD8^+$ subset. Cancer Res. 1987;47:3317–3321.

Berd D, Mastrangelo MJ. Active immunotherapy of human melanoma exploiting the immunopotentiating effects of cyclophosphamide. Cancer Invest. 1988;6(3):337–349.

Bernards R, Schrier PI, Houweling A, et al. Tumorigenicity of cells transformed by adenovirus type 12 by evasion of T cell immunity. Nature. 1983;305:776–779.

Brickwell PM, Latchman DS, Murphy D, Willison K, Rigby PWJ. Activation of a Qa/T/a class I major histocompatibility antigen gene is a general feature of oncogenesis in the mouse. Nature. 1983;306:756–760.

Brocker EB, Zwadlo G, Holzmann B, Macher E, Sorg C. Inflammatory cell infiltrates in human melanoma at different stages of tumor progression. Int J Cancer. 1988;41:562–567.

Bukowski RM, Deodhar S, Hewlett JS, Greenstreet R. Randomized controlled trial of transfer factor in stage II malignant melanoma. Cancer. 1983;51:269–272.

Cahan LD, Irie RF, Singh R, Cassidenti A, Paulson JC. Identification of a human neuroectodermal tumor antigen (OFA-1-2) as ganglioside GD2. Proc Natl Acad Sci USA. 1982; 79:7629–7633.

Camacho ES, Pinksky CM, Braun DW, et al. DNCB reactivity and prognosis in 419 patients with malignant melanoma. Cancer. 1981;47:2446–2450.

Cascinelli N, Vaglini M, Nava M, et al. Prognosis of skin melanoma with regional node metastases. J Surg Oncol. 1984;25:240–247.

Cassel WA, Murray DR. Viral oncolysate in the treatment of regional metastases of melanoma. Symposium on head and neck cancer, MD Anderson Hospital and Tumor Institute, March 1985. In: Cancer in the Neck. Evaluation and Treatment. New York, NY: MacMillan; 1986.

Cassel WA, Murray DR, Phillips HS. A phase II study on the postsurgical management of stage II malignant melanoma with a Newcastle disease virus oncolysate. Cancer. 1983;52:856–860.

Chang A, Metz DH. Further investigation of the mode of entry of vaccinia virus into cells. J Genet Virol. 1976;32:275–282.

Cheresh DA, Reisfeld RA, Varki AP. O-acetylation of disialoganglioside GD3 by human melanoma cells creates a unique antigenic determinant. Science. 1984;225:844–846.

Dales S, Oldstone MBA. Localization at high resolution of antibody-induced mobilization of vaccinia virus hemagglutinin and the major histocompatibility antigens on the plasma membrane of infected cells. J Exp Med. 1982;156:1435–1447.

Dye ES, North RJ. Specificity of the T cells that mediate and suppress adoptive immunotherapy of established tumors. J Leukocyte Biol. 1984;36:27–37.

Fareed GC, Mendiaz E, Sen A, Juillard GJF, Weisenburger TH, Totanes T. Novel antigenic markers of human tumor regression. J Biol Resp Mod. 1988;7:11–23.

Farram E, Nelson M, Nelson DS, Moon DK. Inhibition of cytokine production by a tumour cell product. Immunology. 1982;46:603.

Freedman RS, Bowen JM, Herson J, Wharton JT, Rutledge FN, Hamberger AD. Virus modified homologous tumor-cell extract in the treatment of vulvar carcinoma. Cancer Immunol Immunother. 1980;8:33–38.

Freedman RS, Rutledge FN, Wharton JT. Adjunctive immunotherapy with virus modified tumor cell extract in patients with high risk squamous carcinoma of the uterine cervix. Am J Clin Oncol: Cancer Clinical Trials. 1983;6:155–156.

Fujiwara H, Shimizu Y, Takai Y, et al. The augmentation of tumor-specific immunity by virus help. I. Demonstration of vaccinia virus-reactive helper T cell activity involved in enhanced induction of cytotoxic T lymphocyte and antibody responses. Eur J Immunol. 1984;14:171–175.

Greenberg PD, Cheever MA. Treatment of disseminated leukemia with cyclophosphamide and immune cells. Tumor immunity reflects long-term persistence of tumor-specific donor T cells. J Immunol. 1984;133:3401–3407.

Hersey P. Current status of active specific immunotherapy of melanoma. In: Rümke K, ed. Therapy of advanced malignant melanoma. Pigment cell. Vol. 10. Basel: S Karger AG; 1990:183–200.

Hersey P. Active immunotherapy with viral lysates of micrometastases following surgical removal of high risk melanoma. World Surg. 1992; in press.

Hersey P, Bindon C, Czerniecki M, Spurling A, Wass J, McCarthy WH. Inhibition of interleukin 2 production by factors released from tumor cells. J Immunol. 1983a;131:2837–2842.

Hersey P, Edwards A, Murray E, McCarthy WH, Milton GW. Prognostic significance of leukocyte-dependent antibody activity in melanoma patients. J Natl Cancer Inst. 1983b;71:45–53.

Hersey P, Balch CM. Current status and future prospects for adjuvant therapy of melanoma. Austr NZ J Surg. 1984;54:303–316.

Hersey P, Murray E, Grace J, McCarthy WH. Current research on immunopathology of melanoma: analysis of lymphocyte populations in relation to antigen expression and histological features of melanoma. Pathology. 1985;17:385–391.

Hersey P, Edwards A, D'Alessandro G, MacDonald M. Phase II study of vaccinia melanoma cell lysates (VMCL) as adjuvant to surgical treatment of stage II melanoma. II. Effect on cell mediated cytotoxicity and leukocyte dependent antibody activity. Cancer Immunol Immunother. 1986;22:221–231.

Hersey P, Edwards A, Coates A, Shaw H, McCarthy WH, Milton GW. Evidence that treatment with vaccinia melanoma cell lysates (VMCL) may improve survival of patients with stage II melanoma. Cancer Immunol Immunother. 1987;25:257–265.

Hersey P, MacDonald M, Werkman H. Western blot analysis of antigens on melanoma cells recognized by cytotoxic T cells. J Natl Cancer Inst. 1988;80:826–835.

Hersey P, Werkman H, Edwards A. Western blot analysis of serological responses following immunization with vaccinia viral lysates of melanoma cells. Int J Cancer. 1990;46:612–617.

Hilal EY, Pinksky CM, Hirshaut Y, et al. Surgical adjuvant therapy of malignant melanoma with *Corynebacterium parvum*. Cancer. 1981;48:245–251.

Hill GJ, Moss SE, Golumb FM, et al. DTIC and combination therapy for melanoma. III. DTIC (NSC45388) surgical adjuvant study COG protocol 7040. Cancer. 1981;47:2556–2562.

Hoon DSB, Bowker RJ, Cochran AJ. Suppressor cell activity in melanoma-draining lymph nodes. Cancer Res. 1987;47:1529–1533.

Howard JC. Immunological help at last. Nature. 1985;314:494–495.

Jones PC, Sze LL, Liu PY, Morton DL, Irie RF. Prolonged survival for melanoma patients with elevated IgM antibody to oncofetal antigen. J Natl Cancer Inst. 1981;66:249–254.

Koprowski H, Love R, Koprowska I. Enhancement of susceptibility to viruses in neoplastic tissues. Texas Rep Biol Med. 1957;15:559.

Krzych U, Fowler AV, Miller A, Sercarz EE. Induction of helper and suppressor T cells by nonoverlapping determinants on the large protein antigen, β galactosidase. FASEB J. 1988; 2:141–145.

Lindenmann J. Viruses as immunological adjuvants in cancer. Biochimica et Biophysica Acta. 1974;355:49–75.

Lindenmann J, Klein PA. Viral oncolysis: increased immunogenicity of host cell antigen associated with influenza virus. J Exp Med. 1967;126:93.

Livingston PO, Albino AP, Chung TJC, et al. Serological response of melanoma patients to vaccines prepared from VSV lysates of autologous and allogeneic cultured melanoma cells. Cancer. 1985a;55:713–720.

Livingston PO, Jones M, Deleo AB, et al. The serologic response to meth A sarcoma vaccines after cyclophosphamide treatment is additionally increased by various adjuvants. J Immunol. 1985b;135:1505–1511.

Livingston PO, Cunningham-Rundles S, Marfleet G, et al. Inhibition of suppressor-cell activity by cyclophosphamide in patients with malignant melanoma. J Biol Resp Mod. 1987;6:392–403.

Mallon V, Domber EA, Holowczak JA. Vaccinia virus proteins on the plasma membranes of infected cells. II. Expression of viral antigens and killing of infected cells by vaccinia virus-specific cytotoxic T cells. Virology. 1985;145:1–23.

McGovern VJ. Spontaneous regression of malignant melanoma. In: Blaustein A, ed. Melanoma: histological diagnosis and prognosis. New York, NY: Raven Press; 1982:138–147.

Mehra V, Brennan PJ, Rada E, Convit J, Bloom BR. Lymphocyte suppression in leprosy induced by unique *M. leprae* glycolipid. Nature. 1984;308:194–196.

Milich DR. T- and B-cell recognition of hepatitis B viral antigens. Immunol Today. 1988;9:380–386.

Mitchell MS, Kan-Mitchell J, Kempf RA, Harel L, Shawu H, Lind RN. Active specific immunotherapy for melanoma: phase I trial of allogeneic lysates and a novel adjuvant. Cancer Res. 1988;48:5883–5893.

Morton DL, Nizze JA, Gupta RK, Famatiga E, Hoon DSB, Irie RF. Active specific immunotherapy of malignant melanoma. In: Kim JP, Kim BS, eds. Current status of cancer control and immunobiology. Seoul: JG Park.

Mukherji B, Wilhelm SA, Guha A, Ergin MT. Regulation of cellular immune response against autologous human melanoma. I. Evidence for cell-mediated suppression of in vitro cytotoxic immune response. J Immunol. 1986a;136:1888–1892.

Mukherji B, Nashed AL, Guha A, Ergin MT. Regulation of cellular immune response against autologous human melanoma. II. Mechanism of induction and specificity of suppression. J Immunol. 1986b;136:1893–1898.

Mukherji B, Guha A, Loomis R, Ergin MT. Cell-mediated amplification and down regulation of cytotoxic immune response against autologous human cancer. J Immunol. 1987;138: 1987–1991.

Mukherji B, Guha A, Chakraborty NG, et al. Clonal analysis of cytotoxic and regulatory T cell responses against human melanoma. J Exp Med. 1989;169:1961–1976.

Polla BS. A role for heat shock proteins in inflammation. Immunol Today. 1988;9:134–137.

Portoukalian J, Carrel S, Dore JF, Rumke P. Pilot study of immunotherapy with melanoma-associated gangliosides in high-risk melanoma patients. 2nd International Conference on Melanoma. 1989;322. Abstract.

Preddie E, Hartmann D, Lewis MG. Human tumor specific antigens (1) An allogeneic antigen from patient "PY" melanoma tumor cell plasma membranes. Cancer Biochem Biophys. 1978;2:161–167.

Pross HF, Baines MG. Spontaneous human lymphocyte-mediated cytotoxicity against tumour target cells. I. The effect of malignant disease. Int J Cancer. 1976;18:593–604.

Real FX, Furukawa KS, Mattes MJ, et al. Class 1 (unique) tumor antigens of human melanoma: identification of unique and common epitopes on a 90-kDa glycoprotein. Proc Natl Acad Sci USA. 1988;85:3965–3969.

Roses DF, Provet JA, Harris MN, Gumport SL, Dubin N. Prognosis of patients with stage II cutaneous malignant melanoma. Ann Surg. 1985;201:103–107.

Sacks H, Chalmers TC, Smith H. Randomized versus historical controls for clinical trials. Am J Med. 1982;72:233–238.

Savage HE, Rossen RO, Hersh EM, Freedman RS, Bowen JM, Plager C. Antibody development to viral and allogeneic tumor cell-associated antigens in patients with malignant melanoma and ovarian carcinoma treated with lysates of virus infected tumor cells. Cancer Res. 1986;46:2127–2133.

Schirrmacher V. Postoperative activation of tumor-specific T-cells as a means to achieve control of minimal residual disease. In: Fortner JG, Roads JE, eds. General Motors Research Foundation "Accomplishments in cancer research 1986". Philadelphia, Pa: JB Lippincott; 1987:218–232.

Shimizu Y, Fujiwara H, Ueda S, Wakamiya N, Kato S, Hamaoka T. Eur J Immunol. 1984;14:839–843.

Sinkovics JG, Papadopoulos NE, Plager C. Viral oncolysate in immunotherapy of human tumors. In: Yohn DS, Blakeslee JR, eds. Advances in comparative leukemia research, International Symposium for Comparative Research on Leukemia and Related Diseases. New York, NY: Elsevier North Holland; 1981:613–615.

Srivastava PK. gp96 antigens are cell surface-displayed stress proteins. 7th International Congress of Immunology. 1989;101–28. Abstract.

Tai T, Paulson JC, Cahan CD, Irie RF. Ganglioside GM2 as a human tumor antigen (OFA-1-1). Proc Natl Acad Sci USA. 1983;80:5392–5396.

Van Waes C, Urban JL, Rothstein JL, Ward PL, Schreiber H. Highly malignant tumor variants retain tumor-specific antigens recognized by T helper cells. J Exp Med. 1986;164:1547–1565.

Veronesi U, Adamus J, Aubert C, et al. WHO study group trial No. 6. A randomized trial of adjuvant chemotherapy and immunotherapy in cutaneous melanoma. New Engl J Med. 1982;307:913–916.

Vlock DR, DerSimonian R, Kirkwood JM. Prognostic role of antibody reactivity to melanoma. J Clin Invest. 1986;77:1116–1121.

Vlock DR, Scalise D, Meglin N, Kirkwood JM, Ballou B. Isolation and partial characterization of melanoma-associated antigens identified by autologous antibody. J Clin Invest. 1988; 81:1746–1751.

Wallack MK. Specific immunotherapy with vaccinia oncolysates. Cancer Immunol Immunother. 1981;12:1–4.

Wallack MK, McNally KR, Leftheriotis E, et al. A southeastern cancer study group phase I/II trial with vaccinia melanoma oncolysates. Cancer. 1986;57:649–655.

Wallack MK, Bash JA, Leftheriotis E, et al. Positive relationship of clinical and serologic responses to vaccinia melanoma oncolysate. Arch Surg. 1987;122:1460–1463.

Watanabe T, Pukel CS, Takeyama H, et al. Human melanoma antigen AH is an autoantigenic ganglioside related to GD2. J Exp Med. 1982;156:1884–1889.

Widmer M, Bach F. Antigen driven helper cell-independent cloned cytolytic T lymphocytes. Nature. 1981;294:750.

Wilton S, Gordon J, Dales S. Identification of antigenic determinants by polyclonal and hybridoma antibodies induced during the course of infection by vaccinia virus. Virology. 1986;148:84–96.

Wise KS. Vesicular stomatitis virus-infected L1210 murine leukemia cells: increased immunogenicity and altered surface antigens. J Natl Cancer Inst. 1977;58:83–90.

CHAPTER 14

ACTIVE SPECIFIC IMMUNOTHERAPY OF CANCER: THERAPEUTIC VACCINES ("THERACCINES") FOR THE TREATMENT OF DISSEMINATED MALIGNANCIES

Malcolm S. Mitchell

The presentation of an antigen to $CD4^+$ helper T lymphocytes is the central process in any specific immune response such as the specific response to a tumor, upon which all the other elements depend. That presentation leads to activation of the helper T cells, as well as the macrophages, with consequent release of cytokines from both. Proliferation and activation of macrophages, helper T cells, and killer T cells then occur after stimulation by the released cytokines. Finally, specific effector cells such as killer T cells and nonspecific effector cells such as activated macrophages interact with, and kill, the tumor targets.

Active specific immunotherapy is the attempt to reintroduce tumor-associated antigens (TAA) in a form in which they will be more immunogenic, to utilize what is the most powerful pathway for rejecting microbial invaders in the attack on more insidious enemies. The aim is to try to achieve rejection of the tumor, or at least to initiate that process by significantly augmenting the patient's own potential immunity. If that potential for a stronger immunity against the tumor were realized, a number of subsequent types of immunotherapy would be rendered far more effective, particularly adoptive immunotherapy: reintroduction of the host's autologous antitumor helper and killer T cells after further stimulation ex vivo.

In this chapter, we will discuss active specific immunotherapy, or what has often been called treatment with cancer vaccines. However, the term "vaccine" has usually implied a preventive against disease, as in prophylaxis against viruses or protozoa, whereas cancer investigators have always treated patients who have either gross or microscopic deposits of tumor. Thus we have frequently substituted the phrase "therapeutic vaccine," or the contraction "theraccine" (coined at Ribi ImmunoChem Research, Inc.) to describe cancer vaccines. When the etiology of a particular cancer is established, a true vaccination to prevent its occurrence may in fact be possible.

We will mainly focus here on the use of active immunotherapy to treat disseminated, macroscopically measurable tumor masses. Approaches to developing immunogens effective in causing immunologically mediated rejection of autologous tumors have ranged from the use of killed autologous tumor cells, or extracts derived from autologous tumors, to the use of killed allogeneic or occasionally xenogeneic mate-

TABLE 14-1
ALLOGENEIC MATERIALS (E.G., LYSATES) AS IMMUNOGENS: THEORETICAL DRAWBACKS

Objection	Comment
1. There may be considerable batch-to-batch variation and, thus, irreproducible responses.	1. Variability of a standard preparation is less than with cultured autologous materials. Presence of particular antigens could be standardized with probes for antigenic determinants such as monoclonal antibodies.
2. Alloimmunization (against HLA class I or class II antigens) might predominate, or even preempt, the response.	2. Alloimmunization may potentiate immunological reactivity against tumor antigens, i.e., improve the immunogenicity of histotype-specific (common) TAA. Clinical trials in patients with measurable lesions indicate that an antitumor response is obtainable even in the face of alloimmunization.
3. "Too many" TAA different from those on the autologous tumor might dilute those common to the autologous tumor.	3. If only one or a few immunodominant epitopes characterize a histotype of tumor, immunization with a standard (i.e., allogeneic) preparation may be relatively simple.
4. A standard (allogeneic) preparation requires that there be common TAA within a histological class.	4. Such common TAA may well exist, as demonstrated by work with murine and human monoclonal antibodies.
5. Autologous TAA might be recognized by CTL only with self-MHC. Immunization with allogeneic lysates might cause recognition of TAA only in context of allo-MHC, precluding recognition of autologous tumor.	5. It is equally plausible that processing of the antigen will occur in context of self and lead to self-MHC–restricted response. Also, some human cytotoxic T cells may recognize TAA without self-MHC restriction.
6. A state of tolerance might exist, precluding any attempt at active immunotherapy.	6. Potent adjuvants and/or the use of inhibitors of suppressor T cells might overcome tolerance.

CTL, cytotoxic T lymphocytes; MHC, major histocompatibility complex; TAA, tumor-associated antigens.

TABLE 14-2
ALLOGENEIC MATERIALS (E.G., LYSATES) AS IMMUNOGENS: POTENTIAL ADVANTAGES

1. Standard material to treat large groups of patients at several centers.
2. Permits treatment of patients with microscopic residual disease, to prevent recurrence.
3. Does not presuppose the overriding importance of any one antigen in eliciting rejection.
4. Might improve immune response to weakly immunogenic common TAA by presenting them in a "foreign" context.
5. All antigens of cell, including internal ones, are immediately available for presentation to the recipient's immune system.
6. Batches readily producible from frozen stocks (vs autologous, fresh tumor).
7. Ultimately, affords the possibility of prevention during the preneoplastic stage.

rials. Nonspecific active immunotherapy (adjuvants) has often been added to the regimen. While the issue is far from settled, there are theoretical advantages and disadvantages to the use of either autologous or allogeneic materials. We have summarized these issues in Tables 14-1 and 14-2. The points and counterpoints mentioned in the tables will be discussed in this chapter. Since our approach to treatment has been with allogeneic tumor materials, we have constructed the tables from that perspective. We will cite studies on TAA derived from autologous and allogeneic sources without attempting to settle the controversy over which is superior.

Although the administration of well-defined TAA (preferably fully synthesized epitopes made by recombinant DNA technology) would be ideal, our knowledge of which antigens are immunogenic to human beings and would thus be most relevant to include in vaccines is incomplete. For that reason, we will emphasize work attempting to define those antigens with materials derived from patients who are subjects for immunization.

AUTOLOGOUS THERACCINES

Studies in Animal Models

Virally Altered Tumor Cells in Mice Schirrmacher and colleagues have contributed significantly to our understanding of active specific immunotherapy. They have incisively studied the mechanisms by which syngeneic tumor cells can be made more immunogenic in mice through alterations by mutagens or especially viruses. With the highly metastatic variant ESb 289 of the chemically induced T lymphoma Eb 288 (derived from L5178Y lymphoma), these investigators have shown that infecting the tumor with Newcastle disease virus (NDV) significantly augments its immunogenicity and can prevent metastatic spread (Heicappell et al., 1986). Tumor-specific cytotoxic T lymphocytes (CTL) against ESb were augmented at least threefold in the spleen by this approach (Von Hoegen et al., 1988). $CD4^+$ and $CD8^+$ cells directed against TAA appeared to cooperate in the spleen (Schild et al., 1989).

Cytotoxic T lymphocytes specific for the virus were not detected, and the NDV modification appeared to act as a "second signal" for specific antitumor immunity.

This was presumably accomplished by stimulating helper T cells to produce more cytokines in the milieu of tumor-specific CTL, which was the mechanism suggested by Hamaoka and colleagues for augmentation produced by vaccinia-altered tumor cells (Yoshioka et al., 1986). In fact, increased interleukin-2 (IL-2) production was found with NDV-treated spleen cells in Schirrmacher's experiments (Schild et al., 1989), even though that group could not directly demonstrate $CD4^+$ cells recognizing viral antigens.

Based on these careful observations, clinical trials in patients with various tumors have recently begun, with results not yet available, although conditions for inducing delayed hypersensitivity (DTH) to various TAA have been established (Schirrmacher et al., 1989).

Making a tumor more foreign to the host, or "xenogenization," as Kobayashi (1979) has called it, has also involved in vitro treatments with viruses other than NDV, particularly vaccinia (see also Chapter 13 on this subject) of haptens (Prager and Gordon, 1978) or adjuvant substances such as muramyl dipeptide (MDP) (Yoshioka et al., 1986). It should be kept in mind that alloantigens might conceivably serve the same purpose: to provide a potent second signal to the host's immune system and augment the response to relatively weak common TAA.

Butanol-Extracted Antigens in Mice Kahan, Pellis, LeGrue, and their colleagues have performed a series of experiments with 2.5% 1-butanol–extracted antigens, which remove surface-membrane antigens but leave the tumor cells intact. They have shown that three weekly injections, without an adjuvant, can specifically prevent the outgrowth of a methylcholanthrene (MCA)-induced fibrosarcoma in mice (LeGrue et al., 1980; Kahan et al., 1980, 1982). The development of an antigenically dissimilar MCA-induced tumor was unaffected. Prevention of subsequent metastasis was accomplished after treatment of mice was begun following resection of a primary tumor. Moreover, true immunotherapy was accomplished with macroscopic (4-mm) tumor nodules when cyclophosphamide (CY) was used preceding the inoculation of butanol extracts (Kahan et al., 1982). Cyclophosphamide alone was only partially successful, but long-term survival was achieved only when butanol-extracted antigens were added. Since the immunogenicity of this chemically induced tumor is higher than that of most spontaneous human tumors, whether the same approach will succeed in humans (particularly without an adjuvant) remains to be established. Nevertheless, these experiments are among the few to treat advanced tumors, rather than preventing the "take" of recently inoculated tumor cells, and were among the first to try to develop a method for isolating TAA for more precisely defined vaccines.

Defined Tumor-Associated Antigens as Immunogens Several investigators have attempted to define important TAA that might serve as specific immunogens for patients and to optimize their immunization schemes using these antigens. Livingston et al. have chosen gangliosides GM_2 and GD_2 for particular study in mice because antibodies to those gangliosides have been produced in patients immunized with whole-cell vaccines (Livingston, 1989a, 1989b; Livingston et al., 1989). They have decided to select schedules of administration to mice that lead to the highest titers of antibodies against these gangliosides (Livingston et al., 1989). The greater immunogenicity of GM_2 and GD_2, rather than GD_3, in humans is probably because of the lesser expression of the first two gangliosides on human tissues compared to the last. This is, incidentally, in direct contrast to the situation in the mouse. There are much higher concentrations of all three gangliosides on melanoma cells than in normal human tissues, other than the brain (Tsuchida et al., 1987). One might question the strategy of choosing to optimize schedules and select adjuvants based upon antibody formation, which may not be the closest correlate of clinical responses (v.i.). Furthermore, as Livingston himself has noted, because of differences in expression of the various gangliosides in the mouse compared to humans, direct comparisons of immunogenicity between the two species is impossible. Nevertheless, the selection of important gangliosides as immunogens, at least one of which is present on a given melanoma cell, should be tested. Clinical trials comparing various schemes of immunization with each ganglioside have already begun.

The gene for a 97-kDa glycoprotein related to the transferrin receptor that is present on human melanoma cells has recently been transfected into mouse melanoma K-1735 in C3H mice (Estin et al., 1989) in order to establish a treatment model more closely related to human melanoma. This glycoprotein was the target antigen detected by several mouse monoclonal antibodies in different laboratories and thus is thought to be an important antigenic structure on the melanoma cell. Whether it is an important immunogen for humans should be determined shortly, since the glycoprotein has been produced by complementary DNA (cDNA) cloning and is now entering clinical trials.

Guinea Pigs Hanna and colleagues have worked for some time on a model of line 10 hepatoma in guinea pigs, with which they established principles that have since been applied to human studies. In particular, the importance of viable *Mycobacterium bovis* (strain bacillus Calmette-Guérin [BCG]) as an adjuvant, at an optimal ratio to tumor cells of 1:1 and of a dose of 1×10^7 irradiated, nonreplicating but still viable tumor cells was emphasized (Hanna et al., 1979). Only three injections were required in these studies for optimal effect in preventing the tumor from growing beyond a small inoculum. One particularly interesting observation with potential application to human trials is that in the treatment of existing tumor nodules, vaccines of line 10 + BCG appeared to alter the integrity of the vascular bed in tumors, increasing the ingress of chemotherapeutic agents (Hanna and Key, 1982). This biological effect constitutes one of a limited number of situations in which a rationale can be presented for giving immunotherapy before chemotherapy rather than afterward.

Studies in Humans

From serological studies with a patient's autologous serum and with mouse monoclonal antibodies (Albino et al., 1981; Old, 1981), "private" antigens unique to a given patient were often found. It therefore seemed that the only reasonable approach to immunizing patients was with their own tumor cells. Several investigators have, in fact, attempted to use autologous irradiated melanoma cells to treat patients with advanced melanoma or renal cell carcinoma, or microscopic residual colon cancer. Except for large primary tumors such as colonic, rectal, and renal tumors an immunotherapy with autologous cells is necessarily limited to patients with advanced disease. Under those circumstances, there are sufficient numbers of cells to permit a series of injections over several weeks or months.

Melanoma For the past 8 years, Berd, Maguire, and Mastrangelo have used low-dose CY followed by irradiated melanoma and BCG as an active specific immunotherapeutic regimen (Berd et al., 1984, 1986, 1990; Berd and Mastrangelo, 1988). Clinical responses have been elicited in 5 (12.5%) of 40 patients with measurable advanced melanoma, 4 of which were complete remissions (CR) lasting several years. On the whole, immunological reactivity measured by DTH skin reactions to irradiated autologous melanoma cells has been far more commonly developed by the regimen (61% of 43 patients, at some time during treatment) than was a clinical regression. Nevertheless, of 10 patients with some degree of regression, 8 had DTH. The CY was found to be important for this immunological reactivity, but since the response rate is low, its role in causing clinical remissions is uncertain. More recently, this group has tried to alter the immunogenicity of the autologous cells by adding haptens such as dinitrophenol, causing a greater degree of inflammatory response at tumor sites (Berd et al., 1989).

Livingston and colleagues have used both autologous and allogeneic melanoma cells in attempts at therapeutic immunization, usually in early-stage melanoma (Livingston et al., 1983; Livingston, 1989a). Autologous cells have usually been treated with viruses or "xenogenized" in other ways to try to improve their immunogenicity. Specific humoral responses against melanoma antigens were rare, but those that were present were against gangliosides GM_2 or GD_2. Current trials are directed toward immunization with the purified gangliosides together with an adjuvant and low-dose CY as an immunorestorative agent. Early data with GM_2 given with low-dose CY and BCG suggest that patients with AJCC stage III melanoma who have titers of antibody $\geq$1:40 have had a longer disease-free survival ($P = .03$) than patients with lower titers (Livingston, 1989b). Whether successful immunization reflected, rather than caused, the increased survival will be determined in a randomized trial.

Renal Cell Carcinoma Among the first to attempt active immunotherapy in patients with renal cell carcinoma were Tykka and his colleagues, who have recently summarized a 13-year follow-up of patients receiving treatment for advanced disease after a palliative nephrectomy (Tallberg et al., 1984). Polymerized autologous tumor tissue was used together with immunological adjuvants in this trial of 71 patients. Results were compared with a nonrandomized control group receiving conservative treatment of various kinds. Life expectancy in the immunotherapy group is 44.5 months versus 19 months. In an earlier report on these patients, Tykka and colleagues indicated that measurable pulmonary lesions regressed or remained stable in many of the patients (Tykka et al., 1974).

Clinical trials in patients with measurable lesions have been performed by two different investigative groups, one of which is still actively pursuing this approach. In a study attempting to reproduce the results of Tykka et al. (1974), Neidhart and colleagues (1980) treated 30 patients at Ohio State University with polymerized autologous tumor cells treated with ethylchlorformiate. Two complete and 2 partial remissions (PR) were elicited, while 11 patients had stability of disease for a prolonged period. It is interesting that the 2 CR occurred in stable-disease patients whose autologous tumor had been exhausted and who were then switched to allogeneic cells. A follow-up trial by the Southwest Oncology Group entirely with autologous tumor cells gave a lower response rate (1 CR and 1 PR in 27 patients) with entirely autologous cells (Fazekas de St. Groth, 1982). McCune and colleagues (McCune et al., 1981; Sahasrabudhe et al., 1986) have treated groups of 14 and 20 patients with autologous irradiated renal cell carcinoma cells, together with *Propionobacterium acnes (C. parvum)*. In the first trial (McCune et al., 1981), 4 of 14 patients (28.5%) had PR, with 1 long-term stability, and in the second (Sahasrabudhe et al., 1986), which added low-dose CY preceding the course, 1 CR and 4 PR (25%) were elicited. McCune et al. are now attempting to combine active immunotherapy with lymphokines to try to improve their results.

Overall, these data suggest that a proportion of patients with renal cell carcinoma treated with irradiated or polymerized autologous tumor cells shows regression of metastatic tumors, especially in the lung or bone. Another group of patients may experience stability of tumor masses, but in renal cell carcinoma that is not an infallible criterion of success unless the duration of stability is several years.

Colon Carcinoma Hanna, Hoover, and colleagues have been conducting clinical trials of active specific immunotherapy in colorectal carcinoma since the early 1980s (Hanna and Hoover, 1985; Hoover et al., 1985). These studies were based on the earlier work cited with the line 10 guinea pig hepatoma and BCG. Their results, in a randomized trial after primary surgery with irradiated autologous tumor cells and BCG versus observation have indicated that the vaccinated group has fared better than the controls. After a 6-year follow-up, the recurrence rate was significantly lower in the treated group, with 3 of 20 relapses (15%) versus 9 of 20 (45%) in controls, who were just observed. Those vaccinated patients who have relapsed have tended to have local recurrences that were resectable, and so none had died within 6 years. In contrast, control patients have usually had recurrences at metastatic sites, and 4 of the 9 had succumbed to their illness. However, this form of treatment has not been successful in treating a small number of patients with metastatic colorectal carcinoma (Hanna, personal communication).

ALLOGENEIC THERACCINES

It may theoretically be desirable to use autologous immunization to ensure that all immunologically relevant TAA, especially private antigens, are included in a vaccine.

Nevertheless, the limited number of tumor cells present in a small primary melanoma nodule or regional node makes this approach impractical for those patients who might benefit most from it: those with microscopic residual disease. The issue of unique antigens notwithstanding, there is considerable evidence to suggest that allogeneic theraccines are effective in treating solid tumors. Since monoclonal antibodies from mice and humans have indicated antigens held in common by a histotype of tumor, a theraccine may be constructed from one individual's cells or from cell lines derived from several individuals. In fact, allogeneic theraccines have several potential advantages over autologous tumor preparations, as indicated in Table 14-2.

Melanoma

Shed Antigens in Supernatant Fluids Bystryn and co-workers have treated patients for several years with supernatant fluids from cultures of four different melanoma cell lines, three from humans and one from a hamster. The latter was discovered by cytogenetic analysis of the ostensibly human cell lines, but has purposely been retained since it did not cause adverse reactions and might conceivably be useful as a xenogeneic line. No adjuvant other than alum has been used, in order to see the immunological effects of tumor-derived antigens alone. A clinical response was elicited in 1 of 13 patients with measurable tumor masses, with another showing stability (Bystryn et al., 1986). When the preparation was used in patients after surgery of primary and regional melanoma (AJCC stage IB-III) in an uncontrolled trial, an improved survival (median, >38 months) was found in those patients in whom a DTH response to the melanoma supernates was induced by vaccination, versus 13.5 months in those who had no DTH induced (Bystryn et al., 1989). These interesting data need to be confirmed in a controlled trial with larger numbers of subjects.

Viral Oncolysates This topic is the subject of Chapter 13, but it is appropriate to mention that vaccinia, influenza, and NDV have each been used in human as well as in mouse trials. Viral oncolysates have not been used to treat established metastatic melanomas but have instead been given after surgery for early-stage disease to try to prevent systemic recurrences. Cassel and co-workers (1983) were among the early investigators in this field, obtaining strong suggestive evidence for improved disease-free survivals after treatment with NDV melanoma lysates. Confirmatory data have come from Wallack and colleagues (1989) in uncontrolled trials with stage III melanoma. Wallack et al. (1989) recently reported that 39 patients treated with a vaccinia oncolysate of melanoma cells had an improved disease-free survival, compared with 39 matched historical controls. After a mean follow-up of 17 months, only 14 patients (36%) had relapsed, whereas approximately 20 relapses (50%) would have been expected. A randomized, controlled adjunctive-therapy trial has begun in melanoma patients with stage III disease (positive lymph nodes) after resection, in which patients will receive either vaccinia alone or the vaccinia oncolysate. This trial should definitively settle the issue of whether this form of treatment can improve the disease-free interval and overall survival.

Of immediate relevance and importance to the subject of this chapter is the therapy of disseminated ovarian cancer tumors. Freedman et al. (1988) have successfully treated ovarian carcinoma patients, who had ascites and/or pleural effusions, with viral oncolysates derived from two cultured lines of ovarian carcinoma cells. Influenza A/PR8/34 (PR8) was used to lyse the carcinomas. Treatment was given regionally, that is, intraperitoneally and/or intrapleurally, which led to disappearance of ascites in 7 of 31 patients. One had disappearance of a pleural effusion as well. Two other patients without ascites had a reduction in tumor masses. The duration of response ranged from 3 to 19 months. Evidence for an increase in nonspecific cytotoxicity in the peritoneum was found, indicating a regional immune response (Furukawa et al., 1989). T cell–mediated cytotoxicity was not extensively studied. Freedman et al. (1989) have also used viral oncolysates of squamous-cell carcinoma cells (SW756 cell lines) as an adjunct to radiation therapy for treating carcinoma of the uterine cervix. Unfortunately, no dramatic evidence for prolongation of either the progression-free interval or median survival time was detected in the patients receiving viral oncolysates in addition to radiation, compared with radiation alone.

Irradiated Allogeneic Melanoma Cell Theraccine Morton and associates have for some time been studying irradiated "whole-cell melanoma vaccines" given with BCG and other materials as adjuvants, mainly in the treatment of AJCC stage III melanomas. More recently, they have also reported (Morton et al., 1989) responses in 5 of 27 patients (18.5%) with advanced, measurable melanomas. Like other studies with viral oncolysates, purified gangliosides, and allogeneic supernates, an improved disease-free survival relative to historical controls has been achieved. Prospective trials are clearly warranted here, too. It is of interest that antibodies to GM_2 and GD_2 were produced in those patients who achieved long disease-free survivals, which suggested to the investigators and others that these gangliosides might be useful immunogens.

Studies with Allogeneic Melanoma Lysates and the Novel Adjuvant DETOX™

Our group has reported three different trials with immunizing preparations of mechanical homogenates (lysates) of melanoma cell lines combined with a novel adjuvant called DETOX™ (Mitchell et al., 1988, 1990a, 1990b). DETOX™ consists of a combination of monophosphoryl lipid A, or "detoxified" endotoxin (from which its name is derived) and mycobacterial cell-wall skeletons in a squalane (saturated squalene) oil base containing Tween-20 as an emulsifier. The schema of preparation of this theraccine is shown in Figure 14-1.

Two cell lines, MSM-M-1 (M-1) and MSM-M-2 (M-2), derived from individual biopsies of subcutaneous nodules from two female patients were mechanically disrupted in a Polytron stainless steel homogenizer and then freeze-thawed in order to kill

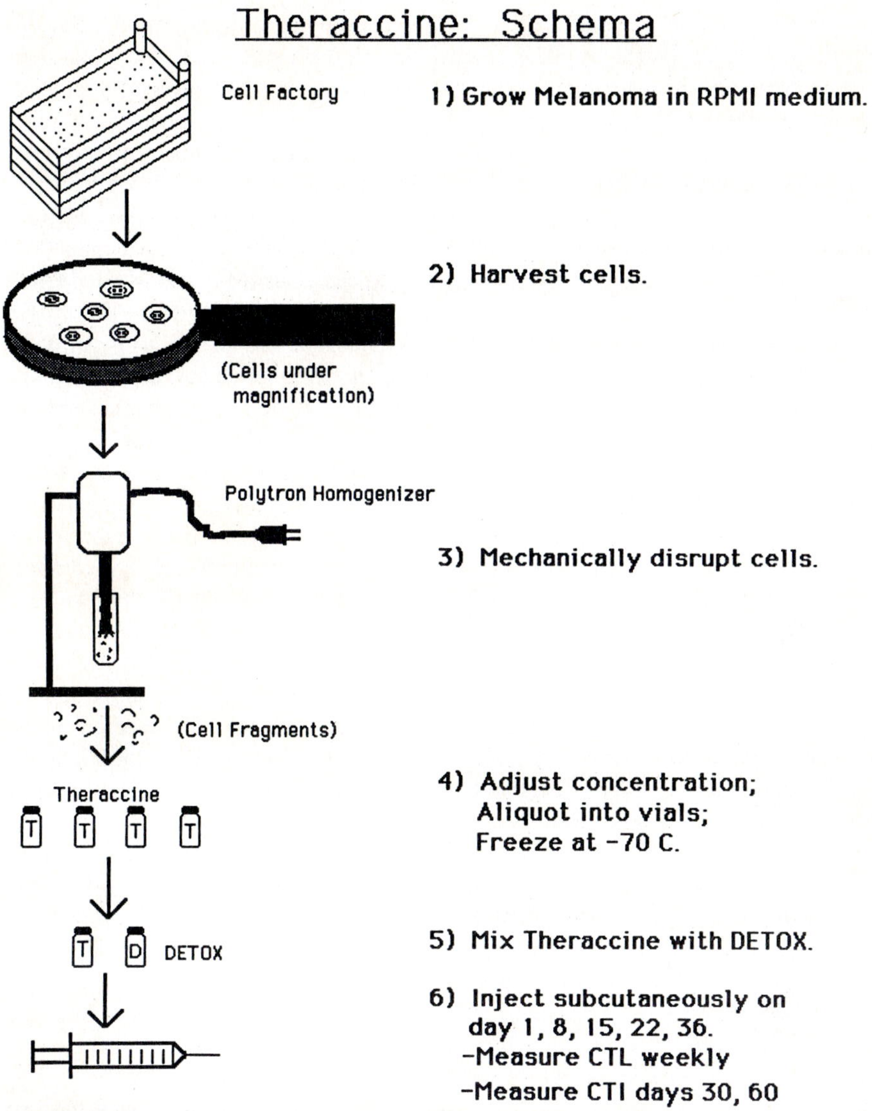

FIGURE 14-1
Schema of preparation of melanoma theraccine. CTL, cytotoxic T lymphocytes; CTI, cold target inhibition (competition) assay.

them without the use of irradiation, enzymes, or mitomycin C, which might conceivably alter their immunogenicity. The potent new adjuvant was used, and in an early study low-dose CY was also given as pretreatment. From the first patient on the phase I trial, it was obvious that not only could immunity be elicited but also that clinical responses occurred as a result of immunization with the allogeneic materials (Mitchell et al., 1988). We have thus far completed six separate clinical trials with various batches of melanoma theraccine (Mitchell et al., 1988, 1990a, 1990b, 1991). MAC 1, 3, and 4 lysates were produced in our laboratory from the same set of cell lines (M-1 and M-2); MAC 5 was produced from two different cell lines (M-3 and M-4). MAC 6 (frozen) and MAC 6 lyophilized lysates were produced by Ribi ImmunoChem Research from our cell lines M-1 and M-2 mixed in the same proportion as in our MAC 4 trial. In all of the studies we have found a subgroup of melanoma patients with disseminated disease in whom we could elicit a PR or CR by active specific immunotherapy. Our most recent analysis of those studies is shown in Tables 14-3 and 14-4.

We have been able to immunize 65 of 111 patients (58%), judging from an increase in precursors of CTL (pCTL) in the peripheral blood directed against melanoma-associated antigens (MAA). Antibody production has been detected by enzyme immunoassay (EIA) in 44%, but when the specificity was carefully checked only a minority of the patients had antibodies reactive only against melanomas. Inexplicably, we have been generally unable to induce DTH reactivity to our materials, at least over the course of 2 months.

Of the immunized patients, approximately one third of them (20% of all patients treated) have shown significant shrinkage of their tumor masses. Five percent of the patients have had CR of disease, and 15% have had PR thus far. From our data, we anticipate that 15% to 25% (95% confidence interval) of patients will have a major clinical response by this procedure.

It is clear that at least one third of the patients who experience a clinical response have had an improved survival as a direct result. As shown in Table 14-5, all 10 patients with a PR or CR (or in one instance, a long-term stability of disease) lasting more than 6 months have lived more than a year, six of whom have survived at least 2 years. Three lived more than 4 years, with two of the three still alive and fully functional. All have received continual booster injections of the theraccine, but have had no other form of treatment. A PR in which there was disappearance of most lesions, rather than >50% shrinkage of each, appears to be useful, not only a CR. In contrast to these results, only CR with chemotherapy generally improve survival, and in melanoma specifically even CR usually do not. Overall survival for the group may also have been improved, judging from an analysis of our data by others (Von Eschen K, unpublished data on file at Ribi ImmunoChem Research, Inc.), but it is far too early to make that assertion with any authority.

There have been major clinical responses to each new batch of theraccine we have produced from frozen stocks of the melanoma cell lines, as well as to lots produced at Ribi ImmunoChem Research, Inc. Therefore, the lot-to-lot variation that is a theoret-

TABLE 14-3
MELANOMA THERACCINE: IMMUNOLOGICAL RESPONSES

	Number of patients/total tested	
Trial	pCTL	Antibodies
Phase I		
(MAC 1 + 3)	12/22	5/22
(MAC 5)	8/18*	12/17†
Phase II		
(MAC 4)	14/21	11/25‡
(MAC 6)	13/20	N.D.
(MAC 6 lyophilized)	8/15	N.D.
(CY + MAC 6 lyophilized)	10/15	N.D.
Total	65/111 (58%)	28/64 (44%)

"MAC n" designates melanoma antigen from cultured cells, nth batch; pCTL, precursors of cytolytic T lymphocytes; CY, cyclophosphamide.

*Dose-response noted: titers increased in 2 of 6, 1 of 6, and 5 of 6 patients, respectively given 5, 10, or 20×10^6 tumor-cell equivalents of lysate per dose.

†No dose-response noted; specificity not tested by absorptions.

‡Only 2 of 11 specific for melanoma on absorption.

TABLE 14-4
MELANOMA THERACCINE: CLINICAL RESPONSES

	Number of patients			
Trial	CR	PR	Minor	Total
Phase I				
(MAC 1 + 3)	2	3	2	17
(MAC 5)	0	1	1	6*
Phase II				
(MAC 4)	1	4†	2	25
(MAC 6)	0	3	1	20‡
(MAC 6 lyophilized)	1	1	2	19‡
(CY + MAC 6 lyophilized)	1	3	1	19‡
Total	5 (4.7%)	15 (14.1%)	9 (8.5%)	106 (100%)

*Only 20×10^6 tumor-cell equivalent level tabulated.

†Includes a patient with 17-month stability who lived >3 years.

‡Melanoma theraccine used in these three trials was produced by Ribi ImmunoChem Research, Inc.

CR, complete response; PR, partial response.

TABLE 14-5
CURRENT STATUS OF PATIENTS RESPONDING >6 MONTHS

Patient	Original response	Date of last follow-up	Duration of survival	Status
L.A.	CR 7/30/86	12/91	>65 mo	Alive. No evidence of disease. Brain metastasis resected 8/21/88.
H.H.	PR 4/8/87	7/91	51 mo	Relapsed in brain 7/90. Died 7/91.
S.H.	PR 7/7/87 CR 3/8/88	10/91	>50 mo	Alive. Single, stable 8–10 mm lung nodule since 9/88.
L.R.	Stable from 9/8/87	12/90	39 mo	Relapsed in brain 1/89. Died 12/90. His metastases were slowly progressive from 1/89.
P.D.	PR 12/2/87 (CR ileum)	12/89	24 mo	Died 12/89. Ileal lesions never recurred.
R.B.	CR 12/27/89	12/91	>24 mo	Alive. No evidence of disease.
K.R.	PR 11/30/89	12/91	>25 mo	Alive. Three 5-mm s.c. nodules remain. No visceral disease.
G.W.	PR 9/5/90 (CR of omental mass, 10/30/90)	12/91	>15 mo	Alive
J.S.	PR 6/27/90	12/91	>16 mo	Alive
C.K.	PR 10/28/90	12/91	>14 mo	Alive. Progressed at local site 10/91.

All patients have received booster doses of theraccine monthly and/or semiannually.

ical drawback to any biological preparation has not been a major problem thus far. Even lyophilized theraccine has been effective, which should permit most hospital pharmacies to store the material conveniently at refrigerator temperature.

Possible Immunological Mechanisms Involved in the Stimulation of Antiautologous Tumor Immunity by Allogeneic Theraccines

The Roles of Cyclophosphamide and DETOX™ We have pretreated approximately one half of our patients with a low dose of CY (300 mg/m^2) 4 to 7 days before beginning immunization. In our phase I study (Mitchell et al., 1988) we found no obvious difference in clinical responders, with 5 patients distributed "equally" between the CY+ and CY− groups. However, 8 of 11 patients pretreated with CY had an increase in pCTL, while 3 of 11 without CY had an increase. Cyclophosphamide was not necessary to achieve clinical responses in our phase II trial (Mitchell et al., 1990a), where it was omitted entirely as part our several attempts to simplify the regimen. Cyclophosphamide may have improved the response to MAC 6 lyophilized theraccine produced by Ribi ImmunoChem Research (Table 14-4), but the difference was slight. For the moment, we are including CY in all theraccine protocols, to give every potential advantage to our patients, some of whom may have excessive levels of suppressor T cells or humoral suppressor factors. Berd and co-workers (1984, 1986, 1988, 1990) have emphasized the importance of CY in autologous immunization, which may be a very different type of situation.

Similarly, the role played by the adjuvant DETOX™ has not been definitively established. Because MAA are only weakly immunogenic, we have used the adjuvant in all of our studies with allogeneic lysates. DETOX™ alone has never caused systemic responses in its phase I trials, given by the intradermal (intratumoral) route, making it unlikely that it alone caused the clinical responses we observed.

Correlation of Clinical Response with Precursors of Cytolytic T Lymphocytes in the Blood The strongest correlate of a major clinical response to melanoma theraccine has been an increase in pCTL. T lymphocytes capable of becoming cytotoxic against melanomas were measured by a limiting dilution mixed lymphocyte–tumor cell essay. Patients have had approximately 1 pCTL in 10,000 to 50,000 lymphocytes at baseline. After immunization the mean peak rise has been 5- to 10-fold, to a level of approximately 1 pCTL in 2,500 to 5,000 lymphocytes. That peak has occurred approximately 3 to 6 weeks after beginning treatment with the theraccine (mode = 4 weeks), with a decline toward baseline thereafter.

Patients who have failed to generate CTL against at least one component of the theraccine have uniformly failed to have a clinical response. There has been only one response in 33 patients in which we did not detect pCTL. Assays in that patient (K.R.) were considered unreliable due to technical problems, with low frequencies in all assays during that 4-month span of time. Furthermore, we have since derived active CTL clones from that patient's blood. Of those who have generated pCTL, approximately one third have had an objective remission. Fisher's exact tests for correlations between success or failure to generate CTL and "clinical responses" (including CR, PR, minor responses, and 1 long-term stability) have been significant at a *P* value of approximately .05 in each of the individual clinical studies.

Cytolytic T lymphocytes from the peripheral blood of these melanoma patients have reacted not only against the immunizing melanomas but against a variety of our melanoma cell lines. Cold target competition assays, in which unlabeled ("cold") tumor cells are added to compete with chromium 51 (^{51}Cr)-labeled targets, have shown no inhibition of the killing of melanoma cells by other types of tumor or by allogeneic lymphoblasts (Mitchell et al., 1988, 1990a). However, cold target competition assays with various types of cell lines showed that all seven melanoma cell lines we tested blocked the reactivity of the T cells against the M-1 or M-2 target cell. All of our melanoma cell lines fortuitously shared the HLA-A2 allele or the cross-reactive HLA-A28, although they differed from each other at other loci. Thus, it is likely that HLA class I-restricted CTL recognized melanoma epitopes in the context of the important HLA-A2/A28 presenting molecule (Darrow et al., 1989; Wolfel et al., 1989).

Antibody responses were frequently detected, but there was no correlation between the ability to form antibodies and a clinical response to the theraccine. We have concluded that the major effector mechanism after active immunotherapy in melanoma is cell-mediated rather than humoral, and that any antibody responses are an epiphenomenon. Under other circumstances, of course, such as when lymphokine-activated killer cells with Fc receptors have been created, monoclonal antibodies purposely administered, or perhaps antibodies produced endogenously, may have beneficial antitumor effects.

Cloning of CD4$^+$ and CD8$^+$ Cytolytic T Lymphocytes from Immunized Patients

In order to study more accurately the interaction of CTL from patients with MAA, we have cloned CTL from the peripheral blood at several times during the process of immunization. CTL appear to be at their peak in the blood at some time between 2 and 6 weeks after the first injection. We have obtained CTL of CD4$^+$ and CD8$^+$ phenotypes, respectively, by several different methods. CD4$^+$ cells appear to be favored by the presence of antigen-presenting cells (APC) and mixed lymphocyte tumor cell (MLTC) interaction, while CD8$^+$ cells can be sorted directly from the blood without previous augmentation by MLTC and generally without APC. Since most of our in vitro stimulations involve one or both of the allogeneic melanomas used to immunize the patient, rather than autologous melanoma cells, our results may have been skewed toward broadly reactive CTL as opposed to entirely self-restricted CTL as classically described in the mouse, and in cultures of tumor-infiltrating lymphocytes. Regardless, we have found CD8$^+$ CTL that kill all melanomas that share an HLA class I allele, almost always HLA-A2 with our patients and cell lines. Only a small proportion of CD8$^+$ CTL in our hands has been completely self-restricted (Kan-

Mitchell et al., submitted for publication). This confirms data alluded to earlier from Wolfel et al. (1989) and Darrow et al. (1989). In some instances, we have also encountered $CD8^+$ clones that lyse HLA class I negative melanomas (Harel et al., submitted for publication). Vanky et al. (1989) have found cytolytic lymphocytes that can be induced to attack tumor cells lacking class I MHC molecules by intensive immunization in vitro with MHC-positive tumor cells.

It is of considerable interest to us that we have cloned $CD4^+$ CTL that are HLA class I restricted. Such $CD4^+$ CTL clones have lysed HLA class II negative melanomas. Furthermore several independent investigators in our laboratory have blocked the activity of $CD4^+$ CTL with monoclonal antibodies to framework determinants of HLA class I but not class II, or in some instances with both (Harel et al., submitted for publication; Goedegebuure et al., submitted for publication; LeMay et al., submitted for publication). $CD4^+$ CTL require for their detection a longer assay, somewhat higher ratios of lymphocytes to melanoma cells, and, most importantly, pretreatment of the melanoma cells overnight with interferon-gamma to upregulate HLA, accessory and MAA molecules. HLA class I-restricted human $CD4^+$ CTL have been observed by other investigators in humans (Herlyn D, Vanky F, personal communications, 1990, 1991).

Thus, it is imperative that we not be limited in our thinking by dogmas generated in mouse experiments when considering types and restriction elements of human CTL.

HLA Phenotypes of Responding Patients We have HLA-typed the lymphocytes from 70 patients given melanoma theraccine, as well as the melanoma cell lines used as for immunization and as the immunological targets in our in vitro assays (Mitchell et al., 1992). We hypothesized that either similarity or disparity between the HLA antigens on the immunizing melanoma lysates and the patients was correlated with clinical response. An association was found between certain HLA class I alleles and a clinical response, but it is open to two different interpretations. HLA-A2 and HLA-28, B12 "split" (including HLA-B12, HLA-B44, and HLA-B45), and HLA-C3, particularly in combination, are overrepresented in responders. Patients who expressed C3 and one other class I tissue type found in the vaccine (either A2/A28 or B12) had an increased chance of responding, possibly as high as 60% to 70%. There were no responders in the group of 22 patients who expressed neither A2/A28 nor B12, while 26% of the 47 patients expressing either A2/A28 or B12 responded. Only one patient responded in the group of 21 patients who expressed neither A2/A28 nor C3, while 28% of 36 patients expressing either A2/A28 or C3 responded. Thirty-eight percent of patients with two or three of these alleles had a response, nearly double the percentage in the overall group.

We are not certain whether patients whose HLA alleles matched those in the theraccine responded because of the match, or because those alleles enabled the patient's CTL to respond better. HLA-A2 is known to be an important presenting molecule for MAA (Darrow et al., 1989; Wolfel et al., 1989) and may permit CTL from patients sharing that allele to recognize and kill melanoma cells most efficiently, after immunization with the allogeneic theraccine. Our data would suggest that the other two molecules, the HLA-B12 group and HLA-C3, are also important restriction elements for HLA class I-restricted CTL. In fact, data from Hom et al. (1991) have recently indicated the importance of HLA-B44 in vitro.

Immunological Implications of Immunotherapy with Allogeneic Materials As we have mentioned, there already existed evidence for a common antigen or antigens characterizing a histotype of tumor from monoclonal antibody serology. That allogeneic melanomas can immunize a patient against his own tumor adds further support to this concept. Beyond that, the data may confirm the concepts generated in mice about the need for a "second (helper) signal" in generating immunity of weak TAA. A second group of $CD4^+$ helper T cells may be recruited, reacting against the additional antigen on the tumor cell, whether that antigen be a hapten, a viral antigen, or an alloantigen. Those additional helper T cells then may generate lymphokines such as IL-2 and IL-4 in the immediate vicinity of helper T cells and pCTL programmed to respond to the TAA. This would necessarily increase the proliferation and elicitation of cytotoxicity in the tumor-specific component of the response. The addition of an adjuvant also seems to be essential, judging from the weaker responses elicited with supernatants alone, and may serve the same function as an additional antigen included on the tumor cells. Interleukin-1 stimulated by the adjuvant (Mitchell et al., 1973; Mokyr and Mitchell, 1975) may also play a role in eliciting subsequent helper T cells and cytotoxic cells.

This concept is shown schematically in Figure 14-2. We are indebted to a similar schema presented by Forni, Hamaoka, and colleagues as the model for our own (Forni et al., 1988). Hersey (see Chapter 13) has independently chosen a very similar model to explain results with vaccinia oncolysates. After we drew our schema, we found that $CD8^+$ CTL proliferate in vitro in the absence of APC, if the melanoma has MHC class I molecules with which to present melanoma epitopes. The portion of the diagram showing macrophages presenting TAA to $CD8^+$ cells is therefore unnecessary, if not incorrect.

The recognition of the autologous tumor in vivo may well be through the "classical" corecognition of MHC class I histocompatibility antigen and TAA by $CD8^+$ cells. In addition, $CD4^+$ killer cells, recognizing tumor-derived epitopes in the context of HLA class I or II molecules might be effector cells. It is particularly interesting in this regard that a subunit gp160 vaccine given to human immunodeficiency virus (HIV)-seronegative volunteers induced cytolytic $CD4^+$ T cells that were capable of recognizing HIV-infected leukocytes in vitro (Orentas et al., 1990). This finding reinforces our contention that at least some endogenously synthesized antigens can be recognized by $CD4^+$ CTL, which are the type of T cell that exogenously administered (soluble) protein antigens stimulate preferentially.

Immunohistology of Rejection We have conducted immunohistological studies on frozen sections from six patients whose subcutaneous melanoma nodules were in

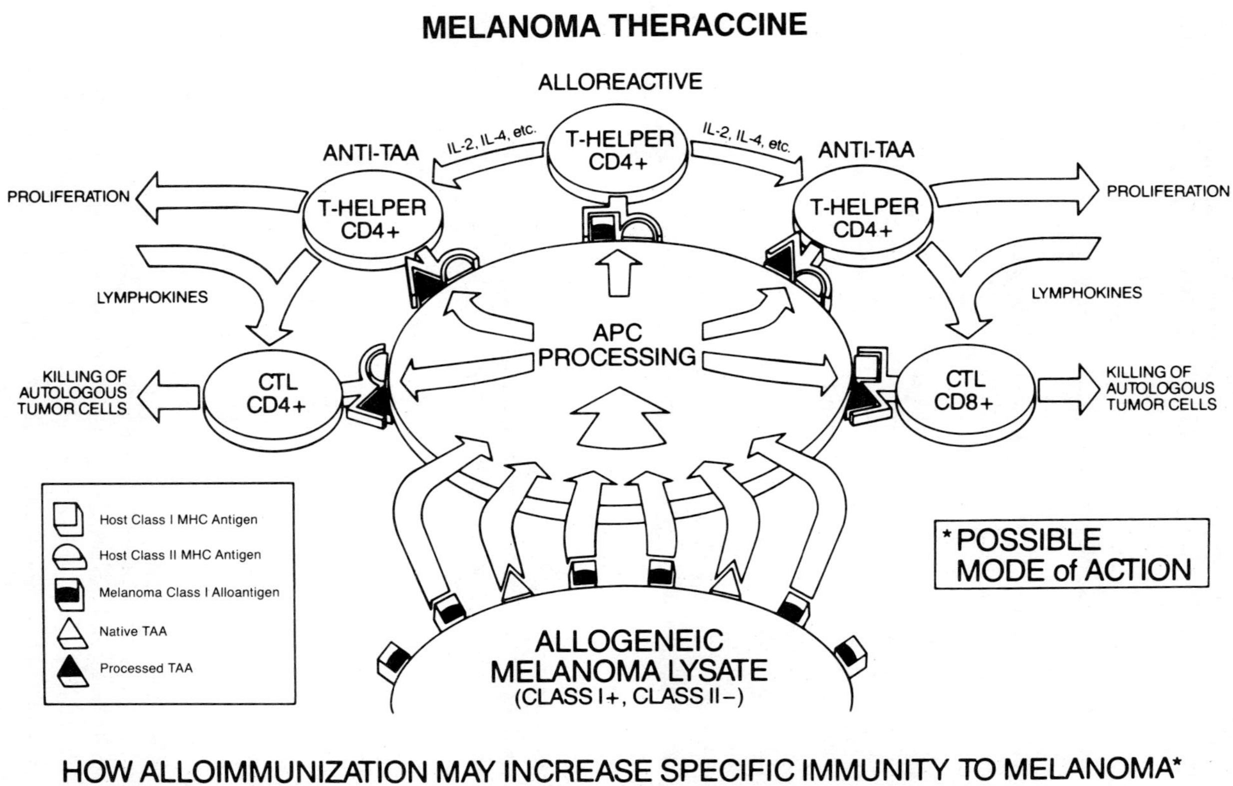

FIGURE 14-2
Schema of possible additive effects of allogeneic materials with tumor-associated antigens (TAA) in active specific immunotherapy. Our hypothesis is that the participation of alloreactive helper T cells leads to (nonspecific) amplification of specific reactivity to TAA. Note that, for symmetry, the possible reactivity of CD8 CTL with macrophages bearing class I antigens and TAA is illustrated. That interaction is not a necessary part of this lymphokine-mediated amplification hypothesis, nor is it proven to occur in vivo.

the process of being rejected after theraccine treatment (Mitchell et al., manuscript in preparation). Four of the six patients were studied on at least two occasions. The consistent findings were of a peripheral and particularly *perivascular* accumulation of $CD3^+$ (T) lymphocytes rather than a profound infiltration of T cells throughout the tumor site. Macrophages were the predominant cells in all lesions, and they were most often present throughout the tumor. Interestingly, $CD4^+$ lymphocytes predominated 3:1 or 3:2 over $CD8^+$ lymphocytes, with activated class II+ T cells and macrophages present in abundance. Cells with natural killer cell (NK) markers such as CD16 were absent, and those with the Leu 7 marker found on both NK and T cells were rare. There were no B lymphocytes except in lesions that had undergone complete regression some time previously. The tumor cells had the appearance of a "cloudy swelling."

Lesions from untreated control melanoma patients have had the same amount of lymphocytes or perhaps even somewhat more, equal in the proportion of $CD4^+$ and $CD8^+$ cells, but those were scattered throughout the lesion and the macrophages were unactivated in their appearance.

These results using sensitive immunohistochemistry are different from those with conventional stains, which have indicated few cells in untreated lesions. Since tumor-infiltrating lymphocytes have usually been recovered from *untreated* melanomas, it has always been logical that there were more cells present than hematoxylin-eosin staining showed.

Our data suggest a DTH lesion, where activated macrophages are the mediators of rejection, rather than one where CTL were the predominant effector cells. Lymphokines and monokines released into the lesion may have caused the death of the tumor cells, or tumor cell death may have been by ischemia due to the perivascular accumulation of host cells. Whether direct killing by cytolytic T cells played a major role was uncertain from the histological appearance, but we did not take the biopsies until several weeks after impending rejection was first evident and have not done serial biopsies. It is also possible that if CTL were involved, they were $CD4^+$ rather than $CD8^+$ CTL.

In vitro correlations notwithstanding, one cannot yet conclude that cytolytic T cells of any kind, $CD4^+$ or $CD8^+$, were more important than helper T cells acting perhaps in a DTH reaction to cause in vivo rejection.

Attempts to Produce Melanoma-Associated Antigens by cDNA Cloning Results obtained with whole melanoma cells, lysates, or extracts of various purity should be considerably improved when pure MAA immunogenic to humans are isolated. Efforts are in progress in several laboratories to determine which antigens stimulate human lymphocytes. Hersey et al. (1988) have used Western immunoblotting and subsequent stimulation of proliferation to identify MAA in the range of 45 to 50 kDa that are consistently recognized by $CD4^+$ clones. While we have also found a stimulatory peptide in that molecular weight range, at least one other of approximately 91 kDa is also stimulatory to one of our $CD4^+$ CTL clones (Harel et al., 1990).

We are attempting to produce more specific theraccines by synthesizing MAA directly by cDNA technology. Twenty-three genes with novel, previously unreported, base sequences have been isolated by molecular subtraction of mRNA from a lung squamous cell carcinoma from melanoma cDNA. Full details on six of the genes are provided in a recent paper (Hutchins et al., 1991). One of the genes, gene 50, appears to encode a MAA, judging by the ability of a 17 amino acid peptide synthesized from a portion of the molecule to cause proliferation of $CD4^+$ T lymphocytes from four of five patients immunized with melanoma theraccine. From one of those patients, four $CD4^+$ noncytolytic clones have been derived that specifically respond to the peptide but not to an irrelevant 20 amino acid peptide control. We have not yet detected an epitope of the gene 50 protein that sensitizes autologous cells for cytotoxicity by CTL from those patients. Van der Bruggen et al. (1991) have recently reported a gene isolated from mutagenized melanoma cell lines detected by CTL from immunized melanoma patients. We are hopeful that within the next few years a wholly synthetic melanoma theraccine can be assembled, where each component is preselected for potent immunogenicity.

Analysis of T-cell receptor gene rearrangements on clones specifically reactive against melanoma will give clues about the number of epitopes recognized. If there are relatively few V_α and V_β sequences utilized, as in ocular melanoma (Nitta et al., 1990), then the task of deriving antigens by cDNA methods may not be overwhelming. The number of components of the immunizing "cocktail" of MAA must not be very large, to avoid dilution of an important immunogen by the others.

Active Immunotherapy of Ocular Melanomas It may be possible to apply the same approach we have outlined to the treatment of ocular (uveal), as well as cutaneous, melanomas. Adjunctive therapy after definitive surgery or irradiation of the ocular primary may be justified, in an attempt to prevent metastases to the liver. Furthermore, in an 82-year-old man, we have successfully reduced a primary choroidal melanoma from 4.2 to 2.3 mm within 6 weeks, which has persisted for >18 months with no dissemination to the liver. A second man, 65 years old, had no change in his very large extrascleral melanoma over a 6-month period. We are not advocating routine treatment of primary ocular melanoma with active immunotherapy. In fact, both of the cited patients were blind in the nontumorous eye and were referred for immunological treatment because enucleation was contraindicated. In selected cases, this medical approach to the primary tumor may have some validity and, in any case, does not of itself preclude subsequent surgery or irradiation.

APPLICATION OF ACTIVE IMMUNIZATION TO ADOPTIVE IMMUNOTHERAPY

Each type of immunotherapy (see the introduction to this section: Types of Biological Therapy) may benefit from another. One sequence that makes eminent theoretical sense is active specific immunization preceding adoptive immunotherapy with specific activated CTL. Whether CTL are obtained from the site of a tumor, as tumor-infiltrating lymphocytes, or from the peripheral blood, both $CD4^+$ and $CD8^+$ CTL can be selected with reactivity to the patient's own tumor. Active immunotherapy can raise the number of CTL found in the peripheral blood, at least transiently, after which those cells presumably migrate to the tumor as well as recirculating among the lymphoid tissues of the body. Shu, Chang, and their co-workers have shown in animals (Shu et al., 1986; Chou et al., 1988) and in preliminary human experiments (Chang and Shu, 1990) that vaccination in vivo followed by secondary restimulation in vitro led to potent CTL. In mice, specific CTL with the ability to affect experimental pulmonary metastases were generated with the "weakly immunogenic" MCA 105 sarcoma and 1000 Cetus U/mL (6000 IU/mL) of IL-2 (Shu et al., 1986). This high concentration of IL-2 generated lymphokine-activated killer cells as well as expanding T cells. Nevertheless, low concentrations of IL-2 (2–10 Cetus U/mL, or 12–60 IU/mL) also expanded killer cells, which in fact had higher therapeutic efficacy than those from higher concentrations of IL-2 (Chou et al., 1988). In humans, in vivo specific immunotherapy has recently been begun with an adaptation of the same methods. Autologous tumor cells and BCG were given intradermally to six patients (Chang and Shu, 1990). Lymphoid cells were harvested from the draining lymph node and were reeducated with irradiated tumor cells. This led to CTL, which were nearly all (>80%) $CD4^+$. In two patients, there was specific antiautologous tumor reactivity, but in four others there was broader reactivity. Peripheral blood lymphocytes activated in the same manner were tested from two patients. There was broad reactivity against the same histotype as the patient's tumor, and not simply the autologous tumor, in both of these patients.

While the clinical efficacy of lymphocytes derived from in vivo immunization and further in vitro sensitization has not yet been tested after reinfusion into patients, the animal experiments suggest that they will be more potent than lymphocytes from unimmunized individuals.

It is possible that ex vivo restimulation may not be essential after active immunization, if one administers IL-2 to expand CTL after in vivo immunization. We have begun to explore this possibility in a preliminary trial of melanoma theraccine on days 1 and 8, preceded by CY on day −3, and accompanied by a 10-day series of IL-2 15-minute infusions on days 1 to 5 and 8 to 12. The entire treatment series was repeated twice more with a 1-week respite between each 2-week cycle. No responses were seen at the 3×10^6 BRMP U/m^2 level (approximately 7.5×10^6 IU/m^2) in six patients, but in nine patients at 4.5 and 6.0 million BRMP U/m^2 (11.25 and 15 million IU/m^2, respectively), there were a total of 3 partial remissions. In addition, 2 n cm liver lesions disappeared in one patient, but reappeared after a month of "vacation" from the program, and another patient had a PR of skin nodules, but had brain metastases that caused termination of the study. The most significant problem to this approach of IL-2 administration immediately after immunization with theraccine and DETOX™ has been an inordinately high incidence of neurological toxicity. Mental depression and brief periods of unconsciousness have occurred in four patients, all given 4.5 million BRMP U/day or more. Whether the endotoxin component of DETOX™ makes the neurological effects of IL-2 greater remains to be determined, but it is known that in mice endotoxin can increase the entrance of IL-2 into the central nervous system.

THE PROBLEM OF BRAIN METASTASES

The most serious obstacle to be overcome in the immunotherapy of melanomas is central nervous system, particularly brain, metastases (see also Chapter 8). As can be seen in Table 14-5, and as we have reviewed elsewhere (Mitchell, 1989), patients who have had dramatic, long-term responses to active immunotherapy, or treatment with IL-2, have often relapsed in the brain. When single small lesions are discovered, stereotactic radiotherapy can cause significant, often complete, regressions. If there is a single large lesion, as is not infrequently the case, it can be resected. Several resections of individual lesions in a single patient have been accomplished without significant morbidity. If many lesions are present, whole brain radiation is often used, but is rarely effective in prolonging useful life.

It would be far preferable to prevent brain metastases in patients who have otherwise rejected their melanoma systemically, but there seems to be a functional "blood–brain barrier" that prevents full immunity from being expressed in the central nervous system. Our histological observations on fixed sections from seven resected single brain metastases indicate that lymphocytes do cross into the brain, as do macrophages. However, there seems to be a lack of activation, such that the macrophages look small and quiescent, and the astrocytes that ordinarily process and present antigens in the brain to T cells are also wispy and unactivated appearing.

Evidence from a newly developed mouse model with B16 melanoma indicates that if the level of immunization is sufficiently high, even brain metastases may be preventable (Staib et al., manuscript in preparation). Syngeneic C57BL/6 mice immunized by five weekly doses of a theraccine composed of a mixture of irradiated B16 and Cloudman melanoma cells (simulating our human theraccine) resisted systemic challenge with viable B16 melanoma. Moreover, these demonstrably immune mice, who also had CTL in their spleen, resisted a challenge of 200 viable B16 melanoma cells injected intracerebrally, whereas unimmunized controls and mice given very low doses of mouse theraccine succumbed within 4 weeks.

There is hope that even this dreaded complication may be overcome purely through a biological approach to the melanoma.

PERSPECTIVE

Identifying the most important TAA recognized by humans and then synthesizing them by cDNA cloning are clearly major objectives to be pursued in all of the investigations involving active specific immunotherapy. The crude materials with which all of us have worked must be replaced by well-defined antigens to achieve consistent, reproducible results in large-scale trials. Nevertheless, even the crude preparations have established that at least some patients can respond to this form of immunotherapy. Since it causes minimal, if any, toxicity, active specific immunotherapy already has one major advantage over many other regimens associated with very similar response rates. Its lack of toxicity also commends it as an adjunctive (surgical adjuvant) therapy in the early stages of disease.

While active specific immunotherapy, like all other forms of immunotherapy, will probably serve best as part of a combination regimen, it must be validated as an entity by itself before it is randomly combined with other forms. Such future combinations will undoubtedly include theraccines with IL-2, to maximally stimulate helper and cytolytic T cells, and perhaps preceding the further in vitro expansion and subsequent reinfusion of those T cells into the patient. Indeed, it is arguable that active specific immunotherapy can serve as a cornerstone for most combinations, by stimulating the host's intrinsic immunity before adding other effective forms of treatment.

REFERENCES

Albino AP, Lloyd KO, Houghton AN, Oettgen HF, Old LJ. Heterogeneity in surface antigen and glycoprotein expression of cell lines derived from different melanoma metastases of the same patient. J Exp Med. 1981;154:1764–1778.

Berd D, Mastrangelo MJ. Active immunotherapy of human melanoma exploiting the immunopotentiating effects of cyclophosphamide. Cancer Invest. 1988;6:337–349.

Berd D, Maguire HC, Jr, Mastrangelo MJ. Potentiation of human cell-mediated and humoral immunity by low-dose cyclophosphamide. Cancer Res. 1984;44:5439–5443.

Berd D, Maguire HC, Jr, Mastrangelo MJ. Induction of cell-mediated immunity to autologous melanoma cells and regression of metastases after treatment with a melanoma cell vaccine preceded by cyclophosphamide. Cancer Res. 1986;46:2572–2577.

Berd D, Mastrangelo MJ, Green C, Clark C, Hart E. Tumor inflammatory response induced by immunization with autologous melanoma cells conjugated to dinitrophenol (DNP). Proc Am Assoc Cancer Res. 1989;30:382. Abstract.

Berd D, Maguire HC, Jr, McCue P, Mastrangelo MJ. Treatment of metastatic melanoma with an autologous tumor cell vaccine: clinical and immunological results in 64 patients. J Clin Oncol. 1990;8:1858–1867.

Bystryn JC, Jacobsen S, Harris M, Roses D, Speyer J, Levin M. Preparation and characterization of a polyvalent human melanoma antigen vaccine. J Biol Resp Mod. 1986;5:211–224.

Bystryn J-C, Dugan M, Oratz R, Speyer J, Harris MN, Roses DF. Vaccine immunotherapy of human malignant melanoma: relationship between method of immunization, immunogenicity, and tumor progression. In: Metzgar RS, Mitchell MS, eds. Human tumor antigens and specific tumor therapy. New York, NY: Alan R. Liss; 1989:307–315.

Cassel WA, Murray DR, Phillips HS. A phase II study on the postsurgical management of stage II malignant melanoma with a Newcastle disease virus oncolysate. Cancer. 1983;52:856–86.

Chang AE, Shu S. Generation of in vitro sensitized T lymphocytes for adoptive immunotherapy. Proc Am Soc Clin Oncol. 1990;9:197. Abstract.

Chou T, Chang AE, Shu S. Generation of therapeutic T lymphocyte from tumor-bearing mice by in vitro sensitization. Culture requirements and characterization of immunologic specificity. J Immunol. 1988;140:2453–2461.

Darrow TL, Slingluff CL, Jr, Seigler HF. The role of HLA Class I antigens in recognition of melanoma cells by tumor-specific cytotoxic T lymphocytes. Evidence for shared tumor antigens. J Immunol. 1989;142:3329–3335.

Estin CD, Stevenson U, Kahn M, Hellstrom I, Hellstrom KE. Transfected mouse melanoma lines that express various levels of human melanoma-associated antigen p97. J Natl Cancer Inst. 1989;81:445–448.

Fazekas de St. Groth FS. The evaluation of limiting dilutions assays. J Immunol Methods. 1982;49:R11–R23.

Finn OJ, Barnd DL, Kerr LA, Miceli MC, Metzgar RS. Specific recognition of human tumor associated antigens by non-MHC-restricted CTL. In: Metzgar RS, Mitchell MS, eds. Human tumor antigens and specific tumor therapy. New York, NY: Alan R. Liss; 1989:157–166.

Forni G, Fujiwara H, Martino F, et al. Helper strategy in tumor immunology: expansion of helper lymphocytes and utilization of helper lymphokines for experimental and clinical immunotherapy. Cancer Metastasis Rev. 1988;7:289–309.

Freedman RS, Edwards CL, Bowen JM, et al. Viral oncolysates in patients with advanced ovarian cancer. Gynecol Oncol. 1988;29:337–347.

Freedman RS, Bowen JM, Atkinson EN, et al. Randomized comparison of viral oncolysate plus radiation and radiation alone in uterine cervix carcinoma. Am J Clin Oncol. 1989;12:244–250.

Furukawa K, Lotzova E, Freedman RS, Bowen JB, Edwards CL, Wharton JT. Effect of virus-modified tumor cell extracts, autologous mononuclear cell infusions and interleukin-2 on oncolytic activity of effector cells of patients with advanced ovarian cancer. Cancer Immunol Immunother. 1989;30:126–132.

Hanna MG, Jr, Key ME. Active specific immunotherapy of metastases enhances subsequent chemotherapy. Science. 1982;217:367–369.

Hanna MG, Jr, Hoover HC, Jr. Active specific immunotherapy as an adjunct to the treatment of metastatic solid tumors. In: Reif AE, Mitchell MS, eds. Immunity to cancer. Orlando, FL: Academic Press; 1985:429–440.

Hanna MG, Jr, Brandhorst JS, Peters LC. Active specific immunotherapy of residual micrometastases. An evaluation of sources, doses and ratios of BCG with tumor cells. Cancer Immunol Immunother. 1979;7:165–173.

Harel W, Li VA, Morse AC, Kan-Mitchell J, Ewoldsen MA, Mitchell MS. Generation of melanoma-reactive T cell clones from patients treated with active specific immunotherapy. Proc Am Assoc Cancer Res. 1990;31:253. Abstract.

Heicappell R, Schirrmacher V, von Hoegen P, Ahlert T, Appelhans B. Prevention of metastatic spread by postoperative immunotherapy with virally modified autologous tumor cells. I. Parameters for optimal therapeutics effects. Int J Cancer. 1986;37:569–577.

Hersey P, MacDonald M, Werkman H. Western blot analysis of antigens on melanoma cells recognized by cytotoxic T cells. J Natl Cancer Inst. 1988;80:826–835.

Hom SS, Topalian SL, Simonis T, Mancini M, Rosenberg SA. Common expression of melanoma tumor-associated antigens recognized by human tumor infiltrating lymphocytes: analysis by human lymphocyte antigen restriction. J Immunother. 1991;10:153–164.

Hoover HC, Jr, Surdyke MG, Dangel RB, Peters LC, Hanna MG, Jr. Prospectively randomized trial of adjuvant active-specific immunotherapy for human colorectal cancer. Cancer. 1985;55:1236–1243.

Hutchins JT, Deans RJ, Uchiwara C, Mitchell MS, Kan-Mitchell J. Novel sequences expressed by human melanoma cells identified by molecular subtraction. Cancer Res. 1991;51:1418–1425.

Kahan BD, Tanaka T, Pellis NR. Immunotherapy of a carcinogen-induced murine sarcoma with soluble tumor-specific transplantation antigens. J Natl Cancer Inst. 1980;65:1001–1004.

Kahan BD, Pellis NR, LeGrue SJ, Tanaka T. Immunotherapeutic effects of tumor specific transplantation antigens released by 1-butanol. Cancer. 1982;49:1168–1173.

Kobayashi H. Viral xenogenization of intact tumor cells. Cancer Res. 1979;30:279–299.

LeGrue SJ, Kahan BD, Pellis NR. Extraction of a murine tumor-specific transplantation antigen with 1-butanol. I. Partial purification by isoelectric focusing. J Natl Cancer Inst. 1980; 65:191–196.

Livingston PO. Experimental and clinical studies with active specific immunotherapy. In: Mitchell MS, ed. Immunity to cancer. II. New York, NY: Alan R. Liss; 1989a:309–321.

Livingston PO. The basis for ganglioside vaccines in melanoma. In: Metzgar RS, Mitchell MS, eds. Human tumor antigens and specific tumor therapy. New York, NY: Alan R. Liss; 1989b:287–296.

Livingston PO, Takeyama H, Pollack MS, et al. Serological responses of melanoma patients to vaccines derived from allogeneic cultured melanoma cells. Int J Cancer. 1983;31:567–575.

Livingston PO, Ritter G, Calves MJ. Antibody response after immunization with the gangliosides GM1, GM2, GM3, GD2, and GD3 in the mouse. Cancer Immunol Immunother. 1989;29:179–184.

Lopez de Castro JA. HLA-B27 and HLA-A2 subtypes: structure, evolution and function. Immunol Today. 1989;10:239–246.

McCune CS, Schapira DV, Henshaw EC. Specific immunotherapy of advanced renal carcinoma: evidence for the polyclonality of metastases. Cancer. 1981;47:1984–1987.

Mitchell MS. Relapse in the central nervous system in melanoma patients successfully treated with biomodulators. J Clin Oncol. 1989;7:121–129.

Mitchell MS. Attempts to optimize active specific immunotherapy for melanoma. Int Rev Immunol. 1991;7:331–347.

Mitchell MS, Kirkpatrick D, Mokyr MB, Gery I. On the mode of action of BCG. Nature (New Biol). 1973;243:216–218.

Mitchell MS, Kan-Mitchell J, Kempf RA, Harel W, Shau H, Lind S. Active specific immunotherapy for melanoma: phase I trial of allogeneic lysates and a novel adjuvant. Cancer Res. 1988;48:5883–5893.

Mitchell MS, Harel W, Kempf RA, et al. Active-specific immunotherapy for melanoma. J Clin Oncol. 1990a;8:856–869.

Mitchell MS, Harel W, Kempf RA, et al. Phase I trial of a new combination of allogeneic melanoma lysates: evidence for a dose-response relationship. Proc Am Soc Clin Oncol. 1990b;9:283. Abstract.

Mitchell MS, Harel W, Groshen S. Association of HLA phenotype with response to active specific immunotherapy of melanoma. J Clin Oncol. 1992;10:in press.

Mokyr MB, Mitchell MS. Activation of lymphoid cells by BCG in vitro. Cell Immunol. 1975;15:264–273.

Morton DL, Nizze A, Famatiga E, Hoon DSB, Gupta R, Irie R. Clinical results of a trial of active specific immunotherapy with melanoma cell vaccine and immunomodulator in metastatic melanoma. Proc Am Assoc Cancer Res. 1989;30:383. Abstract.

Neidhart JA, Murphy SG, Hennick LA, Wise HA. Active specific immunotherapy of stage IV renal carcinoma with aggregated tumor antigen adjuvant. Cancer. 1980;46:1128–1134.

Nitta T, Oksenberg JR, Rao NA, Steinman L. Tumor infiltrating lymphocytes in uveal melanoma predominantly express the T cell receptor gene, Va 7. Science. 1990;249:672–674.

Old LJ. Cancer immunology: the search for specificity. GHA Clowes Memorial Lecture. Cancer Res. 1981;41:361–375.

Orentas RJ, Hildreth JEK, Obah E, et al. Induction of $CD4^+$ human cytolytic T cells specific for HIV-infected cells by a gp160 subunit vaccine. Science. 1990;248:1234–1237.

Prager MD, Gordon WC. Enhanced response to chemoimmunotherapy and immunoprophylaxis with the use of tumor-associated antigens with a lipophilic agent. Cancer Res. 1978;38:2052–2057.

Sahasrabudhe DM, de Kernion JB, Pontes JE, et al. Specific immunotherapy with suppressor function inhibition for metastatic renal cell carcinoma. J Biol Resp Mod. 1986;5:581–594.

Schild H, von Hoegen P, Schirrmacher V. Modification of tumor cells by a low dose of Newcastle disease virus. II. Augmented tumor-specific T cell response as a result of $CD4^+$ and $CD8^+$ immune T cell cooperation. Cancer Immunol Immunother. 1989;28:22–28.

Schirrmacher V, von Hoegen P, Schlag P, et al. Active specific immunotherapy with autologous tumor cell vaccines modified by Newcastle disease virus: experimental and clinical studies. In: Schirrmacher V, Schwartz-Albiez R, eds. Cancer metastasis. New York, NY: Springer-Verlag; 1989:157–170.

Shu S, Chou T, Rosenberg SA. In vitro sensitization and expansion with viable tumor cells and interleukin 2 in the generation of specific therapeutic effector cells. J Immunol. 1986; 136:3891–3898.

Tallberg T, Tykka H, Mahlberg K, et al. Active specific immunotherapy with supportive measures in the treatment of palliatively nephrectomized, renal adenocarcinoma patients. A thirteen-year followup study. Eur Urol. 1984;11:233–243.

Tsuchida T, Saxton RE, Irie RF. Gangliosides of human melanoma: GM2 and tumorigenicity. J Natl Cancer Inst. 1987;78:55–59.

Tykka H, Hjelt L, Oravisto KJ, Turunen M, Tallberg T. Disappearance of lung metastases during immunotherapy in 5 patients suffering from renal carcinoma. Scand J Resp Dis. 1974; 89(suppl):123.

Van der Bruggen C, Traversari C, Chomez P, et al. A gene encoding an antigen recognized by cytolytic T lymphocytes on a human melanoma. Science. 1991;254:1643–1647.

Vanky F, Stuber G, Rotstein S, Klein E. Auto-tumor recognition following in vitro induction of MHC antigen expression on solid human tumors: stimulation of lymphocytes and generation of cytotoxicity against the original MHC-antigen-negative. Cancer Immunol Immunother. 1989;28:17–21.

Von Hoegen P, Weber E, Schirrmacher V. Modification of tumor cells by a low dose of Newcastle disease virus. Augmentation of the tumor-specific T cell response in the absence of anti-viral response. Eur J Immunol. 1988;18:1159–1166.

Wallack MK, Bash J, Bartolucci A. Improvement in disease-free survival of melanoma patients in conjunction with serologic response in a phase Ia/Ib Southeastern Cancer Study Group trial of vaccinia melanoma oncolysate. Am Surg. 1989;55:243–247.

Wolfel T, Klehmann E, Muller C, et al. Lysis of human melanoma cells by autologous cytolytic T cell clones. Identification of human histocompatibility leukocyte antigen A2 as a restriction element for three different antigens. J Exp Med. 1989;170:787–810.

Yoshioka T, Fukuzawa M, Takei Y, et al. The augmentation of tumor specific immunity by virus help: III. Enhanced generation of tumor-specific lyt 1+2− T cells is responsible for augmented tumor immunity in vivo. Cancer Immunol Immunother. 1986;21:193–198.

CHAPTER **15**

SYSTEMIC ACTIVATION OF MACROPHAGES FOR ERADICATION OF CANCER METASTASES

Jerald J. Killion
Isaiah J. Fidler

The most devastating aspect of cancer is the spread of tumor cells from the primary neoplasm to distant organs and the resulting growth of secondary tumors, that is, metastases. Despite the advances of the last decade in our understanding of cancer biology in general patient care, surgical techniques, and adjuvant therapies, the majority of deaths from cancer are still caused by the growth of metastases that are resistant to conventional therapies. There are several reasons why treatment is unsuccessful. First, efforts to inhibit the establishment of metastasis are most likely destined to fail because, in the majority of patients, metastasis probably occurs by the time of diagnosis of primary malignant neoplasms (Fidler et al., 1978). Second, the anatomical location and number of metastases limit the effective dose of a therapeutic agent that can be delivered to the lesion without producing unacceptable side effects to the patient. Third, the heterogeneous nature of malignant neoplasms, manifested by the continuous emergence of variant tumor subpopulations, presents a formidable barrier to successful therapy.

To produce a metastasis, a tumor cell must complete a series of steps that are potentially lethal to it. The outcome of this process is therefore dependent on the responses of the host, intrinsic properties of the tumor cells, and the microenvironment of the metastatic lesion (Poste and Fidler, 1979; Talmadge and Fidler, 1982; Weiss, 1985). Metastasis begins with the detachment of tumor cells from the primary lesion. After they invade the blood vessels and the lymphatics, single tumor cells or multicell emboli circulate and eventually reach the capillary bed of distant organs where they arrest. The viable cells must be able to extravasate into the organ parenchyma and proliferate in order to manifest as secondary lesions.

By the time of diagnosis of the primary tumor, malignant neoplasms contain multiple cell populations that are heterogeneous with respect to a variety of biological properties, including cell-surface characteristics and architecture, antigenicity, immunogenicity, growth rate, karyotype, sensitivity to various chemotherapeutic drugs, and the ability to invade and metastasize (Fidler and Poste, 1985; Fidler and Balch, 1987; Nicholson, 1984, 1987; Poste and Fidler, 1979). The existence of these heterogeneous subpopulations of cells presents a dilemma for the clinician. The emergence of drug-resistant variants during, or subsequent to, chemotherapy has been documented, as have differences in the response of primary and metastatic tumors to therapeutic agents (Fidler and Poste, 1985). The obstacle to therapy that heterogeneity imposes on chemotherapy may also affect the likelihood of success of immunotherapy or biological response modification (Kerbel, 1979; Killion and Kollmorgen, 1976; Killion and Fidler, 1989; Miller, 1982). Biological heterogeneity is equally likely among the tumor cells of the metastatic lesion. This continual evolution of diversity may result from the genetic progression of the tumor (Nicholson, 1987).

Recent data from tumor models provide some explanation for these observations. The process of metastasis is selective (Fidler and Balch, 1987; Talmadge and Fidler, 1982), and cancer metastases result from the nonrandom spread of unique subpopulations of cells that preexist within the primary tumor (Fidler and Kripke, 1977). Metastases can be clonal in their origin, and different metastases within the same organ can originate from different progenitor cells (Hu et al., 1987; Kerbel et al., 1987; Talmadge et al., 1982; Talmadge and Zbar, 1986). Indeed, a single metastasis can originate from one cell (Fidler and Talmadge, 1986). These data provide an explanation for the clinical observations that, within the same patient, different metastases can exhibit different susceptibilities to immunotherapy, chemotherapy, and radiotherapy (Fidler and Balch, 1987; Weiss, 1985). The problem of heterogeneity is compounded by the finding that, in general, metastatic cells are genetically unstable and, therefore, can readily become resistant to chemotherapy (Cifone and Fidler, 1980). For these reasons, it is clear that the successful treatment of neoplastic disease is, in fact, the treatment of metastatic disease, which will require the development of new modalities and therapeutic strategies that can circumvent both the existing cellular heterogeneity of tumors and overcome the development of cells that are resistant to therapy.

The role of macrophages in host defense against neoplasms has attracted increasing attention over the past few years. This stems, in part, from a growing body of experimental evidence that macrophages are important effector cells in the host defense against metastatic tumors (Fidler, 1985, 1986b; Fidler and Poste, 1982). Most important, activated, tumoricidal macrophages are able to kill phenotypically diverse tumor cell populations, so this property may be exploited in order to circumvent the heterogeneity of neoplasms. We shall review the mechanisms of macrophage activation, their ability to eradicate spontaneous metastases, and the rationale for, and development of, liposomes to achieve systemic activation of macrophages.

MACROPHAGES AS EFFECTOR CELLS AGAINST NEOPLASTIC DISEASE

Mononuclear phagocytes are an important physiological component of normal homeostasis. Cells of the macrophage-histiocyte series are involved in processes of tissue turnover such as tissue remodeling during embryogenesis, tissue destruction and repair subsequent to injury, and tissue renewal following the removal of damaged or senescent cells (Fidler, 1985; Fidler and Schroit, 1986). In adult animals, the primary function of macrophages is the phagocytosis and disposal of effete cells (Duvall et al., 1985), such as damaged red blood cells (Solanki, 1985), cellular debris, and serum proteins. These cells are also involved in the metabolism of lipids (Chait, 1983) and iron (Custer et al., 1982), in host response to injury, in defense against microbial infections (Hahn, 1983; Schaffner et al., 1982) and parasitic infestations (Nogueira, 1984), and in the afferent and efferent arms of the immune system. Finally, macrophages are critical to host defense against neoplasms (Fidler, 1986b; Gregoriadis and Allison, 1980).

Macrophages can recognize tumor cells in vivo (Fidler, 1985, 1986b; Fidler and Poste, 1982) and, therefore, may play a role in host surveillance against autochthonous transformed neoplastic cells (Hibbs, 1974a, 1974b; Hibbs et al., 1972). Studies on skin carcinogenesis induced by ultraviolet radiation (UV) in mice support this hypothesis (Norbury and Kripke, 1979). At low doses of UV, treatment of mice with a macrophage stimulant (pyran copolymer) prolonged the latent period of tumor development and protected the animals against this form of carcinogenesis. Conversely, treatment of mice with macrophage toxins (e.g., carrageenan or silica) shortened the latent period of skin cancer induction by UV light. Similarly, in transplantable tumor systems, the impairment of macrophage function by agents such as carrageenan or silica was associated with an increase in the incidence of spontaneous (Jones and Castro, 1977; Sadler et al., 1979) and experimental (Mantovani et al., 1980) metastasis. There are also published reports regarding the efficacy of macrophages in the inhibition of metastasis. Syngeneic mouse macrophages activated in vitro and then injected intravenously into mice reduced the formation of B16 melanoma metastases (Fidler, 1974; Fidler et al., 1979), and the intravenous injection of nonspecifically activated macrophages prevented the formation of spontaneous metastasis by a fibrosarcoma growing subcutaneously (Liotta et al., 1977). Macrophages activated in vitro and then injected in vivo have also been shown to inhibit the growth of tumors at primary sites (Den Otter et al., 1977). Recent evidence has shown that blood monocytes may cross the intact blood–brain barrier and infiltrate metastatic brain lesions (Schackert et al., 1988).

ACTIVATION OF MACROPHAGES TO THE TUMORICIDAL STATE

Macrophage activation has been defined by different morphological and biochemical observations of changes in their adherence to glass, increased mobility, increased phagocytic capability, or increased enzymatic activity (Fidler, 1984; Fidler et al.,

1981a). We shall use the term "macrophage activation" to mean the process whereby noncytotoxic macrophages acquire tumoricidal properties (Fidler, 1985, 1986b; Fidler and Poste, 1982).

There are two major pathways to produce macrophage activation in vivo. Macrophages can become activated subsequent to interaction with microorganisms or their products such as endotoxins and bacterial cell-wall components. Although this interaction is very common, intentional attempts to activate macrophages systemically by administering microorganisms or their products were limited by major side effects such as allergic reactions and granuloma formations (Allison, 1974, 1979). For this reason, the field did not progress until the discovery of muramyl dipeptide (MDP), a defined component of the bacterial cell wall (Chedid et al., 1978; Lederer, 1980) that is capable of activating the immune system. Muramyl dipeptide is a water soluble, low molecular weight (M_r = 495), synthetic moiety of *N*-acetyl-muramyl-*L*-alanyl-*D*-isoglutamine; it has potent effects on a variety of host-defense cells, including macrophages (Chedid et al., 1978; Fogler and Fidler, 1984). Recently, a lipophilic MDP derivative, *N*-acetyl-muramyl-*L*-alanyl-*D*-isoglutamyl-*L*-alanyl-2-(1′,2′-dipalmitoyl)-*sn*-glycero-3′-phosphoryl-ethylamide (MTP-PE), has also been synthesized (Gisler et al., 1979). Although muramyl peptides influence several macrophage functions in vitro, comparable effects have not been observed in vivo because they are rapidly cleared after parenteral administration (Fogler and Fidler, 1984; Fogler et al., 1985; Parant et al., 1979). Even when injected at very high doses, muramyl peptides fail to induce significant macrophage-mediated antitumor activity (Fidler et al., 1982, 1983; Fogler and Fidler, 1984).

Macrophages can also be activated by their interaction with lymphokines. Mitogen- and antigen-stimulated T lymphocytes release diffusible mediators that interact with specific receptors on target cells. A family of lymphokines, referred to as macrophage-activating factors (MAF) (Fidler, 1984; Kleinerman and Fidler, 1983; Kleinerman et al., 1983), are able to render macrophages tumoricidal. These include the interferons—interferon-gamma (IFN-γ), which is able to prime macrophages for activation following the induction of a second signal (such as suboptimal concentrations of MDP) (Saiki and Fidler, 1985; Saiki et al., 1985), interferon-alpha (IFN-α), and interferon-beta (IFN-β)—which also prime macrophages in a synergistic fashion with IFN-γ (Pace, 1988). There is evidence that IFN-γ–mediated priming of macrophages renders them sensitive to tumoricidal activation by tumor necrosis factor (TNF) and interleukin-1 (IL-1), demonstrating that interactions of lymphocyte and macrophage products (interferons and interleukins) with macrophage receptors can lead to both transitory and sustained tumoricidal activity (Hori et al., 1989). In addition, chemotactic peptides, such as *N*-formyl-methionyl-leucyl-phenylalanine, activated macrophages to the tumoricidal state when the peptide was presented to the macrophages incorporated into liposomes, suggesting that intracellular targets for activating molecules may be reached by encapsulation of the proper molecule in liposomes (Morikawa et al., 1988). Evidence indicates that the priming stimulus delivered to macrophages by IFN-γ (or complete activation by MAF) involves the binding and subsequent internalization of specific receptors at the macrophage cell membrane, since liposome encapsulation of these lymphokines allows macrophage priming using mouse IFN-γ on human monocytes and human IFN-γ on mouse macrophages, a process that is species-specific using free-form lymphokines (Fidler et al., 1985; Kleinerman et al., 1985; Poste et al., 1979c).

Regardless of how they are activated, rodent and human tumoricidal macrophages acquire the ability to recognize and destroy neoplastic cells, while leaving nonneoplastic cells unharmed. The mechanisms appear to be nonimmunological in nature and to require cell-to-cell contact (Bucana et al., 1976, 1983; Fidler, 1978; Fidler and Kleinerman, 1984; Hibbs, 1974a; Hibbs et al., 1972). The data generated in rodent and human systems indicate that, at least in vitro, tumoricidal macrophages can discriminate between neoplastic and nonneoplastic cells by a process that is independent of transplantation antigens, species-specific antigens, tumor-specific antigens, cell cycle time, or various phenotypes associated with transformation (Fidler, 1978; Fidler and Kleinerman, 1984). In vitro macrophage lysis of tumor cells appears to be nonselective (Fogler and Fidler, 1985). This conclusion is based on our attempts to select in vitro tumor cell variant lines with absolute resistance to macrophage-mediated lysis. We used techniques similar to those used previously to select a B16 melanoma tumor cell line resistant to lysis by cytotoxic T-lymphocytes (CTL) (Fidler et al., 1976) or UV-2237 fibrosarcoma cells resistant to natural killer (NK) cell–mediated lysis (Hanna and Fidler, 1980). Despite repeated in vitro selections (Fogler and Fidler, 1985) in eight different tumor cell lines, we failed to isolate tumor cells with increased resistance to macrophage-mediated lysis.

SYSTEMIC ACTIVATION OF MACROPHAGES TO THE TUMORICIDAL STATE

Earlier studies have shown that the intravenous injection of nonspecifically activated macrophages into mice bearing metastases inhibited tumor growth both in the primary site (Den Otter et al., 1977) and in metastases (Fidler, 1974; Fidler et al., 1979; Liotta et al., 1977). For clinical use, however, this strategy has two serious shortcomings: the transfusion of a large number of histocompatible or autologous macrophages is required, and most intravenously injected macrophages, especially those in clumps, are likely to be arrested in the capillary bed of the lung, producing pulmonary spasms.

Early attempts to activate macrophages in vivo specifically in order to enhance host defense against cancer have been unsuccessful. Until the isolation and purification of IFN-γ, the therapeutic use of lymphokines was hindered by a lack of purified preparations. But even with IFN-γ, activation of macrophages in vivo did not succeed because lymphokines injected intravenously have an extremely short half-life (Kleinerman et al., 1986; Poste et al., 1979a), only a small fraction of the reticuloendothelial system (RES) can respond to free lymphokines (Poste et al., 1979a), macrophages can be activated by lymphokines only within a relatively short period of time following their extravasation from the peripheral circulation to the tissues (Poste et al.,

1979a); the tumoricidal properties of lymphokine-activated macrophages are short-lived, and the cells become refractory to reactivation by free lymphokines (Poste et al., 1979b). Even under ideal conditions, at least an 8-hour interaction between human monocytes and free lymphokines is required for successful activation (Cameron and Churchill, 1979; Fidler, 1984; Kleinerman et al., 1983). For all these reasons, the systemic administration of soluble lymphokines does not result in monocyte/macrophage activation.

Efforts to activate macrophages in vivo by treatment with agents that stimulate T lymphocytes to produce lymphokines have also been disappointing. We have shown that the lymphocytes of animals bearing large, progressively growing tumors are deficient in their ability to release lymphokines that can recruit and activate macrophages (Kripke et al., 1976). Indeed, if such a defect is found to be common to all tumor-bearing hosts, administration of soluble agents to augment production of lymphokines in situ may be of little value.

Advances in liposome technology may provide a mechanism for activating macrophages in situ. During the last few years, considerable attention has been focused on the use of synthetic phospholipid vesicles, the liposomes, to target various drugs to different organ sites in vivo (Alving, 1983; Daoud et al., 1989; Fidler, 1988; Gregoriadis, 1988; Hwang, 1987; Ostro, 1988; Papahadjopoulos, 1989; Poste et al., 1984; Schroit et al., 1983b). Most attempts to target liposomes to solid neoplasms have failed because these phospholipid vesicles are unable to extravasate from the circulation and are rapidly taken up by circulating and fixed phagocytic cells. We have utilized this natural fate of liposomes to target immunomodulators encapsulated within liposomes to cells of the RES, thus activating these phagocytic cells to the tumoricidal state (Daoud et al., 1989; Fidler, 1980, 1981; Fidler and Raz, 1981; Fidler et al., 1982b; Koff and Fidler, 1985; Mehta et al., 1982; Nayar and Schroit, 1985; Poste et al., 1982; Schroit et al., 1983a). Preferential delivery of the liposome-encapsulated substances can be achieved in vivo because mainly phagocytic cells are exposed to the liposome-entrapped agents. Once phagocytosed, biologically active materials are released into the cytoplasm of the phagocyte, thereby avoiding the problems of dilution, serum protein binding, and rapid clearance and minimizing the elicitation of undesirable side effects (Hart et al., 1981; Poste et al., 1982; Schroit and Fidler, 1982; Schroit et al., 1983a). The natural localization pattern also allows efficient targeting of liposomes and their contents to various macrophage compartments in the body.

In order for liposomes to serve as effective carriers for macrophage activators, they must retain the entrapped compound until the contents are released into intracellular compartments. The liposomes must avidly bind macrophages and be easily internalized by the cytoplasm, either by phagocytosis or by fusion with the lipids of the plasma membranes. Ideally, liposomes should be capable of localizing in a myriad of tissues, and for clinical application of this technology, the liposome preparation should be easy to prepare in a reproducible manner and have a long shelf life.

Through the systemic evaluation of multilamellar vesicles (MLV) with different phospholipid composition, we and others have identified certain classes of phospholipids that are preferentially recognized by macrophages. Specifically, the inclusion of negatively charged phospholipids such as phosphatidylserine (PS) and phosphatidylglycerol (PG) in MLV consisting of phosphatidylcholine (PC) greatly enhances their binding to, and phagocytosis by, macrophages (Fidler, 1980; Fidler et al., 1982b; Mehta et al., 1982; Nayar and Schroit, 1985; Poste et al., 1982, 1984; Schroit and Fidler, 1982). In contrast, neutral MLV composed exclusively of PC are not efficiently bound by macrophages. In fact, the inclusion of PS within PC MLV leads to recognition of these liposomes by every cell of the RES. Thus, enhancement of phagocytosis has been shown to occur in mouse peritoneal macrophages (Poste et al., 1982; Raz et al., 1981; Schroit and Fidler, 1982; Schroit et al., 1983a), mouse Kupffer's cells (Daemen et al., 1986, 1989; Xu and Fidler, 1984), rodent alveolar macrophages (Sone and Fidler, 1980, 1981), human peripheral blood monocytes (Kleinerman and Fidler, 1983; Kleinerman et al., 1983a; Lopez-Berestein et al., 1983; Saiki et al., 1985; Sone et al., 1984, 1986), and human alveolar macrophages (Sone and Tsubura, 1982).

IN VITRO ACTIVATION OF MACROPHAGES BY LIPOSOMES CONTAINING IMMUNOMODULATORS

A series of studies have defined the optimal parameters associated with in vitro activation of mouse macrophages. For example, MAF encapsulated in liposomes of differing size, surface charge, and lipid composition can successfully activate macrophages, but activation is more efficient when large MLV or reverse evaporation vesicle (REV) liposomes are used, rather than small unilamellar vesicles. In addition, activation occurs more rapidly with negatively charged MLV (PC/PS) than with neutral (PC) liposomes (Fidler, 1988; Fidler et al., 1981a; Raz et al., 1981). Although the latent time for activation of macrophages by liposome-encapsulated MAF is longer than that observed using free MAF, their use produces greater tumoricidal activity and requires the exposure of macrophages to less MAF (Kleinerman and Fidler, 1983; Kleinerman et al., 1983a). Efficient in vitro activation of macrophages has been achieved by employing liposomes containing entrapped MDP, MTP-PE, IFN-γ, or MAF.

The early studies on liposome-encapsulated MAF demonstrated two important principles in the use of liposome-encapsulated immunomodulators. First, it is important to recognize that the total amount of free MAF added to the macrophages greatly exceeded the amount of MAF presented to the macrophages in liposomes. Dilution experiments demonstrated that macrophages could be activated by a 10,000-fold dilution of the effective dose of free MAF supernatant (Fidler et al., 1981a; Raz et al., 1981). Second, evidence indicates that entrapped MAF is delivered to intracellular compartments of the macrophage, bypassing the requirement for specific cell-surface receptors, much as liposome-encapsulated IFN-γ is (Fidler et al., 1985b; Kleinerman et al., 1985; Poste et al., 1979c).

Further evidence that liposome-entrapped MAF activates macrophages via an intracellular mechanism comes from activation experiments in which normal macrophages were incubated with either free MAF or liposome-encapsulated MAF in the presence of several compounds known to inhibit MAF binding to the macrophage surface. Liposome-encapsulated MAF, but not free MAF, activated tumoricidal properties in macrophages concomitantly treated with α-L-fucosidase, which removes surface receptors for MAF, or with fucose-binding plant lectins (*Ulex europeaus I* and *Lotus tetragonolobus*), which compete for binding to the MAF receptor on macrophages. Moreover, populations of nontumoricidal inflammatory tissue macrophages, which were inherently unresponsive to free MAF, could be rendered tumoricidal in vitro by incubation with liposome-encapsulated MAF (Poste et al., 1979b, 1979c; Raz et al., 1981). Finally, liposome-encapsulated MAF activated the tumoricidal properties of macrophages obtained from endotoxin-nonresponsive C3H/HeN mice, whereas free MAF did not (Fogler et al., 1983).

By using the local anesthetic dibucaine to impair the endocytic uptake of liposomes (without affecting liposome binding to the macrophage surface), we have demonstrated that activation by liposome-encapsulated MAF requires internalization of the liposomal carrier (Fidler et al., 1981a; Raz et al., 1981). These experiments demonstrate that the activation of macrophages is not caused by MAF leaking from liposomes adsorbed to the cell surface and then binding to surface MAF receptors. Moreover, macrophages exposed to latex beads and free MAF in quantities equivalent to MAF encapsulated in liposomes do not become activated even though the endocytic activity induced by the beads promotes the endocytosis of MAF (Fidler et al., 1981a; Raz et al., 1981).

These initial investigations on the activation of tumoricidal properties in rodent macrophages by liposome-encapsulated MAF have now been expanded to human mononuclear cells with similar results. Liposome-encapsulated human MAF was at least 800 times more efficient than free MAF in rendering human blood monocytes cytotoxic to allogeneic tumor cells in vitro (Kleinerman and Fidler, 1983; Kleinerman et al., 1983a). In addition, the activation of human monocytes by human MAF does not require the binding of this lymphokine to putative monocyte surface receptors (Kleinerman and Fidler, 1983; Kleinerman et al., 1983a).

The mechanism by which MDP activates human monocyte/macrophage function has been investigated in both rodent (Tenu et al., 1982) and human (Fogler and Fidler, 1986) systems with radiolabeled glycopeptides. Collectively, the results indicate the absence of cell-surface MDP receptors and suggest that the activation of tumoricidal properties in mononuclear phagocytes by muramyl peptides occurs as the result of an intracytoplasmic event following pinocytosis of the glycopeptide. In contrast to the activation of macrophages by lymphokines, naturally occurring MDP is liberated following the phagocytosis of bacteria and the breakdown of bacterial cell walls within the macrophage cytoplasm (Chapes and Haskill, 1982; Fogler et al., 1983). In nature, therefore, MDP are presented to the macrophage through an intracellular pathway where MDP can bind to intracellular receptors (Fogler and Fidler, 1984). In this regard, several laboratories have documented this ability of liposome-encapsulated MDP (and various analogues) to activate tumoricidal properties in both rodent (Fidler et al., 1981b, 1982a, 1982b, 1983; Fogler et al., 1983; Lopez-Berestein et al., 1984; Phillips et al., 1985; Schroit and Fidler, 1982; Sone and Fidler, 1980, 1981) and human (Fidler, 1988; Fidler et al., 1981a; Fogler et al., 1983; Lopez-Berestein et al., 1983; Sone and Tsubura, 1982; Sone et al., 1984, 1986) macrophages following phagocytosis of the phospholipid vesicle. In contrast to free MDP, macrophage activation by liposome-encapsulated MDP requires only a 2-hour interaction, and maximum tumoricidal capacity is achieved after an 8-hour incubation (Fogler and Fidler, 1984; Fogler et al., 1985; Kripke et al., 1976). In addition, the duration of macrophage activation obtained with liposomes containing entrapped MDP is significantly prolonged (Daemen et al., 1986), and the required dose of liposome-delivered MDP is at least 400 times lower than that required for free MDP to achieve similar levels of macrophage activation (Fogler and Fidler, 1984). Recent studies have demonstrated that liposome-encapsulated IFN-γ (Fidler et al., 1985b; Saiki and Fidler, 1985; Saiki et al., 1985) and MTP-PE (Kleinerman et al., 1983a) did not require binding of the molecules to the macrophage surface.

As stated above, in several experimental systems, macrophages have been shown to recognize and lyse neoplastic cells without regard to their phenotypic diversity. Tumoricidal macrophages lyse cultures of tumor cells but not cultures of nontumorigenic cells (review, Fidler and Schroit, 1988). This selective destruction of neoplastic cells could be advantageous for treatment of disseminated cancer. Therefore, we wished to determine whether human blood monocytes activated to the tumoricidal state by interaction with liposomes containing immunomodulators could also discriminate between tumorigenic and nontumorigenic allogeneic target cells under cocultivation conditions. In common with other mammalian macrophages, human blood monocytes that were activated in vitro by interaction with liposomes containing MAF selectively lysed neoplastic cells in mixed cultures. Where possible, we attempted to pair tumor cells with physiologically normal counterparts. We therefore used both epithelial cells and fibroblasts as normal controls for tumors of endodermal, ectodermal, and mesenchymal origin. In all assays, we used a monocyte-to-target ratio at which nonactivated blood monocytes are not cytotoxic to susceptible tumorigenic targets, whereas activated monocytes are. The selective lysis of tumorigenic cells was not due merely to an inherent resistance of normal cells to lysis mediated by immune cells, but was associated with activated monocytes (Fidler and Kleinerman, 1984; Fidler and Schroit, 1988). We base this conclusion on the findings that both tumorigenic and nontumorigenic cells were equally susceptible to in vitro lysis mediated by mitogen-stimulated peripheral blood mononuclear leukocytes (Fidler and Schroit, 1988). Hence, activated human blood monocytes can lyse neoplastic cells while sparing normal cells, making this form of therapy attractive for the in situ eradication of metastatic disease.

IN SITU ACTIVATION OF MURINE MACROPHAGES

Since the lung is a major site of disseminated metastatic disease, we identified those liposomes with increased efficiency for localization to the lung parenchyma following intravenous injection of radiolabeled liposomes. Large MLV (>0.1 μm) were retained in the lungs more efficiently than were small unilamellar liposomes of identical lipid composition. In addition, liposomes of the same structural class were more efficiently retained in the lungs when they contained negatively charged lipids (PS) than when they contained only neutral lipids (PC) (Fidler et al., 1980; Schroit and Fidler, 1982).

Subsequent studies indicated that murine blood monocytes can extravasate out of the circulation and differentiate into alveolar macrophages (AM). This was shown by the intravenous injection of PC/PS (7:3 molar ratio) MLV that contained trace amounts of a fluorescent lipid analog, N-NBD-PE, into mice and recovery of AM by lung lavage 24 hours later (Key et al., 1982). About 12% to 15% of the total AM population (as identified by the formation of rosettes between opsonized erythrocytes and macrophages) contained fluorescent MLV, suggesting that the PC/PS liposomes were effective vehicles for the delivery of encapsulated compounds to blood monocytes (Gregoriadis, 1988; Papahadjopoulos, 1989).

The intravenous injection of PC/PS MLV containing MDP or MTP-PE immunomodulators results in the in situ activation of mouse AM. However, any potential therapeutic modality for metastatic disease must provide sustained activity. In order to assess whether AM activated by liposomes containing MDP maintained their tumoricidal properties over an extended period of time, the AM were harvested and assayed for tumoricidal activity 1, 2, 3, or 4 days after injecting a single dose of MLV containing MDP, MTP-PE, or a combination of both. On day 1, AM harvested from all the mice that received MLV with hydrophilic MDP exhibited less than 20% cytotoxicity; at every other time point, AM harvested from mice that received MLV containing MTP-PE consistently exhibited significantly higher levels of tumoricidal activity (Fidler et al., 1982b, 1983; Fogler and Fidler, 1984).

The in situ activation of macrophages by IV administration of liposomes containing macrophage activators resulted from the direct interactions of these liposomes with macrophages. It did not occur by an indirect action of the immunomodulator on T cells and a consequent release of lymphokines that activate macrophages (Fidler, 1981). This conclusion is based on data from experiments in which AM of mice with impaired T-cell function—mice exposed to UV radiation, thymectomized adult mice exposed to X-rays, and athymic nude mice—were all rendered tumoricidal by the systemic administration of liposome-encapsulated MTP-PE but not by control liposome preparations (Fidler, 1981).

ERADICATION OF MURINE MELANOMA METASTASES BY ACTIVATED MACROPHAGES

The systemic activation of macrophages by liposomes containing allogeneic MAF (Fidler, 1980), MDP (Fidler et al., 1982b, 1983; Fogler and Fidler, 1984), MTP-PE (Fidler et al., 1981b, 1982b, 1983; Fogler and Fidler, 1984), recombinant IFN-γ (r-IFN-γ) with MTP-PE (Fidler et al., 1989), or MDP with MAF (Fidler, 1986b) results in destruction of well-established lung and lymph node metastases produced by primary subcutaneous melanoma. The major tumor model for these studies has been the B16-BL6 melanoma cell line, which is syngeneic to C57BL/6 mice. After implantation in the footpad, this tumor metastasizes to lymph nodes and the lungs in more than 90% of the mice (Fidler, 1980; Fidler et al., 1978). Each of the C57BL/6 mice was given an intrafootpad injection of melanoma cells, and 4 to 5 weeks later, when the tumors had reached 10 to 12 mm, the leg bearing the tumor, including the popliteal lymph node, was amputated. Three days later, the mice were injected intravenously with MLV containing immunomodulators or a placebo preparation. Both test and control groups were treated twice weekly for 4 weeks (eight IV injections). Once again, we used PC/PS liposomes because they are not toxic at the dose used (Schroit et al., 1983a) and because they are arrested efficiently in the lungs as well as in organs of the RES following IV injection (Fidler et al., 1980; Schroit et al., 1982, 1983a).

Spontaneous metastases in the lungs and lymph nodes were well established at the time liposome treatment began. Many individual metastases could be seen macroscopically. All mice treated with saline, free lymphokines, free MDP, or liposomes containing placebo died by day 90 of the experiment, that is, 60 days after the amputation of the tumor-bearing leg. Significantly, 70% of mice injected intravenously with liposome-encapsulated lymphokines and 60% of mice injected with liposome-encapsulated MDP were alive when the experiments were terminated at 200 days. In this tumor system, we estimate that the metastases contained 10^7 cells at the beginning of the liposome treatment. Since the median survival time of mice injected with as few as 10 viable B16 cells (admixed with 10^6 dead cells) was 40 to 50 days, we speculate that the residual tumor burden of the surviving mice must have been reduced to less than 10 viable cells. Further studies revealed that the degree of success in this tumor model depended upon the timing of the first treatment with liposome-encapsulated MTP-PE. In animals initially inoculated in the footpad with B16-BL6 melanoma cells, the first injection of liposomes was given either 3 days, 7 days, or 10 days after hind limb amputation. Optimal therapy consisted of early treatment, that is, beginning 3 days after surgery. Moreover, in a separate study, a group of mice with metastatic melanoma was treated with varying schedules of liposome administration. The most effective schedule for treatment of lung metastases was twice weekly injection for 4 weeks: 68% of the mice were alive on day 200 of the experiment ($P<.001$) (Fidler, 1986a).

Collectively, these results demonstrate that the most efficient schedule of liposome administration is twice weekly for 8 weeks and that small metastases (micrometastases) are most susceptible to this form of therapy. Successful treatment of metastases by the intravenous injection of liposomes containing immunomodulators has been reported for mouse fibrosarcoma (Deodhar et al., 1981, 1982; Eppstein et al., 1986; Fidler, 1986b; Lopez-Berestein et al., 1984), melanomas (Phillips and Tsao, 1989; Phillips et al., 1985), lung carcinoma (Brodt et al., 1989), and colon carcinoma (Thrombre and Deodhar, 1984).

Several lines of evidence indicate that the eradication of established metastases following the systemic administration of liposomes containing immunomodulators was due to activation of macrophages to the tumoricidal state. First, the injection of macrophage-activating agents encapsulated within liposomes that were not retained in the lung microvasculature failed to activate lung macrophages, and no regression of lung metastases was observed. Second, the pretreatment of tumor-bearing animals with agents that are toxic for macrophages (silica, carrageenan, hyperchlorinated drinking water) before systemic therapy with liposome-encapsulated immunomodulators abrogated the response to liposome therapy, and the animals soon died of metastatic disease (Fidler et al., 1982a). Third, IV injection of macrophages activated in vitro by incubation with liposomes containing MAF reduced the metastatic burden to an extent comparable to that achieved by systemic administration of liposome-encapsulated activators (Fidler et al., 1982a). Fourth, morphological and functional analysis of macrophages isolated from pulmonary metastases of mice given IV injections of liposomes containing lipophilic MDP revealed that macrophages containing phagocytosed liposomes infiltrate and localize within pulmonary metastases. Furthermore, once localized, macrophages that engulfed liposomes containing MDP, but not those macrophages that engulfed liposomes containing control substances, were tumoricidal against the melanoma cells (Key et al., 1982).

THERAPY OF NATURAL CANINE OSTEOGENIC SARCOMA LUNG METASTASES

Like the disease in humans, the natural behavior of canine osteosarcoma involves progressive growth of the primary tumor, with the dog dying of distant visceral (lung) metastasis (Brodey and Abt, 1976; Gillete, 1982). Surgical resection of the primary neoplasm produces a median survival time of 3 to 6 months, with only 10% of the dogs surviving 1 year or longer (Brodey and Abt, 1976; Gillete, 1982). In a recent randomized study of the therapeutic efficacy of liposome-MTP-PE for metastasis in dogs (MacEwen et al., 1989), 27 dogs were studied. All animals had histologic confirmation of osteosarcoma and complete amputation of the affected limb. Immediately following surgery, dogs were randomized to receive either liposomes containing MTP-PE or liposomes containing saline (placebo), in twice weekly IV infusions for 8 weeks (total of 16 treatments). The dose per treatment was 2 mg/m^2 of MTP-PE (500 mg of phospholipids). Fourteen dogs were treated with active liposome-MTP-PE, and 13 dogs received liposome-saline. The median survival time of dogs treated with liposome-saline was 77 days, a survival that does not differ from surgery alone (Brodey and Abt, 1976; Gillete et al., 1982). In marked contrast, the median survival of dogs treated with liposome-MTP-PE was 222 days ($P<.002$). Moreover, 4 dogs in this group were alive and free of metastasis 1 year after surgery. The treatment did not produce toxic effects and was well tolerated (Brodey and Abt, 1976). A major limitation for eradication of metastases by macrophages is the tumor burden (Fidler, 1985, 1986b, 1988). It is possible that in some dogs, the tumor burden (in micrometastases) exceeded the level that can be destroyed by macrophages. In this (Brodey and Abt, 1976), as well as other preclinical studies (Fidler, 1986b; Hisano and Fidler, 1982), it was recommended that systemic macrophage activation follow other cytoreductive therapies.

CLINICAL STUDIES

Activation of Tumoricidal Properties in Blood Monocytes of Patients with Colorectal Cancer

Before systemic therapy of metastases can be tried in humans, several questions must be answered. These include: (1) Do cancer patients have sufficient numbers of blood monocytes? (2) Can blood monocytes obtained from cancer patients be rendered cytotoxic in vitro against allogeneic tumor targets such as colon carcinoma cells? (3) Does the stage of disease influence the responsiveness of blood monocytes to activation stimuli? (4) Do different patients' monocytes respond differently to different activators? (5) Can monocytes of cancer patients be rendered tumoricidal, that is, able to destroy tumor cells, but not normal cells?

We first studied these questions with blood monocytes obtained from patients with colorectal carcinoma and from normal donors. All blood monocytes were incubated for 24 hours in vitro with free and liposome-encapsulated lymphokines and free and liposome-encapsulated muramyl peptides (MDP, MTP-PE). Monocytes incubated in medium alone served as negative controls, and monocytes incubated with endotoxin (lipopolysaccharide) served as positive controls. The cytotoxic properties of each patient's monocytes were tested against several allogeneic-tumorigenic, and allogeneic-nontumorigenic cells (Fidler et al., 1986).

Monocytes obtained from 11 cancer patients were at levels found for normal donors. Blood monocytes of the cancer patients did not exhibit spontaneous cytotoxicity against any of the target cells. But these same monocytes, upon in vitro activation with any of the free or liposome-entrapped agents, became tumoricidal, that is, they lysed neoplastic cells, but not normal cells. Moreover, the level of monocyte-mediated tumor lysis was comparable to that observed with blood monocytes obtained from normal donors. These data showed that blood monocytes of patients with local or disseminated colorectal carcinoma can be activated in vitro to become tumoricidal by interaction with free and liposome-encapsulated immunomodulators (Fidler et al., 1986).

Activation of Tumoricidal Properties in Blood Monocytes of Patients with Osteogenic Sarcoma

Studies in rodent tumor systems have suggested that systemic macrophage activation could be an attractive approach for destroying tumor cells resistant to conventional chemotherapy (Fidler and Kleinerman, 1984; Hisano and Fidler, 1982). The outcome of macrophage–tumor interaction in vivo is regulated by factors such as the ratio of macrophages to target cells, the state of activity of the macrophages, and the rate of tumor cell proliferation. The major limitation to treatment of disseminated metastases by the systemic activation of macrophages, however, appears to be the tumor burden (Fidler, 1985; Hisano and Fidler, 1982).

Potential therapeutic regimens to stimulate the antitumor properties of macrophages will have to be used in combination with other treatments such as chemotherapy, which could first reduce the tumor burden to allow activated macrophages to destroy the surviving tumor cells regardless of their drug sensitivity (Fidler, 1985). For systemic macrophage activation in cancer patients treated with a chemotherapeutic agent to be successful, the chemotherapy per se cannot be toxic to the macrophage system. For this reason, we investigated whether systemic administration of doxorubicin hydrochloride (Adriamycin [ADR]) to patients with osteosarcoma interferes with the response of their blood monocytes to activation by liposomes containing MTP-PE (Hudson et al., 1988; Kleinerman and Hudson, 1989; Kleinerman et al., 1983b). Human peripheral blood monocytes were isolated from normal donors and preincubated with ADR (0.5 to 500 ng/mL) for 1 hour before the addition of free or liposome-encapsulated activators, or incubated with ADR for 24 hours in the presence of free or liposome-encapsulated immunomodulators. Monocyte-mediated antitumor cytotoxicity was assessed by an in vitro assay. At the concentrations used, ADR did not inhibit the ability of blood monocytes to respond to immunomodulators.

We next determined whether similar results could be obtained with monocytes from osteosarcoma patients treated with ADR (75 mg/m^2). We collected blood monocytes from nine patients at the time of diagnosis and 1 month after systemic therapy with ADR. The monocytes were incubated in vitro with liposomes containing MTP-PE (or other immunomodulators), and their ability to lyse tumorigenic targets in vitro was measured. The data clearly demonstrated that monocytes of osteogenic sarcoma patients treated with ADR could be activated to the tumoricidal state by liposome-encapsulated agents at levels equal to, or greater than, pretherapy levels. In fact, peripheral blood monocytes isolated from four patients as early as 1 day after ADR therapy were readily activated by liposome-encapsulated agents. Collectively, these studies indicated that the monocyte function of osteosarcoma patients treated with ADR is intact and that systemic administration of liposome-encapsulated immunomodulators is not contraindicated for the treatment of metastatic pulmonary osteogenic sarcoma (Hisano and Fidler, 1982).

Phase I Trial of Liposome-Encapsulated MTP-PE in Cancer Patients

Synthetic MTP-PE is a lipophilic analogue of MDP that by its nature can be incorporated into liposomes at a high efficiency (95%) (Van Hoogevest and Fankhauser, 1989). Freeze-dried liposomes containing MTP-PE were produced at Ciba-Geigy, Ltd. (Basel, Switzerland) by mixing MTP-PE with synthetic phospholipids (palmitoyl, oleoyl PC and dioleoyl PS, 7:3 molar ratio) followed by lyophilization (Schumann et al., 1989; Van Hoogevest and Fankhauser, 1989). Prior to administration, 2.5 mL of CA^{2+}- and Mg^{2+}-free phosphate-buffered saline are added to each vial containing lyophilized lipids and 1 mg of MTP-PE. The MTP-PE:phospholipid ratio in the final preparation was a constant 1:250. After hydration, the vials were vortexed for 1 minute at high speed. The resulting suspension was stable and could be stored at 4°C for 24 hours. This commercial preparation of liposomal MTP-PE has been used with success to activate human blood monocytes in vitro (Fogler and Fidler, 1986; Sone et al., 1986) and mouse macrophages under both in vitro and in vivo conditions (Deodhar et al., 1982a; Fidler, 1981). Moreover, this liposome–MTP-PE preparation has also been shown to activate rat lung macrophages subsequent to intranasal administration (Brownbill, 1985) to produce systemic activation of murine macrophages subsequent to oral administration (Fidler et al., 1987), and to eradicate spontaneous metastases in a murine melanoma system (Fidler, 1981) and in dogs with autochthonous osteogenic sarcoma metastases (MacEwen et al., 1989).

This liposome–MTP-PE preparation was evaluated for safety in several species. Species variability for toxicity was revealed (Fidler et al., 1985a; Schumann et al., 1989). In the mouse and rat (the least sensitive), doses of 10 mg/kg (of MTP-PE) were well tolerated. This is about 50 times the biological dose needed to activate macrophages in situ (Fidler, 1981; Fidler et al., 1981b). In rabbits and dogs (the sensitive species), doses of 0.1 mg/kg administered daily for 90 days did not produce any measurable toxicity (Schumann et al., 1989).

This stable pharmaceutical preparation of liposome–MTP-PE was then studied in a multicenter phase I trial in cancer patients (Creaven et al., 1989; Hanagan et al., 1989; Murray et al., 1989a). The main objectives of the study were to determine the toxicity and the maximum tolerated dose of liposome–MTP-PE and to examine the immunomodulating activity of this preparation. The results obtained from the two parallel phase I trials were similar (Hanagan et al., 1989); hence, details will be given for the study at the University of Texas M. D. Anderson Cancer Center (Murray et al., 1989b).

The study included 28 adults older than 18 years of age with histologic confirmation of metastatic cancer who were unresponsive to all previous therapies. Patients had to have an estimated performance status of 0-2 using Zubrod's criteria (Zubrod et al., 1960) and an estimated life span of $\geq$12 weeks. All patients gave written informed consent to participate in the study in accordance with established guidelines from the surveillance committee at the M. D. Anderson Cancer Center. All previous therapy had been discontinued for a minimum of 3 weeks prior to study. To be eligible for study, patients had to have a Hgb of $\geq$9 mg/100 mL, a white blood cell count of $\geq$4,000/mm^3, a granulocyte count of $\geq$2,000/mm^3, and a platelet count of $\geq$100,000/mm^3. Serum bilirubin had to be $\leq$1.5 mg/100 mL, serum glutamyl pyruvate transaminase (SGPT) $\leq$75 mg/100 mL, blood urea nitrogen (BUN) $\leq$30 mg/100 mL, and creatinine $\leq$1.5 mg/100 mL. Since high levels of free unencapsulated MTP-PE have been associated with dose-dependent vasculitis in dogs (Schumann et al., 1989), patients with a previous history of autoimmune disease or vasculitis were excluded from the study. Finally, the extent of disease was evaluated in all patients by physical examination, X-rays, computerized tomography (CT) scans, and other tests.

Liposome–MTP-PE was administered intravenously over 1 hour twice weekly for a total duration of 9 weeks. The first three patients in the study received liposome–MTP-PE at a dose of 0.05 mg/m^2 MTP-PE. After 3 weeks of biweekly infusions, the dose was escalated to the next level (0.1 mg/m^2) and subsequently to a third and final level of 0.25 mg/m^2 MTP-PE (MTP-PE:phospholipid, 1:250). When no major toxicity was observed, an additional three patients were entered at a dose one level higher than the initial starting level for the previous group and were escalated every 3 weeks. The doses of MTP-PE thus administered were 0.05, 0.10, 0.25, 0.50, 1.0, 1.5, 2.0, 3.0, 4.0, 6.0, 9.0, and 12.0 mg/m^2. Patients could continue to receive liposome–MTP-PE at the highest level reached by the end of 9 weeks provided the disease was stable and the patients were without side effects.

Patients underwent a physical examination, routine chest X-ray, and electrocardiography, and blood was drawn every 3 weeks to determine immunological parameters, which included monocyte-mediated tumor cell lysis in vitro. Complete blood counts with differential and platelet count and serum chemistry were determined weekly, 72 hours and, occasionally, 24 hours after IV infusion of liposomes. Serum cholesterol, triglycerides, antinuclear antibodies, and rheumatoid factor assays were also performed once weekly. Samples were also collected 24 hours after IV infusion of liposomes for monocyte-mediated cytotoxicity assay. Finally, at the end of 9 weeks, X-rays, CT scans, and other tests were repeated to evaluate tumor status.

The following immunological parameters were examined: lymphocyte surface markers, in vitro monocyte tumoricidal activity, serum IL-1 levels, and acute phase reactants (including fibrinogen, ceruloplasmin, β_2-microglobulin, and C-reactive protein). All tests were performed prior to infusion of liposome–MTP-PE and at 3-week intervals. In addition, skin tests for seven recall antigens were performed prior to infusion and at 8 weeks of treatment.

The major findings from this phase I trial were: At the dose and schedule described, liposome–MTP-PE was safe. Major dose-limiting side effects were chills and fever (80% of the patients), fatigue (60%), nausea and vomiting (55%), and headaches (20%). Hypo- or hypertension was also observed, but these were self-limiting. In four patients, liposome–MTP-PE treatment was de-escalated due to severe malaise and recurrent fever exceeding 38.8 °C. Toxicity was not cumulative and the maximal tolerated dose of liposome–MTP-PE was 6 mg/m^2.

In accordance with the preclinical data in rodents and dogs, we observed a consistent increase in absolute white blood cells and granulocytes. This finding was significant in patients infused with $\geq$2 mg/m^2 of MTP-PE–liposomes regardless of whether, at 24 hours after infusion, data were analyzed alone or combined with data obtained at 72 and 96 hours after infusion. This could have been due to production of colony-stimulating factors (CSF) by activated monocytes, in particular granulocyte-CSF (G-CSF) given alone or in combination with IL-1β (Moore et al., 1987; Shah et al., 1977).

The IV administration of liposome–MTP-PE activated tumoricidal properties in the monocytes of 24 of the 28 patients. This increased antitumor activity could not be explained by simple fluctuations in cytotoxic function because monocyte-mediated antitumor cytotoxicity in both normal donors and cancer patients did not change when sequentially studied over time (Murray, 1982).

Because the protocol schema called for each patient to have two-dose escalations, the data were difficult to analyze. We therefore employed three different analyses to determine the optimal dose. The optimal biological dose of liposome–MTP-PE was less than the maximum tolerated dose (liposome–MTP-PE, MTD = 6 mg/m²/dose). Monocytes isolated from patients receiving doses of liposome–MTP-PE that exceeded the optimal dose could still be activated in vitro to lyse tumor cells and secrete IL-1 and TNF. This is in contrast to monocytes obtained from patients receiving r-IFN-γ at doses above the optimal biological dose, where no response to in vitro stimuli could be generated (Kleinerman, 1986). We therefore conclude that liposome–MTP-PE was not toxic to the monocytes at doses as high as 12 mg/m², the highest dose administered in this study (Kleinerman, 1989), and that the optimal dose of liposome–MTP-PE for rendering monocytes tumoricidal ranged from 0.5 to 2.0 mg/m².

Patients with increased granulocyte count exhibited a significant decrease in serum cholesterol ($P<.01$). A decrease in serum cholesterol has previously been reported in patients with marked granulocytosis such as in leukemia (Bases and Krakoff, 1965), as well as in patients treated with granulocyte-macrophage CSF (Nimer et al., 1988). The mechanisms for the reduction in serum cholesterol in this trial may be related to activation of Kupffer's cells leading to increased cholesterol excretion (Cai et al., 1988) or to actual uptake and metabolism of cholesterol by activated blood monocytes (Goldstein et al., 1979). The exact nature, however, remains unclear.

Activated human monocytes are known to produce numerous cytokines such as TNF, IL-1β, and IL-6 (Fey and Fuller, 1987). Indeed, we observed increases in serum IL-1β in 6 of 10 patients serially followed prior to, and at 1 hour after, infusion.

Significant elevations in C-reactive protein, β_2-microglobulin, and ceruloplasmin were frequently observed. Whether these were due to the generation of IL-6 (Fey and Fuller, 1987) is not clear at present.

The biodistribution and pharmacokinetics of liposome–MTP-PE were studied in four patients subsequent to IV infusion of technetium 99m (^{99m}Tc)-labeled MLV. At 6 hours following injection of ^{99m}Tc-labeled liposomes containing 1 mg MTP-PE, radioactivity was found in the liver, spleen, nasopharynx, thyroid, and, to a lesser extent, the lungs. This radioactivity partially cleared by 24 hours. In two of the four patients studied, lung metastases were imaged presumably by tumor-associated macrophages laden with liposomes. These data are comparable with other published reports with liposomes (Lopez-Berestein et al., 1985; Perez-Soler et al., 1985; Richardson et al., 1979), with the exception that the PC:PS liposomes appeared to clear more rapidly from lung than those containing phosphatidylglycerol (Lopez-Berestein et al., 1985). The differences in tumor imaging from other studies may reflect differences in liposome composition, charge, and size (Richardson et al., 1978). A rapid alpha phase and slower beta phase half-life could represent immediate targeting to liver and other tissues followed by a slow reequilibration in plasma and circulating monocytes.

In this particular trial, unlike the other phase I trials (Fidler et al., 1985a, 1987), absolute regression of metastatic lesions was not observed. Three patients had stable disease while on treatment for a mean duration of 17 weeks (range 14.5–22 weeks). The average number of doses of liposome–MTP-PE given over this time period was 32 (range 24–43). In the remaining 21 patients, the disease progressed at 9 weeks. The lack of tumor regression in patients treated with liposome–MTP-PE was not unexpected since clinical studies indicate that systemic macrophage activation is effective only against minimal disease; large tumor burdens are not amenable to this treatment (Fidler, 1985, 1986b; Fidler and Poste, 1982). Hence, phase II trials in patients with minimal tumor burdens and trials of its use as an adjuvant need to be performed before the full range of antitumor activity of liposome–MTP-PE is determined.

In summary, the systemic administration of liposome–MTP-PE rendered blood monocytes of cancer patients with advanced disease cytotoxic to tumor cells (Schumann et al., 1989). Since liposome–MTP-PE has no direct antiproliferative effects on tumor cells, the objective of this therapy is to activate the host's monocytes to kill the tumor cells. The results recommend that future trials be conducted with a dose of 0.5 to 2.0 mg/m^2 rather than the maximum tolerated dose of 6 mg/m^2.

CONCLUSIONS

The continuous emergence of variant subpopulations of tumor cells from both the primary and metastatic lesions implies that the successful therapy of disseminated cancer will have to include a modality that will overcome the cellular heterogeneity of tumors that ultimately lead to resistance to therapy. Macrophages activated to become tumoricidal by interaction with liposomes containing immunomodulators may be one such treatment modality. Tumoricidal macrophages recognize and destroy neoplastic, but not normal, cells in vitro and in vivo. Moreover, evidence indicates that macrophage destruction of tumor cells is not associated with the development of tumor cell resistance.

Intravenously administered liposomes are cleared from the circulation by phagocytic cells and the endocytosis of these liposomes containing appropriate immunomodulators generates cytotoxic macrophages in situ. Multiple administration of such liposomes has been shown to bring about eradication of cancer metastases in several murine tumor systems and in spontaneous canine osteosarcoma. These host antitumor responses do not require the participation of functional T lymphocytes or NK cells. Rather, the destruction of established metastases after the multiple systemic administration of liposome-encapsulated immunomodulators seems to be directly mediated by activated macrophages.

Liposomes containing MTP-PE can activate tumoricidal properties in blood monocytes of cancer patients. The results of phase I clinical trials indicate that at the minimum dose sufficient to produce biological effects, these liposomes are well tolerated. The cytolytic effects of macrophages in vivo are regulated by factors such as the ratio of macrophages to target cells, the state of activity of the macrophages, and the rate of tumor cell proliferation. The treatment of metastases by macrophages, therefore, would be most successful when the metastases are small or slow to proliferate and are infiltrated by a large number of tumoricidal macrophages. However, the major limitation to treatment of disseminated metastases by the systemic activation of macrophages appears to be the tumor burden. Thus, the therapeutic stimulation of macrophage-mediated antitumor activity will be unsuccessful for treatment of large or numerous metastatic nodules. For this reason, potential therapeutic regimens designed to stimulate host immunity must be used in combination with other treatment modalities such as chemotherapy, in order to reduce the tumor burden; the activated macrophages may then lyse tumor cells that are resistant to the chemotherapy. A heterogeneous disease such as cancer cannot be treated by a single modality: systemically activated macrophages should add one more modality to our regimens for the eradication of cancer metastases.

REFERENCES

Allison AC. On the role of mononuclear phagocytes in immunity against viruses. Prog Med Virol. 1974;18:15–31.

Allison AC. Mode of action of immunological adjuvants. J Reticuloendothel Soc. 1974;26:619–630.

Alving CR. Delivery of liposome-encapsulated drugs to macrophages. Pharmacol Ther. 1983;22:407–424.

Bases RE, Krakoff IH. Studies of serum cholesterol levels in leukemia. J Reticuloendothel Soc. 1965;2:8–14.

Brodey RS, Abt DA. Results of surgical treatment in 65 dogs with osteosarcoma. J Am Vet Med Assoc. 1976;168:1032–1038.

Brodt P, Blore J, Philips NC, Munzer JS, Rioux JD. Inhibition of murine hepatic tumor growth by liposomes containing a lipophilic muramyl dipeptide. Cancer Immunol Immunother. 1989;28:54–60.

Brownbill AF, Braun DG, Dukor P, Schumann G. Induction of tumoricidal leukocytes by the intranasal application of MTP-PE, a lipophilic muramyl peptide. Cancer Immunol Immunother. 1985;20:11–18.

Bucana C, Hoyer LL, Hobbs B, Breesman S, McDaniel M, Hanna MG Jr. Morphological evidence for the translocation of lysosomal organelles from cytotoxic macrophages into the cytoplasm of tumor target cells. Cancer Res. 1976;36:4444–4458.

Bucana CD, Hoyer LC, Schroit AJ, Kleinerman ES, Fidler IJ. Ultrastructural studies of the interaction between liposome-activated human blood monocytes and allogeneic tumor cells in vitro. Am J Pathol. 1983;112:101–111.

Cai HJ, He ZG, Ding YN. Effects of monocyte macrophage stimulation on hepatic lipoprotein receptors. Biochim Biophys Acta. 1988;959:334–342.

Cameron DJ, Churchill WH. Cytotoxicity of human macrophage for tumor cells: enhancement by human lymphocyte mediators. J Clin Invest. 1979;63:977–984.

Chait A. The role of lipoprotein in lipid transport and in the pathogenesis of the hyperproteinemias. Spec Top Endocrinol Metab. 1983;5:1–53.

Chapes SK, Haskill S. Role of *Corynebacterium parvum* in human blood monocytes by muramyl peptides requires a specific intracellular interaction. J Immunol. 1982;136:2311–2316.

Chedid L, Audibert F, Johnson AG. Biological activities of muramyl dipeptide, a synthetic glycopeptide analogous to bacterial immunoregulating agents. Prog Allergy. 1978;25:63–80.

Cifone MA, Fidler IJ. Correlation of patterns of anchorage-independent growth with in vivo behavior of cells from a murine fibrosarcoma. Proc Natl Acad Sci USA. 1980;77:1039–1043.

Creaven PJ, Brenner DE, Cowens JW, et al. Initial clinical trial of muramyl tripeptide derivative (MTP-PE) encapsulated in liposomes: an interim report. In: Lopez-Berestein G, Fidler IJ, eds. Liposomes in the therapy of infectious diseases and cancer, new series. Vol. 89. New York, NY: Alan R. Liss; 1989:297–303.

Custer A, Ballerzak S, Rinehart J. Human macrophage hemoglobin-iron metabolism in vitro. Am J Hematol. 1982;13:23–36.

Daemen T, Veninga A, Scherphof GL, Roerdink FH. The activation of Kupffer cells of tumor cytotoxicity with immunomodulators encapsulated in liposomes. In: Kirn A, Knook DL, Wisse E, eds. Cell of the hepatic sinusoid. Rijswijk, The Netherlands: The Kupffer Cell Foundation; 1986:379–383.

Daemen T, Veninga A, Roerdink FH, Scherphof GL. The in vitro activation of rat liver macrophages to tumoricidal activity by free or liposome-encapsulated muramyl dipeptide. Cancer Res. 1989;46:4330–4335.

Daoud SS, Hume LR, Juliano RL. Liposomes in cancer therapy. Adv Drug Deliv Rev. 1989;3:405–418.

Den Otter W, Dullens Hub JJ, Can Lovern H, Pels E. Antitumor effects of macrophages injected into animals: a review. In: James K, McBride B, Stuart A, eds. The macrophage and cancer. Edinburgh: Econoprint; 1977:119–141.

Deodhar SD, Barna BP, Edinger M, Chiang T. Inhibition of lung metastases by liposomal immunotherapy in a murine fibrosarcoma model. J Biol Resp Mod. 1982a;1:27–34.

Deodhar SR, James K, Chiang T, Edinger M, Barna B. Inhibition of lung metastases in mice bearing a malignant fibrosarcoma by treatment with liposomes containing human C-reactive protein. Cancer Res. 1982b;42:5084–5091.

Duvall E, Wyllie AH, Morris RG. Macrophage-recognition of cells undergoing programmed cell death (apoptosis). Immunology. 1985;56:351–358.

Eppstein DA, Van der Pas MA, Fraser-Smith EB, et al. Liposome-encapsulated muramyl dipeptide analogue enhances non-specific host immunity. Int J Immunother. 1986;2:115–126.

Fey GH, Fuller GM. Regulation of acute phase gene expression by inflammatory mediators. Mol Biol Med. 1987;4:323–338.

Fidler IJ. Inhibition of pulmonary metastasis by intravenous injection of specifically activated macrophages. Cancer Res. 1974;34:1074–1078.

Fidler IJ. Recognition and destruction of target cells by tumoricidal macrophages. Israel J Med Sci. 1978;14:177–191.

Fidler IJ. Therapy of spontaneous metastases by intravenous injection of liposomes containing lymphokines. Science. 1980;208:1469–1471.

Fidler IJ. The in situ induction of tumoricidal activity in alveolar macrophages by liposomes containing muramyl dipeptide is a thymus-independent process. J Immunol. 1981;127:1719–1720.

Fidler IJ. The MAF dilemma. Lymphokine Res. 1984;3:51–54.43.

Fidler IJ. Macrophages and metastasis—a biological approach to cancer therapy: presidential address. Cancer Res. 1985;45:4714–4726.

Fidler IJ. Optimization and limitation of systemic treatment of murine melanoma metastases with liposomes containing muramyl tripeptide phosphatidylethanolamine. Cancer Immunol Immunother. 1986a;21:169–173.

Fidler IJ. Immunomodulation of macrophages for cancer and antiviral therapy. In: Tomlinson E, Davis SS, eds. Site-specific drug delivery. New York, NY: John Wiley; 1986b:111–135.

Fidler IJ. Targeting of immunomodulators to mononuclear phagocytes for therapy of cancer. Adv Drug Deliv Rev. 1988;2:69–106.

Fidler IJ, Kripke ML. Metastasis results from preexisting variant cells within a malignant tumor. Science. 1977;197:893–895.

Fidler IJ, Raz A. The induction of tumoricidal capacities in mouse and rat macrophages by lymphokines. In: Pick E, ed. Lymphokines. New York, NY: Academic Press; 1981:345–363.

Fidler IJ, Poste G. Macrophage-mediated destruction of malignant tumor cells and new strategies for the therapy of metastatic disease. Springer Semin Immunopathol. 1982;5:161–174.

Fidler IJ, Kleinerman ES. Lymphokine-activated human blood monocytes destroy tumor cells but not normal cells under cocultivation conditions. J Clin Oncol. 1984;2:937–943.

Fidler IJ, Poste G. The cellular heterogeneity of malignant neoplasms: implications for adjuvant chemotherapy. Semin Oncol. 1985;12:207–222.

Fidler IJ, Schroit AJ. Macrophage recognition of self from nonself: implications for the interaction of macrophages with neoplastic cells. In: Kripke ML, Frost P, eds. Immunology and cancer. Austin: University of Texas Press; 1986:183–207.

Fidler IJ, Talmadge JE. Evidence that intravenously derived murine pulmonary melanoma metastases can originate from the expansion of a single tumor cell. Cancer Res. 1986;46:5167–5171.

Fidler IJ, Balch CM. The biology of cancer metastasis and implications for therapy. Curr Probl Surg. 1987;24(3):131–209.

Fidler IJ, Gersten DM, Budmen MB. Characterization in vivo and in vitro of tumor cells selected for resistance to syngeneic lymphocyte-mediated cytotoxicity. Cancer Res. 1976;36:3160–3165.

Fidler IJ, Gersten DM, Hart IR. The biology of cancer invasion and metastasis. Adv Cancer Res. 1978;28:149–259.

Fidler IJ, Fogler WE, Connor J. The rationale for the treatment of established experimental micrometastases with the injection of tumoricidal macrophages. In: Terry WD, Yamamura Y, eds. Immunobiology and immunotherapy of cancer. New York, NY: Elsevier; 1979:361–375.

Fidler IJ, Raz A, Fogler WE, Kirsh R, Bugelski P, Poste G. The design of liposomes to improve delivery of macrophage-augmenting agents to alveolar macrophages. Cancer Res. 1980; 40:4460–4466.

Fidler IJ, Raz A, Fogler WE, Hoyer LC, Poste G. Role of plasma membrane receptors and the kinetics of macrophage activation by lymphokines encapsulated in lipsomes. Cancer Res. 1981a;41:495–504.

Fidler IJ, Sone S, Fogler WE, Barnes ZL. Eradication of spontaneous metastases and activation of alveolar macrophages by intravenous injection of liposomes containing muramyl dipeptide. Proc Natl Acad Sci USA. 1981b;78:1680–1684.

Fidler IJ, Barnes Z, Fogler WE, Kirsh R, Bugelski P, Poste G. Involvement of macrophages in the eradication of established metastases following intravenous injection of liposome containing macrophage activators. Cancer Res. 1982a;42:496–501.

Fidler IJ, Sone S, Fogler WE, et al. Efficacy of liposomes containing a lipophilic muramyl dipeptide for activating the tumoricidal properties of alveolar macrophages in vivo. J Biol Resp Mod. 1982b;1:43–55.

Fidler IJ, Fogler WE, Tarcsay L, Schumann G, Graun DG, Schroit AJ. Systemic activation of macrophages and treatment of cancer metastases by liposomes containing hydrophilic or lipophilic muramyl dipeptide. Immunopharmacology. 1983;2:235–353.

Fidler IJ, Brown NO, Hart IR. Species variability for toxicity of free and liposome-encapsulated muramyl peptides administered intravenously. J Biol Resp Mod. 1985a;4:298–309.

Fidler IJ, Fogler WE, Kleinerman ES, Saiki I. Abrogation of species specificity for activation of tumoricidal properties in macrophages by recombinant mouse or human gamma interferon encapsulated in liposomes. J Immunol. 1985b;135:4289–4294.

Fidler IJ, Jessup JM, Fogler WE, Staerkel R, Mazumder A. Activation of tumoricidal properties in peripheral blood monocytes of patients with colorectal carcinoma. Cancer Res. 1986; 44:994–998.

Fidler IJ, Fogler WE, Brownbill AF, Schumann G. Systemic activation of tumoricidal properties in mouse macrophages and inhibition of melanoma metastases by the oral administration of MTP-PE, a lipophilic muramyl dipeptide. J Immunol. 1987;138:4509–4514.

Fidler IJ, Schroit AJ. Recognition and destruction of neoplastic cells by activated macrophages: discrimination of altered self. Biochim Biophys Acta. 1988;948:151–172.

Fidler IJ, Fan D, Ichinose Y. Potent in situ activation of murine lung macrophages and therapy of melanoma metastases by systemic administration of liposomes containing muramyltripeptide phosphatidylethanolamine and interferon gamma. Inv Metastasis. 1989;9:75–88.

Fogler WE, Fidler IJ. Modulation of the immune response by muramyl dipeptide. In: Chirigos MA, Fenichel RL, eds. Immune modulation agents and their mechanisms. New York, NY: Marcel Dekker; 1984:499–512.

Fogler WE, Fidler IJ. Nonselective destruction of murine neoplastic cells by syngeneic tumoricidal macrophages. Cancer Res. 1985;45:14–18.

Fogler WE, Fidler IJ. The activation of tumoricidal properties in human blood monocytes by muramyl peptides requires a specific intracellular interaction. J Immunol. 1986;136:2311–2316.

Fogler WE, Talmadge J, Fidler IJ. The activation of tumoricidal properties in macrophages of endotoxin responder and nonresponder mice by liposome-encapsulated immunomodulators. J Reticuloendothel Soc. 1983;33:165–173.

Fogler WE, Wade R, Brundish DE, Fidler IJ. Distribution and fate of free and liposome-encapsulated [^{3}H]nor-muramyl dipeptide and [^{3}H]muramyl tripeptide phosphatidylethanomine in mice. J Immunol. 1985;135:1372–1377.

Gillete EL. Spontaneous canine neoplasms as models for therapeutic agents. In: Fidler IJ, White RJ, eds. Design of models for testing cancer therapeutic agents. Van Nostrand-Reinhold; New York, NY: 1982:185–192.

Gisler RH, Dietrich FM, Baschang G, et al. In: Turk JL, Danker D, eds. Immune responsiveness. London: Macmillan; 1979:133–160.

Goldstein JL, Ho YK, Basu SK, Brown D. Binding site of macrophages that mediates uptake and degradation of acetylated low density lipoprotein, producing massive cholesterol deposition. Proc Natl Acad Sci USA. 1979;76:333–337.

Gregoriadis G, ed. Liposomes as drug carriers: recent trends and progress. New York, NY: John Wiley & Sons; 1988.

Gregoriadis G, Allison AC, eds. Liposomes in biological systems. New York, NY: Wiley-Interscience; 1980.

Hahn H. Antibacterial defense mechanisms. Infection. 1983;11:5112–5118.

Hanagan JR, Trunet P, LeSher D, Andrejcio K, Frost H. Phase I development of CGP 19835A lipid (MTP-PE encapsulated in liposomes). In: Lopez-Berestein G, Fidler IJ, eds. Liposomes in the therapy of infectious diseases and cancer. New York, NY: Alan R. Liss; 1989:305–315.

Hanna N, Fidler IJ. Relationship between metastatic potential and resistance to natural killer cell–mediated cytotoxicity in three murine tumor systems. J Natl Cancer Inst. 1980;66:1183–1190.

Hart IR, Fogler WE, Poste G, Fidler IJ. Toxicity studies of liposome-encapsulated immunomodulators administered intravenously into dogs and mice. Cancer Immunol Immunother. 1981;10:157–166.

Hibbs JB Jr. Discrimination between neoplastic and nonneoplastic cells in vitro by activated macrophages. J Natl Cancer Inst. 1974a;53:1487–1492.

Hibbs JB Jr. Heterocytolysis by macrophages activated by bacillus Calmette-Guérin: lysosome exocytosis into tumor cells. Science. 1974b;184:468–471.

Hibbs JB Jr, Lambert LH, Remington JS. Control of carcinogenesis: a possible role for the activated macrophage. Science. 1972;177:998–1000.

Hisano G, Fidler IJ. Systemic activation of macrophages by liposme-entrapped muramyl tripeptide in mice pretreated with the chemotherapeutic agent Adriamycin. Cancer Immunol Immunother. 1982;14:61–66.

Hori K, Mihich E, Ehrke MJ. Role of tumor necrosis factor and interleukin 1 in γ-interferon-promoted activation of mouse tumoricidal macrophages. Cancer Res. 1989;49:2606–2614.

Hu F, Wang RY, Hsu TC. Clonal origin of metastasis in B-16 murine melanoma: a cytogenetic study. J Natl Cancer Inst. 1987;78:315–320.

Hudson MM, Snyder JS, Jaffe N, Kleinerman ES. In vitro and in vivo effect of Adriamycin therapy on monocyte activation by liposome-encapsulated immunomodulators. Cancer Res. 1988;48:5256–5263.

Hwang KJ. Liposome pharmacokinetics. In: Ostro MJ, ed. Liposomes from biophysics to therapeutics. New York, NY: Marcel Dekker; 1987:109–156.

Jones PDE, Castro JE. Immunological mechanisms in metastatic spread and the antimetastatic effects of *C. parvum*. Br J Cancer. 1977;35:519–527.

Kerbel RS. Implications of immunological heterogeneity in tumors. Nature. 1979;280:358–360.

Kerbel RS, Waghorne C, Man MS, Elliot B, Breitman ML. Alteration of the tumorigenic and metastatic properties of neoplastic cells is associated with the process of calcium phosphate-mediated DNA transfection. Proc Natl Acad Sci USA. 1987;84:1263–1267.

Key ME, Talmadge JE, Fogler WE, Bucana C, Fidler IJ. Isolation of tumoricidal macrophages from lung melanoma metastases of mice treated systemically with liposomes containing a lipophilic derivative of muramyl dipeptide. J Natl Cancer Inst. 1982;69:1189–1198.

Killion JJ, Kollmorgen GM. Isolation of immunogenic tumor by cell-affinity chromatography. Nature. 1976;259:674–676.

Killion JJ, Fidler IJ. The biology of tumor metastasis. Semin Oncol. 1989;16:106–115.

Kleinerman ES, Fidler IJ. Production and utilization of human lymphokines containing macrophage-activating factor (MAF) activity. Lymphokine Res. 1983;2:7–12.

Kleinerman ES, Hudson MM. Liposome therapy: a novel approach to the treatment of childhood osteosarcoma. In: Lopez-Berestein G, Fidler IJ, eds. Liposomes in the therapy of infectious diseases and cancer. Vol. 89. New York, NY: Alan R. Liss; 1989:71–80.

Kleinerman ES, Erickson KL, Schroit AJ, Fogler WE, Fidler IJ. Activation of tumoricidal properties in human blood monocytes by liposomes containing lipophilic muramyl tripeptide. Cancer Res. 1983a;43:2010–2014.

Kleinerman ES, Schroit AJ, Fogler WE, Fidler IJ. Tumoricidal activity of human monocytes activated in vitro by free and liposome-encapsulated human lymphokines. J Clin Invest. 1983b;72:1–12.

Kleinerman ES, Fogler WE, Fidler IJ. Intracellular activation of human and rodent macrophages by human lymphokines encapsulated in liposomes. J Leukocyte Biol. 1985;37:571–584.

Kleinerman ES, Kurzrock R, Wyatt D, Quesada JR, Gutterman JU, Fidler IJ. Activation or suppression of the tumoricidal properties of monocytes from cancer patients following treatment with human recombinant γ-interferon. Cancer Res. 1986;46:5401–5405.

Kleinerman ES, Murray JL, Snyder JS, Cunningham JE, Fidler IJ. Activation of tumoricidal properties in monocytes from cancer patients following intravenous administration of liposomes containing muramyl tripeptide phosphatidylethanolamine. Cancer Res. 1989;49: 4665–4670.

Koff WC, Fidler IJ. The potential use of liposome-mediated antiviral therapy. Antiviral Res. 1985;228:495–497.

Kripke ML, Budmen MB, Fidler IJ. Production of specific macrophage-activating factor by lymphocytes from tumor-bearing mice. Cell Immunol. 1976;30:341–348.

Lederer E. Synthetic immunostimulants derived from the bacterial cell wall. J Med Chem. 1980;23:819–825.

Liotta LA, Gattozzi C, Kleinerman J. Reduction of tumor cell entry into vessels by BCG-activated macrophages. Br J Cancer. 1977;36:639–641.

Lopez-Berestein G, Mehta K, Mehta R, Juliano RL, Hersh EM. The activation of human monocytes by liposome-encapsulated muramyl dipeptide analogues. J Immunol. 1983;130:1500–1504.

Lopez-Berestein G, Milas L, Hunter N, et al. Prophylaxis and treatment of experimental lung metastases in mice after treatment with liposome-encapsulated 6-0-steroyl-*N*-acetylmuramyl-*L*-amino-butryl-*D*-isoglutamine. Clin Exp Metastasis. 1984;2(2):366–367.

Lopez-Berestein G, Kasi L, Rosenblum MG, et al. Clinical pharmacology of ^{99m}Tc-labeled liposomes in patients with Hodgkin's disease. J Nucl Med. 1985;26:743–749.

MacEwen EG, Kurzman ID, Rosenthal RC, et al. Therapy for osteosarcoma in dogs with intravenous injection of liposome-encapsulated muramyl tripeptide. J Natl Cancer Inst. 1989; 81:935–938.

Mantovani A, Giavazzi R, Polentanitti N, Spreafico F, Garattini S. Divergent effects of macrophage toxins on growth of primary tumors and lung metastases in mice. Int J Cancer. 1980;25:617–624.

Mehta K, Lopez-Berestein G, Hersh EM, Juliano RL. Uptake of liposomes and liposome-encapsulated muramyl dipeptide by human peripheral blood monocytes. J Reticuloendothel Soc. 1982;32:155–164.

Miller FR. Intratumor immunologic heterogeneity. Cancer Metastasis Rev. 1982;1:319–335.

Moore MAS, Warren DJ. Synergy of interleukin-1 and granulocyte colony stimulating factor: in vivo stimulation of stem cell recovery and hematopoietic regeneration following 5-fluorouracil treatment of mice. Proc Natl Acad Sci USA. 1987;84:7134–7138.

Morikawa K, Nayar R, Fidler IJ. In vitro activation of tumoricidal properties in mouse macrophages using the chemotactic peptide *N*-formyl-methionyl-leucyl-phenylalanine (FMLP) incorporated in liposomes. Cancer Immunol Immunother. 1988;27:1–6.

Murray JL. Prostaglandin E_2 modulation of human monocyte antibody-dependent cell-mediated cytotoxicity against human red blood cells. Cell Immunol. 1982;71:196–201.

Murray JL, Kleinerman ES, Tatom JR, et al. A pilot phase I trial of liposomal *N*-acetyl-muramyl-*L*-alanyl-*D*-isoglutaminyl-*L*-alanyl-phosphatidyl-ethanolamine (MTP-PE, CGP 19835A) in cancer patients. In: Lopez-Berestein G, Fidler IJ, eds. Lipsomes in the therapy of infectious diseases and cancer. Vol. 89. New York, NY: Alan R. Liss; 1989a:329–342.

Murray JL, Kleinerman ES, Cunningham JE, et al. Phase I trial of liposomal muramyl-tripeptide-phosphatidyl-ethanolamine [MTP-PE (CGP19835A)] in cancer patients. J Clin Oncol. 1989b;7:1915–1925.

Nayar R, Schroit AJ. Generation of pH-sensitive liposomes: use of large unilamellar vesicles containing *N*-succinylphosphatidylethanolamine. Biochemistry. 1985;24:5967–5971.

Nicolson GL. Generation of phenotypic diversity and progression in metastatic tumors. Cancer Metastasis Rev. 1984;3:25–42.

Nicolson GL. Tumor cell instability, diversification and progression to the metastatic phenotype: from oncogenes to oncofetal expression. Cancer Res. 1987;47:1473–1488.

Nimer SD, Champlin RE, Golde DW. Serum cholesterol-lowering activity of granulocyte-macrophage colony-stimulating factor. JAMA. 1988;260:3297–3300.

Nogueira N. Intracellular mechanisms of killing. Contemp Topics Immunobiol. 1984;12:53–69.

Norbury KC, Kripke ML. Ultraviolet-induced carcinogenesis in mice treated with silica, trypan blue or pyran copolymer. J Reticuloendothel Soc. 1979;26:827–837.

Ostro MJ. Liposomes. Sci Am. 1988;256:102–111.

Pace JL. Synergistic interactions between IFN-γ and IFN-β in priming murine macrophages for tumor cell killing. J Leukocyte Biol. 1988;44:514–520.

Papahadjopoulos D. Liposomes in drug delivery: from serendipity to tumor targeting. In: Lopez-Berestein G, Fidler IJ, eds. Liposomes in the therapy of infectious diseases and cancer. New York, NY: Alan R. Liss; 1989:135–155.

Parant M, Parant F, Chedid L, Yapo A, Petit JF, Lederer E. Fate of the synthetic immunoadjuvant, muramyl dipeptide (^{14}C-labelled) in the mouse. Int J Immunopharmacol. 1979;1:35–41.

Perez-Soler R, Lopez-Berestein G, Kasi LP, et al. Distribution of technetium-99m-labeled multilamellar liposomes in patients with Hodgkin's disease. J Nucl Med. 1985;26:743–749.

Phillips NC, Tsao M. Inhibition of experimental liver tumor growth in mice by liposomes containing a lipophilic muramyl dipeptide. Cancer Res. 1989;49:936–940.

Phillips NC, Mora ML, Chedid L, Lefrancier P, Bernard JM. Activation of tumoricidal activity and eradication of experimental metastases by freeze-dried liposomes containing a new lipophilic muramyl dipeptide derivative. Cancer Res. 1985;45:128–134.

Poste G, Fidler IJ. The pathogenesis of cancer metastasis. Nature. 1979;283:139–146.

Poste G, Kirsh R, Fidler IJ. Rapid decay of tumoricidal activity and loss of responsiveness to lymphokines in inflammatory macrophages. Cancer Res. 1979a;39:2582–2590.

Poste G, Kirsh R, Fidler IJ. Cell surface receptors for lymphokines. Cell Immunol. 1979b; 44:71–88.

Poste G, Kirsh R, Fogler W, Fidler IJ. Activation of tumoricidal properties in mouse macrophages by lymphokines encapsulated in liposomes. Cancer Res. 1979c;39:881–892.

Poste G, Bucana CD, Raz A, Bugelski P, Kirsh R, Fidler IJ. Analysis of the fate of systemically administered liposomes and implications for their use in drug delivery. Cancer Res. 1982;42:1412–1422.

Poste G, Kirsh R, Bugelski P. Liposomes as a drug delivery system in cancer therapy. In: Sunkara P, ed. Novel approaches to cancer chemotherapy. New York, NY: Academic Press; 1984:323–335.

Raz A, Bucana C, Fogler WE, Poste G, Fidler IJ. Biochemical, morphological and ultrastructural studies on the uptake of liposomes by murine macrophages. Cancer Res. 1981;41:487–494.

Richardson VJ, Jeyaingh K, Jewkes RF, Ryman BE, Tattersall MNH. Possible tumor localization of Tc99m-labeled liposomes: effect of lipid composition, charge, and liposome size. J Nucl Med. 1978;19:1049–1054.

Richardson VJ, Ryman BE, Jewkes RF, et al. Tissue distribution and tumor localization of ^{99m}Technetium-labeled liposomes in cancer patients. Br J Cancer. 1979;40:35–43.

Sadler TE, Jones DDE, Castro JE. The effects of altered phagocytic activity on growth of primary and metastatic tumors. In: Mcbride JF, Stuart A, eds. The macrophage and cancer. Edinburgh: Econoprint; 1979:115–163.

Saiki I, Fidler IJ. Synergistic activation by recombinant mouse interferon-gamma and muramyl dipeptide of tumoricidal properties in mouse macrophages. J Immunol. 1985;135:684–688.

Saiki I, Sone S, Fogler WE, Kleinerman ES, Lopez-Berestein G, Fidler IJ. Synergism between human recombinant gamma-interferon and muramyl dipeptide encapsulated in liposomes for activation of antitumor properties in human blood monocytes. Cancer Res. 1985;45:6188–6193.

Schackert G, Simmons RD, Buzbee TM, Hume DA, Fidler IJ. Macrophage infiltration into experimental brain metastases: occurrence through an intact blood–brain barrier. J Natl Cancer Inst. 1988;80:1027–1034.

Schaffner T, Keller HV, Hess MW, Cottier H. Macrophage functions in antimicrobial defense. Klin Wochenschr. 1982;60:720.

Schroit AJ, Fidler IJ. Effects of liposome structure and lipid composition on the activation of the tumoricidal properties of macrophages by liposomes containing muramyl dipeptide. Cancer Res. 1982;42:161–167.

Schroit AJ, Galligioni E, Fidler IJ. Factors influencing the in situ activation of macrophages by liposomes containing muramyl dipeptide. Biol Cell. 1983a;47:87–94.

Schroit AJ, Hart IR, Madsen J, Fidler IJ. Selective delivery of drugs encapsulated in liposomes: natural targeting to macrophages involved in various disease states. J Biol Resp Mod. 1983b;2:97–100.

Schumann G, van Hoogevest P, Fankhauser P, et al. Comparison of free and liposomal MTP-PE: pharmacological, toxicological and pharmacokinetic aspects. In: Lopez-Berestein G, Fidler IJ, eds. Liposomes in the therapy of infectious diseases and cancer. Vol. 89. New York, NY: Alan R. Liss; 1989:191–203.

Shah RG, Caporale LH, Moore MAS. Characterization of colony-stimulating activity produced by human monocytes and phytohemagglutanin-stimulated lymphocytes. Blood. 1977;50: 811–821.

Solanki DL. Erythrophagocytosis in vivo in sickle cell anemia. Am J Hematol. 1985;20:353–357.

Sone S, Fidler IJ. Synergistic activation by lymphokines and muramyl dipeptide of tumoricidal properties in rat alveolar macrophages. J Immunol. 1980;125:2454–2460.

Sone S, Fidler IJ. In vitro activation of tumoricidal properties in rat alveolar macrophages by synthetic muramyl dipeptide encapsulated in liposomes. Cell Immunol. 1981;130:1500–1504.

Sone S, Tsubura E. Human alveolar macrophages: potentiation of their tumoricidal activity by liposome-encapsulated muramyl dipeptide. J Immunol. 1982;129:1313–1317.

Sone S, Mutsuura S, Ogawara M, Tsubura E. Potentiating effect of muramyl dipeptide and its lipophilic analog encapsulated in liposomes on tumor cell killing by human monocytes. J Immunol. 1984;132:2105–2110.

Sone S, Utsugi T, Tandon P, Ogawara M. A dried preparation of liposomes containing muramyl tripeptide phosphatidylethanolamine as a potent activator of human blood monocytes to the anticancer state. Cancer Immunol Immunother. 1986;22:191–196.

Talmadge JE, Fidler IJ. Cancer metastasis is selective or random depending upon the parent cell population. Nature. 1982;27:593–596.

Talmadge JE, Zbar B. Clonality of pulmonary metastases from the bladder 6 subline of the B16 melanoma studies by Southern hybridization. J Natl Cancer Inst. 1986;78:315–320.

Talmadge JE, Wolman SR, Fidler IJ. Evidence for the clonal origin of spontaneous metastases. Science. 1982;217:361–363.

Tenu JP, Roche AC, Yapo A, Kieda C, Monsigny M, Petit JF. Absence of cell surface receptors for muramyl peptides in mouse peritoneal macrophages. Biol Cell. 1982;144:157–162.

Thombre P, Deodar SD. Inhibition of liver metastases in murine colon adenocarcinoma by liposomes containing C-reactive protein or crude lymphokine. Cancer Immunol Immunother. 1984;16:145–150.

Van Hoogevest P, Fankhauser P. An industrial liposomal dosage form for muramyl-tripeptide-phosphatidylethanolamine (MTP-PE). In: Lopez-Berestein G, Fidler IJ, eds. Liposomes in the therapy of infectious diseases and cancer. Vol. 89. New York, NY: Alan R. Liss; 1989:453–466.

Weiss L. Principles of metastasis. Orlando, Fla: Academic Press; 1985.

Xu ZL, Fidler IJ. The in situ activation of cytotoxic properties in murine Kupffer cells by the systemic administration of whole *Mycobacterium bovis* organisms or muramyl tripeptide. Cancer Immunol Immunother. 1984;18:118–122.

Zubrod CG, Schneiderman M, Frei E, et al. Appraisal of methods for the study of chemotherapy of cancer in man: comparative therapeutic trial of nitrogen mustard and triethylene thiophosphoramide. J Chron Dis. 1960;11:7–33.

CHAPTER **16**

ADOPTIVE CELLULAR IMMUNOTHERAPY OF CANCER

Joshua T. Rubin
Michael T. Lotze

Immunotherapy represents a fourth cancer treatment modality that employs biological reagents to effect the immune-mediated rejection of a patient's tumor. Unlike surgery and radiation therapy, it is suited for the treatment of systemic malignancy and, unlike chemotherapy, it offers the theoretical advantage of tumor-specific toxicity. Various reagents have been evaluated, including tumor vaccines, recombinant cytokines, immunoreactive cells, and antibodies. This review will focus on recent clinical experiences with adoptive cellular immunotherapy using lymphokine-activated killer (LAK) cells or tumor-infiltrating lymphocytes (TIL) with an emphasis on trials conducted in the Surgery Branch of the National Cancer Institute. Seminal observations leading to the development of these protocols will also be reviewed.

EVOLUTION OF IMMUNOTHERAPY

Our current immunotherapeutic efforts evolved from observations made in the first half of this century, establishing that certain transplantable tumors engender an immune response in animals that leads to tumor regression or tumor immunity. Until that time, it had been argued that genetic differences between the tumor and the host or that nonimmunological mechanisms, including decreased tumor viability, were operative in models of tumor rejection. The latter idea was challenged as early as 1925 by Woglom (1925), who reported that multiple tumors simultaneously transplanted to immune rats regressed. He argued cogently that changes within the host induced by the transplanted tumor underlay tumor regression. However, it was not until inbred strains of mice became available that the immune response to transplanted tumors could be definitively demonstrated.

In 1943, Gross (1943) reported that inbred mice, having rejected a small intradermal inoculation of a syngeneic methylcholanthrene (MCA)-induced sarcoma, were subsequently resistant to rechallenge with the same tumor, yet they were susceptible to spontaneous mammary carcinomas. These observations made alloreactivity a less tenable explanation for tumor rejection. Foley (1953) confirmed these observations and, by using early passages of transplanted MCA-induced and spontaneous tumors, established that a state of tumor-specific immunity could be generated in mice that was unrelated to alloreactivity or antigenic drift of serially transplanted tumors. Any lingering skepticism about the existence of a tumor-specific immune response in mice was dispelled by Prehn and Main (1957), who extended Gross's and Foley's observations to other inbred strains of mice using second transplant generation MCA-induced sarcomas. They went on to show that there was little cross-immunity between sarcomas and no cross immunity between tumors and normal tissues. Finally, Révész (1960) and Klein et al. (1960) corroborated these findings using irradiated tumor and normal tissue to immunize mice. The existence of tumor-specific immunity in carefully defined animal models was now beyond dispute.

The focus of attention shifted to lymphocytes as mediators of tumor immunity when Mitchison (1953, 1955) demonstrated that lymphocytes from draining lymph nodes could confer immunity against transplantable tumors by their adoptive transfer to non-tumor-bearing mice. This effect was long lasting in syngeneic mice and was directly related to the number of transferred lymphocytes.

While one could not gainsay the importance of these findings, no immunological maneuver had yet been demonstrated that led to the regression of established tumors. The first successful application of adoptive immunotherapy was reported by Delorme and Alexander (1964), who induced partial regression of a benzpyrene-induced fibrosarcoma by the adoptive transfer of thoracic duct lymphocytes from syngeneic rats immunized with irradiated tumors. A similar model was successfully used by Alexander (1967) to treat mice bearing a 2-day-old intraperitoneal lymphoma. Borberg et al. (1972) demonstrated the efficacy of adoptively transferred in vivo sensitized lymphocytes in mice bearing a 7-day-old transplanted sarcoma. Like others before them, they noted the need for large numbers of lymphocytes and discussed the relevance of this observation to the immunotherapy of human tumors.

Attempts to apply these principles to the therapy of cancer in humans were reported as early as 1966, when Nadler and Moore (1966) cross-transplanted histologically similar tumors between 13 pairs of patients. The subsequent transfer of lymphocytes between these patients was reported to be associated with tumor regression in 6 of 23 patients with metastatic melanoma (MM). Frenster and Rogoway (1968, 1970) treated 5 patients with lymphocytes activated in vitro with phytohemagglutinin (PHA) and reported that 3 patients manifested a reduction in the size of pulmonary nodules. A pervasive problem in these studies was the inability to generate large numbers of lymphocytes.

Since in vivo sensitized lymphocytes were not readily available for the treatment of human cancer, Rouse et al. (1972) applied specifically lytic T cells generated in vitro to the treatment of transplanted tumor lines in sublethally irradiated mice. While they used allosensitized cytotoxic T lymphocytes (CTL), Röllinghoff and Wagner (1973) used lymphocytes stimulated by syngeneic tumors in a mixed lymphocyte tumor culture to prevent tumor growth. Treves et al. (1975) extended these observations by using in vitro sensitized T cells to prevent lung metastases and to prolong survival in mice following excision of a primary Lewis lung carcinoma. This may be the earliest report of successful adjuvant cellular immunotherapy.

Fefer et al. (1976) addressed the problem of generating large numbers of cells to treat established tumors in mice. They were able to cure mice bearing a disseminated Friend retrovirus–induced murine leukemia, FBL-3, using significantly fewer in vivo sensitized lymphocytes by pretreating the mice with cyclophosphamide. An alternative approach, described by Bernstein (1977), utilized a secondary in vitro sensitization (IVS) to expand cytolytic cells from populations of in vivo sensitized splenocytes. Using this approach, he was able to prevent tumor growth in rats by the simultaneous inoculation of lymphocytes with tumor. Fernandez-Cruz et al. (1979) reported curing rats of palpable 8-day-old sarcomas using a similar approach.

By demonstrating that cytotoxic T cells could be generated in vitro against unique tumor antigens and subsequently be used in vivo to eradicate tumors in rodents, these animal models had established a rational basis for the immunotherapy of cancer in humans. The extrapolation of these principles to clinical trials was hindered by the apparent requirement for large numbers of tumor-specific, cytotoxic lymphocytes. Long-term culture and expansion of human T cells had been achieved only in repetitive allogeneic mixed-lymphocyte cultures (MLC) (Svedmyr, 1975; Dennert and De Rose, 1976). Similar attempts using autologous Epstein-Barr virus (EBV)-transformed B-cell lines were not successful. However, in 1976, Morgan, Ruscetti, and Gallo (1976) described a factor produced by PHA-stimulated lymphocytes that supported the long-term growth and expansion of bone marrow–derived cell suspensions. They further characterized the cells proliferating in response to this growth factor as T cells (Ruscetti et al., 1977). Helper and cytotoxic T cells expanded in this T-cell growth factor maintained their in vitro and in vivo activity (Gillis and Smith, 1977; Strausser and Rosenberg, 1978; Tees and Schreier, 1980; Rosenberg et al., 1978). These observations were extended by Cheever et al. (1981, 1982) and Eberlein et al. (1982), who showed that T-cell lines sensitized in vitro and expanded with interleukin-2 (IL-2) were effective either alone or in combination with chemotherapy against advanced localized and micrometastatic FBL-3 leukemia.

There were practical and theoretical shortcomings to the use of in vitro, IL-2-expanded T cells in cancer therapy. Many murine and presumably human tumors were nonimmunogenic and could not be used to generate specific T cells for therapy. Demonstrations of antigenic heterogeneity between primary tumors and their metastases suggested that specifically lytic T cells would be too narrow in their antitumor spectrum (Fidler et al., 1976; Fogel et al., 1979). Finally, human tumors were often not readily available for the in vitro restimulation of lymphocytes.

In 1980, Yron (1980) demonstrated that murine splenocytes incubated in IL-2 developed lytic activity against fresh, autologous tumor. Mills and Paetkau (1980) reported that they also lysed a variety of cultured tumor lines in a non-major histocompatibility complex (MHC)–restricted fashion. These observations were extended to humans by Lotze et al. (1981), who showed that IL-2–activated peripheral blood mononuclear cells (PBMC) from patients with cancer developed lytic activity against both autologous and allogeneic fresh tumors. A similar phenomenon was documented by Mazumder et al. (1982) using lectins to activate human lymphocytes.

These LAK- and PHA-activated killer (PAK) cells were subsequently shown to be effective antitumor agents in a variety of mouse models. Mills et al. (1980) first reported the in vivo efficacy of LAK cells using iodine 131 (^{131}I)-labeled tumor cell lines and retained radioactivity as an indirect measure of tumor killing. Mazumder and Rosenberg (1984) showed that LAK cells reduced the number of lung metastases and prolonged the survival of mice bearing 3-day metastatic B16 melanoma. Mulé et al. (1984) demonstrated that immunogenic and nonimmunogenic pulmonary micrometastatic sarcomas were sensitive to therapy with LAK cells in combination with intraperitoneal IL-2. These and other tumors were also shown to be responsive in both pulmonary and hepatic 3-day micrometastatic models (Lafreniere and Rosenberg, 1985a, 1985b; Papa et al., 1986).

The ease with which activated killer cells could be generated in large numbers, and their documented efficacy in mice anticipated large-scale clinical trials of adoptive immunotherapy in humans. The subsequent cloning of the IL-2 gene (Taniguchi et al., 1983) and its expression in *Escherichia coli* (Devos et al., 1983; Rosenberg et al., 1984) assured an unlimited supply of pure recombinant human IL-2 for these efforts.

THERAPY WITH IL-2 AND LAK CELLS

IL-2 by Intermittent IV Bolus

Preclinical studies of adoptive immunotherapy in mice defined principles that were extrapolated to human trials (Mulé et al., 1984, 1985, 1986a, 1986b; Rosenberg et al., 1985b; Lafreniere and Rosenberg, 1985a, 1985b). Although LAK cells and IL-2 were each capable of mediating the regression of micrometastatic tumors, the combination of the two was usually more potent. The therapeutic response was directly related to the dose of IL-2 and the number of infused LAK cells. A 3-day incubation of splenocytes or PBMC in 6×10^3 IU/mL of IL-2 was optimal for generating LAK-cell activity.

Our early phase I trials evaluating adoptive cellular immunotherapy in patients with cancer utilized PHA-activated lymphocytes since the supply of IL-2 was limited (Mazumder et al., 1984). As many as 1.7×10^{11} cells were safely infused with minimal toxicity. There were no clinical responses noted. Following the development of recombinant IL-2, phase I trials were initiated that defined the toxicity, pharmacology, and immune modulating effects of IL-2 and LAK cells (Lotze et al., 1984, 1985a, 1985b, 1986b, 1987; Rosenberg, 1984).

Phase II trials of IL-2 and LAK cells began in 1984. In 1985, we reported that 11 of 25 patients with advanced disseminated cancer treated with systemic high-dose IL-2 and LAK-cell infusions manifested clinically significant tumor regression (Rosenberg et al., 1985a). Susceptible malignancies included MM, renal cell carcinoma (RCC), and colorectal carcinoma (CRC). Subsequently, responses were seen in patients treated with IL-2 alone (Lotze et al., 1986a).

In 1989, we reported the results of a trial in which 307 patients were treated with Cetus IL-2 either alone or in combination with LAK cells (Rosenberg et al., 1989). All patients had advanced malignancy with measurable disease and no conventional treatment available to them. Any patient with pulmonary, cardiovascular, or renal insufficiency as well as central nervous system (CNS) metastases, was ineligible for therapy. All patients had an Eastern Cooperative Oncology Group performance status of 0 to 2 (Table 16-1). Patients were to receive 10^5 U/kg (6×10^5 IU/kg) of IL-2 by IV bolus every 8 hours from days 1 to 5 up to a maximum of 14 doses. Patients who were randomized to receive LAK cells underwent leukaphoresis on days 8 to 11. All patients were treated again with IL-2 in the same fashion on days 12 to 16. Lymphokine-activated killer cells were administered on days 12, 13, and 15. Doses of IL-2 were withheld as needed so that LAK-cell infusions could be performed, and LAK-cell infusions were occasionally withheld depending on patient tolerance. Most recently, LAK cells were generated by culturing PBMC in a closed, automated system using serum-free medium and 10^3 U/mL (6×10^3 IU/mL) of IL-2. Ficoll-Hypaque separation of PBMC has been eliminated (Aebersold et al., 1988). Patients were reevaluated 1 and 2 months after therapy, and those with stable or regressing disease were retreated as many as five times at 3-month intervals.

Seven of the 85 patients who were to receive LAK cells did not receive them due to complications during their first cycle of IL-2. The median number of doses tolerated

TABLE 16-1
GUIDELINES FOR PATIENT SELECTION

1. Clearly measurable disease.
2. Normal pulmonary, renal, and hepatic function.
3. Noninvasive cardiac evaluation in patients over 50 years old or with documented cardiac risk factors.
4. No other tumor therapy for 1 month preceding treatment.
5. No requirement for immunosuppressive agents such as steroids.
6. No known or suspected sites of infection.
7. No known bleeding abnormalities or evidence of pulmonary, renal, or gastrointestinal sources of bleeding.
8. Normal brain CT within 1 month of therapy (no cerebral metastases).
9. ECOG performance status of 0–2 with an estimated survival of ≥3 months.
10. No effective conventional therapy.

in the first and second cycles of treatment was 10 and 6 for IL-2 and LAK-cell therapy and 10 and 7 for IL-2 alone. The median number of LAK cells administered was 10^{11}. There were 14 complete responses (CR) and 30 partial responses (PR) among 177 patients who received IL-2 and LAK cells (Table 16-2). One of 7 patients who did not receive LAK cells due to complications that occurred during the first cycle of therapy, sustained a CR. There were 4 CR and 18 PR among 130 patients treated with IL-2 alone. The most susceptible malignancies were MM and RCC. Lesional regression was seen in soft tissue, nodal, osseous, and visceral sites (Figs. 16-1 and 16-2). The overall response rates in both treatment groups were not statistically different. The responses have been durable with many continuing beyond 24 months (Table 16-3). Toxicity included myocardial depression, pulmonary edema, renal insufficiency, hypotension, and altered mentation. Increased capillary permeability probably underlies much of this. The degree and spectrum of toxicity were similar in both treatment groups. Seven of the patients died of treatment-related complications. Five of these deaths were due to myocardial infarctions that occurred early in this study, before all patients older than 50 years of age or with significant risk factors were required to undergo a noninvasive cardiac evaluation.

The results of this trial are similar to those recently reported by the National Cancer Institute Extramural IL-2/LAK Working Group (EWG). Dutcher et al. (1989) observed 1 CR and 5 PR among 36 patients with MM, and Fisher et al. (1988) reported 2 CR

TABLE 16-2
RESULTS OF IL-2–BASED IMMUNOTHERAPY IN PATIENTS WITH ADVANCED CANCER

	IL-2*			IL-2 + LAK†			IL-2 + TIL		
Diagnosis	**Total**	**CR**	**PR**	**Total**	**CR**	**PR**	**Total**	**CR**	**PR**
Renal cell carcinoma	54	4	8	72	8	17	—	—	—
Melanoma	42	0	10	48	4	6	20	1	10
Colorectal carcinoma	12	0	0	30	1	4	—	—	—
Non-Hodgkin's lymphoma	11	0	0	7	1	3	—	—	—
Breast carcinoma	3	0	0	—	—	—	—	—	—
Other	8	0	0	20	0	0	—	—	—
Total	130	4	18	177	14	30	20	1	10

Adapted from Rosenberg et al., 1989. Patients were accrued as of March 1989 except for TIL-treated patients who were accrued as of December 1988. CR, complete response; PR, partial response.

*Includes all treated patients except 4 who died of therapy and 21 treated in adjuvant setting.

†Includes all treated patients except 1 lost to follow-up, 1 who died of therapy, and 35 treated in the adjuvant setting.

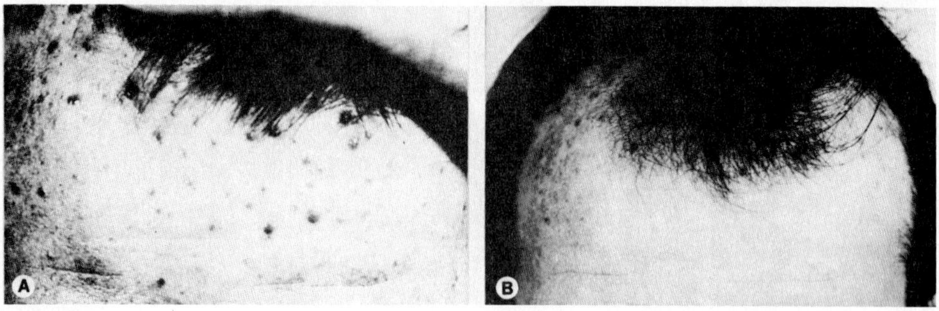

FIGURE 16-1
(A) Multiple cutaneous metastatic melanoma deposits on a patient's forehead; (B) completely regressed after therapy with IL-2 and LAK cells.

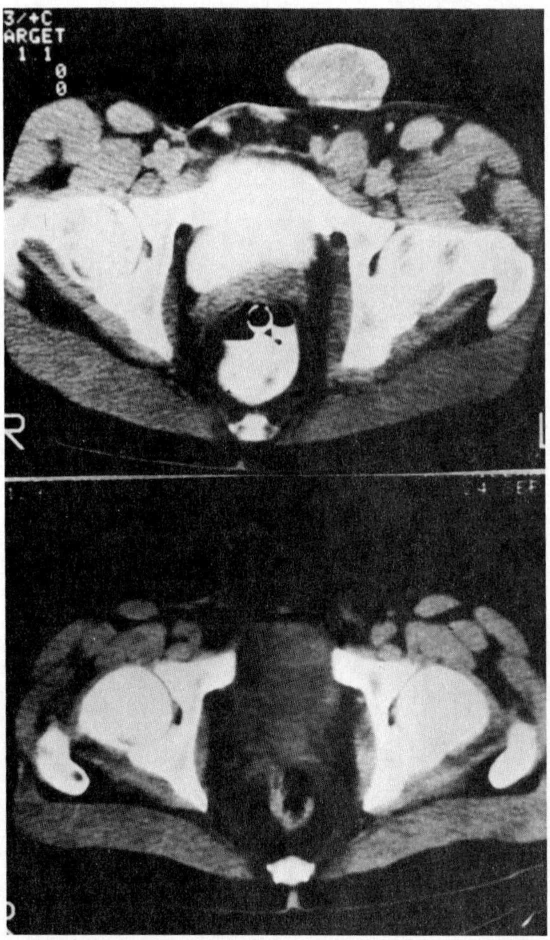

FIGURE 16-2
A large, tumor-bearing, left inguinal lymph node in a patient with metastatic melanoma (top) regressed after therapy with IL-2 and LAK cells (bottom).

TABLE 16-3
DURATION OF RESPONSES

	Treatment					
	IL-2		IL-2 + LAK		IL-2 + TIL	
Diagnosis	CR	PR	CR	PR	CR	PR
Renal cell carcinoma	34+,28+,27+,25+	27+,27+,25+,21+, 21+,19+,15+,3+	30+,27+,23+,15, 13,11,9,6	36+,21+,19,13, 11,11,9,7,7,6, 6,6,6,3,2,1,1	—	—
Melanoma	0	41+,15,12,11, 10,8,7,5,3,2	52+,32+,18+,13	30+,6,6,3,2,2	13+	9,7,7,6,4,4,4, 3,3,2
Colorectal carcinoma	0	0	21	11,6,6,2	—	—
Non-Hodgkin's lymphoma	0	0	10	31+,20,8+	—	—

Adapted from Rosenberg et al., 1989. Patients were accrued as of March 1989 except for TIL-treated patients who were accrued as of December 1988. CR, complete response; PR, partial response; TIL, tumor-infiltrating lymphocytes; +, persistent response at last date of follow-up.

and 3 PR among 35 patients with RCC. The amount of IL-2 administered in these trials was a little higher, with a mean of 13 doses during the first cycle and 10 doses during the second. The amount of LAK cells administered, about 9×10^{10} per patient, was the same. Responses were durable, especially for patients with complete regression of tumor. Fisher et al. (1988) also reported that selected patients with a PR potentially benefited from the resection of remaining disease and could remain disease-free for prolonged periods of time. Tumor regression was observed in all sites except the CNS. A review of response data compiled by Fisher et al. (1988) suggests that patients with RCC do not respond to treatment if they have a mass greater than 100 cm^2 or a primary kidney tumor in place. Toxicity was comparable between these studies, and treatment was well tolerated (Margolin et al., 1989). All but 10 of 93 patients accrued by the EWG received at least one infusion of LAK cells. Five patients received only one cycle due to toxicity. There was one treatment-related death due to myocardial infarction. In addition to documenting the efficacy of immunotherapy in selected patients, these studies demonstrated that this therapy could be safely administered in settings other than the National Cancer Institute.

The protocols developed by the Surgery Branch of the National Cancer Institute that employ high doses of IL-2 (6×10^5 IU/kg every 8 hours) and LAK cells were based on murine models that demonstrated a correlation between response and both the dose of IL-2 and the number of adoptively transferred cells. The in vivo activity of LAK cells is enhanced by the concomitant administration of IL-2 in these models, presumably by inducing proliferation (Ettinghausen et al., 1985). In our protocols, the amount of IL-2 administered with LAK cells has been limited by the toxicity associated with high doses. Consequently, others have used protocols with different doses, schedules, and routes of administration to decrease toxicity and maximize efficacy (Table 16-4).

Eberlein et al. (1988) were reportedly able to decrease toxicity and significantly increase the number of IL-2 doses given with LAK cells during the second cycle of treatment by using only 3×10^4 IU/kg of Amgen IL-2 administered every 8 hours in a protocol similar to those described above. Even though LAK cells were generated in 10^3 IU/mL of IL-2 and the mean number of LAK cells infused was only 4×10^{10}, they reported 4 CR and 9 PR among 29 patients treated, including complete regression of ovarian cancer in 1 such patient. However, Stahel et al. (1989) treated 26 patients in the same fashion, using Amgen IL-2, and reported only 4 PR and significant toxicity that required dose reductions during the second cycle. Finally, Cascinelli et al. (1989) used Glaxo IL-2 to treat 15 patients with MM. The dose of IL-2 was 9.2×10^5 IU/m^2 tid and LAK-cell infusions were administered during the second cycle. No responses were noted. The average number of LAK cells infused was only 3.5×10^{10}.

IL-2 by Continuous IV Infusion

West et al. (1987, 1989) have treated patients with 3×10^6 U/m^2 (18×10^6 IU/m^2) per day of Cetus IL-2 by continuous infusion using a variety of schedules.

TABLE 16-4
IL-2 AND LAK-CELL PROTOCOLS USING BOLUS INJECTION OF IL-2

Author	Source	IL-2 Dose	IL-2 Schedule (D = day)	Response				Date
				DX	PR	CR	Total* (%)	
Rosenberg	Cetus	10^5 U/kg q8h	IL-2: D1-5,D12-16	MM	6	4	48 (21)	1989
		(6×10^5 IU/kg)	LAK: D12,13,15	RCC	17	8	72 (35)	
				CRC	4	1	30 (17)	
				NHL	3	1	7 (57)	
Dutcher	Cetus	10^5 U/kg q8h	IL-2: D1-5,D12-16	MM	5	1	32 (19)	1989
		(6×10^5 IU/kg)	LAK: D12,13,15					
Fisher	Cetus	10^5 U/kg q8h	IL-2: D1-5,D12-16	RCC	3	2	32 (16)	1988
		(6×10^5 IU/kg)	LAK: D12,13,15					
Eberlein	Ortho	3×10^4 U/kg q8h	IL-2: D1-5, D12-19	MM	4	1	10 (50)	1988
	(Amgen)	(3×10^4 IU/kg)	LAK: D12,13,15	RCC	4	1	10 (50)	
				CRC	0	0	4 (0)	
				NHL	0	1	2 (50)	
Stahel	Ortho	3×10^4 U/kg q8h	IL-2: D1-5, D12-19	MM	1	0	7 (14)	1989
	(Amgen)	(3×10^4 IU/kg)	LAK: D12,13,15	RCC	3	0	14 (21)	
Cascinelli	Glaxo	9.2×10^5 U/m^2 tid	IL-2: D1-4,D10-16	MM	0	0	15 (0)	1989
		(9.2×10^5 IU/m^2)	LAK: D10,11,13					
Mittleman†	Roche	$1–30 \times 10^5$ U/m^2 tid	IL-2: D1,D5-23	MM	1	0	4 (25)	1989
		($1–30 \times 10^5$ IU/m^2)	LAK: D8-13,D15-20	RCC	1	0	12 (8)	
				CRC	0	0	8 (0)	

*Includes all patients who received at least one LAK-cell infusion.
†Escalating dose protocol.
DX, diagnosis; PR, partial response; CR, complete response; MM, melanoma; RCC, renal cell cancer; CRC, colorectal cancer; NHL, non-Hodgkin's lymphoma.

They recently reported that among 114 treated patients, 8 of 22 with MM and 7 of 23 with RCC manifested a response that was generally durable. The spectrum of toxicity was similar to that reported for intermittent bolus IL-2. Other reported trials of continuous infusion IL-2 differ in their dose, schedule of administration, and technique of LAK-cell generation, but the results are comparable to those of West (Table 16-5). Philip et al. (1989) treated 17 patients with RCC in a fashion similar to West et al. and reported 3 PR. Paciucci et al. (1989) reported 3 PR among 25 patients treated with weekly 6-day infusions of IL-2 and 1-day cultured LAK cells. There were 4 PR among 8 patients who started treatment at the highest dose escalation.

Additional modifications in the schedule of IL-2 administration have been studied in an attempt to lessen the toxicity and enhance the efficacy of therapy. One such paradigm, the "hybrid" regimen, employed 9 rather than 14 doses of IL-2 prior to leukapheresis. LAK cells were subsequently administered with a continuous infusion of IL-2 at a dose of 18×10^6 IU/m^2/day for as long as 144 hours. This approach was based on observations suggesting that the tumoricidal activity of LAK cells in vivo is IL-2–dependent and that continuous infusions of IL-2 are better tolerated. No advantage to the use of this regimen for the treatment of patients with MM, RCC, or lymphoma has been demonstrated in recently reported clinical trials (Bar et al., 1990; Margolin et al., 1991; Parkinson et al., 1990).

Regional Infusion or Local Infiltration of IL-2 and LAK Cells

Some groups have used regional infusion or local infiltration to treat a variety of malignancies. Grimm (1987) safely infiltrated IL-2 and LAK cells into the brain following excision of malignant glioma but without demonstrated efficacy. Yoshida et al. (1988) treated 23 patients who had recurrent malignant glioma with intratumoral LAK cells and IL-2. Although response criteria were ill-defined, 6 patients appear to have manifested some degree of tumor regression. Steis et al. (1990) reported PR in 2 of 10 patients with ovarian cancer and 5 of 22 patients with CRC limited to the abdomen following intraperitoneal administration of IL-2 and LAK cells. There are several reports describing the hepatic-arterial infusion of IL-2 and LAK cells for treatment of hepatocellular carcinoma (Fagan et al., 1989; Hsieh et al., 1987; Ichida et al., 1989; Onishi et al., 1989); however, these studies involve small numbers of patients, are poorly documented, and lack appropriate controls. Ishikawa et al. (1989) reported that 3 of 6 patients with maxillary or lingual cancer had reduction of tumor after the regional infusion of PBMC sensitized in vitro to allogeneic tumor and cultured with 2 U/mL of Takeda IL-2. Finally, Adler et al. (1984) injected PBMC that had been stimulated in culture with the supernatant of PHA-activated PBMC into MM lesions without effecting significant responses.

Means to Enhance LAK-Cell Activity

Besides altering the dose of IL-2 or the route of administration, attention has also focused on generating more potent or increased numbers of effector cells. Sodium

TABLE 16-5
IL-2 AND LAK-CELL PROTOCOLS USING CONTINUOUS IV INFUSION OF IL-2

Author	Source	IL-2 Dose	IL-2 Schedule	Response				Date
				DX	PR	CR	Total* (%)	
West	Cetus	3×10^6 U/m²/D (18×10^6 IU/m²/D)	IL-2: D1-5, D10-15 LAK: D10,11,13	MM	8	0	22 (36)	1987
				RCC	5	2	23 (30)	1989
				CRC	0	0	22 (0)	
				NHL	2	0	5 (40)	
Philip	Euro-Cetus	3×10^6 U/m²/D (18×10^6 IU/m²/D)	IL-2: D1-5,D12-15 LAK: D12,13,15	RCC	3	0	15 (20)	1989
Paciucci†	Cetus	$1–5 \times 10^6$ IU/m²/D ($6–30 \times 10^6$ IU/m²/D)	IL-2: D2-6,D9-14, D16-21,D23-28 LAK: D2,9,16,23	MM	1	0	5 (20)	1989
				RCC	1	0	9 (11)	
Wang	Cetus	$3–5 \times 10^4$ U/kg/D ($1.8–3 \times 10^5$ IU/kg/D)	IL-2: D1-5,D8-12, D15-19 LAK: D3,5,8,9,12, 15,17,19 LAK: D10,12,15, 17,19,22	RCC	5	2	32 (22)	1989

*Includes all patients who received at least one LAK-cell infusion.
†Escalating dose protocol.
MM, melanoma; RCC, renal cell cancer; CRC, colorectal cancer; NHL, non-Hodgkin's lymphoma.

periodate is an oxidizing mitogen that regulates the expression of high-affinity IL-2 receptors on T cells, and in concert with IL-2, it has been purported to generate more potent LAK cells (Wang et al., 1986). Wang et al. (1989) reasoned that these cells could enhance the efficacy of treatment and, by their increased sensitivity to IL-2, allow for lower doses and less toxicity. They recently reported the results of a phase II protocol under which 40 patients with RCC were treated. Patients received 6 to 8 LAK-cell infusions over 3 weeks and a continuous infusion of Cetus IL-2 that varied between 3 to 5 $\times$ 10^4 U/kg (1.8–3 $\times$ 10^5 IU/kg) per day based on toxicity. Most patients were also treated with maintenance interferon-alpha (IFN-α) alone or with monthly IL-2 and LAK-cell infusions. No patient required vasopressors for blood pressure control. Otherwise, toxicity was similar to other reported trials and included 2 treatment-related deaths. Four patients were removed from the protocol due to rapid progression of disease. There were only 2 CR and 5 PR among the remaining 34 patients.

Osband and Krane (1988) reported the results of treating 80 patients using infusions of autologous in vitro conditioned lymphocytes. They argued that small numbers of lymphocytes are adequate for adoptive therapy if suppressor lymphocytes defined by the H_2 histamine receptor are depleted by panning with cimetidine. Peripheral blood mononuclear cells were depleted of H_2-receptor–bearing lymphocytes and subsequently cultured for 5 days in medium supplemented with the supernatant from cultures of autologous lymphocytes stimulated with allogeneic cells or, more recently, with the mitogenic monoclonal antibody (mAb) OKT3. When available, autologous tumor-cell digestate purportedly containing relevant tumor antigens was added to the cultures. Before infusion, the lymphocytes were irradiated with 100 rad to eradicate contaminating suppressor cells. Therapy was well tolerated, but was associated with only a 10% PR rate in RCC. Of 5 patients with MM who were treated, 1 CR and 1 PR were reported. Other malignancies, including carcinoma of the colon, bladder, and pancreas, were not responsive. More recently, Osband et al. (1990) reported the results of a prospective, randomized trial comparing the efficacy of autolymphocyte therapy with cimetidine alone for metastatic RCC. There was a 21% PR rate among 39 patients treated with cells. There were 2 PR among 41 patients treated with cimetidine. Therapy with lymphocytes was reported to prolong survival 2.5-fold compared to therapy with cimetidine alone. Survival data were not stratified according to tumor response. The response data and reported survival data are difficult to interpret given the small number of patients treated, use of radiation therapy to treat new brain and symptomatic bone metastases following therapy, and the disproportionate number of poor-risk patients in the cimetidine arm of this study. The results of this trial, which was sponsored by a commercial firm, are provocative, but will require confirmation from independent investigators.

Melder et al. (1988) extended previous observations in rodent models (Gunji et al., 1989) to humans by demonstrating that CD16$^+$ CD56$^+$ CD57$^+$–enriched, adherent PBMC proliferate vigorously and develop non-MHC–restricted lytic activity against fresh tumor when cultured with IL-2. Cells are prepared by monocyte depletion followed by plastic adherence and then culture in medium supplemented with 6×10^3 IU/mL of IL-2. These cells are about five times more lytic than IL-2–stimulated, unseparated PBMC on a per cell basis. Fourteen patients have been treated at the Pittsburgh Cancer Institute with adherent LAK cells and IL-2. Two patients with MM were noted to have an objective, clinical response (unpublished data). The application of this therapy has been limited by the observation that mononuclear cells from patients with cancer did not generate large numbers of adherent LAK cells (Sedlmayr et al., 1991). Preliminary observations suggest that a shorter period of plastic adherence and addition of lectin-stimulated, autologous, irradiated PBMC to these cultures will allow greater numbers of adherent LAK cells to be recovered. Clinical trials are now in progress.

Mittleman et al. (1989) reported that PBMC cultured in 10^3 IU/mL of IL-2 developed increasing lytic activity against natural killer (NK)-cell–sensitive and NK-cell–resistant cultured tumor lines that was maximal by day 14. This extended period of culture in a low dose of IL-2 also allowed for significant expansion of cell number. Based on these observations, he conducted a phase I trial using escalating doses of Hoffmann-LaRoche IL-2 and LAK cells cultured for 5 to 17 days. Among 24 treated patients, 1 with MM and 1 with RCC manifested a PR. The responding patient with RCC was treated with only 10^5 IU/m^2 tid. Toxicity was significant at the highest doses of IL-2 used.

Ochoa et al. (1987) generated larger numbers of LAK cells with increased lytic activity by culturing PBMC at low cell density with frequent medium changes using high concentrations of IL-2. Additional enhancement of proliferation and LAK-cell activity was realized by treating the PBMC with anti-CD3 monoclonal antibody during the first 2 days of culture and adding IL-1 to the culture 48 hours before harvesting the cells. Beckner and Farrar (1988) have suggested that a lower dose of IL-2 could be used to sustain LAK-cell activity and proliferation in vivo if it was administered with drugs that upregulate protein kinase C or down regulate adenylate cyclase. This was based on their finding that the development of LAK activity from PBMC and the IL-2–induced proliferation of T cells are mediated to some degree by the level of intracellular cyclic adenosine monophosphate (AMP) that, in turn, is regulated by adenylate cyclase and two guanosine triphosphate (GTP)-binding regulatory proteins. McCrady et al. (1988) found that the increased protein kinase C activity induced by certain phorbol esters was associated with augmented IL-2–induced LAK-cell activity, presumably by decreasing levels of intracellular adenylate cyclase and cyclic AMP. By expanding mononuclear cells in culture with phorbol dibutyrate and ionomycin, and then culturing the cells in IL-2, they could enhance LAK-cell generation. Other reagents that have been found to synergize with low concentrations of IL-2 to generate LAK-cell activity include tumor necrosis factor-alpha (TNF) (Blay et al., 1989; Chouaib et al., 1988; Yang et al., 1989) and swainsonine (Bowlin et al., 1989). Finally, nonspecific lytic activity has been induced by IFN-α and interferon-gamma (IFN-γ), but the level is below that seen with 6×10^3 IU/mL of IL-2 (Ellis et al., 1989). None of these methods has been tested in therapeutic models.

Another approach to improving LAK-cell therapy has focused on the use of mouse-antihuman monoclonal antibodies. We have shown that LAK cells can mediate antibody-dependent cellular cytotoxicity (ADCC) (Eisenthal and Rosenberg, 1989), and in mice bearing hepatic or pulmonary metastatic B16 melanoma, the administration of an antimelanoma antibody with IL-2 and LAK cells led to significantly increased efficacy of therapy (Eisenthal et al., 1988). However, we did not observe any clinical responses among 10 patients with CRC who were treated with LAK cells, IL-2, and the mouse-antihuman CRC mAb L-6 (Hellström et al., 1986a, 1986b; Lotze, unpublished observations).

IL-2 AND TUMOR-INFILTRATING LYMPHOCYTES

Several years following the observation that lymphocytes infiltrating a tumor could be selectively expanded to large numbers from tumor cell suspensions using IL-2, we reported that these cells were able to mediate the regression of a variety of metastatic tumors in both the liver and lungs of mice (Rosenberg et al., 1986). Unlike LAK cells, however, these were conventional T lymphocytes, and their activity was MHC-restricted. They were more effective in immunosuppressed mice and they were 50 to 100 times more potent on a cell-per-cell basis than LAK cells in mouse models. Subsequent to these observations, we and others generated TIL from patients with a variety of malignancies. When expanded from resected MM metastases using 6×10^3 IU/mL of IL-2, the lymphocytes were specifically lytic for the autologous tumor and not for allogeneic tumors approximately 30% of the time (Muul et al., 1987; Topalian et al., 1989).

Kradin et al. (1987) first reported the results of a trial evaluating the systemic administration of TIL to humans with metastatic lung cancer. Seven patients were safely treated with small numbers of cells expanded over 1 to 4 months from fragments of tumor cultured with 10 U/mL of IL-2 (Genetics Institute, Boston) and irradiated autologous PBMC. No clinical responses were seen, and they suggested that the TIL might be more effective if administered concomitantly with IL-2. More recently, they reported 2 PR in 8 patients with adenocarcinoma of the lung, 1 PR each among 3 patients with RCC and, 3 patients with MM (Kradin et al., 1988). The protocol called for seven TIL infusions and a continuous infusion of Cetus IL-2 at various doses for 13 days. Therapy was well tolerated at the low doses of IL-2 used.

Our first clinical trial, reported in 1988, involved 12 patients treated with escalating doses of cyclophosphamide, IL-2, and from 2×10^8 to 2×10^{11} TIL (Topalian et al., 1988). Two PR were seen. There was no apparent correlation between response and in vitro lytic activity against the autologous tumor or phenotype of the TIL. More recently, we reported our experience treating an additional 20 patients with MM, 55% of whom had an objective response to therapy (Rosenberg et al., 1988a) (Fig. 16-3). Two of these responses were seen in a group of 5 patients who had previously failed another IL-2–based therapy. Seventeen additional patients who underwent tumor resection in anticipation of receiving TIL were never treated, either because the cells

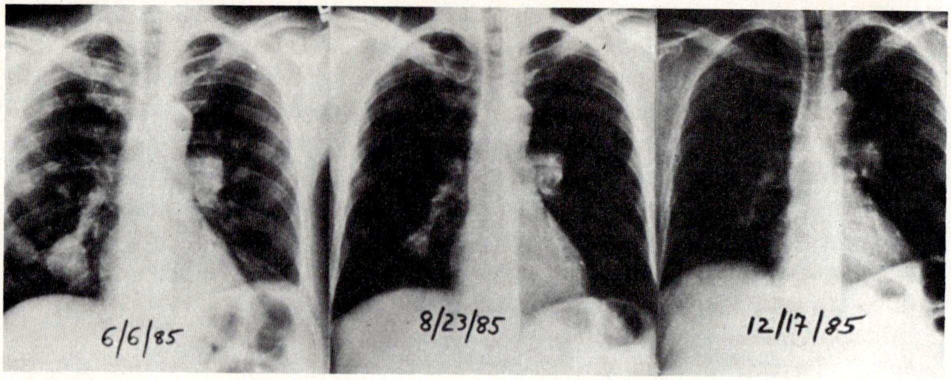

FIGURE 16-3
Sequential chest radiographs obtained prior to (left) and following (center and right) therapy with IL-2 and tumor-infiltrating lymphocytes (TIL) demonstrate regression of pulmonary metastatic melanoma.

grew poorly (8 patients), their disease progressed too rapidly (7 patients), or their cultures became contaminated (2 patients). Responses ranged from 2 to 13 months, averaging 6 months.

More recently, Aoki et al. (1991) have reported their experience using TIL to treat patients with advanced ovarian cancer. Seven patients were treated with from 1.5 to 4.1×10^{10} TIL 48 hours following a 200-mg bolus of cyclophosphamide. Three of these patients manifest a PR.

In an effort to make this therapy more efficacious, we have modified our TIL trial based on observations made in murine models and in vitro that suggest tumors can be rendered more vulnerable to lysis and that more effective TIL can be generated by modifying the culture conditions. Cameron et al. (1990) reported a series of studies demonstrating that TIL and IL-2 are more effective when their administration is preceded by local tumor irradiation. Their results suggest that the effect of irradiation is probably not mediated through the eradication of suppressor T cells. In mice pretreated with cyclophosphamide and irradiation of only one half of the liver before immunotherapy, regression of liver metastases was noted only in the irradiated side. Consequently, a direct tumoricidal effect of irradiation or enhanced trafficking of TIL to the tumor probably underlies this phenomenon. Based on these observations, we treated selected patients with localized tumor radiation therapy followed by TIL and IL-2 infusions. We did not observe enhanced systemic or local responses among 28 patients treated in this fashion (Lange, unpublished data).

Rosenberg et al. (1988b) demonstrated marked synergy between TIL, IFN-α, and IL-2 in mice bearing either 3- or 10-day lung metastases. Mice were rendered nearly tumor free by cells and cytokines at doses much less than otherwise required when using TIL and IL-2 alone. It was suggested that the effect seen with concomitant IFN-α is mediated through enhanced recognition and expression of tumor-associated antigen (TAA) or MHC class I antigen. We are now treating patients with a combination of TIL, IL-2, and IFN-α.

In murine models of adoptive immunotherapy, enhanced lytic specificity of transfused CTL translates into more significant in vivo tumor reduction and prolonged survival (Greenberg et al., 1988). Efforts to generate specifically lytic CTL from murine TIL have included the use of lower concentrations of IL-2, which presumably preferentially expand cells that have already been activated by tumor antigen and express high-affinity IL-2 receptors (Barth et al., 1990; Chou et al., 1988; Shu et al., 1989; Yang et al., 1990). However, T-cell expansion in low concentrations of IL-2 is limited and must be enhanced by restimulating cultures with irradiated tumor. This upregulates expression of the IL-2 receptor on murine CTL and renders them more efficacious in some murine models (Matis et al., 1986). In generating human melanoma TIL, we have found that 10^3 U/mL of IL-4 also enhances proliferation of $CD3^+$ $CD56^-$ lymphocytes in concert with low concentrations of IL-2 (Kawakami et al., 1988). This is consistent with previous observations that IL-4 inhibits IL-2–induced LAK-cell differentiation from unstimulated PBMC, while also serving as a potent T-cell growth factor for cells previously stimulated with antigen, mitogen, or IL-2 (Higuchi et al., 1989; Kawakami et al., 1989). The CTL usually have more specific lytic activity than cells cultured without IL-4. As noted above for mice, the addition of irradiated tumors enhances proliferation. By culturing TIL in medium containing only 120 IU/mL of IL-2 and 10^3 U/mL of IL-4 and by restimulating with irradiated tumor, we hope to generate greater numbers of specifically reactive CTL that will manifest enhanced therapeutic efficacy. Additionally, by using lower doses of IL-2 and fewer cells with LAK-like activity, we may lessen the toxicity associated with this therapy.

Finally, we have begun to treat patients with TIL into which a gene of bacterial origin has been inserted using a retroviral vector (Kasid et al., 1990; Rosenberg et al., 1990). The gene codes for neomycin phosphotransferase (NPT), which inactivates G418, a neomycin analog toxic to mammalian cells (Southern and Berg, 1982; Wagman et al., 1974). The transduced TIL can be detected by assays for NPT, by continued growth in G418, by Southern blot, or by polymerase chain reaction. These cells have been detected in the blood and have been recovered from tissue biopsies obtained from treated patients for up to 2 months after therapy. These studies will provide insight into patterns of TIL recirculation, trafficking, and longevity and will provide a basis for treating patients with TIL transduced with genes of potential therapeutic interest, including TNF and other cytokines.

TOXICITY

We have administered 679 courses of high-dose IL-2 either alone or with adoptively transferred cells to 435 patients with advanced cancer (Rosenberg et al., 1989) (Table 16-6). Infusions of as many as 7.5×10^{11} activated cells were well tolerated, and the observed toxicity appeared to be directly related to the dose of IL-2 utilized. Most patients have been treated with acetaminophen, indomethacin, and antiemetics to de-

TABLE 16-6
TOXICITY OF TREATMENT WITH IL-2*

	IL-2 Alone	IL-2 + LAK	IL-2 + TIL	Total
Number of patients	155	214	66	435
		Number of courses		
	236	348	95	679
Chills	75	191	33	299
Pruritus	53	82	6	141
Necrosis	3	—	—	3
Anaphylaxis	—	—	—	0
Mucositis (requiring liquid diet)	6	12	2	20
Alimentation not possible	1	2	—	3
Nausea and vomiting	162	263	48	473
Diarrhea	144	250	38	432
Hyperbilirubinemia (maximum/mg %)				
2.1 − 6.0	126	190	46	362
6.0 − 10.0	49	72	26	147
10.1 +	26	40	8	74
Oliguria				
<80 mL/8 h	81	114	25	220
<240 mL/24 h	19	12	5	36
Weight gain (% body weight)				
0.0–5.0	106	117	49	272
5.1–10.0	78	148	26	252
10.1–15.0	43	62	15	120
15.1–20.0	7	15	3	25
20.1 +	2	6	2	10
Elevated creatinine (maximum/mg %)				
2.1–6.0	148	237	54	439
6.1–10.0	21	34	12	67
10.1 +	5	2	1	8

crease the chills, fever, nausea, and vomiting that are frequently seen. Cardiovascular side effects included hypotension in 60% of treatment courses that was managed with IV fluid or phenylephrine. Dysrhythmias requiring treatment were seen infrequently, were usually supraventricular, and were rarely life-threatening. Myocardial infarctions were noted in 5 patients. All patients manifested fluid retention and weight gain secondary to a documented vascular leak. This phenomenon probably contributes to the hypotension noted above, as well as to the pulmonary congestion seen in most of our patients. The latter previously led to respiratory distress or endotracheal intubation in about 5% of treatment courses. This complication has become exceedingly rare as a

TABLE 16-6
(Continued)

	IL-2 Alone	IL-2 + LAK	IL-2 + TIL	Total
Hematuria (gross)	—	—	—	2
Edema (symptomatic nerve or vessel compression)	4	7	—	11
Tissue ischemia	—	1	—	1
Respiratory distress				
Not intubated	17	28	7	52
Intubated	15	12	5	32
Bronchospasm	2	4	—	6
Pleural effusion (requiring thoracentesis)	4	8	1	13
Somnolence	29	45	8	82
Coma	9	8	5	22
Disorientation	52	89	10	151
Hypotension (requiring pressors)	119	259	45	423
Angina	5	8	—	13
Myocardial infarction	4	1	—	5
Arrhythmias	15	39	6	60
Anemia requiring transfusion (number units transfused)				
1.5	77	176	40	293
6–10	22	53	9	84
11–15	4	15	4	23
16+	1	11	1	13
Thrombocytopenia (minimum/mm^3)				
<20,000	28	71	19	118
20,001–60,000	53	79	22	154
Central line sepsis	13	36	2	51
Death	4	3	2	9

*Adapted from Rosenberg et al., 1989. TIL, tumor-infiltrating lymphocytes.

result of more judicious use of IV fluids and more liberal use of vasopressors. Other side effects included anemia requiring transfusion in about 61% of treatment courses and thrombocytopenia (less than 20,000) in about 17% of treatment courses. Seventy-six percent of treatment courses were accompanied by creatinine elevation and oliguria. Central nervous system toxicity, including disorientation, somnolence, and coma occurred in about 38% of treatment courses. Nausea, vomiting, and diarrhea were not uncommon. All of these side effects began to resolve within several days of the completion of therapy. Atkins et al. (1988) have reported that IL-2 and LAK-cell therapy is associated with hypothyroidism in 20% of patients, which may persist as long as 10 months. We have recently confirmed these findings (Schwartzentruber et al., 1990). Unusual complications of therapy include colon perforation and small bowel necrosis that can present as surgical emergencies (Schwartzentruber et al., 1988; Rahman et al., 1991). We have not observed significant long-term sequelae of IL-2–based immunotherapy. Among these 435 patients, there were 9 treatment-related deaths.

The etiology of many of these side effects has not been precisely determined. The cardiovascular changes associated with therapy, including myocardial depression, vasodilation, and capillary leak (Lee et al., 1989), are also observed during endotoxemia and septic shock. However, we have been unable to detect circulating endotoxin in our patients (unpublished data). Autopsies performed on a small number of patients have revealed an intense lymphocytic infiltrate in most organs, including the heart, but the significance of this is unknown. The role of other cytokines as mediators of toxicity is suggested by the finding of circulating TNF, IFN-γ, and IL-6 in our patients (Jablons et al., 1989; Lotze et al., 1985b). Fraker et al. (1989) have demonstrated that passive immunization against TNF-α abrogates some of the toxicity seen in mice treated with IL-2. However, in a recently published clinical trial, serum levels of IFN-γ, rather than TNF-α, correlated with observed, IL-2–associated, clinical toxicity (Economou et al., 1991).

We have shown that the endothelial activation antigens, endothelial leukocyte adhesion molecule-1 (ELAM-1), intercellular adhesion molecule-1 (ICAM-1), and HLA-DQ are expressed by the endothelial cells lining cutaneous venules in patients treated with IL-2 (Cotran et al., 1988). These molecules are also displayed by the endothelium-lining venules during delayed hypersensitivity reactions. Since IFN-γ is a potent inducer of these antigens in endothelium, it may contribute to the IL-2–induced capillary leak. Lymphokine-activated killer cells have also been implicated as mediators of this syndrome in murine models (Gately et al., 1988). Systemically administered IL-2 in man is also associated with high levels of circulating beta (β)-endorphin (Denicoff et al., 1989), elevated brain water content (Saris et al., 1989), and detectable cerebrospinal fluid (CSF) IL-2 (Saris et al., 1988), although a correlation between these findings and observed CNS toxicity has not been found. Leukotrienes are suspected of mediating some of the renal and gastrointestinal side effects.

MECHANISMS OF RESPONSE TO IL-2–BASED IMMUNOTHERAPY

Substantial effort has been directed toward elucidating the mechanism of response to these IL-2–based immunotherapies. The immune recognition and destruction of tumor cells have usually been classified as cellular, primarily T cell, or humoral, primarily antibody-mediated. The role of other cells such as those with NK-cell, LAK-cell, or ADCC activity and the effect of various cytokines has been suggested by in vitro studies. Little is known about how an effective antitumor response is orchestrated using such disparate effector mechanisms. There is compelling evidence that T cells mediate IL-2–induced tumor regression. In mice, the antitumor effect of high-dose

IL-2 or IL-2 and IFN-α is abrogated by the selective deletion of certain lymphocyte subsets (Mulé et al., 1987; Peace and Cheever, 1989; Rosenberg et al., 1988b). Specifically lytic, Lyt-2^+, class I restricted CTL are highly effective against some murine tumors (Barth et al., 1990). Other evidence includes the demonstration that a class I deficient murine melanoma resistant to IL-2 therapy was rendered susceptible to such therapy by transfection with the gene H2-K^b (Weber et al., 1987).

The cytokine microenvironment generated within tumors by infiltrating T cells may be central to the antitumor immune response. Cytokines that upregulate class I antigen expression on tumors have been reported to synergize with IL-2 in some murine immunotherapy models (Cameron et al., 1988; McIntosh et al., 1988). Barth et al. (1991) demonstrated that both cytolytic and noncytolytic murine CTL are capable of specifically elaborating IFN-γ and TNF-α in response to stimulation with autologous tumor in vitro. These observations were extended to murine micrometastatic tumor models in which the in vivo efficacy of adoptively transferred TIL was more closely associated with specific lymphokine secretion than with in vitro antitumor cytolytic activity.

In humans, the prominence of T cells within tumor-associated infiltrates (Cohen et al., 1987; Kornstein et al., 1983; Rubin et al., 1989; Shimokawara et al., 1982), their presumed association with prognosis (Shimokawara et al., 1982), and the ability of adoptively transferred IL-2–stimulated lymphocytes to traffic to sites of tumor (Fisher et al., 1989; Griffith et al., 1989) suggest that these cells play an important role in the effective antitumor immune response. We have recently reported an immunohistochemical evaluation of biopsied metastatic tumors obtained from patients treated with IL-2–based therapy that showed all regressing lesions were heavily infiltrated with both $CD4^+$ and $CD8^+$ T cells as well as macrophages (Rubin et al., 1989). There were no detectable NKH-1–positive cells in any lesion, arguing against a direct role for cells with NK-cell, LAK-cell, or ADCC activity. Considering these observations, T cells are probably the ultimate effectors of successful antitumor adoptive immunotherapy with IL-2. The potential role of accessory cells and other cytokines remains to be characterized, and the dynamics of lymphocyte trafficking to sites of tumor need to be further clarified.

It follows that antigen processing and presentation to T cells are critical for effective immunotherapy. Unlike antibodies, which recognize the three-dimensional structure of protein antigens, the T-cell receptor (TCR) recognizes peptide motifs in concert with class I or II histocompatibility molecules. These cell-surface molecules belong to the immunoglobulin supergene family and are critical to many cellular immune responses. Class II molecules, including HLA-DR, are required for antigen presentation to $CD4^+$ T cells, while $CD8^+$ T-cell responses are restricted to antigen presented in concert with class I molecules. The processing requisite for T-cell recognition of antigen is thought to involve cleavage or unfolding of the protein, followed by its association with a histocompatibility molecule before export to the cell surface. Until recently, it was thought that this function was performed only by antigen-presenting macrophages. Now it is clear that B cells (Issekutz et al., 1982) and other cells as well (Hirschberg et al., 1982; Geppert and Lipsky, 1987; Lorenz and Allen, 1989) can present antigen to $CD4^+$ T cells. Recently, it has been suggested that primary melanoma cell lines can process and present tetanus toxoid to class II restricted, antigen-specific T-cell clones and that the T-cell proliferative response to autologous melanoma can be blocked by pretreating the tumor with ammonium chloride, which arrests antigen processing (Alexander et al., 1989). The significance of this latter finding is uncertain due to the effects of this reagent on manifold cellular processes (Dean et al., 1984). Finally, there is a reported association between T-cell proliferation and HLA-DR expression by melanoma cell lines *in vitro* (Fossati et al., 1984; Guerry et al., 1984, 1987) and an association between HLA-DR expression by tumors and lesional regression seen in patients treated with IL-2 (Rubin et al., 1989). These findings suggest that some tumors can process and present their own antigens in a class I or II restricted fashion. The ability to do so may be a prerequisite for successful immunotherapy.

SUMMARY AND FUTURE DIRECTIONS

Immunotherapy with adoptively transferred lymphocytes can effect clinically significant responses in selected patients with advanced cancer. The most susceptible malignancies have been MM and RCC. The impact on survival has not been evaluated. Extensive analysis has not identified any variables that consistently correlate with clinical response. Although responses have also been reported in patients with CRC (Rosenberg et al., 1989; Steis et al., 1990), ovarian cancer (Eberlein et al., 1988; Steis et al., 1990), lymphoma (Bernstein et al., 1991b; Margolin et al., 1991; Rosenberg et al., 1989), and lung cancer (Bernstein et al., 1991a), these responses have generally been transient or too infrequent to warrant the use of IL-2 and LAK cells in the treatment of these diseases.

The optimal treatment protocol and technique of LAK-cell generation have yet to be defined. Based on the dose–response relationship seen in murine models, we have used the maximally tolerated dose of IL-2 administered by intermittent IV bolus and reported that 21% of 48 patients with MM and 35% of patients with RCC responded to therapy. Other reported trials using a variety of treatment protocols have generally involved far fewer patients so that meaningful comparisons are difficult to make. Eberlein et al. (1988) reported a significant response rate and apparently reduced toxicity among 29 patients treated with a lower dose of IL-2. A similar trial conducted by Stahel et al. (1989) was associated with greater toxicity and fewer responses. Some of the protocols that employed continuous infusions of IL-2 reported results similar to ours at the highest doses used.

An advantage of therapy with LAK cells and IL-2 compared to therapy with IL-2 alone has yet to be shown. Our nonrandomized trial suggests that the two are equivalent when high doses of IL-2 are used. This was also the conclusion of our recently completed randomized trial (Rosenberg et al., unpublished data). Marked synergy has been demonstrated between LAK cells and lower doses of IL-2 in murine models. An IL-2 dose-sparing effect would be useful in designing future clinical trials since the degree of treatment-associated toxicity appears to be related to the dose of IL-2. Unfortunately, trials that employed lower doses of IL-2 and LAK cells have reported conflicting results and have involved small numbers of patients so that meaningful conclusions cannot yet be drawn.

Efforts to improve adoptive cellular immunotherapy, including the use of monoclonal antibodies, concomitant radiation therapy, and combinations of cytokines, have been abortive. More potent cellular reagents have been developed but their effectiveness remains to be defined. The Pittsburgh Cancer Institute is currently conducting a phase II trial employing high-dose IL-2 and adherent LAK cells. We have reported that TIL and IL-2 infusions are associated with a 55% response rate among patients with MM, but the responses have been of short duration.

Recombinant IL-4 and IL-7 are two additional T-cell growth factors that have recently been made available for large-scale clinical trials. Their potential role in immunotherapy, either alone or with adoptively transferred cells, is an area for future investigation. Finally, we have been treating patients with gene-modified TIL that are resistant to the antibiotic G418. These studies, which are currently being conducted at the Pittsburgh Cancer Institute and at the Surgery Branch of the National Cancer Institute, will assess the safety, longevity, and patterns of trafficking of these cells. These investigations anticipate the use of TIL genetically engineered to produce cytokines of potential therapeutic benefit. Perhaps the local production of these reagents by transduced, antigen-specific TIL that localize in tumor deposits will translate into enhanced efficacy of these cells.

REFERENCES

Adler A, Stein JA, Kedar E, Naor D, Weiss DW. Intralesional injection of interleukin-2-expanded autologous lymphocytes in melanoma and breast cancer patients: a pilot study. J Biol Resp Mod. 1984;3:491–500.

Aebersold P, Carter CS, Hyatt C, et al. A simplified automated procedure for generation of human lymphokine-activated killer cells for use in clinical trials. J Immunol Meth. 1988; 112:1–7.

Alexander MA, Bennicelli J, Guerry D. Defective antigen presentation by human melanoma cell lines cultured from advanced, but not biologically early, disease. J Immunol. 1989; 142:4070–4078.

Alexander P. Immunotherapy of leukemia: the use of different classes of immune lymphocytes. Cancer Res. 1967;27:2521–2526.

Aoki Y, Takakuwa K, Kodama S, et al. Use of adoptive transfer of tumor-infiltrating lymphocytes alone or in combination with cisplatin-containing chemotherapy in patients with epithelial ovarian cancer. Cancer Res. 1991;51:1934–1939.

Atkins MB, Mier JW, Parkinson DR, Gould JA, Berkman EM, Kaplan MM. Hypothyroidism after treatment with interleukin-2 and lymphokine-activated killer cells. New Engl J Med. 1988;318:1557–1563.

Bar MH, Sznol M, Atkins MB, et al. Metastatic malignant melanoma treated with combined bolus and continuous infusion interleukin 2 and lymphokine-activated killer cells. J Clin Oncol. 1990;8:1138–1147.

Barth RJ, Bock SN, Mulé JJ, Rosenberg SA. Unique murine tumor-associated antigens identified by tumor infiltrating lymphocytes. J Immunol. 1990;144:1531–1537.

Barth RJ, Mulé JJ, Spiess PJ, Rosenberg SA. Interferon-gamma and tumor necrosis factor have a role in tumor regressions mediated by murine CD8$^+$ tumor-infiltrating lymphocytes. J Exp Med. 1991;173:647–658.

Beckner SK, Farrar WL. Potentiation of lymphokine-activated killer cell differentiation and lymphocyte proliferation by stimulation of protein kinase C or inhibition of adenylate cyclase. J Immunol. 1988;140:208–214.

Bernstein ID. Passive transfer of systemic tumor immunity with cells generated in vitro by a secondary immune response to a syngeneic rat Gross virus-induced lymphoma. J Immunol. 1977;118:122–128.

Bernstein ZP, Goldrosen MH, Vaickus L, et al. Interleukin 2 with ex vivo activated killer cells: therapy of advanced non-small-cell lung cancer. J Immunother. 1991a;10:383–387.

Bernstein ZP, Vaickus L, Friedman N, et al. Interleukin 2 lymphokine-activated killer cell therapy of non-Hodgkin's lymphoma and Hodgkin's disease. J Immunother. 1991b;10:141–146.

Blay JY, Bertoglio J, Fradelizi D, Chouaib S. Functional interactions of IL-2 and TNF in the differentiation of LGL into LAK effectors. Int J Cancer. 1989;44:598–604.

Borberg H, Oettgen HF, Choudry K, Beattie EJ. Inhibition of established transplants of chemically induced sarcomas in syngeneic mice by lymphocytes from immunized donors. Int J Cancer. 1972;10:539–547.

Bowlin TL, McKown BJ, Kang MS, Sunkara PS. Potentiation of human lymphokine-activated killer cell activity by Swainsonine, an inhibitor of glycoprotein processing. Cancer Res. 1989;49:4109–4113.

Cameron RB, McIntosh JK, Rosenberg SA. Synergistic antitumor effects of combination immunotherapy with recombinant interleukin-2 and a recombinant hybrid α-interferon in the treatment of established murine hepatic metastases. Cancer Res. 1988;48:5810–5817.

Cameron RB, Spiess PJ, Rosenberg SA. Synergistic antitumor activity of tumor-infiltrating lymphocytes, interleukin-2 and local tumor irradiation. Studies on the mechanism of action. J Exp Med. 1990;171:249–263.

Cascinelli N, Belli F, Marchini S, et al. A phase II study of the administration of recombinant interleukin-2 (rIL-2) plus lymphokine activated killer (LAK) cells in stage IV melanoma patients. Tumori. 1989;75:233–244.

Cheever MA, Greenberg PD, Fefer A. Specific adoptive therapy of established leukemia with syngeneic lymphocytes sequentially immunized in vivo and in vitro and nonspecifically expanded by culture with interleukin-2. J Immunol. 1981;126:1318–1322.

Cheever MA, Greenberg PD, Fefer A, Gillis S. Augmentation of the anti-tumor therapeutic efficacy of long-term cultured T lymphocytes by in vivo administration of purified interleukin-2. J Exp Med. 1982;155:968–980.

Chou T, Bertera S, Chang AE, Shu S. Adoptive immunotherapy of microscopic and advanced visceral metastases with in vitro sensitized lymphoid cells from mice bearing progressive tumors. J Immunol. 1988;141:1775–1781.

Chouaib S, Bertoglio J, Blay J, Marchiol-Fournigault C, Fradelizi D. Generation of lymphokine-activated killer cells: synergy between tumor necrosis factor and interleukin-2. Proc Natl Acad Sci USA. 1988;85:6875–6879.

Cohen PJ, Lotze MT, Roberts JR, Rosenberg SA, Jaffe ES. The immunopathology of sequential tumor biopsies in patients treated with interleukin-2. Am J Pathol. 1987;129:208–216.

Cotran RS, Pober JS, Gimbrone MA, et al. Endothelial activation during interleukin-2 immunotherapy. A possible mechanism for the vascular leak syndrome. J Immunol. 1988;140: 1883–1888.

Dean RT, Jessup W, Roberts CR. Effects of exogenous amines on mammalian cells, with particular reference to membrane flow. Biochem J. 1984;217:27–40.

Delorme EJ, Alexander P. Treatment of primary fibrosarcoma in the rat with immune lymphocytes. Lancet. 1964;2:117–120.

Denicoff KD, Durkin TM, Lotze MT, et al. The neuroendocrine effects of interleukin-2 treatment. J Clin Endocrinol Metab. 1989;69:402–410.

Dennert G, De Rose M. Continuously proliferating T killer cells specific for H-2^b targets: selection and characterization. J Immunol. 1976;116:1601–1606.

Devos R, Plaetinck G, Cheroutre H, et al. Molecular cloning of human interleukin-2 cDNA and its expression in *E. coli.* Nucl Acid Res. 1983;11:4307–4323.

Dutcher JP, Creekmore S, Weiss GR, et al. A phase II study of interleukin-2 and lymphokine-activated killer cells in patients with metastatic malignant melanoma. J Clin Oncol. 1989;7:447–485.

Eberlein TJ, Rosenstein M, Rosenberg SA. Regression of a disseminated syngeneic solid tumor by systemic transfer of lymphoid cells expanded in interleukin-2. J Exp Med. 1982;156:385–397.

Eberlein TJ, Schoof DD, Jung S-E, et al. A new regimen of interleukin-2 and lymphokine-activated killer cells. Efficacy without significant toxicity. Arch Intern Med. 1988;148:2571–2576.

Economou JS, Hoban M, Lee JD, et al. Production of tumor necrosis factor-alpha and interferon-gamma in interleukin-2-treated melanoma patients: correlation with clinical toxicity. Cancer Immunol Immunother. 1991;34:49–52.

Eisenthal A, Rosenberg SA. Systemic induction of cells mediating antibody-dependent cellular cytotoxicity following administration of interleukin-2. Cancer Res. 1989;49:6953–6959.

Eisenthal A, Cameron RB, Uppenkamp I, Rosenberg SA. Effect of combined therapy with lymphokine-activated killer cells, interleukin-2 and specific monoclonal antibody on established B16 melanoma lung metastases. Cancer Res. 1988;48:7140–7145.

Ellis TM, McKenzie RS, Simms PE, Helfrich BA, Fisher RI. Induction of human lymphokine-activated killer cells by IFN-α and IFN-γ. J Immunol. 1989;143:4282–4286.

Ettinghausen SE, Lipford EH, Mulé JJ, Rosenberg SA. Recombinant interleukin-2 stimulates in vivo proliferation of adoptively transferred lymphokine-activated killer (LAK) cells. J Immunol. 1985;135:3623–3635.

Fagan EA, Pulley M, Limb A, et al. Adoptive immunotherapy administered via the hepatic artery and intralesional interleukin-2 in hepatocellular carcinoma. Cancer Treat Rev. 1989;16(suppl A):151–160.

Fefer A, Einstein AB, Cheever MA. Adoptive chemoimmunotherapy of cancer in animals: a review of results, principles and problems. Ann N.Y. Acad Sci. 1976;277:492–504.

Fernandez-Cruz E, Halliburton B, Feldman JD. In vivo elimination by specific effector cells of an established syngeneic rat Moloney virus-induced sarcoma. J Immunol. 1979;123:1772–1777.

Fidler IJ, Gersten DM, Budmen MB. Characterization in vivo and in vitro of tumor cells selected for resistance to syngeneic lymphocyte-mediated cytotoxicity. Cancer Res. 1976;36:3160–3165.

Fisher RI, Coltman CA, Doroshow JH, et al. Metastatic renal cancer treated with interleukin-2 and lymphokine-activated killer cells. Ann Intern Med. 108:518–523.

Fisher B, Packard BS, Read EJ, et al. Tumor localization of adoptively transferred indium-111 labeled tumor infiltrating lymphocytes in patients with metastatic melanoma. J Clin Oncol. 1989;7:250–261.

Fogel M, Gorelik E, Segal S, Feldman M. Differences in cell surface antigens of tumor metastases and those of the local tumor. J Natl Cancer Inst. 1979;62:585–588.

Foley EJ. Antigenic properties of methylcholanthrene-induced tumors in mice of the strain of origin. Cancer Res. 1953;13:835–837.

Fossati G, Taramelli D, Balsari A, Bogdanovich G, Andreola S, Parmiani G. Primary but not metastatic human melanomas expressing DR antigens stimulate autologous lymphocytes. Int J Cancer. 1984;33:591–597.

Fraker DL, Langstein HN, Norton JA. Passive immunization against tumor necrosis factor partially abrogates interleukin-2 toxicity. J Exp Med. 1989;170:1015–1020.

Frenster JH, Rogoway WM. In vitro activation and reinfusion of autologous human lymphocytes. Lancet. 1968;2:979–980.

Frenster JH, Rogoway WM. Early clinical trials of activated autologous lymphocytes for human cancer immunotherapy. Proc Am Assoc Cancer Res. 1970;11:28.

Gately MK, Anderson TD, Hayes TJ. Role of asialo-GM_1-positive lymphoid cells in mediating the toxic effects of recombinant IL-2 in mice. J Immunol. 1988;141:189–200.

Geppert TD, Lipsky PE. Dissection of defective antigen presentation by interferon-γ-treated fibroblasts. J Immunol. 1987;138:385–392.

Gillis S, Smith KA. Long term culture of specific cytotoxic T cells. Nature. 1977;268:154–156.

Greenberg PD, Klarnet JP, Kern DE, Cheever MA. Therapy of disseminated tumors by adoptive transfer of specifically immune T cells. Prog Exp Tumor Res. 1988;32:104–127.

Griffith KD, Read EJ, Carrasquillo JA, et al. In vivo distribution of adoptively transferred indium-111-labeled tumor infiltrating lymphocytes and peripheral blood lymphocytes in patients with metastatic melanoma. J Natl Cancer Inst. 1989;81:1709–1717.

Grimm EA. Interleukin-2 activated cytotoxic lymphocytes and their application in the intraoperative immunotherapy of local tumors. Prog Clin Biol Res. 1987;244:185–195.

Gross L. Intradermal immunization of C3H mice against a sarcoma that originated in an animal of the same line. Cancer Res. 1943;3:326–333.

Guerry D, Alexander MA, Herlyn MF, et al. HLA-DR histocompatibility leukocyte antigens permit cultured human melanoma cells from early but not advanced disease to stimulate autologous lymphocytes. J Clin Invest. 1984;73:267–271.

Guerry D, Alexander MA, Elder DE, Herlyn MF. Interferon-γ regulates the T cell response to precursor nevi and biologically early melanoma. J Immunol. 1987;139:305–312.

Gunji Y, Vujanovic NL, Hiserodt JC, Herberman RB, Gorelik E. Generation and characterization of purified adherent lymphokine-activated killer cells in mice. J Immunol. 1989;142: 1748–1754.

Hellström I, Beaumier PL, Hellström KE. Antitumor effects of L6, an IgG2a antibody that reacts with most human carcinomas. Proc Natl Acad Sci USA. 1986a;83:7059–7063.

Hellström I, Horn D, Linsley P, et al. Monoclonal mouse antibodies raised against human lung carcinoma. Cancer Res. 1986b;46:3917–3923.

Higuchi CM, Thompson JA, Lindgren CG, et al. Induction of lymphokine-activated killer activity by interleukin-4 in human lymphocytes preactivated by interleukin-2 in vivo or in vitro. Cancer Res. 1989;49:6487–6492.

Hirschberg H, Braathen LR, Thorsby E. Antigen presentation by vascular endothelial cells and epidermal Langerhans cells: the role of HLA-DR. Immunol Rev. 1982;66:57–77.

Hsieh KH, Shu S, Lee CS, Chu CT, Yang CS, Chang KJ. Lysis of primary hepatic tumors by lymphokine activated killer cells. Gut. 1987;28:117–124.

Ichida T, Higuchi K, Arakawa K, et al. Treatment of hepatocellular carcinoma utilizing lymphokine-activated killer cells and interleukin-2. Cancer Chemother Pharmacol. 1989;23 (suppl):s45–s48.

Ishikawa T, Ikawa T, Eura M, Fukiage T, Masuyama K. Adoptive immunotherapy for head and neck cancer with killer cells induced by stimulation with autologous or allogeneic tumour cells and recombinant interleukin-2. Acta Otolaryngol. 1989;107:346–351.

Issekutz T, Chu E, Geha RS. Antigen presentation by human B cells: T cell proliferation induced by Epstein-Barr virus B lymphoblastoid cells. J Immunol. 1982;129:1446–1450.

Jablons DM, Mulé JJ, McIntosh JK, et al. IL-6/IFN-β-2 as a circulating hormone. Induction by cytokine administration in humans. J Immunol. 1989;142:1542–1547.

Kasid A, Morecki S, Aebersold P, et al. Human gene transfer: characterization of human tumor-infiltrating lymphocytes as vehicles for retroviral-mediated gene transfer in man. Proc Natl Acad Sci USA. 1990;87:473–477.

Kawakami Y, Rosenberg SA, Lotze MT. Interleukin-4 promotes the growth of tumor-infiltrating lymphocytes cytotoxic for human autologous melanoma. J Exp Med. 1988;168:2183–2191.

Kawakami Y, Custer MC, Rosenberg SA, Lotze MT. IL-4 regulates IL-2 induction of lymphokine-activated killer activity from human lymphocytes. J Immunol. 1989;142:3452–3461.

Klein G, Sjögren H, Klein E, Hellström KE. Demonstration of resistance against methylcholanthrene-induced sarcomas in the primary autochthonous host. Cancer Res. 1960;20:1561–1572.

Kornstein MJ, Brooks JSJ, Elder DE. Immunoperoxidase localization of lymphocyte subsets in the host response to melanoma and nevi. Cancer Res. 1983;43:2749–2753.

Kradin RL, Boyle LA, Preffer FI, et al. Tumor-derived interleukin-2-dependent lymphocytes in adoptive immunotherapy of lung cancer. Cancer Immunol Immunother. 1987;24:76–85.

Kradin R, Dubinett S, Mullin J, et al. Treatment of patients with advanced cancer using tumor-infiltrating lymphocytes and interleukin-2. Transplant Proc. 1988;20:336–338.

Lafreniere R, Rosenberg SA. Successful immunotherapy of murine experimental hepatic metastases with lymphokine-activated killer cells and recombinant interleukin-2. Cancer Res. 1985a;45:3735–3741.

Lafreniere R, Rosenberg SA. Adoptive immunotherapy of murine hepatic metastases with lymphokine activated killer (LAK) cells and recombinant interleukin-2 (RIL 2) can mediate the regression of both immunogenic and nonimmunogenic sarcomas and an adenocarcinoma. J Immunol. 1985b;135:4273–4280.

Lee RE, Lotze MT, Skibber JM, et al. Cardiorespiratory effects of immunotherapy with interleukin-2. J Clin Oncol. 1989;7:7–20.

Lorenz RG, Allen PM. Thymic cortical epithelial cells can present self-antigens in vivo. Nature. 1989;337:560–562.

Lotze MT, Grimm EA, Mazumder A, Strausser JL, Rosenberg SA. Lysis of fresh and cultured autologous tumor by human lymphocytes cultured in T-cell growth factor. Cancer Res. 1981;41:4420–4425.

Lotze MT, Robb RJ, Sharrow SO, Frana LW, Rosenberg SA. Systemic administration of interleukin-2 in humans. J Biol Resp Mod. 1984;3:475–482.

Lotze MT, Frana LW, Sharrow SO, Robb RJ, Rosenberg SA. In vivo administration of purified human interleukin-2. I. Half-life and immunologic effects of the Jurkat cell line-derived interleukin-2. J Immunol. 1985a;134:157–166.

Lotze MT, Matory YL, Ettinghausen SE, et al. In vivo administration of purified human interleukin-2. II. Half life, immunologic effects and expansion of peripheral lymphoid cells in vivo with recombinant IL-2. J Immunol. 1985b;135:2865–2875.

Lotze MT, Chang AE, Seipp CA, Simpson C, Vetto JT, Rosenberg SA. High dose recombinant interleukin-2 in the treatment of patients with disseminated cancer. JAMA. 1986a;256:3117–3124.

Lotze MT, Matory YL, Rayner AA, et al. Clinical effects of toxicity of interleukin-2 in patients with cancer. Cancer. 1986b;58:2764–2772.

Lotze MT, Custer MC, Sharrow SO, et al. In vivo administration of purified human interleukin-2 to patients with cancer: development of interleukin-2 receptor positive cells and circulating soluble interleukin-2 receptors following interleukin-2 administration. Cancer Res. 1987;47: 2188–2195.

Margolin KA, Rayner AA, Hawkins MJ, et al. Interleukin-2 and lymphokine-activated killer cell therapy of solid tumors: analysis of toxicity and management guidelines. J Clin Oncol. 1989;7:486–498.

Margolin KA, Aronson FR, Sznol M, et al. Phase II trial of high-dose interleukin 2 and lymphokine-activated killer cells in Hodgkin's disease and non-Hodgkin's lymphoma. J Immunother. 1991;10:214–220.

Matis LA, Shu S, Groves ES, et al. Adoptive immunotherapy of a syngeneic murine leukemia with a tumor-specific cytotoxic T cell clone and recombinant human interleukin-2: correlation with clonal IL-2 receptor expression. J Immunol. 1986;136:3496–3501.

Mazumder A, Rosenberg SA. Successful immunotherapy of natural killer-resistant established pulmonary melanoma metastases by the intravenous adoptive transfer of syngeneic lymphocytes activated in vitro by interleukin-2. J Exp Med. 1984;159:495–507.

Mazumder A, Grimm EA, Zhang HZ, Rosenberg SA. Lysis of fresh human solid tumors by autologous lymphocytes activated in vitro with lectins. Cancer Res. 1982;42:913–918.

Mazumder A, Eberlein TJ, Grimm EA, et al. Phase I study of the adoptive immunotherapy of human cancer with lectin activated autologous mononuclear cells. Cancer. 1984;53:896–905.

McCrady CW, Li F, Grant AJ, Merchant RE, Carchman RA. Alteration of human lymphokine-activated killer cell activity by manipulation of protein kinase C and cytosolic Ca^{2+}. Cancer Res. 1988;48:635–640.

McIntosh JK, Mulé JJ, Merino MJ, Rosenberg SA. Synergistic antitumor effects of immunotherapy with recombinant interleukin-2 and recombinant tumor necrosis factor-α. Cancer Res. 1988;48:4011–4017.

Melder RJ, Whiteside TL, Vujanovic NL, Hiserodt JC, Herberman RB. A new approach to generating antitumor effectors for adoptive immunotherapy using human adherent lymphokine-activated killer cells. Cancer Res. 1988;48:3461–3469.

Mills GB, Paetkau V. Generation of cytotoxic lymphocytes to syngeneic tumor by using co-stimulator (interleukin-2). J Immunol. 1980;125:1897–1903.

Mills GB, Carlson G, Paetkau V. Generation of cytotoxic lymphocytes to syngeneic tumors by using co-stimulator (interleukin 2): in vivo activity. J Immunol. 1980;125:1904–1909.

Mitchison NA. Passive transfer of transplantation immunity. Nature. 1953;171:267–268.

Mitchison NA. Studies on the immunological response to foreign tumor transplants in the mouse. J Exp Med. 1955;102:157–177.

Mittelman A, Savona S, Gafney E, et al. Treatment of patients with advanced cancer using multiple long-term cultured lymphokine-activated killer (LAK) cell infusions and recombinant human interleukin-2. J Biol Resp Mod. 1989;8:468–478.

Morgan DA, Ruscetti FW, Gallo R. Selective in vitro growth of T lymphocytes from normal human bone marrows. Science. 1976;193:1007–1008.

Mulé JJ, Shu S, Schwarz SL, Rosenberg SA. Adoptive immunotherapy of established pulmonary metastases with LAK cells and recombinant interleukin-2. Science. 1984;225:1487–1489.

Mulé JJ, Shu S, Rosenberg SA. The anti-tumor efficacy of lymphokine-activated killer cells and recombinant interleukin 2 in vivo. J Immunol. 1985;135:646–652.

Mulé JJ, Ettinghausen SE, Spiess PJ, Shu S, Rosenberg SA. Antitumor efficacy of lymphokine-activated killer cells and recombinant interleukin-2 in vivo: survival benefit and mechanisms of tumor escape in mice undergoing immunotherapy. Cancer Res. 1986a;46:676–683.

Mulé JJ, Yang J, Shu S, Rosenberg SA. The antitumor efficacy of lymphokine-activated killer cells and recombinant interleukin-2 in vivo: direct correlation between reduction of established metastases and cytolytic activity of lymphokine-activated killer cells. J Immunol. 1986b;136:3899–3909.

Mulé JJ, Yang JC, Lafreniere RL, Shu S, Rosenberg SA. Identification of cellular mechanisms operational in vivo during the regression of established pulmonary metastases by the systemic administration of high-dose recombinant interleukin-2. J Immunol. 1987;139:285–294.

Muul LM, Spiess PJ, Director EP, Rosenberg SA. Identification of specific cytolytic immune responses against autologous tumor in humans bearing malignant melanoma. J Immunol. 1987;138:989–995.

Nadler SH, Moore GE. Clinical immunologic study of malignant disease: response to tumor transplants and transfer of leukocytes. Ann Surg. 1966;164:482–489.

Ochoa AC, Gromo G, Alter BJ, Sondel PM, Bach FH. Long-term growth of lymphokine-activated killer (LAK) cells: role of anti-CD3, β-IL-1, interferon-γ and -β. J Immunol. 1987;138:2728–2733.

Onishi S, Saibara T, Fujikawa M, et al. Adoptive immunotherapy with lymphokine-activated killer cells plus recombinant interleukin-2 in patients with unresectable hepatocellular carcinoma. Hepatology. 1989;10:349–353.

Osband ME, Krane RJ. Autolymphocyte therapy: previous experience and future prospects. Pathol Immunopathol Res. 1988;7:483–493.

Osband ME, Lavin PT, Babayan RK, et al. Effect of autolymphocyte therapy on survival and quality of life in patients with metastatic renal-cell carcinoma. Lancet. 1990;335:994–998.

Paciucci PA, Holland JF, Glidewell O, Odchimar R. Recombinant interleukin-2 by continuous infusion and adoptive transfer of recombinant interleukin-2-activated cells in patients with advanced cancer. J Clin Oncol. 1989;7:869–878.

Papa MZ, Mulé JJ, Rosenberg SA. Antitumor efficacy of lymphokine-activated killer cells and recombinant interleukin-2 in vivo: successful immunotherapy of established pulmonary metastases from weakly immunogenic and nonimmunogenic murine tumors of three distinct histological types. Cancer Res. 1986;46:4973–4978.

Parkinson DR, Fisher RI, Rayner AA, et al. Therapy of renal cell carcinoma with interleukin 2 and lymphokine-activated killer cells: phase II experience with a hybrid bolus and continuous infusion interleukin 2 regimen. J Clin Oncol. 1990;8:1630–1636.

Peace DJ, Cheever MA. Toxicity and therapeutic efficacy of high-dose interleukin-2. J Exp Med. 1989;169:161–173.

Philip T, Mercatello A, Negrier S, et al. Interleukin-2 with and without LAK cells in metastatic renal cell carcinoma: the Lyon first-year experience in 20 patients. Cancer Treat Rev. 1989;16(suppl A):91–104.

Prehn RT, Main JM. Immunity to methylcholanthrene-induced sarcomas. J Natl Cancer Inst. 1957;18:769–778.

Rahman R, Bernstein Z, Vaickus L, et al. Unusual gastrointestinal complications of interleukin 2 therapy. J Immunother. 1991;10:221–225.

Révész L. Detection of antigenic differences in isologous host–tumor systems by pretreatment with heavily irradiated tumor cells. Cancer Res. 1960;20:443–451.

Röllinghoff M, Wagner H. Brief communication: in vivo protection against murine plasma cell tumor growth by in vitro activated syngeneic lymphocytes. J Natl Cancer Inst. 1973; 51:1317–1318.

Rosenberg SA. Immunotherapy of cancer by systemic administration of lymphoid cells plus interleukin-2. J Biol Resp Mod. 1984;3:501–511.

Rosenberg SA, Schwarz S, Spiess PJ. In vitro growth of murine T cells II. Growth of in vitro sensitized cells cytotoxic for allo-antigens. J Immunol. 1978;121:1951–1955.

Rosenberg SA, Aebersold P, Cornetta K, et al. Gene transfer into humans—immunotherapy of patients with advanced melanoma using tumor-infiltrating lymphocytes modified by retroviral gene transduction. New Engl J Med. 1990;323:570–578.

Rosenberg SA, Grimm EA, McGrogan M, et al. Biological activity of recombinant human interleukin-2 produced in *Escherichia coli*. Science. 1984;223:1412–1415.

Rosenberg SA, Lotze MT, Muul LM, et al. Observations on the systemic administration of autologous lymphokine-activated killer cells and recombinant interleukin-2 to patients with metastatic cancer. New Engl J Med. 1985a;313:1485–1492.

Rosenberg SA, Mulé JJ, Spiess PJ, Reichert CM, Schwarz SL. Regression of established pulmonary metastases and subcutaneous tumor mediated by the systemic administration of high-dose recombinant interleukin-2. J Exp Med. 1985b;161:1169–1188.

Rosenberg SA, Spiess P, Lafreniere R. A new approach to the adoptive immunotherapy of cancer with tumor-infiltrating lymphocytes. Science. 1986;233:1318–1321.

Rosenberg SA, Packard BS, Aebersold PM, et al. Use of tumor-infiltrating lymphocytes and interleukin-2 in the immunotherapy of patients with metastatic melanoma. New Engl J Med. 1988a;319:1676–1680.

Rosenberg SA, Schwarz SL, Spiess PJ. Combination immunotherapy for cancer: synergistic antitumor interactions of interleukin-2, alfa interferon and tumor-infiltrating lymphocytes. J Natl Cancer Inst. 1988b;80:1393–1397.

Rosenberg SA, Lotze MT, Yang JC, et al. Experience with the use of high-dose interleukin-2 in the treatment of 652 cancer patients. Ann Surg. 1989;210:474–485.

Rouse BT, Wagner H, Harris AW. In vivo activity of in vitro immunized lymphocytes. J Immunol. 1972;108:1353–1361.

Rubin JT, Elwood LJ, Rosenberg SA, Lotze MT. Immunohistochemical correlates of response to recombinant interleukin-2 based immunotherapy in humans. Cancer Res. 1989;49:7086–7092.

Ruscetti FW, Morgan DA, Gallo RC. Functional and morphologic characterization of human T cells continuously grown in vitro. J Immunol. 1977;119:131–138.

Saris SC, Rosenberg SA, Friedman RB, Rubin JT, Barba D, Oldfield EH. Penetration of recombinant interleukin-2 across the blood-cerebrospinal fluid barrier. J Neurosurg. 1988; 69:29–34.

Saris CS, Patronas NJ, Rosenberg SA, et al. The effect of intravenous interleukin-2 on brain water content. J Neurosurg. 1989;71:169–174.

Schwartzentruber DJ, Lotze MT, Rosenberg SA. Colonic perforation. An unusual complication of therapy with high-dose interleukin-2. Cancer. 1988;62:2350–2353.

Schwartzentruber DJ, Zweig MH, Weintraub BD, White DE, Rosenberg SA. Thyroid dysfunction induced by immunotherapy in cancer patients. Proc ASCO. 1990;9:184.

Sedlmayr P, Rabiniwich H, Elder EM, et al. Depressed ability of patients with melanoma or renal cell carcinoma to generate adherent lymphokine-activated killer cells. J Immunother. 1991;10:336–346.

Shimokawara I, Imamura M, Yamanaka N, Ishii Y, Kikuchi K. Identification of lymphocyte subpopulations in human breast cancer tissue and its significance: an immunoperoxidase study with anti-human T- and B-cell sera. Cancer. 1982;49:1456–1464.

Shu S, Chou T, Sakai K. Lymphocytes generated by in vivo priming and in vitro sensitization demonstrate therapeutic efficacy against a murine tumor that lacks apparent immunogenicity. J Immunol. 1989;143:740–748.

Southern PJ, Berg P. Transformation of mammalian cells to antibiotic resistance with a bacterial gene under control of the SV40 early region promoter. J Mol Appl Genet. 1982;1:327–341.

Stahel RA, Sculier JP, Jost LM, et al. Tolerance and effectiveness of recombinant interleukin-2 (r-met Hu IL-2 [ala-125]) and lymphokine-activated killer cells in patients with metastatic solid tumors. Eur J Cancer Clin Oncol. 1989;25:965–972.

Steis R, Urba W, VanderMolen LA, et al. Intraperitoneal lymphokine-activated killer cell and interleukin-2 therapy for malignancies limited to the peritoneal cavity. J Clin Oncol. 1990;8:1618–1629.

Strausser JL, Rosenberg SA. In vitro growth of cytotoxic human lymphocytes. J Immunol. 1978;121:1491–1495.

Svedmyr E. Long-term maintenance in vitro of human T cells by repeated exposure to the same stimulator cells. Scand J Immunol. 1975;4:421–427.

Taniguchi T, Matsui H, Fujita T, et al. Structure and expression of a cloned cDNA for human interleukin-2. Nature. 1983;302:305–310.

Tees R, Schreier MH. Selective reconstitution of nude mice with long-term cultured and cloned specific helper T cells. Nature. 1980;283:780–781.

Topalian SL, Solomon D, Avis FP, et al. Immunotherapy of patients with advanced cancer using tumor-infiltrating lymphocytes and recombinant interleukin-2: a pilot study. J Clin Oncol. 1988;6:839–853.

Topalian SL, Solomon D, Rosenberg SA. Tumor-specific cytolysis by lymphocytes infiltrating human melanomas. J Immunol. 1989;142:3714–3725.

Treves AJ, Cohen IR, Feldman M. Immunotherapy of lethal metastases by lymphocytes sensitized against tumor cells in vitro. J Natl Cancer Inst. 1975;54:777–780.

Wagman GH, Testa RT, Marquez JA, Weinstein MJ. Antibiotic G-418, a new *Micromonospora*-produced aminoglycoside with activity against protozoa and helminths: fermentation, isolation, preliminary characterization. Antimicrob Agents Chemother. 1974;6:144–149.

Wang J, Suthanthiran M, Walle A, et al. Antitumor properties of lymphocytes activated by the oxidizing mitogens. J Immunol. 1986;136:4735–4739.

Wang JCL, Walle A, Novogrodsky A, et al. A phase II clinical trial of adoptive immunotherapy for advanced renal cell carcinoma using mitogen-activated autologous leukocytes and continuous infusion interleukin-2. J Clin Oncol. 1989;7:1885–1891.

Weber JS, Gilbert J, Tanaka K, Rosenberg SA. Immunotherapy of a murine tumor with interleukin-2. J Exp Med. 1987;166:1716–1733.

West WH, Tauer KW, Yannelli JR, et al. Constant-infusion recombinant interleukin-2 in adoptive immunotherapy of advanced cancer. New Engl J Med. 1987;316:898–905.

West WH. Continuous infusion recombinant interleukin-2 (rIL-2) in adoptive cellular therapy of renal carcinoma and other malignancies. Cancer Treat Rev. 1989;16(suppl A):83–89.

Woglom WH. Regression of the Jensen rat sarcoma. Cancer Res. 1925;9:171–189.

Yang SC, Owen-Schaub L, Grimm EA, Roth JA. Induction of lymphokine-activated killer cytotoxicity with interleukin-2 and tumor necrosis factor-α against primary lung cancer targets. Cancer Immunol Immunother. 1989;29:193–198.

Yang JC, Perry-Lalley D, Rosenberg SA. An improved method for growing murine tumor-infiltrating lymphocytes with in vivo antitumor activity. J Biol Resp Mod. 1990;9:149–159.

Yoshida S, Tanaka R, Takai N, Ono K. Local administration of autologous lymphokine-activated killer cells and recombinant interleukin 2 to patients with malignant brain tumors. Cancer Res. 1988;48:5011–5016.

Yron I, Wood TA, Spiess PJ, Rosenberg SA. In vitro growth of murine T cells. V. The isolation and growth of lymphoid cells infiltrating syngeneic solid tumors. J Immunol. 1980;125:238–245.

CHAPTER **17**

THE CLINICAL BIOLOGY AND MECHANISMS OF ACTION OF SYSTEMICALLY ADMINISTERED IL-2

Stephan D. Voss
Paul M. Sondel

Despite considerable progress in clinical oncology, successful curative treatment for most patients with established malignancies remains a goal yet to be fully realized. Recent efforts have investigated the use of "biological response modifiers" in the treatment of cancers refractory to conventional therapeutic regimens. Biological response modifiers, by definition, primarily exert their effects indirectly, mediating tumor regression by augmenting the host's ability to mount both specific and nonspecific immune responses against invading neoplasms. In addition to their indirect effects, some biological response modifiers such as the interferons and tumor necrosis factor (TNF) also have direct antitumor effects. Recombinant DNA techniques have made it possible to obtain large quantities of a number of biological response modifiers in purified form, thus enabling clinical trials to be initiated evaluating the potential therapeutic efficacy of pharmacological doses of these agents in treating cancer. These clinical trials have documented that antitumor effects can be obtained and are revealing much about the complex interplay that exists between many of these immunomodulatory factors.

CELLULAR IMMUNE REACTIONS TO TUMORS

The recent use of purified recombinant lymphokines and cytokines in cancer therapy is based in part on the demonstration in the mid-1950s that specific immunity to methylcholanthrene (MCA)-induced sarcomas could be induced in syngeneic animals as well as in the original tumor-bearing animal (Prehn and Main, 1957; Klein et al.,

1960). The initial enthusiasm that followed these observations was tempered somewhat by subsequent work demonstrating that, although strong antitumor immune responses could be shown for experimental chemically and virally induced tumors, it was difficult to convincingly and reproducibly demonstrate similar specific immunity to "spontaneously" arising murine tumors (Herberman, 1974; Hewitt, 1978). The failure to demonstrate antitumor immunity to spontaneously arising tumors is believed to be due to the absence of immunogenic components on the surface of tumor cells, either tumor-specific antigens (TSA) or major histocompatibility complex (MHC) molecules that present the TSA, that could stimulate an immune response. Alternatively, the tumor-bearing host may be immunologically unable to recognize these TSA. These spontaneously arising nonimmunogenic tumors observed in experimental animals may be analogous to the majority of tumors arising in humans; thus data obtained in preclinical animal studies involving experimentally induced tumors do not always extrapolate accurately to the clinical setting.

The effector mechanisms involved in antitumor immunity are only beginning to be understood. Both cellular and humoral immune responses have been readily demonstrated for chemically and virally induced immunogenic tumors (Delorme and Alexander, 1964; Gorczynski, 1974; Berenson et al., 1975; Brown et al., 1978). However, demonstrating a specific effector mechanism operative against nonimmunogenic tumors has proven more elusive. Nonspecific effectors include natural killer (NK) cells (Hanna, 1982; Whiteside and Herberman, 1989) and macrophages (Adams and Nathan, 1983; Fidler, 1985), as well as certain cytolytic T cells that mediate non-MHC–restricted recognition of selected tumor cell lines (Thiele and Lipsky, 1989; Hersey and Bolhuis, 1987). Perhaps the best evidence that these nonspecific immune effector mechanisms play a role in immune surveillance protecting against spontaneously arising malignant neoplasms comes from the observation that in certain immune deficient states, such as that seen in patients with Chédiak-Higashi syndrome (characterized by a deficiency of functional NK cells), the incidence of malignant disease is dramatically increased (Dent et al., 1966; Haliotis et al., 1980; Roder et al., 1980). In experimental model systems, beige mice (which display an NK deficiency similar functionally to that seen in Chédiak-Higashi patients) also show increased susceptibility to development of malignant disease (Karre et al., 1980; Talmadge et al., 1980; Haliotis et al., 1985), while athymic nude mice (which have normal NK- but no T-cell function), when housed under aseptic conditions, show little increase in incidence of tumor development (Outzen et al., 1975; Rygaard and Povlsen, 1976; Holland et al., 1978; Stutman, 1979). Thus, it may be that in immunologically normal individuals, spontaneously arising neoplasms are eliminated routinely by a combination of nonspecific and, less frequently, specific immune effector mechanisms. By treating patients with pharmacological doses of agents normally involved in regulating this "routine" antitumor immune surveillance, it is hoped that the apparently quiescent immune effector mechanisms that allowed the development of the malignant disease can be more efficiently "restimulated" to enable mediation of tumor regression.

INTERLEUKIN-2 AND ITS RECEPTORS

Interleukin-2 (IL-2) is a 15-kDa glycoprotein produced by activated helper T cells that has shown great potential in both in vitro and in vivo systems in activating antitumor immune activity (Sondel, 1989; Parkinson, 1988; Lotze and Rosenberg, 1988). Interleukin-2 was originally purified from the heterogeneous mixture of immunomodulatory substances collectively termed T-cell growth factor (TCGF) and was found to be capable of activating and maintaining proliferative and cytolytic responses mediated by both T cells and NK cells. The complementary DNA (cDNA) for IL-2 was cloned, and large quantities of pure IL-2, overproduced in recombinant bacterial strains, soon became available, enabling in depth studies of structure–function relationships of IL-2 and its cell-surface receptors, as well as of the role IL-2 plays in a variety of immune responses (Waldman, 1989; Smith, 1988, 1989). Interleukin-2 as an antitumor agent is a true biological response modifier in that all of its physiological effects appear to be the indirect result of having activated lymphocytes to differentiate, proliferate, and synthesize, and release other immunomodulatory substances.

Interleukin-2 responsive cells are activated by soluble IL-2 following its interaction with specific IL-2 receptors present on the surface of lymphocytes and certain other immune cells. The IL-2 receptor is made up of at least two chains, α (p55, Tac) and β (p70), that noncovalently associate on the cell surface to produce a high-affinity receptor complex capable of binding IL-2 with an equilibrium dissociation constant (K_d) of approximately 10 to 20 pM. Each of the chains comprising the IL-2 receptor complex can bind IL-2 independently of the other, with either low (α, K_d = 5–20 nM) or intermediate (β, K_d = 0.2–1.0 nM) affinity (Waldman, 1989; Smith, 1988, 1989). Other IL-2–binding peptides have been reported by various laboratories (Hermann and Diamantstein, 1987; Saragovi and Malek, 1988; Takeshita et al., 1990), but to date no additional IL-2 receptor subunits have received universal recognition. Both the intermediate-affinity p70 β chain and the high-affinity αβ complex can internalize IL-2 and mediate biological effects (Robb and Greene, 1987; Fung et al., 1988). The p55 α chain, due to its short cytoplasmic domain (13 amino acids), is unable to internalize IL-2 (Weissman et al., 1986; Robb and Greene, 1987), and no biological effect has been attributed to this low-affinity ligand/receptor interaction.

Resting lymphocytes express only very few high-affinity IL-2 receptors and show little to no response to low concentrations (<50–100 pM) of IL-2 in vitro. High-affinity IL-2 receptors appear on T cells following antigen activation (Cantrell and Smith, 1983) and on both T cells and NK cells following in vitro activation with high concentrations of IL-2 (Siegel et al., 1987; Le Thi Bich-Thuy et al., 1987; Tsudo et al., 1987; Kehrl et al., 1988). High-affinity IL-2 receptors have also been detected on a small fraction of the resting NK-cell population (Nagler et al., 1990; Caligiuri et al., 1990). Both resting T cells and NK cells constitutively express low levels of the p70 β chain, with p70 expression being somewhat greater on NK cells than on T cells (Ohashi et al., 1989; Yagita et al., 1989; Phillips et al., 1989). Since the intermediate affinity p70 β chain alone can bind and internalize IL-2 provided the available concentration of IL-2 is high enough, both resting T cells and NK cells can be directly activated by high doses of IL-2. In in vitro studies, direct activation of resting T cells and NK cells with high concentrations of IL-2 leads to increased synthesis of the p55 α chain, followed by association of the α and β chains at the cell surface to form high-affinity receptors. This observation is relevant to the administration of high doses of IL-2 clinically, in that sufficiently high steady-state levels of IL-2 may need to be maintained to insure the activation of cytolytic effector cells.

THE LYMPHOKINE-ACTIVATED KILLER CELL PHENOMENON

In the early 1980s, Rosenberg and colleagues described a cytolytic effector phenomenon that was induced by culturing splenocytes or peripheral blood lymphocytes in high concentrations of IL-2 (Lotze et al., 1981; Grimm et al., 1982, 1983; Rosenstein et al., 1984). The hallmark of this lymphokine activated killer (LAK)-cell phenomenon was the lysis of a wide range of NK-cell–resistant tumor cells. Fresh normal cells were relatively unharmed by this LAK-cell phenomenon, although some destruction of normal tissue could be detected in vitro (Sondel et al., 1986). This cytotoxic reaction induced by IL-2 was found to be mediated by a heterogeneous mixture of cells, including cells bearing phenotypic surface markers characteristic of both NK cells and T cells, with a predominant role for cells bearing the CD56 NK-cell marker (Phillips and Lanier, 1986; Ortaldo et al., 1986; Yang et al., 1986). The common feature shared by these IL-2–activated effector cells has been the ability to lyse a broad range of NK-cell–resistant tumor targets in a non-MHC–restricted manner, making lymphokine-activated killing a functional definition rather than a restrictive definition of a single class of immune effector cells (Reynolds and Ortaldo, 1987).

In Vivo Activity of IL-2 in Tumor-Bearing Mice

The observation that splenocytes or peripheral blood lymphocytes cultured for 3 to 5 days in 100 to 1000 U/mL of IL-2 could develop significant LAK-cell activity led to preclinical testing of IL-2 in mice carrying established experimentally induced non-immunogenic tumors. Little in vivo effect was achieved in these initial studies administering low doses of IL-2 (Chang et al., 1984; Mulé et al., 1985). Pharmacological studies showed this was due to the rapid compartmental equilibration and subsequent clearance of IL-2 (Donohue and Rosenberg, 1983; Donohue et al., 1984). In subsequent studies using higher doses of IL-2 administered by continuous infusion, or repeated IP or depot injections, to maintain higher steady-state IL-2 levels, significant antitumor responses were documented (Rosenberg et al., 1985a; Lafreniere and Rosenberg, 1985; Thompson et al., 1986). These effects were found to be most dependent on the dose and schedule of IL-2 administered (Cheever et al., 1985; Mulé et al., 1985; Ettinghausen and Rosenberg, 1986); and on the extent (size and spread) of the tumor burden (Thompson et al., 1986; Mulé et al., 1987). These observations served as a critical framework for the design of clinical trials.

In most patients with clinically evident tumor, estimated tumor-cell burdens in excess of 10^9 are not uncommon. Treatment of mice with large tumor burdens with high doses of IL-2 has been found to be not nearly as effective as when treatment is administered before the development of measurable disease (Thompson et al., 1986; Mulé et al., 1987). One attempt to provide a greater complement of activated immune effector cells has been to generate LAK cells ex vivo and then to administer them in vivo along with the maximum tolerated dose of IL-2. In mice, treatment with IL-2 + LAK cells had a greater effect than IL-2 alone, in certain rapidly growing tumor models (Mulé et al., 1984; Lafreniere and Rosenberg, 1985; Rosenberg and Lotze, 1986).

These and many similar studies have led to extensive clinical trials of IL-2 alone, IL-2 + LAK cells, IL-2 + tumor infiltrating lymphocytes (TIL), as well as IL-2 + various other antitumor modalities, including other biological response modifiers, chemotherapeutic agents, radiation therapy, and surgery. This review summarizes the results of phase I and II clinical trials underway from our institution and others, and provides an overview of molecular studies aimed at clarifying the in vivo mechanisms through which IL-2 is exerting its immunoregulatory effects.

CLINICAL TRIALS USING IL-2 ALONE

Clinical Effects

Phase I and II clinical trials utilizing IL-2 as the sole therapeutic agent are underway at numerous institutions. Initial reports using recombinant human IL-2 documented increases in the number of circulating lymphocytes following IL-2 therapy, as well as augmented in vitro proliferative responses to IL-2 by these posttherapy lymphocytes (Atkins et al., 1986; Rosenthal et al., 1988; Hank et al., 1988; Sondel et al., 1988; Lotze and Rosenberg, 1988; Sondel, 1989). Pharmacological and toxicity data collected in these pilot studies confirmed the results obtained in preclinical murine models, with rapid distribution and clearance of IL-2 from the circulation (T 1/2 Distribution = 7–13 min, T 1/2 Elimination = 45–240 min [Lotze et al., 1985; Thompson et al., 1987; Kohler et al., 1989; Konrad et al., 1990]), side effects including chills, fever, capillary leakage, pulmonary edema, and weight gain, as well as hepatic and renal dysfunction, all of which rapidly subsided following cessation of IL-2 therapy (Lotze and Rosenberg, 1988; Sondel, 1989).

Subsequent studies have explored various doses and schedules of IL-2 administration in efforts to establish IL-2 treatment regimens that induce significant immunological activation without necessitating severe toxicity (Thompson et al., 1988; Sosman et al., 1988a, 1988b, 1991; Kohler et al., 1989; Goldstein et al., 1989; Caligiuri et al., 1991). The extent to which this is possible remains uncertain, as the toxicity from IL-2 may relate directly to the very immunological activation that is induced by the therapy (Rosenstein et al., 1986; Ettinghausen et al., 1988). A summary of the clinical response data from a number of recently published clinical trials is presented in Table 17-1.

TABLE 17-1
SUMMARY OF PATIENT RESPONSE DATA FROM CLINICAL TRIALS USING IL-2 ALONE

Reference	IL-2 dose	Tumor	No. patients (Total/eval.)	Responses CR	Responses PR
Rosenberg et al., 1989	10^4–10^5 U/kg or 10^6–6×10^6 U/m²/d	Renal/melanoma and others	155/130	4	18
Sondel et al., 1988	1–3×10^6 U/m²/d	Renal/melanoma	11/11	0	1
Sosman et al., 1988a,b	1–3×10^6 U/m²/d	Renal/melanoma	28/28	0	3
Mitchell et al., 1988, 1989	3.6×10^6 U/m²/d	Melanoma	42/39	2	8
Thompson et al., 1988	0.3–3×10^6 U/m²/d	Renal/melanoma and others	23/17	0	0
Javadpour and Lalehzarian, 1988	3×10^6 U/m²/d	Renal	10/9	1	2
Allison et al., 1989	1.5–3×10^6 U/m²/d	Various	35/26	0	3
Ghosh et al., 1989	11×10^6 U/m²/d	Melanoma	31/20	0	4
Marumo et al., 1989	10^6 U/d	Renal	13/11	2	1
Creekmore et al., 1989	10^3–3×10^7 U/m²/d	Melanoma/colon	33/33	0	2
Paciucci et al., 1989	1–5×10^6 U/m²/d	Various	32/32	0	13
Bukowski et al., 1990	10×10^6 U/m²/d	Renal	44/41	1	4
Sosman et al., 1991	1–3×10^6 U/m²/d	Melanoma/renal	25/22	0	1

CR, complete response; PR, partial response.

It is evident from the results of these studies that administration of IL-2 is capable of inducing purely immune-mediated antitumor responses in a minority of patients, yet induces some degree of toxicity in virtually all patients. Further investigations and improvements in the clinical use of IL-2 are needed before it could be considered an effective form of therapy that should be made available for widespread clinical use. However, because clinical responses are observed in only a small fraction of treated patients, it is important in evaluating these early clinical trials to select suitable intermediate endpoints. Such data, while not necessarily serving as a clinical indicator of antitumor activity, may be important in allowing investigators insight into the mechanisms of immunological activation operating in vivo. Furthermore, without monitoring appropriately selected intermediate endpoints, there is little hope of applying knowledge gained from early studies toward improved therapeutic efficacy in subsequent clinical trials.

Data obtained from a number of laboratories have pointed to a reproducible series of events that occur following systemic administration of IL-2. Maximum tolerated doses (not requiring intensive care unit [ICU] monitoring) have been established in several centers at approximately 3.0×10^6 U/m^2/day for 4 to 7 days when administered as a continuous infusion, with continuous infusion being more effective than bolus administration at maintaining constant steady-state levels of IL-2 in the plasma (Lotze et al., 1985). Within hours after starting IL-2 infusion, there is a rapid disappearance of lymphocytes from the peripheral circulation. This transient lymphopenia persists as long as IL-2 is being infused and is followed by a rapid rebound lymphocytosis after stopping IL-2 infusion. We and others have developed a regimen of IL-2 administration that involves 4 days of continuous IL-2 infusion followed by 3 days rest for 4 consecutive weeks. Using this regimen, we have noted continued increases in rebound lymphocyte counts, suggesting a progressive in vivo activation and expansion of lymphocytes throughout the course of IL-2 therapy (Sosman et al., 1988b, 1991; Sondel et al., 1988; Sondel, 1989).

Immunological Effects of IL-2 Therapy

In vitro studies examining the phenotype and functional immunological activity of the lymphocytes obtained during the rebound lymphocytosis have demonstrated that, during the course of IL-2 administration, there is an increase in both the percentage and absolute number of CD56$^+$ NK cells (Phillips et al., 1987; Sosman et al., 1988b, 1991; Goldstein et al., 1989; Weil-Hillman et al., 1989). This is associated with a corresponding decrease in the percentage of circulating CD3$^+$ T lymphocytes, although the degree of lymphocytosis often results in increases in absolute numbers of circulating T lymphocytes when compared to pretherapy levels, despite the decrease in percentage of CD3$^+$ cells. Functionally, brisk proliferative responses to IL-2 in vitro are observed with posttherapy peripheral blood lymphocytes (PBL), while the in vitro response of pretherapy PBL to IL-2 is sluggish by comparison (Hank et al., 1988, 1990a). Augmented LAK-cell activity in vitro is also observed with freshly obtained

PBL following IL-2 therapy (Hank et al., 1988, 1990b; Sondel et al., 1988; Goldstein et al., 1989). This augmented activity cannot be explained simply on the basis of increased numbers of $CD56^+$ NK cells; rather it seems that these cells have been activated in vivo by IL-2 and display a heightened responsiveness to subsequent exposure to IL-2, when tested in either proliferative or cytolytic assays. These responses will be explored more fully later, as our laboratory's efforts to obtain a better understanding of the molecular mechanisms of in vivo IL-2 activation are reviewed.

In addition to monitoring the effect of IL-2 on cellular immune responses, we and others have begun investigating whether soluble serum factors might yield insight into events occurring during the course of IL-2 administration. Increased serum levels of a soluble form of the p55 α subunit of the IL-2 receptor (sTac) have been observed during the course of IL-2 administration, increasing rapidly throughout a given 4-day cycle of IL-2 infusion, and then falling off 24 to 48 hours after IL-2 is stopped (Voss et al., 1989). In vitro evidence suggests that sTac is released from activated lymphocytes (Rubin et al., 1985). Thus, monitoring sTac levels in patients receiving IL-2 is a potential way of assessing total lymphoid mass activation during those periods of IL-2 administration in vivo when significant numbers of lymphocytes are absent from the peripheral circulation. Furthermore, in a multicenter study investigating the sTac levels in the sera of patients receiving varying doses of IL-2, a statistically significant relationship was observed between the dose of IL-2 administered and the level of sTac released into the serum. In this study it was also shown that the level of sTac following a fixed dose of IL-2 correlates with capillary leak toxicity (measured as weight gain and hypotension) (Bogner et al., 1992). These results indicate that sTac monitoring may be important in quality control studies and clinical decision making in multicenter trials. It is unclear whether the high sTac levels in patient plasma have any immunoregulatory role (e.g., decreasing the level of available free IL-2 in the plasma), although experiments in which sTac was removed from posttherapy patient plasma by immunoaffinity chromatography suggested that sTac did not play a role in inhibiting lymphocyte responses to IL-2 (Gambacorti-Passerini et al., 1990).

To date, no single piece of data has turned out to be of predictive value in determining which patients will respond to IL-2 clinically (Hawkins, 1989). In one study (Mitchell et al., 1988, 1989), only patients with elevated LAK-like activity (against an NK-cell–resistant melanoma target) following IL-2 therapy achieved clinical antitumor responses. However, only a fraction of the total number of patients with augmented activity responded (9 of 24 patients) (Mitchell et al., 1989). In addition, others have noted a lack of correlation between peripheral blood LAK-cell activity and clinical responses (Ghosh et al., 1989). In our own studies, virtually every patient treated with $\geq 10^6$ U IL-2/m^2/day shows an increase in their peripheral blood LAK-cell activity (Rosenthal et al., 1988; Hank et al., 1988; Sondel et al., 1988; Sosman et al., 1988b, 1991; Goldstein et al., 1989). As such, we feel that LAK-cell activation may be necessary, but not sufficient, to obtain antitumor responses using IL-2. Other variables must be involved. Thus, at a time when IL-2 is being entered into protocols employing combinations of immunomodulatory agents, it will be important to refer back to the "intermediate endpoint" data collected during administration of IL-2 alone when evaluating patient responses to IL-2 administered in combination with other agents.

CLINICAL TRIALS USING IL-2 + ADOPTIVELY TRANSFERRED LYMPHOCYTES

IL-2 + LAK Cells

Initial preclinical studies utilizing IL-2 established that antitumor responses were dependent primarily on three factors: the extent of tumor burden, the dose of IL-2 administered, and the degree of lymphocyte activation attained (Rosenberg et al., 1985a; Lafreniere and Rosenberg, 1985; Thompson et al., 1986; Mulé et al., 1986; Rosenberg and Lotze, 1986). Subsequent murine studies demonstrated that the adoptive transfer of ex vivo IL-2–activated syngeneic splenocytes, together with concomitantly administered IL-2, produced greater antitumor responses than administration of IL-2 alone in some tumor models (Mulé et al., 1984; Lafreniere and Rosenberg, 1985; Rosenberg and Lotze, 1986). These effects were absolutely dependent on the coadministration of IL-2 to "maintain" the activated state of the adoptively transferred cells.

Clinical trials in humans utilizing a similar regimen of IL-2 + LAK cells (generated from the patients' own lymphocytes by laboratory culture in IL-2) resulted in a number of clinical responses (Rosenberg et al., 1985b, 1987; West et al., 1987), leading to considerable initial enthusiasm. Based on these encouraging results, similar trials were initiated at a number of institutions. Table 17-2 summarizes the results of some of these studies.

Clearly the IL-2 + LAK-cell regimen was producing clinical responses, particularly for patients with renal cell carcinoma or metastatic melanoma. However, at the same time, regimens utilizing IL-2 alone were evolving such that carefully selected dose and administration schedules were resulting in clinical responses to IL-2 (Sosman et al., 1988a, 1988b) (see also Table 17-1). Careful monitoring during the IL-2 + LAK-cell therapy of intermediate endpoints similar to those discussed previously has revealed little that is not attributable to the concomitantly administered IL-2. Thus, while not refuting the clinical significance of the responses observed with IL-2 + LAK-cell regimens, we have noted that such regimens involve considerable laboratory manipulation (making them less attractive for wide-scale use). In addition, the LAK-cell infusions themselves can make this regimen more toxic to the patients than administration of IL-2 alone (Albertini et al., 1990). Even if controlled studies show a slight advantage in tumor responses for administration of IL-2 together with ex vivo activated LAK cells versus administration of IL-2 alone, response rates for both approaches still remain too low and improvements are needed. Further modifications of IL-2 regimens, combined with other approaches, are needed and are underway (Rosenberg et al., 1988; Sosman et al., 1990).

TABLE 17-2
SUMMARY OF PATIENT RESPONSE DATA FROM CLINICAL TRIALS USING IL-2 COMBINED WITH ADOPTIVELY TRANSFERRED IMMUNE CELLS (LAK CELLS)

Reference	IL-2 dose co-administered	Tumor	No. patients (Total/eval.)	Responses CR	Responses PR
Rosenberg et al., 1989	10^4–10^5 U/kg	Renal/melanoma and others	214/177	14	30
Albertini et al., 1990	1–3 × 10/^{6} U/m^2/d	Renal/melanoma	20/18	0	2
Bar et al., 1990	3 × 10^6 U/m^2/d	Melanoma	50/50	1	7
Margolin et al., 1989 Dutcher et al., 1989 Fisher et al., 1988	10^7 U/m^2/d	Renal/melanoma and Colorectal	93/89	4	12
Paciucci et al., 1989	1–5 × 10^6 U/m^2/d	Renal/melanoma	25/25	0	6
Philip et al., 1989	3 × 10^6 U/m^2/d	Renal	20/17	0	3
Schoof et al., 1988 Eberlein et al., 1988	3 × 10^4 U/kg	Renal/melanoma and others	28/28	4	9
Stahel et al., 1989	3 × 10^4 U/kg	Renal/melanoma	26/26	0	4
Thompson et al., 1989	3 × 10^6 U/m^2/d	Renal/melanoma and others	24/23	1	1
West, 1989	3 × 10^6 U/m^2/d	Renal/melanoma	114/102	2	19

CR, complete response; PR, partial response.

IL-2 + TIL

It had been known for some time that single-cell suspensions prepared from resected tumor tissue consisted of both tumor cells and host immune elements, including both B and T lymphocytes and monocytes (for reviews, see Whiteside, 1989; Parmiani et al., 1990). Such populations of TIL were thought to potentially contain tumor-reactive or tumor-specific lymphocytes that had infiltrated the tumor and for unknown reasons failed to mediate effective destruction of the tumor. While trials with IL-2 were progressing, several laboratories were pursuing the hypothesis that activation of these TIL might expand a subpopulation of tumor-specific lymphocytes present within the total TIL population and thus provide a cellular reagent that would be a more potent mediator of tumor destruction. If such TIL could be expanded in the laboratory and then, together with IL-2, be reinfused back into tumor-bearing individuals, antitumor responses might be achieved that were greater than those seen in regimens utilizing IL-2 alone or IL-2 + LAK cells. In vitro, tumor specificity has been seen in some cultured TIL preparations from melanoma patients (Itoh et al., 1986; Muul et al., 1987), but similar culture techniques have not induced analogous T-cell reactivity for most other human tumor types that have been studied (Heo et al., 1987; Belldegrun et al., 1988; Haas et al., 1990; Balch et al., 1990). In vivo, the issue of TIL specificity has been addressed in trafficking studies using either radioisotope-labeled or genetically "labeled" TIL to enable potential recovery of the infused cells. These studies indicate that, for at least some melanoma patients, the adoptively transferred TIL are preferentially infiltrating tumor tissues in vivo (Fisher et al., 1989; Rosenberg et al., 1990).

In murine tumor models, it was shown that adoptively transferred TIL administered concomitantly with IL-2 were 50 to 100 times more potent than LAK cells in mediating regression of established weakly immunogenic pulmonary and hepatic metastases (Rosenberg et al., 1986). Clinical trials have been initiated utilizing this regimen of TIL + IL-2 (Kradin et al., 1987; Topalian et al., 1988). Although antitumor responses have been observed in selected patients (Kradin et al., 1989; Rosenberg et al., 1989), it is not yet apparent that the administration of TIL + IL-2 in humans, as currently being tested, is producing clinical effects that differ from those observed in the initial clinical IL-2 + LAK cell trials (Sondel et al., 1989).

The current inability of TIL to provide significant clinical benefit for the majority of patients who have tumor harvested for TIL culture (even if analyzed only for melanoma) over that seen with IL-2 alone or IL-2 + LAK cells raises important issues regarding how to proceed with the design of future clinical trials (Sondel et al., 1989). At present, relatively few laboratories have been able to successfully and reproducibly generate large enough numbers of TIL to warrant adoptive transfer back into the patient. Furthermore, with the exception of metastatic melanoma, few recurrent or metastatic human tumors are readily accessible for routine surgical excision, and in many instances, the TIL generated are not "tumor-specific," but rather show in vitro cytolytic activity against a broad range of tumor targets and tumor cell lines, making them functionally more like LAK effectors than tumor-specific T cells. More convincing evidence documenting improved in vivo efficacy of TIL regimens will be required before designing clinical trials that include invasive surgical procedures solely for the purpose of obtaining tumor.

COMBINATION THERAPIES WITH IL-2 AND OTHER IMMUNOMODULATORY AGENTS

IL-2 + Cyclophosphamide

Clinical trials combining low-dose cyclophosphamide (Cytoxan) with IL-2 were based on murine models demonstrating synergistic antitumor effects, as well as decreased toxicity, when both agents were coadministered (Papa et al., 1988). The synergism with IL-2 in inducing antitumor activity is most likely due to direct effects of Cytoxan on the tumor rather than elimination of putative suppressor elements (Papa et al., 1988; Cameron et al., 1990), while the decreased toxicity most likely results from the inhibition of immune-mediated damage to normal tissues, particularly endothelial tissue (Rosenstein et al., 1986; Ettinghausen et al., 1988).

In clinical trials, treating melanoma patients with a combination of IL-2 + low-dose Cytoxan, significant antitumor responses have been reported, including two complete remissions (Mitchell et al., 1988, 1989). However, from these modest response rates and the small number of patients evaluated (8 partial responses [PR] and 2 complete responses [CR] among the 39 patients evaluated by Mitchell et al. and 2 PR among the 15 patients evaluated by the National Cancer Institute [NCI] team [Mulé and Rosenberg, 1989]), it is not certain whether the addition of Cytoxan produced response rates that were higher than those to be expected from administration of IL-2 alone.

IL-2 + Other Cytokines

Extensive in vitro and in vivo animal studies have documented that synergistic antitumor effects can be obtained following combination therapy with regimens utilizing IL-2 + interferons (IFN), IL-2 + tumor necrosis factor (TNF) or a combination of all three agents (reviewed by Mulé and Rosenberg, 1989).

The interferons were the first class of recombinant immunomodulatory agents to be purified and entered into clinical cancer testing. Based on considerable clinical and laboratory evidence, it is now clear that interferons can be administered safely and effectively and that significant antitumor responses can be observed in certain groups of patients, most notably in the therapy of patients with hairy-cell leukemia (reviewed in Foon, 1989; Borden and Sondel, 1990). Investigations into the pleiotropic effects of interferons led to studies that suggested the combination of IL-2 and IFN might have synergistic antitumor effects relative to therapy with either agent alone (Mulé and Rosenberg, 1989). Recent clinical trials testing this hypothesis have been encouraging, with reports from some study centers of response rates (including CR and PR) of up to 41% (Lee et al., 1989; Rosenberg et al., 1989; Krigel et al., 1990). Little information, other than that available from preclinical studies, is presently available regarding the potential in vivo mechanisms leading to the augmented in vivo effects that might be obtained. Combination therapy with IL-2 and TNF-α has been less encouraging. Initial in vitro and in vivo animal data suggested that TNF augmented the IL-2–induced generation of cells mediating LAK-cell activity and produced synergistic antitumor effects in mice (Mulé and Rosenberg, 1989). However, in a recent report, the NCI team suggested that TNF may be producing little, if any, antitumor effect beyond that which might be attributable to the actions of IL-2 (Rosenberg et al., 1989).

IL-2 + Monoclonal Antibodies

Another approach to combination therapy with IL-2 has been based on two observations. First, we and others had documented expansion, by administration of IL-2 in vivo, of NK cells throughout the course of therapy, many of which bore the Fc receptor for IgG (Fc receptor, CD16), and should be capable of mediating antibody-dependent cellular cytotoxicity (ADCC) (Phillips et al., 1987; Sondel et al., 1988; Weil-Hillman et al., 1989). Second, several monoclonal antibodies (mAb) characterized by "selective" reactivity with specific types of tumors have recently been characterized (reviewed in: Foon, 1989). It has therefore been postulated that the addition of tumor type–specific monoclonal antibodies to present IL-2 regimens might confer a degree of specificity to the nonspecific effector arm of the immune system (i.e., NK cells) and might offer a means of enhancing the specific targeting of Fc receptor-bearing NK cells to sites of tumor growth, while producing few side effects due to nonspecific immune-mediated damage to normal tissues.

Our laboratory has recently shown that patients receiving in vivo IL-2 have augmented ADCC function relative to fresh PBL (Hank et al., 1990c), confirming results obtained in preclinical animal studies (Kawase et al., 1988; Eisenthal et al., 1988). Clinical trials at several centers are now testing the incorporation of murine or "humanized" chimeric antibodies able to mediate ADCC into IL-2 regimens known to activate ADCC effectors (i.e., Fc receptor–bearing NK cells) in vivo.

Another approach for combination therapy that is currently being tested clinically is based on in vitro and in vivo animal studies showing that anti-CD3 (directed against the CD3 complex, the structure associated with the T-cell receptor [TCR] and responsible for T-cell activation), either alone or together with IL-2, was capable of inducing significant antitumor responses (Ellenhorn et al., 1988; Yang et al., 1990). In addition, provision of anti-CD3, a potent T-cell stimulus, may serve to activate tumor-specific T-cell clones that are present in vivo, but remain functionally inactive. Finally, the trials underway evaluating the combination of anti-CD3 + IL-2 will serve as a basis upon which to model future trials employing bispecific heteroconjugate monoclonal antibodies with dual specificity for target structures present on both the effector- and target-cell populations (Segal and Wunderlich, 1988). These heteroconjugate monoclonal antibodies have the advantage not only of delivering an activating stimulus to effector-cell populations (e.g., via the CD3 complex in the case of T cells), but also of bringing the effectors in close contact with putative tumor targets, potentially allowing more efficient and prolonged effector/target interaction. Furthermore, using bispecific monoclonal antibodies to simultaneously target structures on T cells and tumor cells might offer a means of circumventing the decreased T-cell responses observed following in vivo IL-2 therapy (see below). This approach might also improve attempts to generate in vivo ADCC with conventional monoclonal antibodies as we occasionally observe in some patients only low numbers of circulating Fc receptor–bearing NK cells following IL-2 treatment.

Important in the analysis of these combination protocols will be the clinical monitoring that has been undertaken in the evaluation of therapies involving administration of IL-2 alone. The knowledge gained with regard to the effects of IL-2 therapy on patients will be critical in the evaluation of clinical responses to the combination regimens. Together with a thorough evaluation of the immunological effects induced in vivo by these various agents, the results of these initial combination regimens will serve an important role in the design of subsequent clinical protocols.

MECHANISMS OF ACTION OF IL-2 IN VIVO

Interleukin-2 is currently being administered in various treatment centers in conjunction with many different treatment regimens. Despite this widespread use of IL-2 as an anticancer agent, relatively little information exists regarding the molecular mechanisms of IL-2 action occurring in vivo in patients. The following section summarizes some of the approaches our laboratory has taken to investigate these mechanisms.

Activation of Distinct Lymphocyte Subsets by In Vivo IL-2

As noted earlier, continuous administration of IL-2 in vivo leads to a dramatic expansion of lymphocytes. This activation and expansion are presumably occurring in nonperipheral blood compartments, since relatively few lymphocytes are found in the peripheral circulation during the period of IL-2 infusion (Sondel et al., 1988; Voss et al., 1989). Lymphocytes obtained 24 to 48 hours after the last week of a 4-week course of IL-2 therapy during the period of rebound lymphocytosis are predominantly $CD56^+$ NK cells. A fraction (50%–60%) of these cells also coexpress the Fc receptor III (CD16) molecule and are potentially important in ADCC-mediated antitumor effects (Hank et al., 1990c). Often, it is possible to separate the posttherapy NK-cell population into $CD56^{dim}$ and $CD56^{bright}$ subsets. Cell separation experiments revealed a functional heterogeneity between these two subsets, with a predominant role for the $CD56^{bright}$ population in mediating in vitro proliferative and cytotoxic responses to IL-2 (Weil-Hillman et al., 1989).

Recent studies have shown that $CD56^{bright}$ NK cells isolated from fresh peripheral blood from healthy volunteer donors express high-affinity IL-2 receptors and, in contrast to the CD56^{dim} subset, are capable of responding to low concentrations of IL-2 through this receptor (Nagler et al., 1990; Caligiuri et al., 1990). It is therefore interesting to speculate that the population of CD56^{bright} NK cells recovered following in vivo expansion in IL-2 may have derived from the high-affinity IL-2 receptor-binding CD56^{bright} precursors, the expansion in vivo having been facilitated by the fact that the steady-state plasma IL-2 levels attained during continuous IL-2 infusion (approximately 30 U/mL = 145 pM [Kohler et al., 1989]) are sufficient to saturate the majority of the high-affinity receptors expressed on the cells. However, despite detailed efforts, we have not been able to detect or induce high-affinity IL-2 receptors on these CD56$^+$ NK cells obtained following in vivo IL-2 therapy (Voss et al., 1990) (see below).

The role of the Fc receptor (CD16) on posttherapy NK cells is also of interest since recent experiments have shown that the signal-transducing CD3 ζ subunit of the CD3 complex is present on NK cells obtained from fresh peripheral blood and is associated at the cell surface with CD16 (Lanier et al., 1989; Anderson et al., 1990). Natural killer cells activated in vivo by IL-2 have not yet been examined for the presence of this signal-transducing subunit. The CD3 ζ chain is tyrosine phosphorylated on fresh NK cells following Fc receptor triggering, either with cross-linking monoclonal antibody or ADCC-type effector/target interaction (Vivier et al., 1991; O'Shea et al., 1991). Whether the CD3 ζ chain found on NK cells will be similarly phosphorylated following stimulation of the cells with IL-2 is not known. It also remains to be determined whether CD3 ζ is present on the CD16$^-$ subset of NK cells, obtained either from the fresh peripheral blood or following in vivo IL-2 therapy, and whether it plays a universal role in NK-cell signaling mechanisms, analogous to its function in T cells.

Analysis of T cells obtained following in vivo IL-2 therapy presents a more perplexing set of results. We and others have noted that T cells exposed to IL-2 in vivo have a decreased capacity, relative to pretherapy T cells, to respond either in vitro or in vivo to specific antigenic and polyclonal mitogenic stimuli (Hank et al., 1990a; Wiebke et al., 1988). This does not appear to be due simply to the decreased percentage of peripheral blood T cells obtained following IL-2 therapy (Hank et al., 1990a), although experiments comparing equal numbers of purified pre- and posttherapy T cells must be done to formally exclude this possibility. Supporting this observation of decreased T-cell responsiveness following exposure to IL-2 in vivo is the observation that fluorescence activated cell sorter (FACS)-sorted posttherapy T cells show negligible responses to IL-2, even at concentrations sufficient to saturate both high- and intermediate-affinity receptors (Voss et al., 1990). These T cells, despite the lack of a response to IL-2, express high-affinity IL-2 receptors, as detected in radiolabeled IL-2 receptor binding assays (Voss, unpublished observations). There are a number of possibilities to explain this lack of T-cell responsiveness to IL-2. Interleukin-2, while binding to cell-surface receptors with high-affinity (as measured in equilibrium binding assays) might not be internalized by the cell. Alternatively, the cells may be in a resting G_0 phase of the cell cycle such that IL-2, which normally serves as a progression signal to allow antigen-activated cells to enter into the replication phase of the cell cycle, may not be sufficient to stimulate the cells to proliferate. Second messenger pathways, which remain to be elucidated for IL-2 receptor signaling, may also not be operational. Experiments are underway to investigate these different possibilities.

Of fundamental importance in understanding the mechanisms involved in regulating T-cell responses to IL-2 is determining whether endogenous resting T cells exposed to IL-2 in vivo are in fact active in the in vivo environment. This is especially relevant to studies of TIL, in which it is hypothesized that IL-2 may be able to activate endogenous specific antitumor T-cell responses. The fact that T lymphocytes, which appear to be at least tumor-reactive for some tumors, can be identified in the tumor bed is encouraging. However, the apparent absence of an endogenous T-cell response to the tumor in situ is perplexing. Kradin and colleagues (1990) have recently demonstrated that TIL obtained from biopsies of malignant melanoma, renal cell carcinoma, and small-cell carcinoma of the lung contain a high proportion of cells displaying the surface phenotype of memory T cells rather than naive T cells. The majority of these TIL, however, did not appear to have been recently antigen-activated, based on the low level of surface Tac expression observed. Our studies of T cells obtained from the peripheral blood following treatment with IL-2 confirm earlier work done in in vitro systems and demonstrate that the simple presence of cell-surface IL-2 receptors may not alone dictate the responsiveness of a cell to IL-2. These observations, together with the studies of TIL, make it clear that the presence of lymphocytes in the tumor bed or the expression of appropriate receptors for mitogenic growth factors are only minimal necessary components of an antitumor immune response; other factors, both local and systemic, must be involved. Nevertheless, it remains possible that systemic treatment with IL-2 may activate antigen-reactive T cells that encounter antigen (such as a tumor itself), while decreasing responsiveness of otherwise resting T cells (such as those circulating in the peripheral blood).

In an effort to explain the augmented proliferative and cytotoxic responses observed when posttherapy NK cells are reexposed to IL-2 in vitro (Hank et al., 1990b; Sondel, 1989), we examined these cells for potential increases in IL-2 receptor expression. We had previously noted increased levels of sTac in the sera of patients receiving systemic IL-2 (Voss et al., 1989). Together with the increase in the percentage of $CD56^+$ NK cells observed, we anticipated finding increased levels of high-affinity IL-2 receptors on the posttherapy NK cells. However, when examined by FACS for IL-2 receptor α (Tac) expression, these cells were negative (Weil-Hillman et al., 1990; Voss et al., 1990). In addition, posttherapy NK cells, when cultured in IL-2 in vitro, released negligible quantities of sTac into the culture medium (Weil-Hillman et al., 1990). Proliferative responses to IL-2, as well as radiolabeled IL-2 binding, were unaffected by inclusion of an anti-Tac monoclonal antibody in the assays, confirming that posttherapy NK cells are neither responding through, nor synthesizing and reexpressing, high-affinity IL-2 receptors (Voss et al., 1990).

At the same time we were collecting these results, two independent groups of Japanese investigators reported the isolation of monoclonal antibodies to the p70 β subunit of the IL-2 receptor. Using these monoclonal antibodies to evaluate the expression of the IL-2 receptor β subunit on posttherapy NK cells, we found that p70 β chain expression was dramatically increased relative to its expression on pretherapy cells (Voss et al., 1990) and initially invoked this as the explanation for the augmented responses to IL-2 seen with posttherapy NK cells. However, control experiments using the YT cell line (an NK-cell–like leukemic line bearing a relatively high level of p70-associated intermediate-affinity IL-2 receptor expression [Robb and Greene, 1988]) indicated that despite the high level of p70 expression on the posttherapy NK cells, only low levels of intermediate-affinity IL-2 binding sites were present, as determined in radiolabeled IL-2 binding analyses. We concluded from these studies that the regulation of functional IL-2 receptor formation could not be determined solely by the level of p70 expression at the cell surface and that some other IL-2 receptor subunit may be needed to allow the formation of a functional intermediate-affinity IL-2 receptor. This conclusion was supported by other studies demonstrating a requirement for some other molecules in addition to the p55 α and p70 β chains for the formation of high-affinity IL-2 receptors (Minamoto et al., 1990; Tsudo et al., 1990; Zuraweski et al., 1990; Hatakeyama et al., 1991; Ringheim et al., 1991; Saito et al., 1991). One possibility for this subunit is the p64 γ chain described by Sugamura and co-workers (Takeshita et al., 1990), although their study focused on cells expressing high-affinity IL-2 receptors. In studies performed in our laboratory (Voss et al., submitted), together with Richard Robb at DuPont/Merck, we have used a newly developed monoclonal antibody directed against the p70 IL-2 receptor β chain to demonstrate, in cells bearing only intermediate affinity IL-2 receptors, the association of p64, the putative IL-2R γ chain with the β chain. Examination of p64 expression in posttherapy NK cells, in which only low levels of IL-2 binding were detectable, revealed that p64 was associated with only 10% of the β chains expressed on those cells. This contrasted with approximately equal levels of β chain and p64 expression in control cells that expressed a high level of IL-2 binding. These results together with studies showing a rapid dissociation of IL-2 from isolated β chains expressed at the cell surface (Ringheim et al., 1992) suggest that p64 may regulate functional IL-2 receptor formation by associating with the β chain and allowing IL-2, once bound, to remain stably associated with the receptor. Thus, in adding an additional level of complexity to the structure of the IL-2 receptor, these studies lend further insight into mechanisms whereby lymphocytes might regulate their responsiveness to IL-2.

It is important to note that, despite low levels of intermediate-affinity binding, the posttherapy NK cells responded exclusively through those receptors in functional proliferative assays; an anti-p70 mAb completely inhibited the response of these cells to IL-2 (Voss et al., 1990). What was not known from these studies is what fraction of the NK-cell population is responding to IL-2. Although there appears to be a uniform distribution of IL-2 receptors on these cells, it is important to determine what fraction of the population is responding functionally through these receptors and whether in vivo IL-2 therapy results in globally augmented responses, or whether only a select subset of cells is functionally responsive to IL-2. In experiments aimed at addressing this question, NK cells were purified from five patients who had received in vivo IL-2 therapy. Restimulation of these NK cells with IL-2, followed by analyses of the fraction of cells entering the cell cycle, showed that the majority, if not all, of the posttherapy NK cells were capable of responding to IL-2, entering the cell cycle, and proliferating (Voss S, Bogner M, unpublished observations). While these observations only begin to address IL-2 receptor structure–function relationships operational in vivo, they emphasize the need to choose carefully those parameters from which conclusions relating to in vivo function will be based.

Induction of Gene Transcription by IL-2

In attempts to elucidate a mechanism for IL-2 signaling, numerous groups have investigated changes in proto-oncogene expression following stimulation of cells with IL-2. The most consistent reproducible changes seen have been the early induction of *c-fos, c-myb,* and *c-myc* transcription, followed by induction of Tac and IL-2 messenger RNA (mRNA) synthesis (Reed and Nowell, 1988). Relatively little work has been done to investigate which transcripts are present in in vivo activated NK-cell and T-cell subsets. To date, only one study has looked at mRNA obtained from posttherapy PBL (Kasid et al., 1989). Because the analyses were performed on unseparated populations of PBL, these results are somewhat difficult to interpret. It will be important to determine whether the expression of cell cycle–linked proto-oncogenes such as *c-fos, c-myb,* and *c-myc* provides any insight into the response of posttherapy NK cells (or in the case of T cells, lack of response) to IL-2. In addition, we do not know why the posttherapy NK cells fail to express Tac following exposure to IL-2 or why they have such abundant expression of the p70 IL-2 receptor β chain. Transcriptional, posttranscriptional, and posttranslational mechanisms are all possibilities that must be investigated.

We have noted that posttherapy cells mediate significant LAK-cell activity in the absence of added IL-2, but when IL-2 is added during the course of the 4-hour chromium release assay, the LAK-cell activity is dramatically increased (Hank et al., 1990b). This activity could not be explained by increases in cytoplasmic serine-esterase (BLT esterase; Pasternack et al., 1985) activity (Cannon et al., 1991). An alternative possibility is increased expression of the C9-like pore-forming molecule perforin. Podack and colleagues, as well as Young and co-workers, have isolated the cDNA for the perforin gene and have shown that perforin gene transcription is increased in cytotoxic T lymphocytes (CTL) upon addition of IL-2 (Lowrey et al., 1989; Smythe et al., 1990). Their studies showed constitutive levels of perforin mRNA expressed in fresh NK cells that were unaffected by addition of IL-2. Based on these observations, it will be of interest to examine the posttherapy NK cells for potential induction of perforin gene expression following addition of IL-2, in an effort to explain the rapid augmentation of cytolytic activity in the presence of IL-2.

OTHER FACTORS INFLUENCING IN VIVO RESPONSES TO SYSTEMIC IL-2 THERAPY

One of the more common explanations offered for the failure of significant numbers of cancer patients to respond to immunotherapeutic regimens has been to implicate suppressor T cells in negatively regulating in vivo responses to systemically administered cytokines. Indeed, part of the rationale for combining IL-2 with low-dose Cytoxan was to eliminate potential suppressor T-cell influences prior to initiating IL-2 therapy. Rosenberg and colleagues have recently addressed this issue directly and have shown that the synergistic antitumor effects observed in mice when either Cytoxan or local tumor irradiation are combined with IL-2 are not due solely to elimination of putative suppressor T cells (Cameron et al., 1990). Rather, their data suggest that the antitumor effects observed in these combination therapies include a component that is the direct antitumor effect of Cytoxan or local tumor irradiation on the tumor. Whether these agents are cytostatic, directly cytolytic, or influence the local tumor environment allowing greater access of immune cells to the tumor bed is not clear.

The importance of the local tumor environment on the ultimate generation of antitumor responses has been studied elegantly by Schreiber and colleagues (Perdrizet et al., 1990). Their observations indicate that highly immunogenic tumors are capable of progressing in tumor-bearing hosts, even in the presence of CTL specific for the relevant tumor-associated antigens (TAA), and emphasize the potential importance of local factors at the tumor site in preventing immune-cell access or in modulating immune-cell responses.

Other studies have evaluated the importance of local secretion of cytokines in determining whether immune cells at the tumor site will have antitumor effects. Two recent reports have shown that when poorly immunogenic tumors are engineered, by DNA transfection or retroviral insertion, to produce their own IL-2, both in vitro and in vivo antitumor responses are seen (Fearon et al., 1990; Gansbacher et al., 1990). Animals immunized with IL-2–secreting tumors were also resistant to subsequent challenge with the parental tumor cell, suggesting that the local provision of high concentrations of IL-2 created a paracrine environment that functioned in the absence of effective helper T cells. These data further demonstrate that, while specific tumor-reactive immune cells may be present in the tumor-bearing host, modification of the local tumor environment may be critical in determining whether responses to systemically administered cytokines, with or without adoptively transferred immune cells, will be achieved.

CONCLUSIONS

Understanding the complexity of the immune system and the host immune response to malignancy has proven to be a far more formidable task than initially imagined. There is little dispute that cancer has been cured in the culture dish. Immune cells capable of destroying tumor cells in vitro have been described by countless groups of investigators. Furthermore, under certain experimentally controlled circumstances, immune-mediated antitumor responses can be reproducibly documented and extremely effective in animal models. However, most current regimens using IL-2, alone or in combination with other biological agents, have demonstrated response rates (CR and PR) of less than 30%, and only for certain types of malignant disease, as currently tested for patients with widespread metastases. Accumulating evidence suggests that all of the necessary components for an antitumor immune response are present in the tumor-bearing individual. The challenge that remains is activating these effector elements and targeting them to the tumor tissue. It is unlikely that any one systemically administered therapeutic modality will be universally effective in such activation and delivery of tumor-reactive immune effectors to the tumor site. Combination therapies employing both nonspecific and tumor-specific (i.e., monoclonal antibodies, certain chemotherapeutic agents, local tumor irradiation) treatment regimens, as well as the use of biological response modifiers in the adjuvant setting when tumor burdens are relatively small, are examples of efforts aimed at modifying both the tumor and the tumor-bearing host. Whether these efforts, and those to follow, will prove fruitful or whether the coming decade will reveal more twists along the already tortuous path toward the application of immunotherapy to the successful treatment of cancer remains to be determined.

ACKNOWLEDGMENTS

This work was supported by NIH contracts CM-47669, CM-87290, NIH grants CA 32685, RR-03186, and American Cancer Society grant CH-237. S.D. Voss is supported by a Lutheran Brotherhood/Life and Health Insurance Medical Research Fund M.D./Ph.D. training fellowship and NCI training grant 5T32-CA09471.

REFERENCES

Adams DO, Nathan CF. Molecular mechanisms in tumor-cell killing by activated macrophages. Immunol Today. 1983;4:166–170.

Albertini MA, Sosman JA, Hank JA, et al. The influence of autologous lymphokine activated killer cell infusions on the toxicity and antitumor effect of repetitive cycles of interleukin 2. Cancer. 1990;66:2457–2464.

Allison MAK, Jones SE, McGuffey P. Phase II trial of outpatient interleukin 2 in malignant lymphoma, chronic lymphocytic leukemia and selected solid tumors. J Clin Oncol. 1989;7:75–80.

Anderson P, Caligiuri M, O'Brien C, Manley T, Ritz J, Schlossman SF. Fcγ receptor type III (CD16) is included in the ζ NK receptor complex expressed by human natural killer cells. Proc Natl Acad Sci USA. 1990a;87:2274–2278.

Atkins MB, Gould JA, Allegretta M, et al. Phase I evaluation of recombinant interleukin 2 in patients with advanced malignant disease. J Clin Oncol. 1986;4:1380–1391.

Balch CM, Riley LB, Bae YJ, et al. Patterns of human tumor-infiltrating lymphocytes in 120 human cancers. Arch Surg. 1990;125:200–205.

Bar MH, Sznol M, Atkins MB, et al. Metastatic malignant melanoma treated with combined bolus and continuous infusion interleukin-2 and lymphokine-activated killer cells. J Clin Oncol. 1990;8:1138–1147.

Belldegrun A, Muul LM, Rosenberg SA. Interleukin 2 expanded tumor infiltrating lymphocytes in human renal cell cancer: isolation, characterization, and antitumor activity. Cancer Res. 1988;48:206–214.

Berenson JR, Einstein AB, Fefer A. Syngeneic adoptive immunotherapy and chemoimmunotherapy of a Friend leukemia: requirement for T cells. J Immunol. 1975;115:234–238.

Bogner MP, Voss SD, Bechhofer R, et al. Serum soluble CD25 T levels during interleukin 2 therapy: dose dependence and correlation with clinical toxicity and lymphocyte surface CD25 expression. J Immunother. 1992;11:111–118.

Borden EC, Sondel PM. Lymphokines and cytokines as cancer treatment. Immunotherapy realized. Cancer. 1990;65:800–814.

Brown JP, Klitzman JM, Hellstrom I, Nowinski RC, Hellstrom KE. Antibody response of mice to chemically induced tumors. Proc Natl Acad Sci USA. 1978;75:955–958.

Bukowski RM, Goodman P, Crawford ED, Sergi JS, Redman BG, Whitehead RP. Phase II trial of high dose intermittent interleukin 2 in metastatic renal cell carcinoma: a Southwest oncology group study. J Nat Cancer Inst. 1990;82:143–146.

Caligiuri MA, Zmudidzinas A, Manley TJ, Levine H, Smith KA, Ritz J. Functional consequences of interleukin 2 receptor expression on resting human lymphocytes. Identification of a novel natural killer cell subset with high affinity receptors. J Exp Med. 1990;171:1509–1526.

Caligiuri MA, Murray C, Soiffer RJ, et al. Extended continuous infusion low dose recombinant interleukin-2 in advanced cancer: prolonged immunomodulation without significant toxicity. J Clin Oncol. 1991;9:2110–2119.

Cameron RB, Spiess PJ, Rosenberg SA. Synergistic antitumor activity of tumor-infiltrating lymphocytes, interleukin 2, and local tumor irradiation. J Exp Med. 1990;171:249–263.

Cannon A, Hank JA, Sondel PM. BLT esterase activity following in vitro and in vivo activation of human lymphocytes with interleukin-2. Biotherapy. 1991;3:253–260.

Cantrell DA, Smith KA. Transient expression of interleukin 2 receptors. Consequences for T cell growth. J Exp Med. 1983;158:1895–1911.

Chang AE, Hyatt CL, Rosenberg SA. Systemic administration of recombinant human interleukin 2 in mice. J Biol Resp Mod. 1984;3:561–572.

Cheever MA, Thompson JA, Kern DE, Greenberg PD. Interleukin-2 (IL-2) administered in vivo: influence of IL-2 route and timing on T cell growth. J Immunol. 1985;134:3895–3899.

Creekmore SP, Harris JE, Ellis TM, et al. A phase I clinical trial of recombinant interleukin 2 by periodic 24 hours intravenous infusions. J Clin Oncol. 1989;7:276–284.

Darzynkiewicz Z, Sharpless T, Staino-Coico L, Melamed MR. Subcompartments of G_1 phase of the cell cycle detected by flow cytometry. Proc Natl Acad Sci USA. 1980;77:6696–6699.

Delorme EJ, Alexander P. Treatment of primary fibrosarcoma in the rat with immune lymphocytes. Lancet. 1964;2:117–120.

Dent PB, Fish LA, White JG, Good RA. Chédiak-Higashi syndrome. Observations on the nature of the associated malignancy. Lab Invest. 1966;15:1634–1642.

Donohue JH, Rosenberg SA. The fate of interleukin 2 after in vivo administration. Cancer Res. 1983;130:2203–2208.

Donohue JH, Lotze MT, Robb RJ, et al. In vivo administration of purified Jurkat-derived interleukin 2 in mice. Cancer Res. 1984;44:1380–1386.

Dutcher JP, Creekmore SP, Weiss GR, et al. A phase II study of interleukin 2 and lymphokine-activated killer cells in patients with metastatic malignant melanoma. J Clin Oncol. 1989; 7:477–485.

Eberlein TJ, Schoof DD, Jung S, et al. A new regimen of interleukin 2 and lymphokine activated killer cells: efficacy without significant toxicity. Arch Int Med. 1988;148:2571–2576.

Eisenthal A, Shiloni E, Rosenberg SA. Characterization of IL-2 induced murine cells which exhibit ADCC activity. Cell Immunol. 1988;115:257–272.

Ellenhorn JD, Hirsh R, Schreiber H, Bluestone JA. In vivo administration of anti-CD3 prevents malignant progressor tumor growth. Science. 1988;242:569–571.

Ettinghausen SE, Rosenberg SA. Immunotherapy of murine sarcomas using lymphokine activated killer cells: optimization of the schedule and route of administration of recombinant interleukin 2. Cancer Res. 1986;46:2784–2792.

Ettinghausen SE, Puri RK, Rosenberg SA. Increased vascular permeability in organs mediated by systemic administration of lymphokine activated killer cells and recombinant interleukin 2 in mice. J Natl Cancer Inst. 1988;80:177–188.

Fearon ER, Pardoll DM, Itaya T, et al. Interleukin-2 production by tumor cells bypasses T helper function in the generation of an antitumor response. Cell. 1990;60:397–403.

Fidler IJ. Macrophages and metastasis—a biological approach to cancer therapy: presidential address. Cancer Res. 1985;45:4714–4726.

Fisher B, Packard BS, Read EJ, et al. Tumor localization of adoptively transferred Indium-111 labeled tumor infiltrating lymphocytes in patients with metastatic melanoma. J Clin Oncol. 1989;7:250–261.

Fisher RI, Coltman CA, Doroshow JH, et al. Metastic renal cancer treated with interleukin 2 and lymphokine activated killer cells. Ann Intern Med. 1988;108:518–523.

Foon KA. Biological response modifiers: the new immunotherapy. Cancer Res. 1989;49:1621–1639.

Fung MR, Ju G, Greene WC. Co-internalization of the p55 and p70 subunits of the high affinity human interleukin-2 receptor: evidence for a stable ternary receptor complex. J Exp Med. 1988;168:1923–1928.

Gambacorti-Passerini C, Rovelli F, Ghezzi R., Traversari C, Belli F, Parmiani G. Serum CD25 levels in patients treated with rIL-2 and correlation with in vivo immune activation. J Immunol Res. 1990;2(1):19–24.

Gansbacher B, Zier K, Danials B, Cronin K, Bannerji R, Gilboa E. Interleukin 2 gene transfer into tumor cells abrogates tumorigenicity and induces protective immunity. J Exp Med. 1990;172:1217–1224.

Ghosh AK, Dazzi H, Thatcher N, Moore M. Lack of correlation between peripheral blood lymphokine activated killer (LAK) cell function and clinical response in patients with advanced malignant melanoma receiving recombinant interleukin 2. Int J Cancer. 1989;43:410–414.

Goldstein D, Sosman JA, Hank JA, et al. Repetitive weekly cycles of interleukin 2: effect of outpatient treatment with a lower dose of interleukin 2 on non-major histocompatibility complex–restricted killer activity. Cancer Res. 1989;49:6832–6839.

Gorczynski RM. Evidence for in vivo protection against murine sarcomavirus induced tumors by T lymphocytes from immune animals. J Immunol. 1974;112:533-539.

Grimm EA, Mazumber A, Zhang HZ, Rosenberg SA. Lymphokine-activated killer cell phenomenon. Lysis of natural killer-resistant fresh solid tumor cells by interleukin 2-activated autologous human peripheral blood lymphocytes. J Exp Med. 1982;155:1823–1841.

Grimm EA, Robb RJ, Roth JA, et al. Lymphokine-activated killer cell phenomenon. III. Evidence that IL-2 is sufficient for direct activation of peripheral blood lymphocytes into lymphokine-activated killer cells. J Exp Med. 1983;158:1356–1361.

Haas GP, Solomon D, Rosenberg SA. Tumor infiltrating lymphocytes from nonrenal urological malignancies. Cancer Immunol Immunother. 1990;30:342-350.

Haliotis T, Roder JC, Klein M, Ortaldo J, Fauci AS, Herberman RB. Chédiak-Higashi gene in humans. I. Impairment of natural killer function. J Exp Med. 1980;151:1029–1048.

Haliotis T, Ball JK, Dexter D, Roder JC. Spontaneous and induced primary oncogenesis in natural killer (NK) cell-deficient beige mutant mice. Int J Cancer. 1985;35:505–513.

Hank JA, Kohler PC, Hillman GH, et al. Interleukin 2 (IL-2) dependent human lymphokine activated killer (LAK) cells generated in vivo during administration of human recombinant IL-2. Cancer Res. 1988;48:1965–1971.

Hank JA, Sosman JA, Kohler PC, Bechhofer R, Storer B, Sondel PM. Depressed in vitro T cell responses concomitant with augmented interleukin 2 responses by lymphocytes from cancer patients following in vivo treatment with interleukin 2. J Biol Resp Mod. 1990a;9:5–14.

Hank JA, Weil-Hillman G, Surfus JE, Sosman JA, Sondel PM. Addition of interleukin 2 in vitro augments detection of lymphokine activated killer activity generated in vivo. Cancer Immunol Immunother. 1990b;31:53–59.

Hank JA, Robinson RR, Surfus J, et al. Augmentation of antibody dependent cell mediated cytotoxicity following in vivo therapy with recombinant interleukin 2. Cancer Res. 1990c; 50:5234–5239.

Hanna N. Role of natural killer cell in control of cancer metastasis. Cancer Metastasis Rev. 1982;1:45-64.

Hatakeyama M, Kono T, Kobayashi N, et al. Interaction of the IL-2 receptor with the *src*-family kinase $p56^{lck}$: identification of novel intermolecular association. Science. 1991;252:1523–1528.

Hawkins MJ. IL-2/LAK: current status and possible future directions. Principles and Practice of Oncology: Updates. 1989;3(8):1–14.

Heo DS, Whiteside TL, Johnson JT, Chen K, Barnes EL, Herberman RB. Long term interleukin 2 dependent growth and cytotoxic activity of tumor infiltrating lymphocytes from human squamous cell carcinomas of the head and neck. Cancer Res. 1987;47:6353–6362.

Herberman RB. Cell mediated immunity to tumor cells. Adv Cancer Res. 1974;19:207–263.

Hermann T, Diamantstein T. The mouse high affinity IL-2 receptor complex. I. Evidence for a third molecule, the putative γ chain, associated with the α and/or β chain of the receptor. Immunobiology. 1987;175:145–148.

Hersey P, Bolhuis R. Nonspecific MHC-unrestricted killer cells and their receptors. Immunol Today. 1987;8:233–239.

Hewitt HB. The choice of animal tumors for experimental studies of cancer therapy. Adv Cancer Res. 1978;27:149–200.

Holland JM, Mitchell TJ, Gipson LC, Whitaker MS. Survival and cause of death in aging germfree athymic nude and normal inbred C3Hf/He mice. J Natl Cancer Inst. 1978;61:1357–1361.

Javadpour N, Lalehzarian M. A phase I–II study of high dose human interleukin 2 in disseminated renal cell carcinoma. Semin Surg Oncol. 1988;4:207–209.

Itoh K, Tilden AB, Balch CM. Interleukin 2 activation of cytotoxic T lymphocytes infiltrating into human metastatic melanomas. Cancer Res. 1986;46:3011–3017.

Karre K, Klein GO, Kiessling R, Klein G, Roder JC. Low natural in vivo resistance to syngeneic leukaemias in natural killer-deficient mice. Nature. 1980;284:624–626.

Kasid A, Director EP, Rosenberg SA. Induction of endogenous cytokine mRNA in circulating peripheral blood mononuclear cells by IL-2 administration to cancer patients. J Immunol. 1989;143:736–739.

Kawase I, Komuta K, Hara H, et al. Combined therapy of mice bearing a lymphokine-activated killer-resistant tumor with recombinant interleukin 2 and an antitumor monoclonal antibody capable of inducing antibody-dependent cellular cytotoxicity. Cancer Res. 1988;48:1173–1179.

Kehrl JH, Dukovich M, Whalen G, Katz P, Fauci AS, Greene WC. Novel interleukin 2 (IL-2) receptor appears to mediate IL-2 induced activation of natural killer cells. J Clin Invest. 1988;81:200–205.

Klein G, Sjogren HO, Klein E, Hellstrom KE. Demonstration of resistance against methylcholanthrene-induced sarcomas in the primary autochthonous host. Cancer Res. 1960;20:1561–1572.

Kohler PC, Hank JA, Moore KH, et al. Phase I clinical trial of recombinant interleukin 2: a comparison of bolus and continuous intravenous infusion. Cancer Invest. 1989;7:213–223.

Konrad MW, Hemstreet G, Hersh EM, et al. Pharmacokinetics of recombinant interleukin 2 in humans. Cancer Res. 1990;50:2009–2017.

Kradin RL, Boyle LA, Preffer FI, et al. Tumor-derived interleukin 2 dependent lymphocytes in adoptive immunotherapy of lung cancer. Cancer Immunol Immunother. 1987;24:76–85.

Kradin RL, Lazarus DS, Dubinett SM, et al. Tumour-infiltrating lymphocytes and interleukin-2 in treatment of advanced cancer. Lancet. 1989;1:577–580.

Kradin RL, Xia W, Kurnick J, Lazarus D. Tumor infiltrating lymphocytes display the surface phenotype of T-memory cells in vivo. FASEB J. 1990;4(7):A1948.

Krigel RL, Padavic-Schaller KA, Rudolph AR, Konrad M, Bradley EC, Comis RL. Renal cell carcinoma: treatment with recombinant interleukin 2 plus β interferon. J Clin Oncol. 1990;8:460–467.

Lafreniere R, Rosenberg SA. Successful immunotherapy of murine experimental hepatic metastases with lymphokine-activated killer cells and recombinant interleukin 2. Cancer Res. 1985;45:3735–3741.

Lanier LL, Yu G, Phillips JH. Co-association of CD3 ζ with a receptor (CD16) for IgG Fc on human natural killer cells. Nature. 1989;342:803–805.

Le Thi Bich-Thuy, Dukovich M, Peffer NJ, Fauci AS, Kehrl JH, Greene WC. Direct activation of human resting T cells by IL-2: the role of an IL-2 receptor distinct from the Tac protein. J Immunol. 1987;139:1550.

Lee KH, Talpaz M, Rothberg JM, et al. Concomitant administration of recombinant human interleukin 2 and recombinant interferon α-2A in cancer patients: A phase I study. J Clin Oncol. 1989;7:1726–1732.

Lotze MT, Rosenberg SA. Interleukin 2 as a pharmacologic reagent. In: Smith KA, ed. Interleukin 2. San Diego, Calif: Academic Press; 1988:237–294.

Lotze MT, Grimm EA, Mazumber A, Strausser JL, Rosenberg SA. In vitro growth of cytotoxic human lymphocytes. IV. Lysis of fresh and cultured autologous tumor by lymphocytes cultured in T cell growth factor (TCGF). Cancer Res. 1981;41:4420–4425.

Lotze MT, Matory YL, Ettinghausen SE, et al. In vivo administration of purified human interleukin 2. II. Half life, immunologic effects, and expansion of peripheral lymphoid cells in vivo with recombinant IL-2. J Immunol. 1985;135:2865–2875.

Lowrey DM, Aebischer T, Olsen K, et al. Cloning, analysis, and expression of murine perforin 1 cDNA, a component of cytolytic T cell granules with homology to complement component C9. Proc Natl Acad Sci USA. 1989;86:247–251.

Margolin KA, Rayner AA, Hawkins MJ, et al. Interleukin 2 and lymphokine activated killer cell therapy of solid tumors: analysis of toxicity and management guidelines. J Clin Oncol. 1989;7:486–498.

Minamoto S, Mori H, Hatakeyama M, et al. Characterization of the heterodimeric complex of human IL-2 receptor αβ chains reconstituted in a mouse fibroblast cell line, L929. J Immunol. 1990;145:2177–2182.

Mitchell MS, Kempf RA, Harel W, et al. Effectiveness and tolerability of low dose cyclophosphamide and low dose intravenous interleukin 2 in disseminated melanoma. J Clin Oncol. 1988;6:409–424.

Mitchell MS, Kempf RA, Harel W, et al. Low-dose cyclophosphamide and low-dose interleukin-2 for malignant melanoma. Bull NY Acad Med. 1989;65:128–144.

Mulé JJ, Rosenberg SA. Immunotherapy with lymphokine combinations. In: DeVita VT, Hellman S, Rosenberg SA, eds. Important advances in oncology. Philadelphia, Penn: J B Lippincott; 1989:99–126.

Mulé JJ, Shu S, Schwarz SL, Rosenberg SA. Adoptive immunotherapy of established pulmonary metastases with LAK cells and recombinant interleukin 2. Science. 1984;225:1487–1489.

Mulé JJ, Shu S, Rosenberg SA. The anti-tumor efficacy of lymphokine activated killer cells and recombinant IL-2 in vivo. J Immunol. 1985;135:646–652.

Mulé JJ, Yang J, Shu S, Rosenberg SA. The anti-tumor efficacy of lymphokine-activated killer cells and recombinant interleukin 2 in vivo: direct correlation between reduction of established metastases and cytolytic activity of lymphokine-activated killer cells. J Immunol. 1986;136:3899–3909.

Mulé JJ, Yang JC, Lafreniere R, Shu S, Rosenberg SA. Identification of cellular mechanisms operational in vivo during the regression of established pulmonary metastases by the systemic administration of high dose recombinant interleukin 2. J Immunol. 1987;139:285–294.

Murumo K, Muraki J, Ueno M, et al. Immunologic study of human recombinant interleukin 2 (low dose) in patients with advanced renal cell carcinoma. Urology. 1989;33:219–225.

Muul LM, Spiess PJ, Director EP, Rosenberg SA. Identification of specific cytolytic immune responses against autologous tumor in humans bearing malignant melanoma. J Immunol. 1987;138:989–995.

Nagler A, Lanier LL, Phillips JH. Constitutive expression of high affinity interleukin 2 receptors on human CD16 natural killer cells in vivo. J Exp Med. 1990;171:1527–1533.

Ohashi Y, Takeshita T, Nagata K, Mori S, Sugamura K. Differential expression of the interleukin 2 receptor subunits, p55 and p75, on various populations of primary peripheral blood mononuclear cells. J Immunol. 1989;143:3548–3555.

Ortaldo JR, Mason A, Overton R. Lymphokine-activated killer cells. Analysis of progenitors and effectors. J Exp Med. 1986;164:1193–1205.

O'Shea JJ, Weissman AM, Kennedy ICS, Ortaldo JR. Engagement of the natural killer cell IgG Fc receptor results in tyrosine phosphorylation of the ζ chain. Proc Natl Acad Sci USA. 1991;88:350–354.

Outzen HC, Custer RP, Eaton GJ, Prehn RT. Spontaneous and induced tumor incidence in germfree "nude" mice. J Reticuloendothel Soc. 1975;17:1–9.

Paciucci PA, Holland JF, Ryder JS, et al. Immunotherapy with interleukin 2 by constant infusion with and without adoptive cell transfer and with weekly doxorubicin. Cancer Treat Rev. 1989;16(Suppl A):67–81.

Papa MZ, Yang JC, Vetto JT, Shiloni E, Eisenthal A, Rosenberg SA. Combined effects of chemotherapy and interleukin 2 in the therapy of mice with advanced pulmonary tumors. Cancer Res. 1988;48:122–129.

Parkinson DR. Interleukin 2 in cancer therapy. Semin Oncol. 1988;15(suppl 6):10–26.

Parmiani G, Anichini A, Fossati G. Cellular immune response against autologous human malignant melanoma: are in vitro studies providing a framework for a more effective immunotherapy? J Natl Cancer Inst. 1990;82:361–370.

Pasternack MS, Eisen HN. A novel serine esterase expressed by cytolytic T lymphocytes. Nature. 1985;314:743–745.

Perdrizet GA, Ross SR, Stauss HJ, Singh S, Koeppen H, Schreiber H. Animals bearing malignant grafts reject normal grafts that express through gene transfer the same antigen. J Exp Med. 1990;171:1205–1220.

Philip T, Mercatello A, Negrier S, et al. Interleukin 2 with and without LAK cells in metastatic renal cell carcinoma: the Lyon first-year experience in 20 patients. Cancer Treat Rev. 1989;16(suppl A):91–104.

Phillips JH, Lanier LL. Dissection of the lymphokine-activated killer phenomenon. Relative contribution of peripheral blood natural killer cells and T lymphocytes to cytolysis. J Exp Med. 1986;164:814–825.

Phillips JH, Gemlo BT, Myers WW, Rayner AA, Lanier LL. In vivo and in vitro activation of natural killer cells in advanced cancer patients undergoing combined recombinant interleukin 2 and LAK cell therapy. J Clin Oncol. 1987;5:1933–1941.

Phillips JH, Takeshita T, Sugamura K, Lanier LL. Activation of natural killer cells via the p75 interleukin 2 receptor. J Exp Med. 1989;170:291–296.

Prehn RT, Main JM. Immunity of methylcholanthrene-induced sarcomas. J Natl Cancer Inst. 1957;18:769–778.

Reed JC, Nowell PC. Mechanisms of interleukin 2 action: IL-2 inducible gene expression in T lymphocytes. In: Smith KA, ed. Interleukin 2. San Diego, Calif: Academic Press; 1988:137–162.

Reynolds CW, Ortaldo JR. Natural killer activity: the definition of a function rather than a cell type. Immunol Today. 1987;8:172–174.

Ringheim GE, Freimark BD, Robb RJ. Quantitative characterization of the intrinsic ligand binding affinity of the interleukin 2 β chain and its modulation by the α chain and a second affinity-modulating element. Lymphokine Cytokine Res. 1991;10:219–224.

Robb RJ, Greene WC. Internalization of interleukin 2 is mediated by the β chain of the high affinity interleukin 2 receptor. J Exp Med. 1987;165:1201–1206.

Roder JC, Haliotis T, Klein M, et al. A new immunodeficiency disorder in humans involving NK cells. Nature (Lond). 1980;284:553–555.

Rosenberg SA, Lotze MT. Cancer immunotherapy using interleukin 2 and interleukin 2 activated lymphocytes. Ann Rev Immunol. 1986;4:681–709.

Rosenberg SA, Mulé JJ, Spiess PJ, Reichert CM, Schwarz SL. Regression of established pulmonary metastases and subcutaneous tumor mediated by the systemic administration of high dose recombinant IL-2. J Exp Med. 1985a;161:1169–1188.

Rosenberg SA, Lotze MT, Muul LM, et al. Observations on the systemic administration of autologous lymphokine-activated killer cells and recombinant interleukin 2 to patients with metastatic cancer. New Engl J Med. 1985b;313:1485–1492.

Rosenberg SA, Spiess PJ, Lafreniere R. A new approach to the adoptive immunotherapy of cancer with tumor infiltrating lymphocytes. Science. 1986;1318–1321.

Rosenberg SA, Lotze MT, Muul LM, et al. Observations on the systemic administration of autologous lymphokine-activated killer cells and recombinant interleukin 2 to patients with metastatic cancer. New Engl J Med. 1985b;313:1485–1492.

Rosenberg SA, Lotze MT, Mulé JJ. New approaches to the immunotherapy of cancer using interleukin 2. Ann Intern Med. 1988;108:853–864.

Rosenberg SA, Lotze MT, Yang JC, et al. Experience with the use of high dose interleukin 2 in the treatment of 652 cancer patients. Ann Surg. 1989;210:474–485.

Rosenberg SA, Blaese M, Aebersold P, et al. Immunotherapy of cancer using gene-modified tumor infiltrating lymphocytes. Proc Am Soc Clin Oncol. 1990;9:710.

Rosenstein M, Yron I, Kaufman Y, Rosenberg SA. Lymphokine activated killer cells: lysis of fresh syngeneic NK-resistant murine tumor cells by lymphocytes cultured in interleukin 2. Cancer Res. 1984;44:1946–1953.

Rosenstein M, Ettinghausen SE, Rosenberg SA. Extravasation of intravascular fluid mediated by the systemic administration of recombinant interleukin 2. J Immunol. 1986;137:1735–1742.

Rosenthal NS, Hank JA, Kohler PC, et al. The in vitro function of lymphocytes from 25 cancer patients receiving four to seven consecutive days of recombinant IL-2. J Biol Resp Mod. 1988;7:123–139.

Rubin LA, Kurman CC, Fritz ME, et al. Soluble interleukin 2 receptors are released from activated human lymphoid cells in vitro. J Immunol. 1985;135:3172–3177.

Rygaard J, Povlsen CO. The nude mouse vs. the hypothesis of immunological surveillance. Transplant Rev. 1976;28:43–61.

Saito Y, Tada H, Sabe H, Honjo T. Biochemical evidence for a third chain of the interleukin 2 receptor. J Biol Chem. 1991;266:22186–22191.

Saragovi H, Malek TR. Direct identification of the murine IL-2 receptor p55-p75 heterodimer in the absence of IL-2. J Immunol. 1988;141:476–482.

Schoof DD, Gramolini BA, Davidson DL, et al. Adoptive immunotherapy of human cancer using low dose recombinant interleukin 2 and lymphokine activated killer cells. Cancer Res. 1988;48:5007–5010.

Segal DM, Wunderlich JR. Targeting of cytotoxic cells with heterocrosslinked antibodies. Cancer Invest. 1988;6:83–92.

Seigel JP, Sharon M, Smith PL, Leonard WJ. The IL-2 receptor β chain (p70): role in mediating signals for LAK, NK, and proliferative activities. Science. 1987;238:75–78.

Smith KA. Interleukin 2: inception, impact, and implications. Science. 1988;240:1169–1176.

Smith KA. The interleukin 2 receptor. Annu Rev Cell Biol. 1989;5:397–425.

Smyth MJ, Ortaldo JR, Shinkai Y, et al. Interleukin 2 induction of pore-forming protein gene expression in human peripheral blood $CD8^+$ T cells. J Exp Med. 1990;171:1269–1281.

Sondel PM. Cellular immunotherapy of cancer: preclinical and clinical testing utilizing interleukin 2. In: Lotzova E, Herberman R, eds. IL-2 activated killer cells and cancer treatment. CRC Press; 1989:1–24.

Sondel PM, Hank JH, Kohler PC, Chen BP, Minkoff DZ, Molenda JA. Destruction of autologous human lymphocytes by interleukin 2-activated cytotoxic cells. J Immunol. 1986; 137:502–511.

Sondel PM, Kohler PC, Hank JA, et al. Clinical and immunological effects of recombinant interleukin 2 given by receptive weekly cycles to patients with cancer. Cancer Res. 1988; 48:2561–2567.

Sondel PM, Sosman JA, Hank JA, Kohler PC, Storer B. Tumor infiltrating lymphocytes and interleukin 2 in melanoma (letter). New Engl J Med. 1989;320:1418–1419.

Sosman JA, Kohler PC, Hank JA, et al. Repetitive weekly cycles of recombinant human interleukin 2: responses of renal carcinoma with acceptable toxicity. J Natl Cancer Inst. 1988a;80:60–63.

Sosman JA, Kohler PC, Hank JA, et al. Repetitive weekly cycles of interleukin 2. II. Clinical and immunologic effects of dose, schedule, and addition of indomethacin. J Natl Cancer Inst. 1988b;80:1451–1461.

Sosman JA, Hank JA, Sondel PM. In vivo activation of lymphokine-activated killer activity with interleukin 2: prospects for combination therapies. Semin Oncol. 1990;17:22–30.

Sosman JA, Hank JA, Moore KH, et al. Prolonged interleukin 2 (IL-2) treatment can augment immune activation without enhancing antitumor activity in renal cell carcinoma. Cancer Invest. 1991;9:35–48.

Stahel RA, Sculier JP, Jost LM, et al. Tolerance and effectiveness of recombinant interleukin 2 (r-met Hu IL-2 [ala-125]) and lymphokine-activated-killer cells in patients with metastatic solid tumors. Eur J Cancer Clin Oncol. 1989;25:965–972.

Stutman O. Tumor development after 3-methylcholanthrene in immunologically deficient athymic nude mice. Science. 1979;183:534–536.

Takeshita T, Asao H, Suzuki J, Sugamura K. An associated molecule, p64, with high affinity IL-2 receptor. Int Immunol. 1990;2:477–480.

Talmadge JE, Meyers KM, Prieur DJ, Starkey JR. Role of NK cells in tumour growth and metastasis in beige mice. Nature. 1980;284:622–624.

Thiele DL, Lipsky PE. The role of surface recognition structures in the initiation of MHC-unrestricted "promiscuous" killing by T cells. Immunol Today. 1989;10:375–381.

Thompson JA, Peace DJ, Klarnet JP, Kern DE, Greenberg PD, Cheever MA. Eradication of disseminated murine leukemia by treatment with high dose interleukin 2. J Immunol. 1986;137:3675–3680.

Thompson JA, Lee DJ, Welby Cox W, et al. Recombinant interleukin 2 toxicity, pharmacokinetics, and immunomodulatory effects in a phase I trial. Cancer Res. 1987;47:4202–4207.

Thompson JA, Lee DJ, Lindgren CG, et al. Influence of dose and duration of infusion of interleukin 2 on toxicity and immunomodulation. J Clin Oncol. 1988;6:669–678.

Thompson JA, Lee DJ, Lindgren CG, et al. Influence of schedule of interleukin 2 administration on therapy with interleukin 2 and lymphokine activated killer cells. Cancer Res. 1989;49:235–240.

Topalian SL, Solomon D, Avis FP, et al. Immunotherapy of patients with advanced cancer using tumor infiltrating lymphocytes and recombinant interleukin 2: a pilot study. J Clin Oncol. 1988;6:839–853.

Tsudo M, Goldman CK, Bongiovani KF, et al. The p75 peptide is the receptor for interleukin 2 expressed on large granular lymphocytes and is responsible for the interleukin 2 activation of these cells. Proc Natl Acad Sci USA. 1987;84:5394–5398.

Tsudo M, Karasuyama H, Kitamura F, et al. The IL-2 receptor β chain (p70): ligand binding ability of the cDNA-encoding membrane and secreted forms. J Immunol. 1990;145:599–606.

Vivier E, Morin P, O'Brian C, et al. Tyrosine phosphorylation of the Fc γRIII (CD16): ζ complex in human natural killer cells. Induction by antibody dependent cytotoxicity but not by natural killing. J Immunol. 1991;146:206–210.

Voss SD, Hank JA, Nobis CA, Fisch P, Sosman JA, Sondel PM. Serum levels of the low-affinity interleukin 2 receptor molecule (TAC) during IL-2 therapy reflect systemic lymphoid mass activation. Cancer Immunol Immunother. 1989;29:261–269.

Voss SD, Robb RJ, Weil-Hillman G, et al. Increased expression of the IL-2 receptor β chain (p70) on $CD56^+$ NK cells following in vivo IL-2 therapy: p70 expression does not alone predict the level of intermediate-affinity IL-2 binding. J Exp Med. 1990;172:1101–1114.

Waldmann TR. The multi-subunit interleukin 2 receptor. Ann Rev Biochem. 1989;58:875–911.

Wiebke EA, Rosenberg SA, Lotze MT. Acute immunologic effects of interleukin 2 therapy on cancer patients: decreased delayed type hypersensitivity response and decreased proliferative response to soluble antigens. J Clin Oncol. 1988;1440–1449.

Weil-Hillman G, Fisch P, Prieve AF, Sosman JA, Hank JA, Sondel PM. Lymphokine activated killer activity induced by in vivo interleukin 2 therapy: predominant role for lymphocytes with increased expression of CD2 and Leu19 antigens but negative expression of CD16 antigens. Cancer Res. 1989;49:3680–3688.

Weil-Hillman G, Voss SD, Fisch P, et al. In vivo interleukin 2 induced lymphokine activated killer activity is mediated by Leu19+ cells which maintain the Tac negative phenotype. Cancer Res. 1990;50:2683–2690.

Weissman AM, Harford JB, Svetlik PB, et al. Only high-affinity receptors for interleukin-2 mediate internalization of ligand. Proc Natl Acad Sci USA. 1986;83:1463–1466.

West WH. Continuous infusion recombinant interleukin 2 (rIL-2) in adoptive cellular therapy of renal carcinoma and other malignancies. Cancer Treat Rev. 1989;16(suppl A):83–89.

West WH, Tauer KW, Yannelli JR, et al. Constant infusion recombinant interleukin 2 in adoptive immunotherapy of cancer. New Engl J Med. 1987;316:898–905.

Whiteside TL. Human tumor-infiltrating lymphocytes and their characterization. In: Lotzova E, Herberman R, eds. IL-2 activated killer cells and cancer treatment. CRC Press; 1989:133–151.

Whiteside TL, Herberman RB. The role of natural killer cells in human disease. Clin Immunol Immunopathol. 1989;53:1–23.

Yagita H, Nakata M, Azuma A, et al. Activation of peripheral blood T cells via the p75 interleukin 2 receptor. J Exp Med. 1989;170:1445–1450.

Yang JC, Mulé JJ, Rosenberg SA. Murine lymphokine-activated killer (LAK) cells: phenotypic characterization of the precursor and effector cells. J Immunol. 1986;137:715–722.

Yang SC, Fry KD, Grimm EA, Roth JA. Successful combination immunotherapy for the generation in vivo of antitumor activity with anti-CD3, interleukin 2, and tumor necrosis factor α. Arch Surg. 1990;125:220–225.

Zurawski SM, Imler JL, Zurawski G. Partial agonist/antagonist mouse interleukin-2 proteins indicate that a third component of the receptor complex functions in signal transduction. EMBO J. 1990;9:3899–3905.

CHAPTER **18**

ANTITUMOR EFFECTS OF INTERFERONS: MECHANISMS AND THERAPEUTIC ACTIVITY

Ernest C. Borden
Patricia L. Witt
Donna M. Paulnock
Sidney Grossberg

Interferons play a key role in host response as pleiotropic modulators of cell function. Interferons are a family of more than 20 proteins produced by almost all vertebrate cells after stimulation by antigens, viruses, double-stranded RNA, and low molecular weight compounds. As induced proteins, interferons contrast with other physiological molecules such as corticoids or albumin, which are relatively continuously produced. The cellular actions of interferons include enhancement of monocyte and natural killer (NK)-cell function, augmentation of tumor-associated antigen (TAA) expression, induction of cellular proteins, inhibition of angiogenesis, and antiproliferative effects. Antitumor effects have been suggested principally to be the result of two mechanisms: a direct effect on the functional capacity or antigenic composition of tumor cells or an indirect effect on modulation of immunological effector-cell populations with tumor specificities. Over the past decade, they have been established as effective therapeutic molecules for malignant and viral diseases (Borden, 1984; Finter, 1986; Mihich, 1986; Bonnem and Oldham, 1987; Tyrrell, 1987; Shearer and Taylor-Papadimitriou, 1987). Our goal will be to review those elements of biological response modification that may underlie antitumor effects and highlight some of the effects of interferons in man (Table 18-1).

INTERFERON MOLECULES AND THEIR RECEPTORS

Although evidence pointed to heterogeneity in the interferon family, the existence of as many as 20 distinct proteins was unexpected prior to the development of recombi-

TABLE 18-1
MECHANISMS UNDERLYING ANTITUMOR ACTIVITY OF INTERFERONS

Biological roles of induced proteins
Surface proteins
Intracellular proteins
Immune effector-cell function
Cytotoxic T-lymphocyte activation
Macrophage activation
NK- and LAK-cell activity
Direct cellular effects
Antiproliferative effects
Cell cycle effects
Interferons and growth factors
Oncogene expression
Differentiation
Inhibition angiogenesis
Therapeutic effects in humans
Hematologic malignancies
Solid tumors

nant DNA (rDNA) technology. Interferon-α, also called type I or leukocyte interferon, is now known to consist of at least 14 subtypes. Interferon-β, also a type I interferon, has been produced by incubation of fibroblasts and many other cell types with double-stranded RNA. Interferon-γ, type II or immune interferon, has been generated by incubation of T lymphocytes with mitogens. A new interferon family, IFN-ω, has been distinguished from other interferons.

The families of interferons were initially characterized by their methods of preparation, antigenicity, and physicochemical properties (Finter, 1986). Confirming these studies, differences in amino acid sequence have now been defined (Taniguchi et al., 1980a, 1980b; Mantei et al., 1980; Goeddel et al., 1980, 1981; Pestka, 1986). Human IFN-α have been shown to consist of 165 or 166 amino acids with differences of 20 to 40 amino acids among subtypes (Goeddel et al., 1981). Interferon-β, also 166 amino acids in length, has been determined to share about 30% homology with IFN-α (Taniguchi et al., 1980b; Derynck et al., 1980). A single gene for human IFN-γ has been described that codes for a protein 143 amino acids in length. Little homology has been demonstrated between IFN-γ and either IFN-α, IFN-β, or IFN-ω. Interferon-ω, previously not distinguished from IFN-α, differs by 40% to 50% in primary amino acid sequence from IFN-α (Capon et al., 1985; Baldwin and Sharp, 1987; Adolf, 1987). The genes for IFN-α, IFN-β, and IFN-ω have been found on chromosome 9 and the one for IFN-γ on chromosome 12.

Alterations in structure of interferons have been made by recombinant DNA technology. Recombinant IFN-β had 10-fold lower activity than the natural molecule, attributed to disulfide bridging between cysteine moieties, which has been eliminated with a serine substitution. Interferon-β_{ser}, produced by substitution of serine for cysteine at amino acid 17, has activity similar to naturally produced interferon (Mark et al., 1984; Colby et al., 1986). Hybrid IFN-α molecules incorporating putative desirable parts of the molecule have also been prepared (Fidler et al., 1987; Horisberger and Starilzky, 1987).

Interferon receptors (10^3–10^4 high-affinity sites/cell) have been found on the surface of most cells, although cell lines without receptors have been identified (Shearer and Taylor-Papadimitriou, 1987). Interferon-α and IFN-β share and compete for the same receptor, while IFN-γ binds to a separate receptor, suggesting that the tertiary structures of α and β interferons may be similar, but that these differ from IFN-γ (Branca and Baglioni, 1981; Anderson et al., 1982). Binding of IFN-β to the nuclear membrane has also been observed (Kushnaryov et al., 1985). The gene for the receptor for human IFN-α and IFN-β is on chromosome 21 while chromosome 6 codes for the human IFN-γ receptor (Chany et al., 1975; Tan, 1976; Rashidbaigi et al., 1986; Aguet et al., 1988).

BIOLOGICAL ROLES OF INDUCED PROTEINS

Interferons, like other cytokines and peptide hormones, interact with cell-surface receptors and induce specific responses in the target cell. Differences between the effects of type I or type II interferons include receptor specificities, transduction pathways and regulation of gene transcription and translation (Williams, 1987), and subsequent changes in enzyme activity and expression of cell-surface proteins (Revel and Chebath, 1986; Pestka et al., 1987). Several transduction mechanisms have been implicated but not proven to be involved: activation of protein kinase C in response to IFN-α, IFN-β, and IFN-γ (Yap et al., 1986; Mehmet et al., 1987; Ito et al., 1988) and involvement of cytoskeletal matrix (Pfeffer et al., 1987). After IFN-γ, stimulation of the G_s guanosine triphosphate (GTP)-binding protein implicates adenylate cyclase and cyclic adenosine monophosphate (cAMP), the second messenger common to many hormone response pathways (Gariglio et al., 1988).

Approximately 15 to 20 proteins or messenger RNA (mRNA) induced by interferons have been identified. Dissecting their function will be essential for elucidating the mechanism of antiproliferative, antiviral, and immunomodulatory activities of interferons (Table 18-2). Increases in these proteins have been identified in cultured cells, in peripheral blood cells, and in serum after administration of interferons. In this section, interferon-induced proteins studied in our laboratory and those of others will be discussed. These include surface proteins, e.g., the major histocompatibility complex (MHC) class II proteins HLA-DR, HLA-DQ, and HLA-DP, β_2-microglobulin which is a component of MHC class I, and specific tumor-associated antigens. Several intracellular enzymes have been characterized, including 2′,5′-oligoadenylate synthetase (2-5AS), indoleamine 2,3 dioxygenase (IDO), and other molecules for which a function has not yet been identified.

TABLE 18-2
CHALLENGES FOR PROBING INTERFERON-INDUCED GENE MODULATION IN MAN

Roles of specific proteins
Induction by specific interferons
Kinetics of expression
Dose response
Correlation with biological effects
Predictive roles for therapeutic response

Surface Proteins

MHC Proteins The most effective modulators of MHC class I are interferons, which increase mRNA accumulation and cell-surface expression (reviewed in Tanaka et al., 1988). T cells recognize foreign antigens presented to them in conjunction with MHC molecules ("MHC restriction"), with cytotoxic T cells responding primarily to MHC class I and helper T cells to class II antigens. Increased MHC antigen surface expression could improve recognition of targets by cytotoxic T lymphocytes (CTL). Such increases have been found on tumor cells (Tanaka et al., 1988). Beta$_2$-microglobulin is a small molecular weight protein noncovalently associated with the MHC class I antigens found on the surface of most cells. Beta$_2$-microglobulin is shed or secreted into the serum (Ramadori et al., 1988) and has been shown by sequence and functional homology to be indistinguishable from thymotaxin, a chemotactic protein (Dargemont et al., 1989). There is also evidence that it functions in transport of class I molecules to the cell surface (Williams et al., 1989).

Most cells express class I antigens, and in vitro studies have shown that these antigens can be upregulated by interferons. Wallach et al. (1982) showed that IFN-γ increased both mRNA and protein levels of class I (HLA-A, B, C) antigens and β_2-microglobulin in human cell lines. These increases were correlated both in time course and dependence on interferon concentration. Type I interferons were effective at slightly higher concentrations than IFN-γ. Interferon treatment in vitro of adenovirus-transformed cells was also demonstrated to decrease their subsequent tumorigenicity in mice (Hayashi et al., 1985), supporting the negative correlation between level of class I antigen expression and tumorigenicity.

In clinical trials, significant increases in β_2-microglobulin have been measured in serum 24 and 48 hours after treatment with interferons. Increases in the mean values in serum were observed after IFN-γ (Paulnock et al., 1989), IFN-β (Borden et al., 1988; Goldstein et al., 1989), and IFN-α (Witt et al., 1989). A significant increase in monocyte surface β_2-microglobulin was also measured in patients receiving IFN-β (Spear et al., 1987) and IFN-γ (Paulnock et al., 1989). A correlation has also been identified between increases in β_2-microglobulin and clinical response to IFN-α in patients with Kaposi's sarcoma (Krown et al., 1989).

An important function of monocytes is to present antigen to helper T lymphocytes in complex with MHC class II antigens HLA-DR, HLA-DQ, and HLA-DP. Interferons, primarily IFN-γ, activate a number of macrophage functions, including surface expression of the MHC class II antigens (Basham et al., 1984), which results in increased T-cell proliferation (Becker, 1985). Increased accumulation of an RNA for class II proteins has been observed within 4 hours after exposure of mouse macrophages to IFN-γ (Paulnock et al., 1985).

Surface expression of HLA-DR and HLA-DQ was measured by flow cytometry as percent positive cells (%+) and mean fluorescence intensity (MFI) on monocytes isolated from cancer patients before and after interferon treatment. Treatment with 0.15 to 15 mg/m^2 IFN-γ showed increases in DRMFI, DR%+, and DQ%+ (Paulnock et al., 1989). Significant increases in DQ%+ and DRMFI were observed after treatment with IFN-β but not after IFN-α (Witt et al., 1989). These studies suggest that the antigen-presenting function of macrophages in vivo is enhanced by IFN-β or IFN-γ administration.

Tumor-Associated Antigens A number of surface proteins relatively specific to tumor cells have been identified by developing monoclonal antibodies (mAb) to them, and studying their distribution. The expression of several of these antigens was increased by interferon, thus potentially increasing their recognition as targets by the body's own antitumor activity by macrophages and other cytotoxic cells. In addition, augmentation of TAA by interferons led to increased binding of monoclonal antibodies for both diagnostic and potentially therapeutic purposes (Greiner et al., 1987). Interferon increased the surface expression of carcinoembryonic antigen (CEA), recognized by Col-4 mAb (Kantor et al., 1989), and mRNA content in some tumor lines (Kantor et al., 1989; Guadagni et al., 1990). A glycoprotein (TAG-72) constitutively expressed on a number of human carcinomas was found to be increased by both type I and type II interferons on both breast and colon cell lines, and on adenocarcinoma cells freshly isolated from patients (Greiner et al., 1984; Guadagni et al., 1989). An intracellular adhesion molecule with a high concentration in metastatic tissue (I-CAM) was induced by IFN-γ and interleukin-1 (IL-1) (Dustin et al., 1986), and a 90-kDa protein associated with human breast cancers was induced by IFN-α and occurred at higher levels in the serum of many cancer patients (Iacobelli et al., 1988). A high molecular weight glycoprotein, CA-125, expressed on the surface of coelomic epithelial cells during embryonic development, was also upregulated by interferons (Marth et al., 1989).

A 16-kDa lymphocyte surface antigen (Leu-13), which induces T-cell aggregation and proliferation, was upregulated on human endothelial cells by IFN-γ (Jaffe et al., 1989).

Intracellular Proteins

2′,5′-Oligoadenylate Synthetase The intracellular enzyme 2-5AS synthesizes from adenosine triphosphate (ATP), a polyadenylate that, in turn, activates a ribonuclease. It is induced preferentially by type I interferons and is part of pathways for interferons' antiviral activity (Chebath et al., 1987) and possibly antiproliferative activity (Kimchi et al., 1981; Creasey et al., 1983; Rosenblum et al., 1986). Increased enzyme levels have been measured in peripheral blood cells of individuals with viral infections (Schattner et al., 1982), including acquired immunodeficiency syndrome (AIDS) (Preble et al., 1985; Read et al., 1985). Type I interferons increased enzyme activity in virtually all cultured cell types (Stark et al., 1979).

Significant increases of 2- to 13-fold in 2-5AS activity have been measured after clinical administration of IFN-α or IFN-β to patients with a variety of malignancies (Merritt et al., 1985, 1986; Krown et al., 1987; Rinehart et al., 1987; Borden et al., 1988; Goldstein et al., 1989). Increases after IFN-γ were observed in some studies (Paulnock et al., 1989), but not in others (Rinehart et al., 1986). In a retrospective statistical analysis of approximately 275 patients, IFN-α was a better inducer of 2-5AS than IFN-β, and IFN-β in turn better than IFN-γ (Witt et al., 1989).

Correlations between increases in 2-5AS activity and clinical response have been found in several studies. In a study of 14 patients with chronic myelogenous leukemia (CML), a 10-fold increase in 2-5AS activity was observed in the responding patients compared to a sevenfold increase in those who did not respond (Rosenblum et al., 1986). In a similar study of 10 patients with chronic lymphocytic leukemia (CLL), 2-5AS was induced in all patients responding to therapy, but only minimally in two thirds of patients failing therapy (Talpaz et al., 1987). A correlation between the ability of IFN-α to induce blast transformation and differentiation and 2-5AS induction was identified in malignant cells from 24 patients with CLL (Ostlünd et al., 1986a).

In a study of 35 patients with chronic hepatitis B treated with IFN-α (17) and IFN-β (18) and monitored over 2 years, 2-5AS activity increased more in patients who improved (became negative for HBV DNA polymerase and for HBe antigen) than in patients who did not (Nishiguchi et al., 1989). Patient peripheral blood mononuclear cells (PBMC) were also treated with interferons in vitro and 2-5AS activity was measured, yielding a correlation of 0.68 between in vivo and in vitro increases. Similar results were obtained by Karino et al. (1989). Thus patients' PBMC could be tested in vitro to predict potential response.

Protein Kinase Another protein that, like 2-5AS, is induced by interferons and activated by double-stranded RNA is a protein kinase with a molecular weight of about 68 kDa. This enzyme phosphorylates a subunit of protein synthesis initiation factor eIF-2, inhibiting initiation of protein synthesis in a cell-free system. The time course of phosphorylation has been correlated with establishment of an antiviral state in cells (Samuel, 1979; Samuel and Knutson, 1982). Recently, the *tat* or transactivating protein response (TAR) region of the human immunodeficiency virus (HIV-1) mRNA has been shown to activate this kinase (Edery et al., 1989). A decrease in kinase was observed during HIV infection in HeLa cells. However, responsiveness to interferons in general did not decrease, since induction of 2-5AS was not different in *tat*-positive and *tat*-negative cells (Roy et al., 1990). The *tat*-gene product may in part counter the antiviral state established by the kinase and possibly other interferon-inducible proteins.

Indoleamine 2,3 Dioxygenase The intracellular enzyme IDO, which degrades tryptophan to kynurenine, has been shown to increase in human PBMC in culture after IFN-α, IFN-β, or IFN-γ and interleukin-2 (IL-2), but not tumor necrosis factor-α (TNF-α) (Carlin et al., 1987, 1989b). Induction of IDO was also shown by IFN-γ but not by IFN-α or IFN-β in human cell lines (Takikawa et al., 1988; Werner et al., 1989). The ability of IFN-γ to induce IDO has been correlated with its antiproliferative activity through deprivation of the essential amino acid, L-tryptophan (Ozaki et al., 1988). Interferon-β also induces IDO in patients (Carlin et al., 1989a).

Other Proteins A specific protein induced in mice by type I interferon, which confers resistance to influenza virus in Mx^+ but not Mx^- mice, was identified as having a molecular weight of approximately 78 kDa (Horisberger et al., 1983; Dreiding et al., 1985). Transformation of 3T3 cells with the cloned Mx gene conferred selective resistance to influenza virus (Staeheli et al., 1986), confirming the identity of this gene. A human protein was subsequently purified having molecular weight, pI, amino-acid composition, antigenic determinants, and interferon inducibility similar to those of the mouse protein, although the function remains unknown (Horisberger and Hochkeppel, 1987). This protein was also induced in PBMC isolated from cancer patients treated with IFN-β and IFN-γ (Schiller et al., 1990).

Several other interferon-induced proteins of unknown function have been evaluated. A cytoplasmic guanylate binding protein of 68 kDa is induced in several human cell types in vitro by type I interferons (Cheng et al., 1983, 1985) and induced approximately twofold in vivo after treatment with either IFN-β or IFN-γ (Cheng et al., 1988). In addition, the p78 protein described above was shown to have guanylate-binding properties (Staeheli et al., 1984). A cytoplasmic protein of 56 kDa, induced by all three types of interferons, has also been partially sequenced and an antibody made to it (Cheng et al., 1983, 1985, 1988; Rubin et al., 1988). A protein of 15 kDa was found to be secreted from human or bovine cells treated with type I or II interferons (Korant et al., 1984) and a complementary DNA (cDNA) has been isolated from IFN-β–treated human Daudi cells (Blomstrom et al., 1986). Another protein of 30 kDa of unknown function has been induced in hematopoietic cells (Luster et al., 1988). Studies are continuing to identify the roles of these proteins in the complex action of interferons.

CELLULAR EFFECTS

Interferons are host-protective molecules that should be considered as much "procell" as "antivirus." Interferons have multiple effects on cell physiology, both inhibitory and stimulatory (Table 18-3). The interferon system causes complex network effects that may alter or be altered by other networks, for example, those involving growth factors, hormones in the adrenal–pituitary axis, drug detoxification systems, as well as other cytokines such as tumor necrosis factor (TNF) and the interleukins (reviewed by Grossberg, 1987; Pestka et al., 1987; De Maeyer and De Maeyer-Guignard, 1988; Taylor and Grossberg, 1990).

TABLE 18-3
CELLULAR EFFECTS OF INTERFERONS

Antimicrobial effects
RNA viruses
DNA viruses
Intracellular pathogens
Antiproliferative actions
Retards mitotic cycle time
Enhanced differentiation
Depression oncogenes
Increased cell-surface proteins
Tumor-associated antigens
Major histocompatibility complex
Enzyme induction
2′,5′-oligoadenylate synthetase
Protein kinase
Indoleamine 2,3 dioxygenase
Increased immune effector-cell activity
T cell (MHC-restricted)
Non-MHC–restricted monocyte
Macrophage activation
Toxic oxygen intermediates
Secretion of monokines

Cell Proliferation

In 1962, partially purified interferon preparations were shown to inhibit proliferation of cultured mouse cells (Paucker et al., 1962). More than a decade and a half passed before it was established that highly purified interferons, and not contaminants in impure preparations, were the inhibitory substances. Interferons retard the growth and proliferation of tumor cells, as well as normal cells, by prolonging the cell cycle. There are substantial differences among normal cells and tumor cells in their sensitivity to direct antiproliferative actions, with some being extremely sensitive and others completely resistant (Tsuruo et al., 1982; Taylor et al., 1984). Most studies on the effects of interferons on cell division have utilized continuous lines of tumor cells, but also fibroblasts and normal cells from liver, mammary epithelium, vascular smooth muscle, and endothelium (Frayssinet et al., 1973; Balkwill et al., 1978; Heyns et al., 1985; Schiller et al., 1986). Only a small number of differentiated and undifferentiated normal cells derived from bone marrow and the immune system have been systematically tested for their antiproliferative sensitivity to interferons. The human lymphoblastoid B-cell lines transformed by Epstein-Barr virus (EBV) are extraordinarily sensitive to the antiproliferative action of Hu IFN-α, and IFN-β, but not IFN-γ. Another EBV-transformed lymphoblastoid cell line (Namalwa), a vigorous producer of IFN-α subtypes, is essentially resistant to the action of interferons. Whereas IFN-α and IFN-β appear to act to oppose growth factors and mitogens of different types in a manner resembling the autocrine regulation of cell division, IFN-γ does not seem to be so involved. Interferon-resistant mutant cells can be isolated from interferon-sensitive cell lines (Gresser et al., 1974). Since the resistant mutants can sometimes retain their antiviral sensitivity (Lin et al., 1982), the resistance is not necessarily due to the reduced number, or absence, of interferon receptors, but may point to some other mechanism of growth-inhibitory action. Melanoma cells (both human and murine) initially sensitive to growth inhibition by IFN-α and IFN-β became resistant to these interferons but retained their initial sensitivity to IFN-γ (Fleischmann and Fleischmann, 1988). It is possible that established tumor cell lines become resistant to interferons because of selection during maintenance in vitro or in vivo. However, freshly isolated tumor cells can also be resistant to this interferon effect with a range in sensitivity from complete inhibition to total resistance that does not correlate with tumor cell type.

Cell Cycle Effects

Interferon-α and IFN-β can affect all phases of the cell cycle, that is, the M phase (mitosis and cell division), the G_1 phase (in which there is variable synthetic activity), the S phase (when new DNA synthesis occurs), and the G_2 phase (the period between the completion of DNA synthesis and mitosis). When fibroblasts were stimulated to grow by serum, epidermal growth factor, insulin, or vasopressin, interferon caused a marked prolongation of the G_1 phase, a reduced rate of entry into the S phase, and a lengthening of the S and the G_2 phases (Sokawa et al., 1977; Balkwill and Taylor-Papadimitriou, 1978; Sreevalsan et al., 1979). Human diploid fibroblasts treated with IFN-β were prolonged in all phases in their cell cycle, with doubling time increasing as much as three times. Synthetic rates of protein, RNA, and DNA were minimally affected such that DNA in proteins accumulated and the cells became enlarged (Pfeffer et al., 1979). Mouse mammary tumor cells treated with IFN-α/β were delayed in their G_1 phase, an effect that became more marked with each succeeding generation (D'Hooghe et al., 1977). Similarly, the G_0/G_1 phase of human melanoma cells treated with human leukocyte IFN-α was significantly prolonged, such that the entry into the S phase was delayed (Creasey et al., 1981). Ehrlich ascites tumor cells treated with IFN-α/β prolonged their cell cycle, with little effect on macromolecular synthesis, such that cell size increased and cell separation diminished, resulting in multinucleated cells (Panniers and Clemens, 1981). Human tumor cells of different tissue origins also increased in size after treatment with human lymphoblastoid IFN-α, human leukocyte-α or Hu IFN-β (Shibata and Taylor-Papadimitriou, 1981; Pfeffer and Tamm, 1983). The cumulative effects of the prolongation of the cell cycle of both normal and tumor cells by IFN-α/β can result in cytostasis. In the case of a human lymphoblastoid cell line, the cells not only ceased to proliferate, but began to die (Gewert et al., 1984).

Cytokine Interactions

Combinations of different types of interferons (α or β combined with γ) have been shown to be synergistic in their antiproliferative effects (Fleischmann et al., 1984; Schiller et al., 1986). In contrast, interferons antagonize in a reciprocal fashion the effects of growth factors, the relatively cell-specific proteins that bind to high-affinity cell-surface receptors to stimulate cell growth and division. Interferons block growth factor–induced entry of cells into S phase, and growth factors reverse the antimitotic effects of interferons. The growth of quiescent cells stimulated to undergo DNA synthesis by platelet-derived growth factor (PDGF), epidermal growth factor (EGF), or fibroblast growth factor (FGF), as well as other mitogenic stimuli can be inhibited by IFN-α or IFN-β. This antiproliferative effect has been observed when as many as three different mitogens are used in combination; however, when four or more of such factors are combined, the antiproliferative effects of even high doses of interferons can be overcome (Taylor-Papadimitriou et al., 1981), even when the growth factors are added after interferons. The antiviral action of interferons, however, is not reversed by the addition of the growth factors (Sreevalson et al., 1980; Taylor-Papadimitriou et al., 1981). With low concentrations of serum, which ordinarily contain several mitogens, the addition singly of PDGF, EGF, or FGF was not enough to overcome the antiproliferative effect of IFN-β (Oleszak and Inglot, 1980). On the other hand, interferons can inhibit the mitogenicity of growth factors. Recombinant IFN-α2 inhibited PDGF-stimulated growth of bovine vascular smooth muscle cells and FGF-induced growth of vascular epithelial cells (Heyns et al., 1985). The level of some PDGF-induced mRNA, including c-*myc* mRNA, was slightly enhanced by interferons, whereas the secretion of several PDGF-induced proteins was impaired (Tominaga and Lengyel, 1985; Lin et al., 1986).

Since several growth factors and cytokines induce interferon, late activation of the interferon mechanism may be part of a negative feedback regulation of cell replication. For example, PDGF-stimulated mouse 3T3 fibroblast activated the IFN-β gene as one of several late-activated genes (Zullo et al., 1985). Tumor necrosis factor-α can stimulate the proliferation of human diploid fibroblasts, and the addition of anti–IFN-β antibody enhanced this mitogenic effect (Ruggiero et al., 1989). Tumor necrosis factor can also stimulate interleukin-6 (previously designated IFN-β_2) which in turn can stimulate anti–IFN-β production, so that one or both factors might act as feedback autoregulatory inhibitors of cell division (Kohase et al., 1986; Zilberstein et al., 1986). When bone marrow stem cells were stimulated to proliferate and differentiate by macrophage growth factor CSF-1, the cells produced IFN-α or IFN-β, which could be neutralized by adding anti-interferon antibody (Moore et al., 1984). Interferon-α/β inhibited colony formation of bone marrow–derived macrophages and granulocytes stimulated by colony-stimulating factor (CSF-1) (Klimpel et al., 1982). When anti–IFN-β antibodies were added to cultures of human melanoma cells stimulated by growth factors in fresh serum, the entry of cells into S phase was accelerated (Creasey et al., 1983).

Oncogene Expression

Oncogenes are cellular or viral genes that can cause normal cells to acquire the characteristics of malignantly transformed cells by altering the regulation of cell division or differentiation. Oncogene products include normal or altered growth factors, growth factor receptors, tyrosine or serine/threonine kinases, and nuclear DNA-binding proteins. Proto-oncogenes, cellular genes with a high degree of sequence homology with retroviral oncogenes, may become activated or expressed abnormally as a result of DNA rearrangements, amplification resulting in multiple oncogene copies, chromosomal translocations, point mutations, or insertions of promoters of transcriptional enhancer elements (Bishop, 1987; Klein, 1988; Storms and Bose, 1989).

The cellular *myc* proto-oncogene is the homologue of the avian myelocytomatosis (leukemia) virus oncogene. The c-*myc* gene (present on human chromosome 8) codes for a nuclear dsDNA-binding protein present in avian, murine, and human cells and has been implicated in DNA synthesis. Treatment of cells with PDGF activates a number of competence genes, including c-*myc,* which are in turn inhibited by interferon treatment. Interferons also downregulate c-*myc* expression in Daudi cells from Burkitt's lymphoma (Clemens et al., 1988) in which the c-*myc* gene has been translocated from chromosome 8 to 14. Indeed, endogenous IFN-β acted as an autocrine growth inhibitor during terminal differentiation of hematopoietic cells (Resnitzky et al., 1986) and may be considered as an antioncogene; the inhibitory effects of IFN-γ and TNF on c-*myc* were found to be additive (Kimchi, 1987).

The c-*fos* proto-oncogene, present on human chromosome 14, is constitutively expressed to high levels in bone marrow cells and differentiated macrophages and has been induced by the macrophage-specific growth factor CSF-1 (M-CSF), which itself will induce IFN-α/β (Gonda and Metcalf, 1984; Müller et al., 1985). Platelet-derived growth factor and CSF-1 activated the c-*fos* gene prior to the activation of the IFN-α/β genes. Interferon-α/β rapidly inhibited the increase in c-*fos* mRNA after PDGF stimulation (Einat et al., 1985). This downregulatory effect of interferons on c-*fos* expression suggests a negative feedback regulation.

Four members of the human *ras* gene family are homologous to oncogenes of the murine sarcoma viruses; c-Harvey (Ha)-*ras* has been identified on human chromosome 11, c-Kirsten (Ki)-*ras* on human chromosome 12, and r-*ras* on chromosome 19. All members of the *ras* gene family code for antigenically similar proteins of molecular weights of about 21 kDa. The *ras* genes have been detected in various human cancers and are activated to oncogenes by point mutations, linkage to a long terminal repeat, or amplification of copy number. Mouse 3T3 cells transformed with the human Ha-*ras*-1 gene and cultured continuously in the presence of murine IFN-α/β produced revertant colonies in which transcription of the *ras* gene was inhibited. After interferon treatment, most cells kept the revertant phenotype during many cell generations despite renewed high levels of transcription of the *ras* gene and of p21 *ras* protein (Samid et al., 1986; Samid and Friedman, 1986). Interferon-β decreased expression of c-Ha-*ras* in human bladder carcinoma cells but not the expression of the c-Ki-*ras* gene (Soslau et al., 1984). Expression of the *ras* gene, however, can block antiviral and antiproliferative activities of IFN-γ (Gariglio et al., 1989), as well as its ability to induce MHC class II antigens (Morris et al., 1989). The expression in transformed cells of the *src* gene, introduced by the avian Rous sarcoma virus (which codes for a tyrosine kinase), was reduced by interferons (Lin et al., 1983). Interferon reduced expression of *src* as well as c-Ha-*ras* in RT4 bladder carcinoma cells (Samid et al., 1984).

The c-*mos* proto-oncogene is the cellular homologue of a similar gene of the murine Moloney sarcoma virus present on human chromosome 8. It codes for a cytoplasmic protein with serine/threonine kinase activity. In myeloma cells, the normal c-*mos* gene undergoes rearrangement to become transcriptionally active from a normally quiescent state. Interferon-α/β treatment of Moloney sarcoma virus–transformed mouse fibroblasts selected a cell population that had reverted to a nonmalignant, stable state even after interferon had been withdrawn (Sergiescu et al., 1986). Phenotype reversion from malignancy to a noncancerous state by interferons occurred without extinguishing oncogene expression.

Differentiation

Interferons have altered differentiation of different kinds of cells (Taylor et al., 1984). Growth inhibition of the B-cell lymphoblastoid Daudi cell line by IFN-α was accompanied by plasmacytoid differentiation and the lack of response to autocrine growth factors (Exley et al., 1987). Interferon-α, IFN-β, and IFN-γ induced B-cell blast transformation, as well as plasmacytoid differentiation, in chronic lymphocytic leukemic cells in some patients (Einhorn et al., 1985; Ostlünd et al., 1986b). Treatment of HL-60 promyelocytic leukemia cells with various recombinant IFN-α subtypes alone or in combination with retinoic acid resulted in enhancement of differentiation (Lin and Sartorelli, 1987). When HL-60 cells were stimulated to differentiate with dimethyl sulfoxide (DMSO), they were not only markedly inhibited by IFN-β but also died, a cytocidal effect rarely observed after interferon treatment (Hamburger et al., 1985). Erythroleukemic cells (transformed by Friend murine leukemia virus and treated with DMSO) were inhibited to differentiate by high doses of IFN-α/β, but stimulated to do so by low doses (Affabris et al., 1988). Human IFN-α, given to nude mice bearing xenografts of human osteosarcoma, inhibited tumor growth. In some cases, the sarcoma was replaced by normal bone and marrow, an effect most likely explained by tumor differentiation following blockade of cellular proliferation (Brosjö et al., 1987).

Differentiation of normal, nontransformed cells can also be altered by interferons. Mouse 3T3-L1 fibroblasts that can be stimulated to differentiate into adipocytes by insulin, were inhibited by treatment with IFN-α, IFN-β, or IFN-γ (Keay and Grossberg, 1980); this inhibition could not be correlated with activation of the protein kinase system (Taylor et al., 1988). Interferon-α and IFN-β inhibited maturation of monocytes into macrophages (Lee and Epstein, 1980). Interferon-γ also inhibited the B-cell proliferation and differentiation induced by interleukin-4 (IL-4) (Rousset et al., 1988).

On the other hand, interferons have stimulated cells to differentiate; for example, IFN-α2 treatment of a cytotoxic T lymphocyte (CTL) clone caused rearrangement of the T-cell receptor gene, with T-cell differentiation (Chen et al., 1986a). Further, recombinant IFN-γ treatment of human keratinocytes caused a change from small basal-type cells to large, mature-type keratinocytes, and IFN-α/β stimulated keratin synthesis in cultured mouse epidermal cells (Nikoloff et al., 1986). Thus, the effects of interferon on differentiation may vary with the cell type, as well as with the type and even the dose of interferon.

Several observations have raised the possibility that interferons may progressively cause reversion of the transformed phenotype of some malignant cells treated continuously with interferons. A stepwise progressive reversion of the transformed phenotype to a nontransformed phenotype occurred when X-ray-transformed mouse fibroblasts were cultivated and passaged in the continuous presence of mouse IFN-α/β. The cells no longer produced tumors in nude mice and their morphology changed from fibroblastic to epithelioid. When interferon treatment ceased, they reverted to the transformed phenotype and became tumorigenic again (Brouty-Boye and Gresser, 1981). Further, mouse fibroblasts transformed by murine sarcoma virus that were similarly maintained in the presence of mouse IFN-α/β showed decreased saturation density, formed fewer foci when plated on normal cell monolayers, and became more anchorage-dependent, forming fewer colonies in soft agar (Hicks et al., 1981). Mouse embryonic fibroblasts transformed by Moloney sarcoma virus recovered their normal morphological phenotype, lost their ability to form colonies in agar, and failed to produce tumors in nude mice (Chany-Fournier, 1983; Sergiescu et al., 1986). Murine leukemia Kirstin virus-transformed cells treated with IFN-α/β reverted to a more normal phenotype; however, tumorigenic activity was potentiated (Brouty-Boye, 1986). Tumor cell lines derived from human osteosarcoma, as well as from bladder, colon, and ovarian carcinomas, that were serially passaged in the presence of IFN-α, did not reverse their tumor phenotype as measured by suppressed tumorigenicity in nude mice. Indeed, one line of bladder tumor cells seemed to become more tumorigenic in nude mice than cells not treated with interferon (Brouty-Boye, 1986). Thus, it has not been possible to predict what change in phenotype may occur by long-term in vitro exposure to interferon.

IMMUNE EFFECTOR-CELL FUNCTION

Although components of the cellular immune response that serve as the basis for successful tumor eradication in vivo remain incompletely understood, interferons have positive regulatory effects on three cellular components believed to be involved in antitumor immunity: (1) CTL, which recognize TAA in conjunction with MHC antigens; (2) non-MHC–restricted NK cells and lymphokine-activated (LAK) cells, which do not require prior stimulation by specific antigen for their activity; and (3) macrophages. As a result, efforts at elucidating the mechanisms of action of interferons in vivo have focused on assessment of changes in the functional parameters of these cell types.

Effects on Cytotoxic T Lymphocyte Activation

Studies in the murine system have suggested that a principal effector cell active in host defense against tumors is the antigen-specific CTL. Examples of systems providing evidence in support of this hypothesis are those of mice bearing ultraviolet light (UV)-induced neoplasms (Urban and Schreiber, 1983) and mice inoculated with the B16 melanoma (Talmadge, 1988). In these systems, CTL isolated from tumor-bearing animals were capable of specific tumoricidal activity and were found to be capable of initiating tumor regression in some instances (Urban and Schreiber, 1983; Talmadge, 1988). Similar measurements of cellular responses in patients with a variety of tumors have suggested that tumors also can induce tumor-specific T-cell responses (Mitsuya et al., 1983; DeVries and Spits, 1984). Although the tumor determinants responsible for eliciting these responses in general remain uncharacterized, the question of how the generation of cytotoxicity is regulated in these populations during tumor growth and development merits pursuit.

With regard to the role of interferons in the development of a productive CTL response, a number of recent studies have analyzed both the role of interferons in the activation of T lymphocytes in general and of CTL in particular. The results have suggested multiple activities for this lymphokine family. Initial studies clearly demonstrated that IFN-γ could augment the generation of CTL in vitro and that this activity could be blocked by neutralizing antibody to IFN-γ (Farrar et al., 1981; Landolfo et al., 1985; Simon et al., 1986). However, questions still remain as to which stage of CTL development was directly affected by IFN-γ. Recent studies have suggested that this positive effect on CTL development is the result of two distinct actions of interferons. First, IFN-γ has a direct effect on mature $CD8^+$ T cells (Siegel, 1988). This activity appears restricted to IFN-γ; IFN-α was ineffective. Mechanistically, this effect involved upregulation of the IL-2 receptor α chain by IFN-γ, resulting in augmented proliferative capacity of the $CD8^+$ lymphocytes (Siegel, 1988). In addition to a direct effect on mature CTL, there is evidence in murine models of CTL development for a role for IFN-γ in the differentiation of CTL precursors to mature effector cells (Finke et al., 1983; Gromo et al., 1987; Raulet and Bevan, 1987). Studies with human cells have confirmed that IFN-γ also can play an early role in CTL development (Chen et al., 1986b). Thus, IFN-γ appears to play an important role in both induction and early development of CTL and in expansion and survival of committed cytotoxic cells.

Specifically immune CTL have been shown to be effective in the modulation of tumor growth in animal model systems. However, few clinical trials of interferons have assessed CTL function. This is largely because the MHC-restriction of CTL development and function makes the assays for the presence of CTL difficult on a large-scale basis. Thus, although a role for IFN-γ in potentiating antitumor CTL activity in vivo in humans remains a strong possibility, this has not been explored in clinical trials.

Effects on Macrophage Activation

Macrophages comprise the second key cellular component of effective tumor immunity identified in animal model systems (Urban and Schreiber, 1983; Fernandez-Cruz et al., 1985; Talmadge, 1988). As for most other macrophage functions, an antitumor role for macrophages is dependent on activating functional capacity of these cells. Analysis of the role of interferons in macrophage activation has emphasized assessment of both efferent and afferent macrophages in direct antitumor cytolytic activity and accessory cell function.

Studies in murine systems have defined a series of steps, each requiring a specific signaling ligand for activation of macrophage tumoricidal function (Ruco and Meltzer, 1978). The first activation signal is provided by IFN-γ, which primes macrophages for response to a second signal (Pace et al., 1983). This second signal, which can be provided by bacterial lipopolysaccharide (LPS) and other mediators (Meltzer, 1981), actually triggers cytolytic activity. This activation scheme also has been applied to human monocytes, although the requirement for two signals appears less strict in the human system (Philip and Epstein, 1986). In both man and mouse, activated macrophages exhibit specific lytic activity against a wide variety of tumor cells, using a recognition mechanism that remains undefined. The actual tumoricidal effects result from the secretion by activated cells of one of a number of cytolytic substances (TNF-α, reactive oxygen intermediates, and arginase), each of which may be active on selected tumor target cell types (Hamilton and Adams, 1987). Interferon-α, IFN-β and IFN-γ have priming capacity for murine and human macrophages; however, IFN-γ has the more potent priming signal (Jett et al., 1980; Roberts and Vasil, 1982; Basham et al., 1984). One explanation for differences in potency may lie in the ability of the different interferons to induce distinct signaling mechanisms. Signaling pathways may be controlled at the level of receptor–ligand interactions, as each interferon class binds to a distinct cell-surface receptor (Rubin and Gupta, 1980; Forti et al., 1984 and discussed above). Although the mechanisms associated with interferon-mediated macrophage activation remain largely unknown, the acquisition of macrophage tumoricidal function involves substantial changes in the protein mosaic of the activated cell (Gonwa et al., 1983; MacKay and Russell, 1986; Paulnock and Lambert, 1990). Thus, current efforts toward a more detailed understanding of the activation process are centered on elucidation of the signal transduction mechanisms required for effective macrophage stimulation and on identification of the functional role of induced proteins and genes.

A second role proposed for activated macrophages in the development of tumor immunity is that of an antigen-presenting cell capable of the stimulation of antigen-specific helper T cells. This general accessory cell function of macrophages is enhanced by interferons as a result of induction of expression of MHC-encoded class II antigens on the macrophage cell surface. Increased levels of class II antigen expression ultimately lead to MHC-restricted presentation of tumor antigens to helper T-cell stimulation (Gonwa et al., 1983). Both classes of interferons possess the capacity to induce MHC antigen expression, although in vitro studies of murine and human cells suggest that IFN-γ is more effective (Basham et al., 1984; Wallach et al., 1982). In response to effective macrophage antigen presentation, activated helper T cells both enter a proliferative phase of clonal expansion and begin to produce a variety of lymphokines. These endogenous mediators, which include IFN-γ and IL-2 serve subsequently to activate both non–T-cell effector mechanisms, including tumoricidal macrophages and LAK cells, as well as to aid in CTL development. In this way, effective stimulation of macrophage antigen-presenting cell function would be a key requirement for the development of a productive antitumor immune response composed of multiple cellular elements.

Because macrophages and monocytes exhibit specific cytotoxicity toward malignant cells in vitro, they have been targets for assessment of efficacy of interferons in vivo. Trials have evaluated development of activated macrophages following administration of interferons, using either macrophage functional activity or production of various secreted factors as markers for the activated state (Rhodes et al., 1983; Nathan et al., 1985; Kleinerman et al., 1986; Spear et al., 1987; Maluish et al., 1988; Paulnock et al., 1989). Peripheral blood monocytes obtained from patients receiving IFN-γ were more cytotoxic for tumor cells (Kleinerman et al., 1986). Other studies have suggested that monocyte activity is enhanced in patients receiving IFN-γ, using as markers for activated cells either monocyte-mediated antitumor cytostatic activity (Maluish et al., 1988) or production of hydrogen peroxide (Nathan et al., 1985). With regard to antigen-presenting cell function, several studies suggest that changes in histocompatibility antigen expression can occur in patients in response to IFN-α, IFN-β, and IFN-γ (Rhodes et al., 1983; Spear et al., 1987; Paulnock et al., 1989). Thus, evidence for effective stimulation of multiple aspects of monocyte function by interferons in vivo has been observed, suggesting these cells may be sensitive and important for host response alterations with interferons. Determining whether changes observed in monocyte and macrophage function can be linked to positive therapeutic effects will be an important goal of future studies. However, route, dose, and schedule of interferon administration can affect the nature and extent of cellular modulation achieved with these mediators (Rhodes et al., 1983; Kleinerman et al., 1986; Maluish et al., 1988; Paulnock et al., 1989). Immunomodulatory effects may be obtained at interferon dose levels considerably less than the maximum tolerated dose.

Effects on NK- and LAK-Cell Activity

The role of interferons in potentiating the activity of nonspecific cytotoxic effector cells other than macrophages also has been assessed in dissecting the antitumor potential. Natural killer cell activation has received perhaps the most attention to date. The wide range of target cells susceptible to NK cell–mediated cytolytic activity suggests that their activation may play an important role in some phases of host defense against tumors (Herberman, 1982). Both IFN-α and IFN-γ can stimulate NK-cell activity in murine and human systems. Natural killer cell activity in murine spleen was markedly enhanced by IFN-α administered in vivo or in vitro (Brunda and Rosenbaum, 1984).

Interferon-γ has augmented murine NK-cell activity after administration in vivo or in vitro (Djeu et al., 1979; Kuribayashi et al., 1981); however, this effect has not always been observed (Brunda et al., 1986). Levels of human peripheral blood NK-cell cytotoxicity have also been augmented by interferons; interferons may contribute directly to NK-cell maturation and/or activation. Interferons also have been shown to accelerate the kinetics of lysis and degree of killer cell recycling and to increase production of NK-cell cytotoxic factors (Silva et al., 1980; Gustaffson and Lundgren, 1981; Wright and Bonavida, 1983).

Extension of these in vitro studies to patients receiving interferons has suggested that effects of interferons on NK-cell function are complex. Interferon-α may either augment (Lotzova et al., 1983; Edwards et al., 1984; Hawkins et al., 1984; Neefe et al., 1985) or depress (Lotzova et al., 1983; Maluish et al., 1983) the peripheral blood NK-cell cytotoxicity of cancer patients. Analysis of the dose–response relationship suggests that, as in the case of macrophage function, the dose of interferon administered has differential effects on NK-cell function (Edwards et al., 1985), with lower doses often demonstrating enhanced biological activity. These results once again emphasize the bell-shaped dose–response curve for the in vivo efficacy of these regulatory factors (Talmadge, 1988).

There is a complex relationship between the ability of interferons and IL-2 to modulate natural cytotoxic cell activity, including both NK- and LAK-cell function. Lymphokine-activated killer cells are defined as those cytotoxic cells developing from peripheral blood lymphocytes (PBL) cultured with IL-2, in the absence of any antigen or mitogen (Grimm et al., 1982). Interleukin-2 can stimulate both NK and LAK cells directly (Brunda et al., 1986; Grimm et al., 1982); however, interferons can act with IL-2 to modulate NK- and LAK-cell activity. For example, IFN-γ has been shown to augment IL-2–induced LAK-cell activity (Itoh et al., 1985), while IFN-α and IFN-β appear to inhibit LAK-cell activity and development (Sone et al., 1988). A role for interferon in modulating IL-2 receptor expression has been proposed (Riccardi et al., 1983; Sone et al., 1988). In turn, it also has been proposed that IL-2 enhances NK-cell function through its induction of IFN-γ, perhaps providing a circuit of activation for these two lymphokines (Torres et al., 1982). These interactions may be clinically relevant and of particular importance in the development of effective protocols for therapeutic use of these cytokines (Sedman et al., 1988).

ANTITUMOR ACTIVITY IN HUMANS

Interferons have proven active as single agents in inducing tumor regressions in more than a dozen different neoplasms (for detailed reviews of clinical activity, see Krown, 1986; Goldstein and Laszlo, 1986; Kovach, 1987; Borden, 1988). In general, interferons have had greater therapeutic effectiveness for hematologic malignancies than for solid tumors. Interferon-α2 was the first previously unlicensed therapeutic produced by rDNA technology, to be approved for marketing by the US Food and Drug Administration. Interferons are also the first human proteins to be effective as a cancer treatment modality; we will focus on a limited sample of therapeutic results. However, like other potent physiological products such as glucocorticoids, interferons have toxicities when administered with pharmacological intent (Table 18-4). A detailed review of toxicities has been published (Quesada et al., 1986).

Hematologic Malignancies

In the chronic leukemias, (chronic myelogenous leukemia [CML] and hairy-cell leukemia [HCL]), IFN-α has resulted in therapeutic response in a majority (>75%) of patients. In addition to reduction in leukemic cell mass, IFN-α has resulted in improvements in quality of life. A significant reduction in requirements for red cell and platelet transfusion and a decrease in incidence of infections have resulted (Ratain et al., 1987). In CML, a gradual reduction has occurred in frequency of cells bearing the underlying 9-22 chromosomal translocations (Talpaz et al., 1986; Alimena et al., 1988). Duration of treatment for these disorders remains uncertain. However, the time required to induce objective hematologic response suggests the need for relatively continuous treatment.

In multiple myeloma, optimal doses, schedules, and disease stage for treatment have yet to be identified. Response rates of only 8% to 18% were observed when patients with advanced disease were treated on various schedules (Quesada et al., 1984; Wagstaff et al., 1985; Costanzi et al., 1985). When 27 patients who received 12×10^6 U/m^2 of IFN-α2 IM daily were analyzed according to prior therapy, 7 of 14 (50%) of previously untreated patients had responded (Quesada et al., 1986). Similarly, patients who had received only phenylalanine mustard and prednisone had a 40% response rate (Costanzi et al., 1985). In patients who had a tumor response, levels of serum immunoglobulins were restored, an effect infrequently seen with chemotherapy

TABLE 18-4
CLINICAL SIDE EFFECTS OF INTERFERON*

Acute	Chronic
Chills	Fatigue
Fever	Anorexia
Malaise	Mild neutropenia
Myalgias	Transaminase elevations
Mild neutropenia	Diarrhea
Less common: mental slowing, confusion, hair shedding, thrombocytopenia, nausea, vomiting	Depression

*Summarized in greater detail (Quesada et al., 1986.)

(Quesada et al., 1985b). Some complete responses (CR) persisted for over 2 years (Costanzi et al., 1985; Quesada et al., 1985b), an unusual event in myeloma. Thus, interferons will probably eventually become part of the treatment of various stages of multiple myeloma.

In lymphomas of various histologies and of both B- and T-cell phenotypes, IFN-α may have a therapeutic role. Interferon-α2, 50 × 10^6 units three times per week, was effective in patients with advanced cutaneous T-cell lymphoma (CTCL) (Bunn et al., 1984). Nine objective partial responses (PR) lasting 3 months to >25 months (median, 5 months) occurred in 20 evaluable patients. Interferon may prove to be more effective for CTCL than any other reported agent. An initial report with buffy coat leukocyte IFN-α described three PR in three treated patients with nodular, poorly differentiated B-cell lymphomas (Merigan et al., 1978). A greater than 50% response frequency occurred in a trial of IFN-α2 in 24 evaluable patients of whom 13 (54%) responded (Foon et al., 1984). All responding patients had been heavily pretreated with combination chemotherapy. Responses persisted for 2 to 7 months after cessation of therapy. Three patients who had relapsed after interferon was discontinued subsequently responded to a second course. This latter trial utilized a dose of 50 × $10^6/m^2$ IM three times weekly, a dose that required at least 50% reduction within 4 weeks in all patients. Equivalent effectiveness occurred in a trial with IFN-α2 given subcutaneously at a much lower dose, 2 × 10^6 U/m^2 three times weekly (Wagstaff et al., 1985). Objective responses occurred in 17 of 34 patients and only 1 patient required dose reduction. Thus, as in HCL, objective response can be achieved at a minimum dose. Furthermore, in this latter trial, patients who had had prior chemotherapy responded well (Wagstaff et al., 1985). Previously untreated patients with favorable lymphoma were evaluated at 12 × 10^6 U/m^2 IM three times weekly (O'Connell et al., 1986). Responses occurred in 7 of 16 patients (44%); median duration of response was 5 months. Thus, prior chemotherapy may not substantially influence potential for response in this disease.

Solid Tumors

For some solid tumors, IFN-α has resulted in response rates equivalent to the best chemotherapeutic approaches. Response rates to IFN-α metastatic melanoma have ranged from 2% to 29%; the cumulative response, totaled from 10 recent papers describing various trials involving patients utilizing recombinant or partially purified IFN-α, was 15% (CR + PR) (Retsas et al., 1983; Creagan et al., 1984a, 1984b, 1985; Krown et al., 1984; Goldberg et al., 1985; Hersey et al., 1985; Kirkwood et al., 1985a; Legha, 1986; Dorval et al., 1987), a level comparable to chemotherapeutic results with cytotoxic agents. Response has been correlated with better performance status, no prior chemotherapy, and low volume of visceral disease. Initial studies seemed to show synergy with cimetidine, but recent trials have not confirmed this (Borgstrom et al., 1983; Creagan et al., 1985). Response rates to IFN-γ have been reported between 6% and 11% (Ernstoff et al., 1987; Creagan et al., 1987). For patients at high risk for recurrence of melanoma, national cooperative groups have ongoing randomized trials utilizing interferons as adjuncts to surgery.

Metastatic renal cell carcinoma has a response rate to cytotoxic agents of less than 10%. Response rates from 4% to 26% have been reported in trials of recombinant and purified IFN-α in this disease, with a mean response of 16% (CR + PR) (Quesada et al., 1983, 1985a, 1985b; Neidhart et al., 1984; Vugrin et al., 1985; Kirkwood et al., 1985b; Buzaid et al., 1987; Trump et al., 1987; Muss et al., 1987; Creagan et al., 1988; Fujita et al., 1988). A dose of IFN-α2 as low as 1×10^6 units daily has been effective (Marshall et al., 1989). A more favorable response has been observed in patients who have had resection of bulky primary disease, and lung metastases appear to respond better than disease at other sites. This suggests a possible role for interferon postoperatively as adjuvant therapy. A phase III adjuvant trial for patients with renal cell carcinoma following radical nephrectomy and lymphadenectomy is currently being conducted by the Eastern and Southwestern Cooperative Oncology Groups. In two studies of IFN-γ or combinations of IFN-α and IFN-γ have had response rates of 9% to 33% (CR + PR) in renal cell carcinoma (Aulitzky et al., 1989; Quesada et al., 1987; Recombinant Human Interferon-γ Research Group, 1987). The response rate of 33% occurred in patients receiving IFN-γ at a biologically effective, but low, dose of 1×10^6 units weekly (Aulitzky et al., 1989).

Response rates for recombinant IFN-α2 in Kaposi's sarcoma have ranged from 3% to 45%, with a mean of 33% (Krown et al., 1983; Rios et al., 1985; Real et al., 1986; Volberding et al., 1987; Lane et al., 1988; DeWit et al., 1988). A dose–response effect has been suggested and responses have been seen in patients with visceral and nodal disease. Studies continue with IFN-α2 in combination with zidovudine and other agents, and the response rate has been further improved (Krown et al., 1990; Kovacs et al., 1989).

Clinical trials of IFN-α in endocrine pancreatic tumors have reported a mean objective response rate of 79% (decrease in tumor-produced peptides) (Eriksson et al., 1986, 1987; Oberg et al., 1987). In addition, a decrease in tumor size by more than 50% occurred in approximately one third of patients in these trials. Interferon-α has also been useful in decreasing the severe diarrhea common in pancreatic endocrine tumors (Oberg et al., 1985). Midgut carcinoid tumors, although often behaving in an indolent fashion, produce symptoms such as flushing and diarrhea that may interfere with daily activities (Kvols, 1986). In trials of recombinant IFN-α, a mean response rate (improvement in symptoms or decrease in 5 hydroxyindoleacetic acid [5HIAA]) of 48% has been reported (Oberg et al., 1983, 1986, 1987; Kvols, 1986; Smith et al., 1987). The decrease in 5HIAA has been correlated with lessened symptoms; rebound of 5HIAA levels frequently occurred when interferon was discontinued.

Other solid tumors, such as ovarian and bladder carcinoma, have responded to IFN-α administered regionally (Torti et al., 1984, 1988; Berek et al., 1985). In ovarian carcinoma, IFN-α2 has been used in combination with *cis*-platinum: of 14 evaluable patients, 2 had CR and 3 had PR (Berek et al., 1988). Other solid malignancies show promise of responding to systemic IFN-α2 in combination with chemotherapy. In metastatic colorectal carcinoma, more than 80% of patients responded to a combination of 5-fluorouracil with IFN-α2 (Wadler et al., 1989). Interestingly, interferons used in mice not only increased therapeutic effectiveness, but also protected from lethal toxicities of 5-fluorouracil (Stolfi et al., 1983).

CONCLUSION

Interferons have improved therapeutic approaches for viral diseases and malignancies. Recognition of the potent ability of interferons to modulate cell structure and function has served as the basis for initiation of trials of these cytokines for treatment of human disease. The full spectrum of actions and interactions, mechanism of antitumor effects, and optimal dose, schedule, and type of interferon for specific clinical indications has not yet been fully delineated. Because interferons modulate host response, the traditional emphasis on using compounds at maximally tolerated doses for cancer may need to be shifted to use of doses effective in modifying biological response. This may result in fuller realization of therapeutic potential. Interferons are part of the complex network of interacting lymphokines. Clinical combinations with cytotoxic and biological agents hold promise for the future, and investigation of these combinations continues (Borden and Hawkins, 1986; Schiller and Borden, 1987; Bonnem, 1987). Dose, route, and schedule of administration will be increasingly important in combinations. As with other biologicals, stabilization of disease and minor responses, often seen in patients with advanced disease, may be important. As phase III trials comparing conventional chemotherapy with interferons are completed, it may become apparent that interferons are more effective in patients with a smaller tumor burden and in the adjuvant setting.

Interferons, as a prototype for other biological response modifiers, have opened a new era in oncologic treatment. The groundwork has been laid for use of interferons to modulate specific gene regulation, oncogene expression, cell proliferation and differentiation, and immunological function. In combination with other lymphokines, monoclonal antibodies, and cytoreductive approaches, interferons should continue to

TABLE 18-5
FUTURE CHALLENGES FOR DEVELOPING MORE EFFECTIVE APPLICATION OF INTERFERONS IN CANCER

- Structure–function relationships
- Signal transduction mechanisms
- Function of induced proteins
- Immunomodulatory effects
- Somatic cell effects
- Mechanism antitumor effects
- Combination therapies
- New therapeutic targets

reduce morbidity from cancer. The future challenges are to dissect further mechanisms of antitumor action and optimally effective combinations; this must be complemented by studies dissecting other aspects of interferons' cellular and clinical actions (Table 18-5). With such research, interferons should have much broadened clinical applications in management of patients with malignancy by the year 2000.

ACKNOWLEDGMENTS

Research in our laboratories on interferons is supported by the National Institute of Allergy and Infectious Disease, the National Cancer Institute, American Cancer Society, and Triton Biosciences. E. C. Borden is an American Cancer Society Professor of Clinical Oncology, and S. E. Grossberg, an American Cancer Society Scholar in Cancer Research.

REFERENCES

Adolf GR. Antigenic structure of human interferon ω1 (interferon alpha II1): comparison with other human interferons. J Genet Virol. 1987;68:1669–1676.

Affabris E, Federico M, Romeo G, Coccia EM, Rossi GB. Opposite effects of murine interferons on erythroid differentiation of Friend cells. Virology. 1988;167:185–193.

Aguet M, Dembic Z, Merlin G. Molecular cloning and expression of the human interferon-γ receptor. Cell. 1988;55:273–280.

Alimena G, Morra E, Lazzarino M, et al. Interferon alpha-2b as therapy for Ph′-positive chronic myelogenous leukemia: a study of 82 patients treated with intermittent or daily administration. Blood. 1988;72(2):642–647.

Anderson P, Yip YK, Vilcek J. Specific binding of ^{125}I-human interferon-gamma to high affinity receptors on human fibroblasts. J Biol Chem. 1982;257:11301–11304.

Aulitzky W, Gastl G, Aulitzky WE, et al. Successful treatment of metastatic renal cell carcinoma with a biologically active dose of recombinant interferon-gamma. J Clin Oncol. 1989; 7(12):1875–1884.

Baldwin AS Jr, Sharp PA. Binding of a nuclear factor to a regulatory sequence in the promoter of the mouse H-2KB class I major histocompatibility gene. Mol Cell Biol. 1987;7(1):305–313.

Balkwill F, Taylor-Papadimitriou J. Interferon affects both G1 and S + G2 in cells stimulated from quiescence to growth. Nature. 1978;274:798–800.

Balkwill F, Watling D, Taylor-Papadimitriou J. Inhibition by lymphoblastoid interferon of growth of cells derived from the human breast. Int J Cancer. 1978;22:258–265.

Basham T, Smith W, Lanier L, Morhenn V, Merigan TC. Regulation of expression of class II major histocompatibility antigens on human peripheral blood monocytes and langerhans cells by interferon. Human Immunol. 1984;10:83–94.

Becker S. Interferon-γ accelerates immune proliferation via its effect on monocyte HLA-DR expression. Cell Immunol. 1985;91:301–307.

Berek JS, Hacker NF, Lichtenstein A, et al. Intraperitoneal recombinant alpha-interferon for "salvage" immunotherapy in stage III epithelial ovarian cancer: a Gynecologic Oncology Group study. Cancer Res. 1985;45:4447–4453.

Berek JS, Welander C, Montz FJ, Schink JC, Grossberg H. Treatment of ovarian cancer with intraperitoneal cis-platin and α2β interferon. Proc Am Soc Clin Oncol. 1988;7:138.

Bishop JM. The molecular genetics of cancer. Science. 1987;235:305–311.

Blomstrom DC, Fahey D, Kutny R, Korant BD, Knight E Jr. Molecular characterization of the interferon-induced 15kDa protein: molecular cloning and nucleotide and amino acid sequence. J Biol Chem. 1986;261:8811–8816.

Bonnem EM. Alfa interferon: combinations with other antineoplastic modalities. Semin Oncol. 1987;14(Suppl 2):48–60.

Bonnem EM, Oldham RK. Gamma interferon: physiology and speculation on its role in medicine. J Biol Resp Mod. 1987;6:275–301.

Borden EC. Progress toward therapeutic application of interferons—1979–1983. Cancer. 1984;54:176–182.

Borden EC. Effects of interferons in neoplastic diseases of man. Pharmacol Ther. 1988;37:213–229.

Borden EC, Hawkins MJ. Biologic response modifiers as adjuncts to other therapeutic modalities. Semin Oncol. 1986;13:144–152.

Borden EC, Hawkins MJ, Sielaff KM, Storer BM, Schiesel JD, Smalley RV. Clinical and biological effects of recombinant interferon beta administered intravenously daily in a phase I trial. J Interferon Res. 1988;8:357–366.

Borgstrom S, Von Eyben FE, Flodgren P, Axelsson B, Sjögren HO. Human leukocyte interferon and cimetidine for metastatic melanoma. New Engl J Med. 1983;307:1080–1081.

Branca AA, Baglioni C. Evidence that types I and II interferons have different receptors. Nature. 1981;294:768–770.

Brosjö O, Bauer HCF, Broström LA, Nilsson OS, Reinholt FP, Tribukait B. Growth inhibition of human osteosarcomas in nude mice by human interferon-α: significance of dose and tumor differentiation. Cancer Res. 1987;47:258–262.

Brouty-Boye D. Interferon and the tumour cell phenotype. In: Gresser I, ed. Interferon 7. London: Academic Press; 1986:145–165.

Brouty-Boye D, Gresser I. Reversibility of the transformed and neoplastic phenotype. I. Progressive reversion of the phenotype of x-ray–transformed C3H/10T1/2 cells under prolonged treatment with interferon. Int J Cancer. 1981;28:165–173.

Brunda MJ, Rosenbaum D. Modulation of murine natural killer cell activity in vitro and in vivo by recombinant human interferons. Cancer Res. 1984;44:597–601.

Brunda MJ, Tarnowski D, Davatelis V. Interaction of recombinant interferons with recombinant interleukin-2: differential effects on natural killer cell activity and interleukin-2-activated killer cells. Int J Cancer. 1986;37:787–793.

Bunn PA, Foon KA, Ihde DC, et al. Recombinant leukocyte A interferon: an active agent in advanced cutaneous T-cell lymphomas. Ann Intern Med. 1984;101:484–487.

Buzaid AC, Robertone A, Kisala C, Salmon SE. Phase II study of interferon alfa-2A, recombinant (Roferon®-A) in metastatic renal cell carcinoma. J Clin Oncol. 1987;5:1083–1089.

Capon DJ, Shepard HM, Goeddel DV. Two distinct families of human and bovine interferon-alpha genes are coordinately expressed and encode functional polypeptides. Mol Cell Biol. 1985;5(4):768–779.

Carlin JM, Borden EC, Sondel PM, Byrne GI. Biologic response modifier-induced indoleamine 2,3-dioxygenase activity in human peripheral blood mononuclear cell cultures. J Immunol. 1987;139:2414–2418.

Carlin JM, Borden EC, Byrne GI. Enhancement of indoleamine 2,3-dioxygenase activity in cancer patients receiving interferon-betaser. J Interferon Res. 1989a;9:167–173.

Carlin JM, Borden EC, Sondel PM, Byrne GI. Interferon-induced indoleamine 2,3-dioxygenase activity in human mononuclear phagocytes. J Leukocyte Biol. 1989b;45:29–34.

Chany C, Vignal M, Couillin P, Van Cong N, Boué J, Boué A. Chromosomal localization of human genes governing the interferon-induced antiviral state. Proc Natl Acad Sci USA. 1975;72:3129–3133.

Chany-Fournier F. Rôle de l'interféron dans la réversion phénotypique des cellules transformées: perte du caractère de malignité. Pathol Biol. 1983;31:199–213.

Chebath J, Benech P, Revel M, Vigneron M. Constitutive expression of (2′-5′) oligo A synthetase confers resistance to picornavirus infection. Nature. 1987;330:587–588.

Chen LK, Mathieu-Mahul D, Bach FH, Dausset J, Bensussan A, Sasportes M. Recombinant interferon α can induce rearrangement of T-cell antigen receptor α-chain genes and maturation to cytotoxicity in T-lymphocyte clones in vitro. Proc Natl Acad Sci USA. 1986a; 83:4887–4889.

Chen L, Tourvieille B, Burns GF, et al. Interferon: a cytotoxic T lymphocyte differentiation signal. Eur J Immunol. 1986b;16:767–770.

Cheng Y-SE, Colonno RJ, Yin FY. Interferon induction of fibroblast proteins with guanylate binding activity. J Biol Chem. 1983;258:7746–7750.

Cheng Y-SE, Becker-Manley MF, Chow TP, Horan DC. Affinity purification of an interferon-induced human guanylate-binding protein and its characterization. J Biol Chem. 1985;260: 15834–15839.

Cheng Y-SE, Becker-Manley MF, Rucker RG, Borden EC. Accumulation of guanylate binding proteins in patients treated with interferons. J Interferon Res. 1988;8:385–391.

Clemens MJ, Tilleray VJ, James R, Gewert DR. Relationship of cellular oncogene expression to inhibition of growth and induction of differentiation of Daudi cells by interferons or TPA. J Cell Biochem. 1988;38(4):251–259.

Colby CB, Geigert JH, Ruzicka FJ, et al. In vitro biological assessment of an interferon beta with a site specific amino acid substitution. In: Stewart WE II, Schellekens H, eds. The biology of the interferon system. Amsterdam: Elsevier; 1986:273–278.

Costanzi JJ, Cooper MR, Scarffe JH, et al. Phase II study of recombinant alpha-2 interferon in resistant multiple myeloma. J Clin Oncol. 1985;3:654–659.

Creagan ET, Ahmann DL, Green SJ, et al. Phase II study of low-dose recombinant leukocyte A interferon in disseminated malignant melanoma. J Clin Oncol. 1984a;2:1002–1005.

Creagan ET, Ahmann DL, Green SJ. Phase II study of recombinant leukocyte A interferon (rIFN-alpha-A) in disseminated malignant melanoma. Cancer. 1984b;54:2844–2849.

Creagan ET, Ahmann DL, Green SJ, Long HJ, Frytak S, Itri LM. Phase II study of recombinant leukocyte A interferon (IFN-rA) plus cimetidine in disseminated malignant melanoma. J Clin Oncol. 1985;3:977–981.

Creagan ET, Ahmann DL, Long HJ, Frytak S, Sherwin SA, Chang MN. Phase II study of recombinant interferon-gamma in patients with disseminated malignant melanoma. Cancer Treat Rep. 1987;71:843–844.

Creagan ET, Buckner JC, Hahn RG, Richardson RR, Schaid DJ, Kovach JS. An evaluation of recombinant leukocyte A interferon with aspirin in patients with metastatic renal cell cancer. Cancer. 1988;61:1787–1791.

Creasey AA, Bartholomew JC, Merigan TC. The importance of G_0 in the site of action of interferon in the cell cycle. Exp Cell Res. 1981;134:155–160.

Creasey AA, Eppstein DA, Marsh YV, Khan Z, Merigan TC. Growth regulation of melanoma cells by interferon and (2′-5′) oligoadenylate synthetase. Mol Cell Biol. 1983;3:780–786.

D'Hooghe MC, Brouty-Boye D, Malaise EP, Gresser I. Interferon and cell division: XII. Prolongation by interferon of the intermitotic time of mouse mammary tumor cells in vitro. Microcinematographic analysis. Exp Cell Res. 1977;105:73–77.

Dargemont C, Dunon D, Deugnier M-A, et al. Thymotaxin, a chemotactic protein, is identical to β2-microglobulin. Science. 1989;246:803–805.

De Maeyer E, De Maeyer-Guignard J. The effects of interferons on cell growth and division. In: Interferons and other regulatory cytokines. New York, NY: John Wiley; 1988:134–153.

Derynck R, Content J, Leclerq E. Isolation and structure of a human fibroblast interferon gene. Nature. 1980;285:542–547.

DeVries JE, Spits H. Cloned human cytotoxic T lymphocyte (CTL) lines reactive with autologous melanoma cells. I. In vitro generation, isolation, and analysis to phenotype and specificity. J Immunol. 1984;132:510–519.

DeWit R, Boucher CAB, Veenhof KHN, Schattenkerk JKME, Bakker PJM, Danner SA. Clinical and virological effects of high dose recombinant interferon α in disseminated AIDS-related Kaposi's sarcoma. Lancet. 1988;2:1214–1217.

Djeu JY, Heinbaugh JA, Holden HT, Herberman RB. Augmentation of mouse natural killer cell activity by interferon and interferon inducers. J Immunol. 1979;122:175–181.

Dorval T, Palangie T, Jouve M. Treatment of metastatic melanoma with recombinant interferon alfa-2b. Invest New Drugs. 5(suppl):S61–S64.

Dreiding P, Staeheli P, Haller O. Interferon-induced protein Mx accumulates in nuclei of mouse cells expressing resistance to influenza viruses. Virology. 1985;140:192–196.

Dustin ML, Rothlein R, Bhan AK, Dinarello CA, Springer TA. Induction by IL1 and IFN gamma: tissue distribution, biochemistry and function of a natural adherence molecule (ICAM-1). J Immunol. 1986;137:245–254.

Edery I, Petryshyn R, Sonenberg N. Activation of double-stranded RNA-dependent kinase (dsl) by the TAR region of HIV-1 mRNA: a novel translational control mechanism. Cell. 1986; 56:303–312.

Edwards BS, Hawkins MJ, Borden EC. Comparative in vivo and in vitro activation of human natural killer cells by recombinant alpha interferons differing in antiviral activity. Cancer Res. 1984;44:3135–3139.

Edwards BS, Merritt JA, Fuhlbrigge RC, Borden EC. Low doses of interferon alpha result in more effective clinical natural killer cell activation. J Clin Invest. 1985;75:1908–1913.

Einat M, Resnitzky D, Kimchi A. Inhibitory effects of interferon on the expression of genes regulated by platelet-derived growth factor. Proc Natl Acad Sci USA. 1985;82:7608–7612.

Einhorn S, Robert K-H, Ostlünd L, Juliusson G, Biberfeld P. Interferon induces proliferation and differentiation in primary chronic lymphocytic leukemia cells. In: Kirchner H, Schellenkens H, eds. The biology of the interferon system 1984. Amsterdam: Elsevier Science Publishers; 1985:293–297.

Eriksson B, Alm G, Lundquist G, et al. Treatment of malignant endocrine pancreatic tumours with human leukocyte interferon. Lancet. 1986;2:1307–1309.

Eriksson B, Oberg K, Alm G, et al. Treatment of malignant endocrine pancreatic tumors with human leukocyte interferon. Cancer Treat Rep. 1987;71:31–37.

Ernstoff MS, Trautman T, Davis CA. A randomized phase I/II study of continuous versus intermittent intravenous interferon gamma in patients with metastatic melanoma. J Clin Oncol. 1987;5:1804–1810.

Exley R, Gordon J, Nathan P, Walker L, Clemens MJ. Antiproliferative effects of interferons on Daudi Burkitt lymphoma cells: induction of cell differentiation and loss of response to autocrine growth factors. Int J Cancer. 1987;40:53–57.

Farrar WL, Johnson HM, Farrar JJ. Regulation of the production of immune interferon and cytotoxic T lymphocytes by interleukin 2. J Immunol. 1981;126:1120–1125.

Fernandez-Cruz E, Ulich T, Schreiber RD. In vivo activity of lymphokine-activated macrophages in host defense against neoplasia. J Immunol. 1985;134:3489–3496.

Fidler IJ, Heicappell R, Saiki I, Grutter MG. Direct antiproliferative effects of recombinant human interferon-alpha B/D hybrids on human tumor cell lines. Cancer Res. 1987;47:2020–2027.

Finke JH, Scott J, Gillis S, Hilfiker ML. Generation of alloreactive cytotoxic T lymphocytes: evidence for a differentiation factor distinct from IL-2. J Immunol. 1983;130:763–767.

Finter NB. The classification and biological functions of the interferons. A review. J Hepatol. 1986;3(suppl 2):S157–S160.

Fleischmann CM, Fleischmann WR Jr. Differential antiproliferative activities of IFNs α, β and γ: kinetics of establishment of their antiproliferative effects and the rapid development of resistance to IFNs α and β. J Biol Regul Homeost Agents. 2:173–185.

Fleischmann WR Jr, Schwarz LA, Fleischmann CM. Requirement for IFN-gamma in potentiation of interferon's antiviral and anticellular activities: identity of mouse and human systems. J Interferon Res. 1984;4:265–274.

Foon KA, Sherwin SA, Abrams PB, et al. Treatment of advanced non-Hodgkin's lymphoma with recombinant leukocyte A interferon. New Engl J Med. 1984;311:1148–1152.

Forti RL, Mitchell WM, Hubbard WC, Workman RJ, Forbes JT. Pleiotropic activities of human interferons are mediated by multiple response pathways. Proc Natl Acad Sci USA. 1984; 81:170–174.

Frayssinet C, Gresser I, Tovey M, Lindahl P. Inhibitory effect of potent interferon preparations on the regeneration of mouse liver after partial hepatectomy. Nature. 1973;245:146–147.

Fujita T, Asano H, Naide Y, et al. Antitumor effects of human lymphoblastoid interferon on advanced renal cell carcinoma. J Urol. 1988;139:256–258.

Gariglio M, Franco A, Cavallo G, Landolfo S. Evidence for a GTP-binding protein involved in interferon gamma transduction signal. J Interferon Res. 1988;8:463–472.

Gariglio M, Gribaudo G, Franco A, Pierotti MA, Cavallo G, Landolfo S. Inhibition of interferon-γ antiviral and antiproliferative activities by *ras* oncogene expression. J Natl Cancer Inst. 1989;81:1014–1020.

Gewert DR, Moore G, Tilleray VJ, Clemens MJ. Inhibition of cell proliferation by interferons. 1. Effects on cell division and DNA synthesis in human lymphoblastoids (Daudi) cells. Eur J Biochem. 1984;139:619–625.

Goeddel DV, Yelverton E, Ullrich A. Human leukocyte interferon produced by *E. coli* is biologically active. Nature. 1980;287:411–416.

Goeddel DV, Leung DW, Dull TJ, et al. The structure of eight distinct cloned human leukocyte interferon cDNAs. Nature. 1981;290:20–26.

Goldberg RM, Ayoob M, Silgals R, Ahlgren JD, Neefe JR. Phase II trial of lymphoblastoid interferon in metastatic malignant melanoma. Cancer Treat Rep. 1985;69:813–816.

Goldstein D, Laszlo J. Interferon therapy in cancer: from imaginon to interferon. Cancer Res. 1986;46:4315–4329.

Goldstein D, Sielaff KM, Storer BE, et al. Human biologic response modification by interferon in the absence of measurable serum concentrations: a comparative trial of subcutaneous and intravenous interferon betaserine. J Natl Cancer Inst. 1989;81:1061–1068.

Gonda TJ, Metcalf D. Expression of *myb, myc* and *fos* proto-oncogenes during the differentiation of a murine myeloid leukaemia. Nature. 1984;310:249–251.

Gonwa TA, Picker LJ, Raff HV, Goyert SM, Silver J, Stobo JD. Antigen-presenting capabilities of human monocytes correlates with their expression of HLA-DS, an 1a determinant distinct from HLA-DR. J Immunol. 1983;130:706–711.

Greiner JW, Hand PH, Noguchi P, Fisher PB, Pestka S, Schlom J. Enhanced expression of surface tumor-associated antigens on human breast and colon tumor cells after recombinant human leukocyte alpha-interferon treatment. Cancer Res. 1984;44:3208–3214.

Greiner JW, Guadagni F, Noguchi P, et al. Recombinant interferon enhances monoclonal antibody-targeting of carcinoma lesions in vivo. Science. 1987;235:895–898.

Gresser I, Bandu MT, Brouty-Boye D. Interferon and cell division. IX. Interferon-resistant L1210 cells: characteristics and origin. J Natl Cancer Inst. 1974;52:553–559.

Grimm EA, Mazumder A, Zhang HZ, Rosenberg SA. Lymphokine-activated killer cell phenomenon: lysis of natural killer resistant fresh solid tumor cells by interleukin 2–activated autologous human peripheral blood lymphocytes. J Exp Med. 1982;155:1823–1841.

Gromo G, Geller RL, Inverardi L, Bach FH. Signal requirements in the step-wise functional maturation of cytotoxic T lymphocytes. Nature. 1987;327:424–426.

Grossberg SE. Interferons: an overview of the general biological and biochemical properties. In: Pfeffer LM, ed. Mechanisms of interferon actions. Vol. 1. Boca Raton, Fla: CRC Press; 1987:1–32.

Guadagni F, Schlom J, Johnston WW, et al. Selective interferon-induced enhancement of tumor-associated antigens on a spectrum of freshly isolated human adenocarcinoma cells. J Natl Cancer Inst. 1989;81:502–512.

Guadagni F, Witt PL, Robbins P, Schlom J, Greiner JW. Regulation of carcinoembryonic antigen expression in different human colorectal tumor cells by interferon gamma. Cancer Res. 1990;50:6248–6255.

Gustafsson A, Lundgren E. Augmentation of natural killer cells involves both enhancement of lytic machinery and expression of new receptors. Cell Immunol. 1981;62:367–376.

Hamburger AW, White CP, Siebenlist RE, Sedmak JJ, Grossberg SE. Cytotoxicity of human beta-interferon for differentiating leukemic HL-60 cells. Cancer Res. 1985;45:5369–5373.

Hamilton TA, Adams DO. Mechanisms of macrophage-mediated tumor injury. In: Den Otter W, Ruitenberg EJ, eds. Tumor immunology—mechanisms, diagnosis, therapy. New York, NY: Elsevier; 1987:89–107.

Hawkins MJ, Krown SE, Borden EC, et al. American Cancer Society phase I trial of naturally produced interferon beta. Cancer Res. 1984;44:5934–5938.

Hayashi H, Tanaka K, Jay F, Khoury G, Jay G. Modulation of the tumorigenicity of human adenovirus-12-transformed cells by interferon. Cell. 1985;43:263–267.

Herberman RB. Immunoregulation and natural killer cells. Mol Immunol. 1982;19:1313–1321.

Hersey P, Hasic E, MacDonald M, et al. Effects of recombinant leukocyte interferon (rIFN-αA) on tumour growth and immune responses in patients with metastatic melanoma. Br J Cancer. 1985;51:815–826.

Heyns AP, Eldor A, Vlodavsky I, Kaiser N, Fridman R, Panet A. The antiproliferative effect of interferon and the mitogenic activity of growth factors are independent cell cycle events. Studies with vascular smooth muscle cells and endothelial cells. Exp Cell Res. 1985; 161:297–306.

Hicks NJ, Morris AG, Burke DC. Partial reversion of the transformed phenotype of murine sarcoma virus–transformed cells in the presence of interferon: a possible mechanism for the antitumor effect of interferon. J Cell Sci. 1981;49:225–236.

Horisberger MA, Hochkeppel HK. IFN-alpha induced human 78kD protein: purification and homologies with the mouse Mx protein, production of monoclonal antibodies, and potentiation effect of IFN-gamma. J Interferon Res. 1987;7:331–343.

Horisberger MA, Staritzky K. A recombinant human interferon-α B/D hybrid with a broad host range. J Genet Virol. 1987;68:945-948.

Horisberger MA, Staeheli P, Haller O. Interferon induces a unique protein in mouse cells bearing a gene for resistance to influenza virus. Proc Natl Acad Sci USA. 1983;80:1910-1914.

Iacobelli S, Scambia G, Natoli C, et al. Recombinant human leukocyte interferon alpha2b stimulates the synthesis and release of a 90K tumor-associated antigen in human breast cancer cells. Int J Cancer. 1988;42:182-184.

Ito M, Takami Y, Tanabe F, Shigeta S, Tsukui K, Kawade Y. Modulation of protein kinase C activity during inhibition of tumor cell growth by IFN-β and -γ. Biochem Biophys Res Commun. 1988;150:126-132.

Itoh K, Shiiba K, Shimizu Y, Suzuki R, Kumagai K. Generation of activated killer (AK) cells by recombinant interleukin-2 (rIL-2) in collaboration with interferon-γ (IFN-γ). J Immunol. 1985;134:3124-3129.

Jaffe EA, Armellino D, Lam G, Cordon-Cardo C, Murray HW, Evans RL. IFN gamma and IFN alpha induce the expression and synthesis of Leu-13 antigen by cultured human endothelial cells. J Immunol. 1989;143:3961-3966.

Jett JR, Mantovani A, Herberman RB. Augmentation of human monocyte-mediated cytolysis by interferon. Cell Immunol. 1980;54:425-434.

Kantor J, Tran R, Greiner J, et al. Modulation of carcinoembryonic antigen messenger RNA levels in human colon carcinoma cells by recombinant human gamma interferon. Cancer Res. 1989;49:2651-2655.

Karino Y, Sugawara R, Saga A, et al. Serum 2′-5′ oligoadenylate synthetase as a monitoring marker of anti-viral effect during interferon therapy for chronic type B hepatitis. Gastroenterologia Japonica. 1989;24:164-169.

Keay S, Grossberg SE. Interferon inhibits the conversion of 3T3-L1 mouse fibroblasts into adipocytes. Proc Natl Acad Sci USA. 1980;77:4099-4103.

Kimchi A. Autocrine interferon and the suppression of the c-*myc* nuclear oncogene. In: Interferon. Vol. 8. London: Academic Press; 1987:85-110.

Kimchi A, Shure H, Revel M. Anti-mitogenic function of interferon-induced (2′-5′)oligo (adenylate) and growth-related variations in enzymes that synthesize and degrade this oligonucleotide. Eur J Biochem. 1981;114:5-10.

Kirkwood JM, Ernstoff MS, Davis CA, Reiss M, Farraresi R, Rudnick SA. Comparison of intramuscular and intravenous recombinant interferon in melanoma and other cancers. Ann Intern Med. 1985a;103:32-36.

Kirkwood JM, Harris J, Vera R, et al. A randomized study of low and high doses of leukocyte alpha-interferon in metastatic renal cell carcinoma: the American Cancer Society Collaborative Trial. Cancer Res. 1985b;45:863-871, 1985.

Klein G. Oncogenes and tumor suppressor genes. In: Acta Oncologica, Reviews in Oncology 1. 1988;27:427-437.

Kleinerman ES, Kurzrock R, Wyatt D, Quesada JR, Gutterman JU, Fidler IJ. Activation or suppression of the tumoricidal properties of monocytes from cancer patients following treatment with human recombinant gamma-interferon. Cancer Res. 1986;46:5401-5405.

Klimpel GR, Fleischmann WR Jr, Klimpel KD. Gamma interferon (IFN-γ) and IFN-α/β suppress murine myeloid colony formation (CFU-C): magnitude of suppression is dependent upon level of colony-stimulating factor (CSF). J Immunol. 1982;129:76-80.

Kohase M, Henriksen-DeStefano D, May LT, Vilcek J, Sehgal PB. Induction of β2-interferon by tumor necrosis factor: a homeostatic mechanism in the control of cell proliferation. Cell. 1986;45:659-666.

Korant BD, Blomstrom DC, Jonak GJ, Knight E Jr. Interferon-induced proteins: purification and characterization of a 15,000-dalton protein from human and bovine cells induced by interferon. J Biol Chem. 1984;259:14,835-14,839.

Kovach JS. Current status of recombinant interferon in cancer therapy. Cancer. 1987;59:633-674.

Kovacs JA, Deyton L, Davey R, et al. Combined zidovudine and interferon-α therapy in patients with Kaposi sarcoma and the acquired immunodeficiency syndrome (AIDS). Ann Intern Med. 1989;111:280-287.

Krown SE. Interferons and interferon inducers in cancer treatment. Semin Oncol. 1986;13:207-217.

Krown SE, Real FX, Cunningham-Rundles S, et al. Preliminary observations on the effect of recombinant leukocyte A interferon in homosexual men with Kaposi's sarcoma. New Engl J Med. 1983;308:1071–1076.

Krown SE, Burk MW, Kirkwood J, Kerr D, Morton D, Oettgen HF. Human leukocyte (alpha) interferon in metastatic malignant melanoma: the American Cancer Society Phase II Trial. Cancer Treat Rep. 1984;68:723-726.

Krown SE, Mintzer D, Cunningham-Rundles S, et al. High-dose human lymphoblastoid interferon in metastatic colorectal cancer: clinical results and modification of biological responses. Cancer Treat Rep. 1987;71:39-45.

Krown SE, Niedzwiecki D, Bhalla R, Flomenberg N, Bundow D. Beta-2 microglobulin (β2-m) and neopterin (Neo) in AIDS: association with endogenous interferon production and response of Kaposi's sarcoma (KS) to exogenous IFN-α. J Interferon Res. 1989;9:S117.

Krown SE, Gold JWM, Niedzwiecki D, et al. Interferon-α with zidovudine: safety, tolerance, and clinical and virologic effects in patients with Kaposi sarcoma associated with the Acquired Immunodeficiency Syndrome. Ann Intern Med. 1990;112:812-821.

Kuribayashi K, Gillis S, Kern DE, Henney CS. Murine NK cell cultures: effects of interleukin-2 and interferon on cell growth and cytotoxic reactivity. J Immunol. 1981;126:2321-2327.

Kushnaryov VM, MacDonald HS, Sedmak JJ, Grossberg SE. Murine interferon-beta receptor-mediated endocytosis and nuclear membrane binding. Proc Natl Acad Sci USA. 1985; 82:3281-3285.

Kvols LK. Metastatic carcinoid tumors and the carcinoid syndrome: a selective review of chemotherapy and hormonal therapy. Am J Med. 1986;81:49-55.

Landolfo S, Cofano F, Giovarelli M, Prat M, Cavallo G, Forni G. Inhibition of interferon-gamma may suppress allograft reactivity by T lymphocytes in vitro and in vivo. Science. 1985;229:176-179.

Lane HC, Kovacs JA, Feinberg J, et al. Anti-retroviral effects of interferon-α in AIDS-associated Kaposi's sarcoma. Lancet. 1988;2:1218-1222.

Lee SHS, Epstein LB. Reversible inhibition by interferon of the maturation of human peripheral blood monocytes to macrophages. Cell Immunol. 1980;50:177-190.

Legha SS. Interferons in the treatment of malignant melanoma: a review of recent trials. Cancer. 1986;57:1675-1677.

Lin J, Sartorelli AC. Stimulation by interferon of the differentiation of human promyelocytic leukemia (HL-60) cells produced by retinoic acid and actinomycin D. J Interferon Res. 1987;7:379-387.

Lin SL, Greene JJ, Ts'o POP, Carter WA. Sensitivity and resistance of human tumour cells to interferon and $rI_n \cdot rC_n$. Nature. 1982;297:417-419.

Lin SL, Garber EA, Wang E, et al. Reduced synthesis of $pp60^{src}$ and expression of the transformation-related phenotype in interferon-treated Rous sarcoma virus-transformed rat cells. Mol Cell Biol. 1983;3:1656-1664.

Lin SL, Kikuchi T, Pledger WJ, Tamm I. Interferon inhibits the establishment of competence in G_0/S-phase transition. Science. 1986;233:356-359.

Lotzova E, Savary CA, Gutterman JU, Quesada JR, Hersh EM. Regulation of human natural killer cell cytotoxicity by recombinant leukocyte interferon Clone A. J Biol Resp Mod. 1983;2:482-496.

Luster AD, Weinshank RL, Feinman R, Ravetch JV. Molecular and biochemical characterization of a novel gamma-interferon-inducible protein. J Biol Chem. 1988;263:12,036-12,043.

MacKay RJ, Russell SW. Protein changes associated with stages of activation of mouse macrophages for tumor cell killing. J Immunol. 1986;137:1392-1398.

Maluish AE, Ortaldo JR, Conlon JC, et al. Depression of natural killer cytotoxicity after in vivo administration of recombinant leukocyte interferon. J Immunol. 1983;131:503-507.

Maluish AE, Urba WJ, Longo DL, et al. The determination of an immunologically active dose of interferon-gamma in patients with melanoma. J Clin Oncol. 1988;6:434-445.

Mantei N, Schwarzstein M, Streuli M, Panem S, Nagata S, Weissmann C. The nucleotide sequence of a cloned human leukocyte interferon cDNAs. Gene. 1980;10:1-10.

Mark DF, Lu SD, Creasy AA, Yamamoto R, Lin LS. Site-specific mutagenesis of the human fibroblast interferon gene: a structure-function analysis of the protein. Proc Natl Acad Sci USA. 1984;81:5662-5666.

Marshall ME, Simpson W, Butler K, Fried A, Fer MF. Treatment of renal cell carcinoma with daily low-dose alpha-interferon. J Biol Resp Mod. 1989;8:453-461.

Marth C, Fuith LC, Bock G, Daxenbichler G, Dapunt O. Modulation of ovarian carcinoma tumor marker CA-125 by gamma interferon. Cancer Res. 1989;49:6538-6542.

Mehmet H, Morris CMG, Taylor-Papadimitriou J, Rozengurt E. Interferon inhibition of DNA synthesis in Swiss 3T3 cells: dissociation from protein kinase C activation. Biochem Biophys Res Commun. 1987;145:1026-1032.

Meltzer MS. Macrophage activation for tumor cytotoxicity: characterization of priming and trigger signals during lymphokine activation. J Immunol. 1981;127:179-183.

Merigan TC, Sikora K, Breeden JH, Levy R, Rosenberg SA. Preliminary observations on the effect of human leukocyte interferon in non-Hodgkin's lymphoma. New Engl J Med. 1978;299:1449-1453.

Merritt JA, Borden EC, Ball LA. Measurement of 2′,5′-oligoadenylate synthetase in patients receiving interferon alpha. J Interferon Res. 1985;5:191-198.

Merritt JA, Ball LA, Sielaff KM, Meltzer DM, Borden EC. Modulation of 2′,5′-oligoadenylate synthetase in patients treated with alpha interferon: effects of dose, schedule and route of administration. J Interferon Res. 1986;6:189-198.

Mihich E. Future perspectives for biological response modifiers: a viewpoint. Semin Oncol. 1986;13:234-254.

Mitsuya M, Matis LA, Megson M, et al. Generation of an HLA-restricted cytotoxic T cell line reactive against cultured tumor cells from a patient infected with human T cell leukemia/lymphoma virus. J Exp Med. 1983;158:994-999.

Moore RN, Larsen HS, Horohov DW, Rouse BT. Endogenous regulation of macrophage proliferative expansion by colony-stimulating factor-induced interferon. Science. 1984;223:178-181.

Morris AG, Ward GA, Bateman WJ. Interaction of v-Ki-*ras* oncogene and interferon-γ in the control of histocompatibility antigen expression in mouse fibroblasts. Cell Immunol. 1989;120:470-476.

Müller R, Curran T, Müller D, Guilbert L. Induction of c-*fos* during myelomonocytic differentiation and macrophage proliferation. Nature. 1985;314:546–548.

Muss HB, Costanzi JJ, Leavitt R, et al. Recombinant alfa interferon in renal cell carcinoma: a randomized trial of two routes of administration. J Clin Oncol. 1987;5:286–291.

Nathan CF, Horowitz CR, de la Harpe J, et al. Administration of recombinant interferon-gamma to cancer patients enhances monocyte secretion of hydrogen peroxide. Proc Natl Acad Sci USA. 1985;82:8686–8690.

Neefe JR, Sullivan JE, Ayoob M, Phillips E, Smith FP. Augmented immunity in cancer patients treated with α-interferon. Cancer Res. 1985;45:874–878.

Neidhart JA, Gagen MM, Young D, et al. Interferon α therapy of renal carcinoma. Cancer Res. 1984;44:4140–4143.

Nickoloff BJ, Mahrle G, Morhenn V. Ultrastructural effects of recombinant γ-interferon on cultured human keratinocytes. Ultrastruct Pathol. 1986;10:17–21.

Nishiguchi S, Kuroki T, Otani S, et al. Relationship of the effects of interferon on chronic hepatitis B and the induction of 2′,5′-oligoadenylate synthetase. Hepatology. 1989;10: 29–33.

Oberg K, Funa K, Alm G. Effects of leukocyte interferon on clinical symptoms and hormone levels in patients with mid-gut carcinoid tumors and carcinoid syndrome. New Engl J Med. 1983;309:129–132.

Oberg K, Alm G, Lindstrom H, Lundquist G. Successful treatment of therapy-resistant pancreatic cholera with human leukocyte interferon. Lancet. 1985;1:725–727.

Oberg K, Norheim I, Lind E, et al. Treatment of malignant carcinoid tumors with human leukocyte interferon: long-term results. Cancer Treat Rep. 1986;70:1297–1304.

Oberg K, Eriksson B, Norheim I. Interferon treatment of neuroendocrine gut tumors. Proc Am Soc Clin Oncol. 1987;6:80.

O'Connell MJ, Colgan JP, Oken MM, Ritts RE Jr, Kay NE, Itri LM. Clinical trial of recombinant leukocyte A interferon as initial therapy for favorable histology non-Hodgkin's lymphomas and chronic lymphocytic leukemia. An ECOG Pilot Study. J Clin Oncol. 1986; 4(2):128–136.

Oleszak E, Inglot AD. Platelet-derived growth factor (PDGF) inhibits antiviral and anticellular action of interferon in synchronized mouse or human cells. J Interferon Res. 1980;1:37–48.

Ostlünd L, Einhorn S, Robert KH. Induction of 2′,5′-oligoadenylate synthetase and blast transformation in primary chronic lymphocytic leukemia cells following exposure to interferon in vitro. Cancer Res. 1986a;46:2160–2163.

Ostlünd L, Einhorn S, Robert KH, Juliusson G, Biberfeld P. Chronic B-lymphocytic leukemia cells proliferate and differentiate following exposure to interferon in vitro. Blood. 1986b; 67:152–159.

Ozaki Y, Edelstein MP, Duch DS. Induction of indoleamine 2,3-dioxygenase: a mechanism of the antitumor activity of IFN gamma. Proc Natl Acad Sci USA. 1988;85:1242–1246.

Pace JL, Russell SW, Torres BA, Johnson HM, Gray PW. Recombinant mouse gamma interferon induces the priming step in macrophage activation for tumor cell killing. J Immunol. 1983;130:2011–2013.

Panniers LRV, Clemens MJ. Inhibition of cell division by interferon: changes in cell cycle characteristics and in morphology of Ehrlich ascites tumour cells in culture. J Cell Sci. 1981;48:259–279.

Paucker K, Cantell K, Henle W. Quantitative studies on viral interference in suspended L cells. III. Effect of interfering viruses and interferon on the growth rate of cells. Virology. 1962;17:324–334.

Paulnock D, Sizer KC, Freund YR, Jones PP, Fand Parnes JR. Coordinate induction of Ia, α, β, and I_i mRNA in a macrophage cell line. J Immunol. 1985;135:632.

Paulnock DM, Havlin KA, Storer BM, Spear GT, Sielaff KM, Borden EC. Induced proteins in human peripheral mononuclear cells over a range of clinically tolerable doses of interferon-gamma. J Interferon Res. 1989;9:457–473.

Paulnock DM, Lambert LE. Identification and characterization of monoclonal antibodies specific for macrophages at intermediate stages in the tumoricidal activation pathway. J Immunol. 1990;144:765–773.

Pestka S. Interferon: a decade of accomplishments, foundations of the future in research and therapy. Semin Hematol. 1986;23:27–37.

Pestka S, Langer JA, Zoon KC, Samuel CE. Interferons and their actions. Annu Rev Biochem. 56:727–77.

Pfeffer LM, Tamm I. Comparison of the effects of α and β interferons on the proliferation and volume of human tumor cells (HeLa-S3, Daudi, P_3HR-1). J Interferon Res. 1983;3:395–408.

Pfeffer LM, Murphy JS, Tamm I. Interferon effects on the growth and division of human fibroblasts. Exp Cell Res. 1979;121:111–120.

Pfeffer LM, Donner DB, Arakawa T, Stebbing N, Tamm I. Early events in the interaction of IFN-alpha with IFN-sensitive and IFN-resistant Daudi cells. In: Cantell K, Schellekens H, eds. The biology of the interferon system, 1986. Dordrecht: M. Nijhoff; 1987:99–105.

Philip R, Epstein LB. Tumour necrosis factor as immunomodulator and mediator of monocyte cytotoxicity induced by itself, gamma-interferon and interleukin-1. Nature. 1986;323: 86–89.

Preble OT, Rook AH, Steis R, et al. Interferon-induced 2′-5′ oligoadenylate synthetase during interferon-α therapy in homosexual men with Kaposi's sarcoma: marked deficiency in biochemical response to interferon in patients with acquired immunodeficiency syndrome. J Infect Dis. 1985;152:457–465.

Quesada JR, Swanson DA, Trindade A, Guttermann JU. Renal cell carcinoma: antitumor effects of leukocyte interferon. Cancer Res. 1983;43:940–947.

Quesada JR, Hawkins MJ, Horning S, Alexanian R, Borden EC, Merigan T, Gutterman J. A collaborative Phase I-II study of recombinant DNA-produced leukocyte interferon (clone A) in metastatic breast cancer, malignant lymphoma and multiple myeloma. Am J Med. 1984;77:427–432.

Quesada JR, Rios A, Swanson D, Trown P, Gutterman JU. Antitumor activity of recombinant derived interferon alpha in metastatic renal carcinoma. J Clin Oncol. 1985a;3:1522–1528.

Quesada JR, Swanson DA, Guttermann JU. Phase II study of alpha interferon in metastatic renal cell carcinoma: a progress report. J Clin Oncol. 1985b;3:1086–1092.

Quesada JR, Talpaz M, Rios A, Kurzrock R, Gutterman JU. Clinical toxicity of interferons in cancer patients: A review. J Clin Oncol. 1986;4:234–243.

Quesada JR, Kurzrock R, Sherwin SA, Guttermann JU. Phase II studies of recombinant human interferon γ in metastatic renal cell carcinoma. J Biol Resp Mod. 1987;6:20–27.

Ramadori G, Mitsch A, Rieder H, Meyer Zum Buschenfelde K-H. Alpha- and gamma-interferon (IFNα, IFNγ) but not interleukin-1 (IL-1) modulate synthesis and secretion of β2-microglobulin by hepatocytes. Eur J Clin Invest. 1988;18:343–351.

Rashidbaigi A, Langer JA, Jung V, et al. The gene for the human immune interferon receptor is located on chromosome 6. Proc Natl Acad Sci USA. 1986;83:384–388.

Ratain MJ, Golomb HM, Bardawil RG, et al. Durability of responses to interferon α-2b in advanced hairy cell leukemia. Blood. 1987;69:872–877.

Raulet DH, Bevan MH. A differentiation factor required for the expression of cytotoxic T-cell function. Nature. 1987;296:754–757.

Read SE, Williams BRG, Coates RA, et al. Elevated levels of interferon-induced 2′-5′ oligoadenylate synthetase in generalized persistent lymphadenopathy and the acquired immunodeficiency syndrome. J Infect Dis. 1985;152:466–472.

Real FX, Oettgen HF, Krown SE. Kaposi's sarcoma and the acquired immunodeficiency syndrome: treatment with high and low doses of recombinant leukocyte A interferon. J Clin Oncol. 1986;4:544–551.

Recombinant Human Interferon Gamma (S-6810) Research Group on Renal Cell Carcinoma. Phase II study of recombinant human interferon gamma (S-6810) on renal cell carcinoma: summary of two collaborative studies. Cancer. 1987;60:929–933.

Resnitzky D, Yarden A, Zipori D, Kimchi A. Autocrine β-related interferon controls c-*myc* suppression and growth arrest during hematopoietic cell differentiation. Cell. 1986;46: 31–40.

Retsas S, Priestman TJ, Newton KA, Westbury G. Evaluation of human lymphoblastoid interferon in advanced malignant melanoma. Cancer. 1983;51:273–276.

Revel M, Chebath J. Interferon-activated genes. TIBS. 1986;11:166–170.

Rhodes J, Jones DH, Bleehen NM. Increased expression of human monocyte HLA-DR antigens and Fc γ receptors in response to human interferon in vivo. Clin Exp Immunol. 1983;53:739–743.

Riccardi C, Vose BM, Heberman RB. Modulation of IL 2-dependent growth of mouse NK cells by interferon and T lymphocytes. J Immunol. 1983;130:228–232.

Rinehart JJ, Malspeis L, Young D, Neidhart JA. Phase I/II trial of human recombinant interferon gamma in renal cell carcinoma. J Biol Resp Mod. 1986;5:300–308.

Rinehart JJ, Young D, Laforge J, Colborn D, Neidhart JA. Phase I/II trial of interferon beta-serine in patients with renal cell carcinoma: immunological and biological effects. Cancer Res. 1987;47:2481–2487.

Rios A, Mansell PWA, Newell GR, Reuben JM, Hersh EM, Gutterman JU. Treatment of acquired immunodeficiency syndrome-related Kaposi's sarcoma with lymphoblastoid interferon. J Clin Oncol. 1985;3:506–512.

Roberts WK, Vasil A. Evidence for the identity of murine gamma interferon and macrophage activating factor. J Interferon Res. 1982;2:519–532.

Rosenblum MG, Maxwell BL, Talpaz M, Kelleher PJ, McCredie KB, Gutterman JU. In vivo sensitivity and resistance of chronic myelogenous leukemia cells to α-interferon: correlation with receptor binding and induction of 2′,5′-oligoadenylate synthetase. Cancer Res. 1986;46:4848–4852.

Rousset F, De Waal Malefijt R, Slierendregt B, et al. Regulation of Fc receptor for IgE (CD23) and class II MHC antigen expression on Burkitt's lymphoma cell lines by human IL-4 and IFN-gamma. J Immunol. 1988;140:2625–2632.

Roy S, Katze MG, Parkin NT, Edery I, Hovanessian AG, Sonenberg N. Control of the interferon-induced 68-kilodalton protein kinase by the HIV-1 *tat* gene product. Science. 1990; 247:1216–1219.

Rubin BY, Gupta SL. Differential efficacies of human type I and type II interferons as antiviral and antiproliferative reagents. Proc Natl Acad Sci USA. 1980;77:5928–5932.

Rubin BY, Anderson SL, Lunn RM, Hellermann GR, Richardson NK, Smith LJ. Production of a monoclonal antibody directed against an interferon-induced 56,000-dalton protein and its use in the study of this protein. J Virol. 1988;62:1875–1880.

Ruco LP, Meltzer MS. Macrophage activation for tumor cytotoxicity: development of macrophage cytotoxic activity requires completion of a sequence of short-lived intermediary reactions. J Immunol. 1978;121:2035–2042.

Ruggiero V, Antonelli G, Conciatori G, Gentile M, Van Damme J, Dianzani F. The in vitro antiviral activity of tumor necrosis factor (TNF) in WISH cells is mediated by IFN-β induction. Antiviral Res. 1989;11:77–88.

Samid D, Friedman RM. Transcriptional regulation of *ras* by interferon. In: Friedman RM, Merigan T, Sreevalsan T, eds. Interferons as cell growth inhibitors and antitumor factors. UCLA Symposia on Molecular and Cellular Biology New Series. Vol. 50. New York, NY: Alan R. Liss; 1986:413–422.

Samid D, Chang EM, Friedman RM. Biochemical and biophysical correlates of phenotypic reversion in interferon-treated mouse cells transformed by a human oncogene. Biochem Biophys Res Comm. 1984;119:21–28.

Samid D, Flessate DM, Greene JJ, Chang EH, Friedman RM. Persisting revertants after interferon treatment of oncogene-transformed cells. In: Stewart WE II, Schellekens H, eds. The biology of the interferon system 1985. Amsterdam: Elsevier Science; 1986:327–332.

Samuel CE. Mechanism of interferon action: phosphorylation of protein synthesis initiation factor eIF-2 in interferon-treated human cells by a ribosome-associated kinase possessing site specificity similar to hemin-regulated rabbit reticulocyte kinase. Proc Natl Acad Sci USA. 1979;76:600–604.

Samuel CE, Knutson GS. Mechanism of interferon action. J Biol Chem. 1982;257:11791–11795.

Schattner A, Wallach D, Merlin G, et al. Variation of (2′-5′)OligoA synthetase level in lymphocytes and granulocytes of patients with viral infections and leukemia. J Interferon Res. 1982;2:355–361.

Schiller JH, Borden EC. Potentials for therapeutic applications of interferons with other cell modulating proteins. In: Holcenberg JC, Winkelhake JL, eds. The pharmacology and toxicology of proteins. New York, NY: Alan R. Liss; 1987:273–285.

Schiller JH, Groveman DS, Schmid SM, Willson JKV, Cummings KB, Borden EC. Synergistic antiproliferative effects of human recombinant α54- or β_{ser}-interferon with γ interferon on human cell lines of various histogenesis. Cancer Res. 1986;46:483–488.

Schiller JH, Storer B, Witt PL, et al. Biological and clinical effects of the combination of beta and gamma interferons administered as a five-day continuous infusion. Cancer Res. 1990;50:4588–4594.

Sedman PC, Ramsden CW, Brennan TG, Giles GR, Guillou PJ. Augmentation of lymphokine-activated killer cell activity in patients with gastrointestinal cancer. Br J Surg. 1988;75:591–594.

Sergiescu D, Gerfaux J, Joret AM, Chany C. Persistent expression of v-*mos* oncogene in transformed cells that revert to nonmalignancy after prolonged treatment with interferon. Proc Natl Acad Sci USA. 1986;83:5764–5768.

Shearer M, Taylor-Papadimitriou J. Regulation of cell growth by interferon. Cancer Metastasis Rev. 1987;6:199–221.

Shibata H, Taylor-Papadimitriou J. Effects of human lymphoblastoid interferon on cultured breast cancer cells. Int J Cancer. 1981;28:447–453.

Siegel JP. Effects of interferon-γ on the activation of human T lymphocytes. Cell Immunol. 1988;111:461–472.

Silva A, Bonavida B, Targan S. Mode of action of interferon-mediated modulation of natural killer cytotoxic activity: recruitment of pre-NK cells and enhanced kinetics of lysis. J Immunol. 1980;125:479–484.

Simon MM, Hochgeschwender U, Brugger U, Landolfo S. Monoclonal antibodies to interferon-γ inhibit interleukin 2–dependent induction of growth and maturation in lectin/antigen-reactive cytolytic T lymphocyte precursors. J Immunol. 1986;136:2755–2762.

Smith DB, Scarffe JH, Wagstaff J, Johnston RJ. Phase II trial of rDNA alfa 2b interferon in patients with malignant carcinoid tumor. Cancer Treat Rep. 1987;71:1265–1266.

Sokawa Y, Watanabe Y, Watanabe Y, Kawade Y. Interferon suppresses the transition of quiescent 3T3 cells to a growing state. Nature. 1977;268:236–238.

Sone S, Utsugi T, Nii A, Ogura T. Differential effects of recombinant interferons a, b, and g on induction of human lymphokine (IL-2)-activated killer activity. J Natl Cancer Inst. 1988;80:425–431.

Soslau G, Bogucki AR, Gillespie D, Hubbell HR. Phosphoproteins altered by antiproliferative doses of human interferon-β in a human bladder carcinoma cell line. Biochem Biophys Res Comm. 1984;119:941–948.

Spear GT, Paulnock DM, Jordan RL, Meltzer DM, Merritt JA, Borden EC. Enhancement of monocyte class I and II histocompatibility antigen expression in man by in vivo interferon-beta. Clin Exp Immunol. 1987;69:107–115.

Sreevalsan T, Taylor-Papadimitriou J, Rozengurt E. Selective inhibition by interferon of serum-stimulated biochemical events in 3T3 cells. Biochem Biophys Commun. 1979;87:679–685.

Sreevalsan T, Rozengurt E, Taylor-Papadimitriou J, Burchell J. Differential effect of interferon on DNA synthesis, 2-deoxyglucose uptake and ornithine decarboxylase activity in 3T3 cells stimulated by polypeptide growth factors and tumor promoters. J Cell Physiol. 1980;104:1–9.

Staeheli P, Prochazka M, Steigmeier PA, Haller O. Genetic control of interferon action: mouse strain distribution and inheritance of an induced protein with guanylate-binding property. Virology. 1984;137:135–142.

Staeheli P, Haller O, Boll W, Lindemann J, Weissmann C. Mx protein: constitutive expression in 3t3 cells transformed with cloned Mx cDNA confers selective resistance to influenza virus. Cell. 1986;44:147–158.

Stark GR, Dower WJ, Schimke RT, Brown RE, and Kerr IM. 2-5A synthetase: assay, distribution and variation with growth or hormone status. Nature. 1979;278:471–473.

Stolfi RL, Martin DS, Sawyer RC, Spiegelman S. Modulation of 5-fluorouracil–induced toxicity in mice with interferon or with the interferon inducer, polyinosinic-polycytidylic acid. Cancer Res. 1983;43:561–566.

Storms RW, Bose HR Jr. Viral oncogenes and signal transduction. Virus Res. 1989;12:251–282.

Takikawa O, Kuroiwa T, Yamazaki F, Kido R. Mechanism of interferon-gamma action: characterization of indoleamine 2,3-dioxygenase in cultured human cells induced by IFN gamma and evaluation of the enzyme-mediated tryptophan degradation in its anticellular activity. J Biol Chem. 1988;263:2041–2048.

Talmadge JE. Therapeutic potential of cytokines: a comparison of preclinical and clinical studies. In: Cruse JM, Lewis RE Jr, eds. Progress in experimental tumor research. Vol. 32. Basel: Karger; 1988:154–173.

Talpaz M, Kantarjian HM, McCredie K, Trujillo JM, Keating MJ, Gutterman JU. Hematologic remission and cytogenetic improvement induced by recombinant human interferon alpha(A) in chronic myelogenous leukemia. New Engl J Med. 1986;314(17): 1065–1069.

Talpaz M, Rosenblum M, Kurzrock R, Reuben J, Kantarjian HM, Gutterman J. Clinical and laboratory changes induced by alpha interferon in chronic lymphocytic leukemia—a pilot study. Am J Hematol. 1987;24:341–350.

Tan YH. Chromosome 21 and the cell growth inhibitory effect of human interferon preparations. Nature. 1976;260:141–143.

Tanaka K, Yoshioka T, Bieberich C, Jay G. Role of the major histocompatibility complex class I antigens in tumor growth and metastasis. Ann Rev Immunol. 1988;6:359–380.

Taniguchi T, Mantei N, Schwarzstein M, Nagata S, Muramatsu M, Weissmann C. Human leukocyte and fibroblast interferons are structurally related. Nature. 1980a;285:547–549.

Taniguchi T, Ohno S, Fujii-Kuriyama Y, Muramatsu M. The nucleotide sequence of human fibroblast interferon cDNA. Gene. 1980b;10:11–15.

Taylor JL, Grossberg SE. Recent progress in interferon research: Molecular mechanisms of regulation, action, and virus circumvention. Virus Res. 1990;15:1–26.

Taylor JL, Sabran JL, Grossberg SE. The cellular effects of interferon. In: Came PE, Carter WA, eds. Interferons and their application. New York, NY: Springer-Verlag; 1984:169–204.

Taylor JL, Samuel CE, Grossberg SE. Antiviral and antidifferentiative activities of interferon-β and γ in relation to their induction of double-stranded RNA-dependent protein kinase activity in 3T3-L1 cells. J Biol Chem. 1988;263:1336–1341.

Taylor-Papadimitriou J, Shearer M, Rozengurt E. Inhibitory effect of interferon on cellular DNA synthesis: modulation by pure mitogenic factors. J Interferon Res. 1981;1:401–409.

Tominga SI, Lengyel P. β-Interferon alters the pattern of proteins secreted from quiescent and platelet-derived growth factor-treated BALB/c-3T3 cells. J Biol Chem. 1985;260:1975–1978.

Torres BA, Farrar WL, Johnson HM. Interleukin-2 regulates immune interferon (IFN-g) production by normal and suppressor cell cultures. J Immunol. 1982;128:2217–2219.

Torti FM, Shortliffe LD, Williams RD, et al. Superficial bladder cancers are responsive to alpha-2 interferon administered intravesically. Proc Am Soc Clin Oncol. 1984;3:160.

Torti FM, Shortliffe LD, Williams RD, et al. Alpha interferon in superficial bladder cancer: a Northern California Oncology Group study. J Clin Oncol. 1988;6:476–483.

Trump DL, Elson PJ, Borden EC, et al. High dose lymphoblastoid interferon in advanced renal cell carcinoma: an Eastern Cooperative Oncology Group study. Cancer Treat Rep. 1987; 71:165–169.

Tsuruo T, Iida H, Tsukagoshi S, Oku T, Kishida T. Different susceptibilities of cultured mouse cell lines to mouse interferon. Gann. 1982;73:42–47.

Tyrrell DAJ. Interferons and their clinical value. Rev Infect Dis. 1987;9:243–249.

Urban JL, Schreiber H. Selections of macrophage-resistant progressor tumor variants by the normal host: requirement for concomitant T cell–mediated immunity. J Exp Med. 1983; 157:642–656.

Volberding PA, Mitsuyasu RT, Golando JP, Spiegel RJ. Treatment of Kaposi's sarcoma interferon alfa-2b (Intron A). Cancer. 1987;59:620–625.

Vugrin D, Hood L, Taylor W, Laszlo J. Phase II study of human lymphblastoid interferon in patients with advanced renal carcinoma. Cancer Treat Rep. 1985;69:817–820.

Wadler S, Schwartz EL, Goldman M, et al. Fluorouracil and recombinant alfa-2a interferon: an active regimen against advanced colorectal carcinoma. J Clin Oncol. 1989;7(12):1769–1775.

Wagstaff J, Loynds P, Scarffee JH. Phase II study of rDNA human alpha-2 interferon in multiple myeloma. Cancer Treat Rep. 1985;69:495–498.

Wallach D, Fellous M, Revel M. Preferential effect of gamma interferon on the synthesis of HLA antigens and their mRNAs in human cells. Nature. 1982;299:833–836.

Werner ER, Werner-Felmayer G, Fuchs D, Hausen A, Reibnegger G, Wachter H. Parallel induction of tetrahydrobiopterin biosynthesis and indoleamine 2,3-dioxygenase activity in human cells and cell lines by interferon-gamma. Biochem J. 1989;262:861–866.

Williams BRG. Molecular mechanisms of interferon action. In: Smith RA, ed. Interferon in the treatment of neurological disorders. New York, NY: Marcel Dekker; 1987:43–63.

Williams DB, Barber BH, Flavell RA, Allen H. Role of β_2-microglobulin in the intracellular transport and surface expression of murine class I histocompatibility molecules. J Immunol. 1989;142:2796–2806.

Witt PL, Storer BE, Helgeson DO, Borden EC. Interferon-induced proteins in clinical trials: 2′,5′-oligoadenylate synthetase as a prototype. In: Kawade Y, Kobayashi S, eds. The biology of the interferon system, 1988. Tokyo: Kodansha Scientific; 1989:195–200.

Wright SC, Bonavida B. Studies on the mechanism of natural killer cytotoxicity. III. Activation of NK cells by interferon augments the lytic activity of released natural killer cytotoxic factors (NCKF). J Immunol. 1983;130:2960–2964.

Yap WH, Teo TS, McCoy E, Tan YH. Rapid and transient rise in diacylglycerol concentration in Daudi cells exposed to interferon. Proc Natl Acad Sci USA. 1986;83:7765–7769.

Zilberstein A, Ruggieri R, Korn J, Revel M. Structure and expression of cDNA and genes for human interferon-β2, a distinct species inducible by growth-stimulatory cytokines. EMBO J. 1986;5:2529–2537.

Zullo JN, Cochran BH, Huang AS, Stiles CD. Platelet-derived growth factor and double-stranded ribonucleic acids stimulate expression of the same genes in 3T3 cells. Cell. 1985;43:793–800.

CHAPTER **19**

BIOLOGICAL EFFECTS AND CLINICAL APPLICATIONS OF HUMAN HEMATOPOIETIC GROWTH FACTORS

Janice Lynn Gabrilove
Ann Jakubowski

Colony-stimulating factors (CSF) are a family of glycoproteins that regulate the self-renewal, proliferation maturation, functional integrity, and activation of mature blood cells that are of critical importance in general host defense, oxygen consumption, and hemostasis. Recently, the genes for several human hematopoietic growth factors have been cloned, and recombinant forms of the proteins produced and purified (Souza et al., 1986; Wong et al., 1985, 1987; Kawasaki et al., 1985; Yang et al., 1986; Hirano et al., 1986; Dinarello, 1988).

The major potential clinical applications for hematopoietic growth factors lie in three general areas: (1) restoration of hematopoiesis by either preventing or accelerating recovery from iatrogenic-induced or disease-related myelosuppression; (2) stimulation and production of functionally primed effector cells that have antitumor capability and are also able to augment general host defense; (3) clonal extinction of malignant disease by differentiation induction alone or by recruitment of cells into S phase, allowing them to be rendered more susceptible to killing by cycle-specific agents.

The clinical ramifications and therapeutic evaluation of hematopoietic growth factors are a rapidly moving field that holds great promise for the treatment of a variety of medical illnesses. In addition, an understanding of the mechanism and action of these factors should provide insight into their role in the pathophysiology and clinical manifestations of many diseases. In this chapter, we will (1) provide an overview of the identity of some of the regulatory molecules that affect the process of blood cell development and (2) review those clinical studies that have contributed so far to our understanding of the physiological effects of these factors in man and their utility in the treatment of human disease.

HEMATOPOIETIC GROWTH FACTORS: BIOCHEMICAL, BIOLOGICAL, AND MOLECULAR CHARACTERIZATION

There are at least seven major hematopoietic growth factors involved in the development and functional activation of hematopoietic elements. These are schematically depicted in Figure 19-1. The molecular and biochemical characteristics, major cell targets, and cellular sources for each respective growth factor are outlined in Tables 19-1 and 19-2.

FIGURE 19-1
Regulation of hematopoietic cell development. CFU, colony-forming unit; CFU-GM, CFU granulocyte macrophage; PRO, promyelocyte; MONO, monocyte; GRAN, granulocyte. (Adapted from Griffin, 1988.)

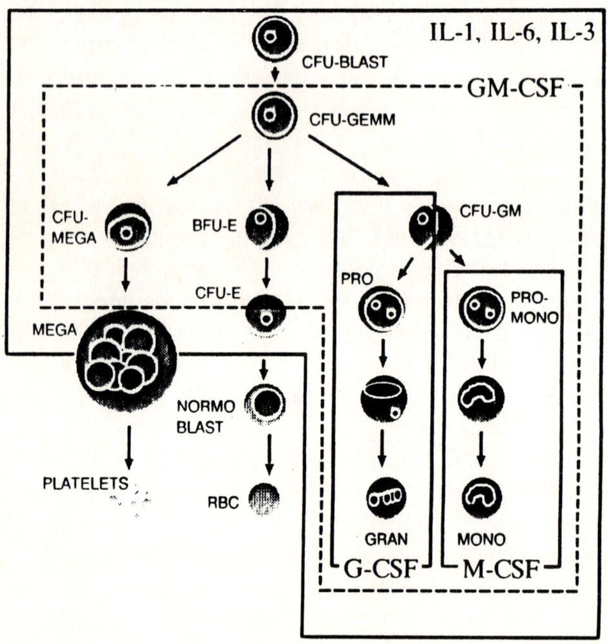

TABLE 19-1
SUMMARY OF THE BIOCHEMICAL AND MOLECULAR CHARACTERISTICS, CELL SOURCES, AND TARGETS OF THE CSF

Factor cell lineage	Chromosomal location	Cell source	mRNA size (kilobases)	Protein size (kDa)	Receptor molecular mass (kDa)
IL-3 (multi-CSF) (n,m,e,b,E.M)	5q23–q31	T Lymphocyte	1.0	14–28	140,000
GM-CSF (n,m,e,b,E.M) +	5q23–q32	Monocyte Fibroblast Endothelial T Lymphocyte Epithelial	1.0	14–35	50,000 130,000–180,000
G-CSF (n)	17q11–q23	Monocyte Endothelial Epithelial	2.0	18	150,000
M-CSF (CSF-1) (m)	5q23–q31	Monocyte Fibroblast Endothelial	4.0 1.8	35–45 (x2) 18–26 (x2)	160,000
IL-1 (Hemopoietin-1)	2q23–q34	Monocyte	2.3	12–19	
IL-4	5q23–q31	T Lymphocyte		20	NK*
IL-6	7p15–p21	Monocytes Fibroblasts T Cells B Cells Endothelial	1.3	26	80,000
Erythropoietin	7q11–q22	Kidney:? Peritubular cells Liver:? cell type	1.8	30.4	100,000 and 85,000

*Not known.

TABLE 19-2
CELL SOURCES OF IL-1–LIKE FACTORS

Monocytes/macrophages and monocyte lines
Langerhans cells
A dendritic cell line
Keratinocytes and epithelial cell lines
Corneal and ginigival epithelium
Melanocyte lines
B lymphocytes and EBV+ cell lines
Large granular lymphocytes (NK cells)
Astrocytes and gliomas
Microglial cells
Mesangial cells
Fibroblasts
Synovial cells
Neutrophils and myelocytic lines
Endothelial cells

IN VITRO ACTIVITY, NORMAL CELLS: GRANULOCYTE COLONY-STIMULATING FACTOR

Human granulocyte colony-stimulating factor (G-CSF) was first purified to homogeneity from the human bladder carcinoma cell line 5637 (Welte et al., 1985). This does not appear to be a reflection of the malignant cell phenotype since the gene is identical to the gene found in normal cells.

The natural protein has a molecular weight on SDS-PAGE of 19.6 kDa. Reduction in the molecular weight to 18.0 kDa, following treatment of the native protein with neuraminidase and O-glyconase suggests that the protein contains neuraminic acid and is minimally O-glycosylated (Zsebo et al., 1986).

The gene for human G-CSF was first cloned from 5637 cells by Souza et al. (Souza et al., 1986). The amino acid sequence has no significant homology to human or murine granulocyte-macrophage CSF (GM-CSF), interleukin-3 (IL-3), or macrophage CSF (M-CSF). A region of amino acid similarity exists between G-CSF and interleukin-6 (IL-6) suggesting that there may be some similarity in the tertiary structure, as well as some functional similarity (Hirano et al., 1986). Blots of messenger RNA (mRNA) isolated from 5637 cells, using a G-CSF–specific oligonucleotide probe reveal a single species of mRNA migrating at 1.65 kDa (Zsebo et al., 1986). Human G-CSF has also been cloned by Nagata et al. (1986) from a squamous carcinoma cell line; however, this clone contained nine additional bases, giving rise to a protein with three additional amino acids. Furthermore, this 177 amino acid species was 100-fold less biologically active in vitro (Zsebo et al., 1986; Nagata et al., 1986). It appears from analysis of genomic sequence that the formation of this 177 amino acid species occurs as the result of splicing at an alternative splice donor site between exons two and three (Zsebo et al., 1986).

The gene for G-CSF has been successfully expressed in *Escherichia coli (E. coli)* and recombinant protein produced (Souza et al., 1986). The molecular weight of recombinant human granulocyte CSF (rhG-CSF) is 18.0 kDa. The difference in molecular weight, compared to the natural protein, reflects the lack of glycosylation in the bacterially derived product; for G-CSF, however, this glycosylation is not required for in vitro or in vivo biological activity.

At the myeloid progenitor cell level, G-CSF stimulates the growth of neutrophilic granulocyte precursors (colony-forming units, granulocyte [CFU-G]) (Souza et al., 1986; Welte et al., 1985; Zsebo et al., 1986; Nagata et al., 1986; Platzer et al., 1985) and supports the survival and expansion in vitro of immature precursors of colony-forming cells (Pre-CFU) (Platzer et al., 1985).

Originally, human G-CSF was thought to be a pluripoietin, since it appeared to support the growth of human burst-forming unit erythroid (BFU-E), and uncommitted progenitors, so-called human "mixed" granulocyte, erythroid macrophage, and megakaryocyte (GEMM) colonies from bone marrow subjected to simple adherence and E rosette depletion of T cells (Souza et al., 1986; Welte et al., 1985; Platzer et al., 1985). However, with further depletion of accessory cells and enrichment of progenitors, G-CSF was found to no longer support the growth of erythroid or multilineage progenitors from this target-cell population (Strife et al., 1987). More recently, G-CSF has been shown to support the growth of megakaryocyte colonies in conjunction with IL-3 (McNiece et al., 1988). Granulocyte CSF also stimulates the growth and transient clonal proliferation of enriched promyelocytes and myelocytes (Begley et al., 1988).

On cells of the mature, postmitotic compartment, G-CSF has been shown to enhance the specific binding of the chemotactic bacterial peptide formyl-methionyl-leucyl-phenyl-alanine (FMLP) (Zsebo et al., 1986), to promote chemotaxis (Zsebo et al., 1986), and to augment neutrophil-mediated antibody-dependent cellular cytotoxicity (ADCC) (Platzer et al., 1986).

One important feature is that human G-CSF is not species-specific in its action and is quite active on myeloid elements of lower species (Welte et al., 1985; Zsebo et al., 1986).

GRANULOCYTE-MACROPHAGE COLONY-STIMULATING FACTOR

Human GM-CSF was first purified by Gasson et al. (1984) and molecularly cloned and expressed in mammalian cells by Wong et al. (1985). Human GM-CSF is highly and variably glycosylated, accounting for a wide range in reported molecular weights. The role of variable glycosylation with regard to cell-specific production, biological activity, or half-life remains to be determined. Although no formal comparison has been performed, both glycosylated and nonglycosylated GM-CSF are biologically active in vitro and in vivo in man. At the present time, three major recombinant forms of GM-CSF are available for clinical use: the characteristics of these preparations are outlined in Table 19-3.

TABLE 19-3
COMPARISON OF DIFFERENT RECOMBINANT GM-CSF PREPARATIONS

Source	Company	Specific activity (U/mg protein)
E. coli	Schering	1×10^8
Yeast	Immunex	4×10^7
Yeast	Immunex/Behringwerke	5×10^7
CHO	Sandoz	8×10^6

Recombinant human GM-CSF supports the growth of both granulocytic and monocytic colonies in semisolid culture (Gasson et al., 1984). However, it is also active at much earlier stages of myeloid development, as evidenced by its ability to produce colonies containing myeloid, erythroid, and megakaryocytic cells when combined with erythropoietin, a late-acting promoter of erythroid development (Gabrilove et al., 1986; Sieff et al., 1985; Metcalf et al., 1986). In the presence of rhGM-CSF, mature macrophages and neutrophils demonstrate enhanced tumoricidal and phagocytic activity, intracellular killing, ADCC, superoxide production, complement-mediated (opsonized) phagocytosis, and responsiveness to chemotactic factors (Weisbart et al., 1985; Lopez et al., 1986). Mature eosinophils also respond to rhGM-CSF with increased ADCC activity (Lopez et al., 1986). Granulocyte-macrophage CSF is an extremely potent inducer of Mo-1, a molecule involved in granulocyte cell-to-cell adhesion, and induces increased granulocyte aggregation in vitro (Lopez et al., 1986; Arnaout et al., 1986). Granulocyte-macrophage CSF has also been shown to inhibit the migration of neutrophil granulocytes in vitro (Gasson et al., 1984) and in vivo, in patients treated with a continuous infusion of GM-CSF (Peters et al., 1988c). The clinical significance of this remains to be determined. Biological effects of rhM-CSF include augmentation of macrophage-mediated and antibody-dependent monocyte-mediated cytotoxicity (ADMC) against human melanoma cell lines, antitumor activity in a mouse B-16 melanoma model, and induction of peripheral blood (PB) monocytosis in primates.

MACROPHAGE COLONY-STIMULATING FACTOR

Macrophage CSF is a heavily glycosylated dimer. Two forms of the glycoprotein exist, due to differential splicing of the gene (Griffin et al., 1984). The larger form encodes a 70,000 kDa glycoprotein, which is the major form of M-CSF in human urine and was first cloned by Wong et al. (1985). A smaller form was first cloned from a human pancreatic cell line by Kawasaki et al. (1985). Both forms of M-CSF are biologically active. Recombinant human M-CSF promotes the growth and maturation of monocyte and macrophage precursors. In addition, M-CSF enhances the phagocytic and tumoricidal activity of human monocyte/macrophages and induces them to secrete a variety of cytokines including tumor necrosis factor (TNF-α), interleukin-1 (IL-1), and CSF (Griffin et al., 1988). The receptor for M-CSF has also been identified and is identical to the proto-oncogene c-*fms* (Scher et al., 1985). Receptors for M-CSF have also been identified on tissue trophoblasts and may play a role in the process of fertilization and/or implantation.

INTERLEUKIN-3

Murine IL-3 was purified and characterized first by Ihle et al. (1982) and was subsequently shown to support the formation of multilineage colonies in vitro. Gibbon and human IL-3 have recently been cloned using expression cloning techniques (Yang et al., 1986). Interleukin-3 is a complex glycoprotein, ranging in size from 14 to 28 kDa. The expected size of the polypeptide is 14 to 15 kDa (Yang et al., 1986). It is interesting to note that the homology of murine IL-3 and human IL-3 at the amino acid level is only 29%, compared with a 93% homology between gibbon IL-3 and human IL-3 (Yang et al., 1986).

Recently, Leary et al. (1987) tested recombinant gibbon IL-3 on the proliferation and differentiation of an enriched population of human hematopoietic progenitors. Recombinant IL-3 supported the formation of various types of single lineage, as well as multilineage colonies by CD34 (My10)-positive bone marrow cells in the presence of erythropoietin. In addition, IL-3 supported the formation of blast-cell colonies with high replating capability (Leary et al., 1987a; Andreeff and Welte, 1989). In these experiments, IL-3 proved to be much more effective than GM-CSF in supporting 21-day colony formation by normal human hematopoietic blasts, and the resulting colonies could be replated to yield secondary colonies with much higher efficiency than that obtained with GM-CSF–derived colonies (Leary et al., 1987; Andreeff et al., 1989). These data suggest that IL-3 is probably the least restricted of the CSF with regard to cell lineage and is also the factor with the greatest variety of action with regard to target cells. Interleukin-3 acts not only at the restricted progenitor cell level, but appears to affect the functional activity of mature granulocytes (Ihle et al., 1982) and monocytes as well.

INTERLEUKIN-6

Human IL-6 (B-cell stimulating factor 2 [BSF2]) was originally identified as a factor in the culture supernatants of mitogen- or antigen-stimulated mononuclear cells, which induced immunoglobulin production in either Epstein-Barr virus (EBV)–transformed B cells lines or in *Staphylococcus aureus* Cowan 1 (SAC)–stimulated normal B cells (Kishimoto, 1989; Muraguchi et al., 1987).

The molecular cloning of the cDNA of IL-6 revealed that this factor was identical to a number of other well-described regulatory molecules with a variety of biological activities (Table 19-4). Thus, it became apparent that the actions of IL-6 were not restricted to B cells, but played an important role in various tissues and cells (Kishimoto, 1989).

Interleukin-6 is a cytokine produced by a variety of normal cells including T and B cells, monocytes, endothelial cells, keratinocytes, astrocytes, fibroblasts, mesangial cells, and bone marrow stromal cells (Table 19-4) (Kishimoto, 1989). In addition, a number of cultured cell lines have been known to produce IL-6, including the monocytic leukemia cells U937 and P388D1, HTLV-1 transformed cells, T24 bladder "epithelial" carcinoma cell line, osteosarcoma (MG63), lung carcinoma (A549) glioblastoma (SKMG4), and astrocytoma (U373) cells (Kishimoto, 1989).

A number of investigators have demonstrated the effect of IL-6 on the hematopoietic system (Kishimoto, 1989; Leary et al., 1988). Most studies have shown a synergistic effect of IL-6 with IL-3 in supporting the formation (increasing both number and size) of multilineage blast colonies in culture suggesting either the recruitment

TABLE 19-4
MOLECULAR EQUIVALENTS AND ACTION OF INTERLEUKIN-6*

Molecules identical to IL-6	Major actions of IL-6
B-cell stimulatory factor 2	Induction of B cell differentiation and/or specific gene expression
Interferon-beta-2	Immunoglobulin induction in B cells, in liver cells including fibrinogen, alpha 1-antichymotypsin, alpha-1-acid glycoprotein, haptoglobin, C-reactive protein 1-antitypsin, and amyloid A.
26-kDa protein	Induction of cytotoxic T-cell differentiation (with IL-2)
Myeloma/plasmacytoma	Induction of neural cell (PC12) differentiation
Induction of acute phase proteins growth factor	Activation of hematopoietic stem cells from G_0 to G_1
Hepatocyte stimulating factor	Stimulation of cell growth
Macrophage-granulocyte inducing factor 2	Induction of the growth of myeloma/plasmacytoma cells
Cytotoxic T-cell differentiation factor	Induction of T-cell growth, activation
	Induction of IL-2 receptors and IL-2 production in mitrogen stimulated T cells.
	Induction of mesangial cell growth
	Supports murine neutrophil/macrophage eosinophils, mast cell and megakaryocyte colonies
	Inhibition of cell growth
	Growth inhibition of myeloid leukemia cells (M1 cells)
	Growth inhibition of breast carcinoma cell lines
	Growth inhibition for human fibroblasts

*Adapted from Kishimoto, 1989.

from G_0 of stem cells or their proliferation (Kishimoto, 1989; Leary et al., 1988). In fact, the synergistic activity of IL-1 with IL-3 in promoting the proliferation of hematopoietic stem cells may be induced and secondary to the induction of IL-6 by IL-1 (Leary et al., 1988). In addition, IL-6 has demonstrated some activity in inducing differentiation of the murine myelomonocytic leukemic cells (M1) into macrophages, as well as enhancing phagocytosis and the expression of Fc and C3d receptors on these same targets (Kishimoto, 1989).

INTERLEUKIN-1

Interleukin-1 is a mediator involved in numerous inflammatory, immunological, and hematologic responses (Miller and Dinarello, 1987). Two forms of IL-1 have been characterized, IL-1 β and IL-1 α, although a few differences in the range of their respective biological activities have been observed and both species apparently bind to the same receptor. Interleukin-1 is a 17.5-kDa protein that is produced by activated monocytes, as well as a variety of other cell types (Table 19-2) (Dinarello, 1988). The major actions of IL-1 are summarized in Table 19-5.

INTERLEUKIN-4

As with most lymphokines, IL-4 has been found to be multifunctional in its regulation of the immune response, acting on different cell lineages and at different stages of development and differentiation (Sideras et al., 1988; Peschel et al., 1987). More recently, it has been shown to have both direct and indirect effects on the regulation of hematopoiesis. The actions of IL-4 are summarized in Table 19-6.

TABLE 19-5
ACTIONS OF IL-1 (ALPHA AND BETA)

Endocrine effects
Stimulation of ACTH secretion
Inhibition of LH + FSH induced differentiation of granulosa cells
Stimulation/inhibition of insulin release
Cytotoxic for pancreatic islet cells
Growth effects
Astroglial cells
IL-2 receptor expression
Hematopoietic effects
Radioprotective
Myeloprotective
Increases procoagulant activity
Potent stimulant of neutrophil chemotaxis

TABLE 19-6
ACTIONS OF INTERLEUKIN-4

Proliferation of human pre-B cells
Induces DNA synthesis in purified B-cell populations
Increases class II antigen (Ag) expression on resting B cells
Induces low-affinity IgE receptors
Increases CD23 Ag expresssion
Costimulant of B-cell activation
Increases I E production
Costimulates growth of T cells
Stimulates growth of CD4, CD8, and CD3 NK cells
Inhibits IL-2–mediated induction of LAK-cell activity
Enhanced activity of Ag-specific cytotoxic T cells
Synergizes with IL-6 and G-CSF to promote growth of high proliferative potential cells from 5-FU–treated mice: interacts with rhG-CSF to enhance proliferation of CFU-GM
Induces mRNA expression for GM-CSF, IL-3, and M-CSF from monocytes, GM-CSF, G-CSF, and M-CSF in endothelial cells.

IN VITRO AND IN VIVO BIOLOGICAL EFFECTS AND PRODUCTION OF CSF BY MALIGNANT HEMATOPOIETIC CELLS

Many investigators have studied the effects of IL-3, GM-CSF, G-CSF, and M-CSF on leukemic cell colony growth (Nara et al., 1988; Kelleher et al., 1987; Griffin et al., 1986; Hoang et al., 1986). These growth factors have been shown to stimulate the proliferation, self-renewal, and differentiation of blast stem cells from patients with acute myeloblastic leukemia in either suspension culture or clonogenic assays (Souza et al., 1986; Nara et al., 1987; Kelleher et al., 1987; Griffin et al., 1986; Hoang et al., 1986; Vallenga et al., 1987; Miyauchi et al., 1987; Lange et al., 1987). Other investigators have shown that the incubation of defective neutrophil granulocytes from patients with either chronic myelogenous leukemia (CML) or myelodysplastic syndrome can repair neutrophil function as measured by superoxide anion production induced by FMLP (Yuo et al., 1987). One problem with the interpretation of the data from these different experiments is that there is no clear evidence of whether one is stimulating residual normal or leukemic progenitors. The use of cytogenetics employing the premature condensation technique or molecular analysis that takes advantage of restriction-length DNA polymorphism should help to clarify in future studies whether or not the normal or leukemic cell clone is being affected in these types of proliferation- and differentiation-inducing experiments.

Several investigators have also demonstrated that leukemic cells may constitutively express message and produce biologically active CSF (Young and Griffin, 1986; Sakai et al., 1987; Cheng et al., 1988; Griffin et al., 1987; Young et al., 1987). Alteration in the structure of both G-CSF and GM-CSF, as detected by Southern analysis, has been reported in two instances (Cheng et al., 1988). In one case, an abnormally large GM-CSF message was observed. Granulocyte-CSF is located in close proximity to the breakpoint on chromosome 17 involved in the 15/17 translocation in acute promyelocytic leukemia; however, no rearrangements of the gene for G-CSF in this disorder have been found (Simmers et al., 1987).

In the 5q- syndrome, the region of variable deletion on chromosome 5 contains the genes for IL-3, GM-CSF, M-CSF, and the receptor for M-CSF (Nimer and Golde, 1988); however, one presumably normal copy of each gene can still be found on the remaining intact chromosome 5. What relationship the disruption or loss of these growth factor genes plays in the natural history of this disease and the evolution to acute leukemia is unknown and remains an area of active investigation.

These hematopoietic growth factors may not only be important physiological regulators in maintaining hematopoiesis and augmenting host defense, but may also play a role in the pathogenesis or observed phenomena associated with disease. A summary of the associations between these CSF as well as IL-3, IL-1, and IL-6 and various physiological and/or disease states, with regard to either expression, production, or detection in vitro or in vivo, is outlined in Table 19-7.

TABLE 19-7
ASSOCIATIONS OF GROWTH FACTOR EXPRESSION, PRODUCTION, DETECTION, AND DISEASE: IN VITRO AND/OR IN VIVO

G-CSF	Endotoxemic/Bacteremia	Increase serum level in vivo
	ANLL blasts	Constitutive mRNA expression, in vitro, in some cells
GM-CSF	ANLL blasts	Constitutive mRNA expression in vitro, in some cells
IL-3	ANLL blasts	Constitutive mRNA expression, in vitro, in come cells
M-CSF		
IL-1	ANLL blasts	Constitutive mRNA expression, in vitro, in some cells
	Diabetes	Islet cell destruction
	Rheumatoid arthritis	Increased levels in synovial fluid
IL-6	Lennert's T-cell lymphoma	IL-6 supports in vitro growth Anti–IL-6 inhibits macrophage-dependent growth of lymphoma
	Cardiac myxoma	Constitutive mRNA and protein by myxoma cells, in vitro
	Myeloma and plasmacytoma	In vitro constitutive production by myeloma cells and cell lines
	Castleman's disease	In vitro responsiveness related to severity of disease
	Rheumatoid arthritis	Increased levels in synovial fluid constitutive production by T cells

PRECLINICAL IN VIVO

In preclinical models, IL-3 (Donahue et al., 1987), GM-CSF (Donahue et al., 1986; Mayer et al., 1987), and G-CSF (Welte et al., 1987a) have been shown to elevate the number of functionally normal leukocytes in nonhuman primates. Following GM-CSF, this elevation is in part due to an increase in circulating eosinophil granulocytes (Donahue et al., 1986), whereas the augmentation in white cell count following G-CSF is due predominantly to an increase in neutrophil granulocytes (Welte et al., 1987a). Interleukin-1 α has also been reported to enhance murine granulopoiesis (Stork et al., 1987). This effect may be due to either the direct action of IL-1 α or to the induction of CSF following IL-1 α administration (Stork et al., 1987). The sequential administration of IL-3 followed by GM-CSF to nonhuman primates has been shown to modestly augment circulating platelet counts as well (Donahue et al., 1987a).

The administration of CSF and IL-1 in the setting of viral-induced pancytopenia or myelosuppression related to either chemotherapy or radiation treatment has also been tested in nonhuman primate and murine models. Granulocyte-macrophage CSF has been shown to augment leukocyte counts in rhesus monkeys infected with a type D retrovirus (Donahue et al., 1986) and to accelerate the recovery of hematopoietic reconstitution following total body irradiation (TBI) and infusion of autologous bone marrow (Nienhuis et al., 1987; Monsoy et al., 1987a). Administration of rhG-CSF has been shown to shorten the period of neutropenia in cynomologous primates treated with either high-dose cyclophosphamide (Welte et al., 1987a), busulfan (Gillio et al., 1987), or TBI in the setting of autologous bone marrow transplantation (BMT) (Neta et al., 1986). Treatment with IL-1 has been observed to accelerate stem-cell recovery in 5-fluorouracil–treated mice and to synergize with lineage-specific factors such as G-CSF in augmenting early hematopoietic reconstitution in the same model system (Warren et al., 1987). In addition, a single injection of IL-1 has been shown to protect against radiation-induced myelosuppression (Neta et al., 1986). More recently, IL-1 (α and β) has been demonstrated to stimulate normal granulopoietic and accelerate platelet recovery when administered to rhesus monkeys after total body irradiation and autologous BMT (Monsoy et al., 1987b).

More recently, Schuening et al. (1989) tested whether administration of rhG-CSF could reverse the otherwise lethal myelosuppressive effect of total body irradiation. The study design included animals treated with either (1) TBI alone (4G4 at 10 cGY/min from two opposing Cobalt 60 [^{60}Co] sources), (2) TBI (day 0) and rhG-CSF (DO [beginning 2 hours after TBI] to day 21), (3) TBI (day 0) and rhG-CSF commencing on day 7 (Schuening et al., 1989). The results demonstrated that rhG-CSF was radioprotective if given immediately following exposure to TBI; however, protection was lost if one waited 7 days to begin administration of the hematopoietic growth factor (Schuening et al., 1989). Although the animals were protected from lethality and myeloid cell recovery did occur, the animals still became profoundly neutropenic for a finite period, suggesting that if one wanted to further accelerate recovery or completely protect the host from neutropenia as well as thrombocytopenia, one would need to employ either a combination of stem-cell and lineage-specific factors with or without the infusion of progenitors (either in the form of blood or marrow) to promote more complete and effective reconstitution.

CLINICAL APPLICATIONS

Until recently, insufficient amounts of CSF were available for definitive in vivo studies. The availability of all the CSF in gram quantities is now allowing the pharmacology and physiology of each factor to be studied in detail.

For the purpose of this review, we will focus the major portion of our attention on those studies employing rhG-CSF and rhGM-CSF, since these two hematopoietic factors have been the most extensively investigated.

ADMINISTRATION OF CSF TO CANCER PATIENTS AND NORMAL VOLUNTEERS NOT RECEIVING MYELOSUPPRESSIVE TREATMENT

Administration of both rhG-CSF and rhGM-CSF to cancer patients either in the absence of, or prior to, myelosuppressive treatment results in a dramatic elevation in circulating neutrophilic and neutrophilic-eosinophilic granulocytes, respectively (Morstyn et al., 1988; 1989a, 1989b; Bronchud et al., 1988; Peters et al., 1988a; Gabrilove et al., 1988a; Jakubowski et al., 1989b; Herrmann et al., 1989a; Rifkin et al., 1988; Lieschke et al., 1989; Clark et al., 1988; Steward et al., 1988; Antman et al., 1989; Phillips et al., 1989; Vadhan-Raj et al., 1988a; Devreux et al., 1988). We will review the use of each growth factor separately in this setting and discuss the physiological effects on (1) neutrophilic granulocyte production and function, (2) other hematopoietic cell lineages, (3) bone marrow cellularity and morphology, (4) bone marrow and circulating progenitor cell development and growth, and (5) pharmacokinetics. We will discuss side effects and safety separately.

Recombinant Human G-CSF

Neutrophilic Granulocytes A number of studies exploring different routes of administration of rhG-CSF, including a twice-daily intravenous (IV) infusion, subcutaneous injection as a bolus, continuous subcutaneous infusions, and continuous IV infusions in the absence of chemotherapy have demonstrated the immediate effect of rhG-CSF to be a decrease in circulating neutrophil counts within 5 minutes (short IV administration) or 1 hour (continuous IV infusion) with the magnitude of the decrease independent of the dose (Morstyn et al., 1988, 1989a, 1989b; Bronchud et al., 1988). After 4 hours, a rise in circulating neutrophils occurred that was near maximal within 24 hours (Morstyn et al., 1988; Bronchud et al., 1988). The basis of the transient fall in neutrophils has not been determined, but does not appear to be due to any selective organ and, in particular, not to pulmonary sequestration (Bronchud et al., 1988; Peters et al., 1988b).

In all studies, a marked increase in circulating neutrophilic granulocytes has been noted. The fold increase in circulating neutrophil counts in one study was identical for patients who had received prior pelvic radiation therapy when compared to their previously nonirradiated cohorts (Gabrilove et al., 1988b). However, in a second study, two of three patients who had received extensive prior chemotherapy or radiotherapy did not exhibit a sustained increase in neutrophil counts (Morstyn et al., 1988, 1989a).

In all studies, the increase in absolute neutrophil count (ANC) was due primarily to an increase in mature segmented polymorphonuclear granulocytes with some increase in band forms (Morstyn et al., 1988, 1989a, 1989b; Bronchud et al., 1988; Peters et al., 1988; Gabrilove et al., 1988a; Jakubowski et al., 1989b). The increase in ANC does not appear to be due to an increase in survival of neutrophilic granulocytes, since PB neutrophils obtained from patients during rhG-CSF treatment exhibit similar survival kinetics to those obtained from normal control volunteers (Bronchud et al., 1988).

In all studies, morphological changes noted in neutrophilic granulocytes included the appearance of Dohle bodies (Morstyn et al., 1988, 1989a, 1989b; Gabrilove et al., 1988a; Jakubowski et al., 1989b), toxic granulations (Gabrilove et al., 1988a; Jakubowski et al., 1989b), a decrease in nuclear lobulation (Gabrilove et al., 1988a; Jakubowski et al., 1989b), and an increase in the leukocyte alkaline phosphatase (LAP) score (Morstyn et al., 1988, 1989a, 1989b; Bronchud et al., 1988; Peters et al., 1988a; Gabrilove et al., 1988a; Jakubowski et al., 1989b).

Neutrophil Function Neutrophilic granulocytes obtained from patients treated with rhG-CSF appear to function normally in vitro and in vivo as measured by phagocytic activity (chemoluminescence) (Bronchud et al., 1988), migration in vitro (chemotaxis) (Gabrilove et al., 1988a; Jakubowski and Gabrilove, 1989b), and in vivo as measured by employing a skin-chambers technique (Toner et al., 1989).

Other Peripheral Blood Hematopoietic Cell Lineages Circulating eosinophilic and basophilic granulocytes remained unchanged following administration of rhG-CSF. Circulating monocyte counts were unchanged in patients treated with lower doses; however, a 10-fold increase in monocytes was noted following 30 to 100 μg of rhG-CSF/μg/day administered as a 30- to 40-minute IV infusion (Gabrilove et al., 1988; Jakubowski and Gabrilove, 1989). A dose-independent twofold increase in lymphocytes was also noted with daily IV administration of rhG-CSF (Gabrilove et al., 1988; Jakubowski and Gabrilove, 1989). No consistent effect on hemoglobin, hematocrit, or platelet counts were noted in any study during the period of rhG-CSF administration (Gabrilove et al., 1988a; Jakubowski and Gabrilove, 1989b).

Bone Marrow An increase in bone marrow myeloid to erythroid (M:E) cell ratio and cellularity was noted in all studies (Morstyn et al., 1988, 1989a, 1989b; Bronchud et al., 1988; Peters et al., 1988a; Gabrilove et al., 1988a; Jakubowski and Gabrilove, 1989b). Gabrilove et al. (1988a) noted that at the 3 μg/kg/day dose level the increase in M:E ratio was due primarily to an increase in the postmitotic compartment (metamyelocytes, bands, and polymorphs), whereas at the 30 to 60 μg/kg dose level, the increase in M:E ratio reflected an increase in the mitotic compartment, with a marked increase in the proportion of promyelocytes. Similar observations were made by Morstyn et al. (1988, 1989a, 1989b).

Hematopoietic Progenitors In two studies, a significant increase in circulating hematopoietic progenitors was noted (Gabrilove et al., 1988a; Duhrsen et al., 1988) with up to a 100-fold dose-related increase in the number of circulating progenitor cells of the granulocyte-macrophage, erythroid, and megakaryocyte type (Duhrsen et al., 1988). In both studies, the frequency of bone marrow progenitors detected remained either unchanged or was decreased per 10^5 bone marrow cells plated (Gabrilove et al., 1988a; Duhrsen et al., 1988). The proportion of cycling bone marrow–derived hematopoietic progenitor cells was only slightly increased by rhG-CSF treatment (Bronchud et al., 1988).

Pharmacokinetics In one study, circulating levels of rhG-CSF were assessed by a solid phase sandwich radioimmunoassay using patient serum samples collected at intervals after administration (Gabrilove et al., 1988a). A subset of five patients receiving rhG-CSF at the 10 to 60 μg/kg/day dose level was studied. For a period of 40 minutes, immediately after cessation of the rhG-CSF infusion, the levels of rhG-CSF remained relatively constant and proportional to the dosage of material administered. After 40 minutes, the serum levels of rhG-CSF decayed logarithmically with time, allowing the calculation of elimination kinetics. Elimination half-lives for five patients were 3.9, 3.9, 6.3, 6.3, and 5.0 hours, respectively, for an average value of 5.1 ± 0.5 hours (standard error) (Gabrilove et al., 1988a). Furthermore, these results indicated that the elimination pathway had not reached saturation for the doses tested (Gabrilove et al., 1988a).

In a second study, the elimination half-life was found to be dose dependent, as measured by bioassay, employing either a clonal agar differentiation assay using WEHI 3B (D^+) myelomonocytic leukemia cells or normal human or murine bone marrow progenitor cell growth. Using these assays, a dose of 0.5 and 1.5 μg/kg/day was found to be cleared with a half-life of 1.4 ± 0.3 hours and doses of 5.0 μg and 30 μg/kg having a half-life of 3.7 ± 1.1 hours. These data suggest that at least one mechanism of clearance becomes saturated at a dose of 5 μg/kg (Morstyn et al., 1988, 1989a).

Following a single-bolus subcutaneous injection, peak serum levels of G-CSF are reached after about 4 hours at the 10 μg/kg/day dose level with levels of detectable G-CSF being maintained for 9 hours or more (Morstyn et al., 1988). When rhG-CSF was administered as a continuous subcutaneous infusion over a 5-day period at 10 μg/kg/day, a plateau serum G-CSF level was expected because the rate of infusion was constant; however, the G-CSF levels fell markedly over the last 2 days of the infusion, apparently because a new clearance mechanism was induced (Morstyn et al., 1988). In another group of patients, a 5-day continuous subcutaneous infusion was given after an injection of melphalan (Morstyn et al., 1988). In this situation, the large fall in serum G-CSF during the infusion was not seen, indicating that a high output of neutrophils from the bone marrow was required for the induced clearance seen in the first group (Morstyn et al., 1988). This method of downregulation of G-CSF may be important in returning neutrophil levels to normal after a crisis such as septicemia (Morstyn et al., 1988). In conclusion, there appear to be at least three mechanisms for the clearance of G-CSF, but the nature of these mechanisms remains to be elucidated (Morstyn et al., 1988).

Other Laboratory Changes In all three studies, a dose-associated increase in alkaline phosphatase (presumably bone in origin), lactate dehydrogenase, and leukocyte alkaline phosphatase has been observed (Morstyn et al., 1988, 1989a, 1989b; Bronchud et al., 1988; Peters et al., 1988a; Gabrilove et al., 1988a; Jakubowski and Gabrilove, 1989b). At higher doses (>30 μg/kg/day IV) an increase in uric acid, most likely related to an increase in leukocyte turnover, has also been noted (Muraguchi et al., 1987; Fukuoka et al., 1988; Gottschall et al., 1987). At the 100-μg dose level (IV), a mild increase in SGOT and GGTP was also observed (Jakubowski and Gabrilove, 1989). All of these values returned to normal or near baseline within 1 to 2 weeks of G-CSF administration. In patients administered 60 to 100 μg/kg/day as a short IV infusion, cholesterol levels demonstrated a decrease over the treatment period with variable changes in triglycerides (Jakubowski and Gabrilove, 1989).

Recombinant Human GM-CSF

Different rhGM-CSF preparations, both bacterial (*E. coli*), yeast, and mammalian (CHO) cell–derived, each with different specific activities, have been administered to hematologically normal and leukopenic cancer patients with success (Herrmann et al., 1989a; Rifkin et al., 1988; Lieschke et al., 1989; Clark et al., 1988; Steward et al., 1988; Antman et al., 1989; Phillips et al., 1989; Vadhan-Raj et al., 1988b).

Neutrophil Counts A dose-dependent increase in neutrophil counts has been reported in most studies (Herrmann et al., 1989a; Rifkin et al., 1988; Lieschke et al., 1989; Clark et al., 1988; Steward et al., 1988; Antman et al., 1989; Phillips et al., 1989; Vadhan-Raj et al., 1988b). Herrmann et al. (1989), however, reported that only 4 of 15 patients had a rise above pretreatment levels in their white blood count (WBC) and segmented neutrophilic granulocytes following IV bolus administration of 120 to 1500 $\mu g/m^2/day \times 5$ days, whereas rhGM-CSF administered by continuous infusion (CI) resulted in a striking dose-related rise in circulating neutrophil counts. Similar findings were reported by Rifkin et al. (1988) in patients with advanced cancer treated with the identical rhGM-CSF preparation. Subcutaneously administered rhGM-CSF (0.3–30 μg/kg/day) for 10 days resulted in up to a 2.2- to 10-fold increase in circulating neutrophilic granulocytes, with an initial dose-dependent response (0.1–3 μg/kg/day) followed by a plateau in the neutrophilic granulocyte response (3–15 μg/kg/day) and, then, once again a further small increment in leukocyte augmentation at the 20 μg/kg/day dose level (Lieschke et al., 1989). In this study, patients who had received previous extensive chemotherapy or radiotherapy had the smallest elevations in circulating leukocytes during rhGM-CSF treatment at the 3, 10, and 15 μg/kg/day subcutaneous dose levels (Lieschke et al., 1989).

Following the start of either glycosylated or nonglycosylated rhGM-CSF administration (either as a short or as a continuous IV infusion), immediate, transient neutropenia, eosinopenia, and monocytopenia, which in one study appeared to be dose-related (Herrmann et al., 1989a) and in two others appeared not to be (Herrmann et al., 1989a; Phillips et al., 1989), have been observed. The time of the maximum nadir was observed at 30 minutes with a rebound in the leukocyte count to baseline or above baseline by 2 hours. This effect was noted even at doses that had no apparent proliferative effect and resulted in no augmentation of the circulating leukocyte count (Morstyn et al., 1988, 1989a; Lieschke et al., 1989). Radionuclide labeling studies, first reported by Devreux et al. (1988), showed that the leukopenia was due to sequestration within the lungs. Subsequently, several groups have confirmed these initial findings (Peters et al., 1988d; Herrmann et al., 1989a). Following subcutaneous administration of nonglycosylated rhGM-CSF, a rapid decrease in circulating leukocytes, with a maximum nadir occurring by 60 minutes and lasting for up to 4 hours, has been observed. This effect appears to be independent of the dose administered.

In all studies, an apparent biphasic response to rhGM-CSF has been noted over time, with an initial plateau in WBC augmentation achieved after 3 to 7 days, depending upon the route of administration, followed by a second increase and plateau thereafter. Two explanations could be proposed to account for the kinetics of the neutrophil response following GM-CSF administration. One explanation would be that it takes 7 days to mature cells from the myeloblast to polymorphonuclear leukocyte stage and 7 more days to see reflected in the circulating counts, the proliferative effects of rhGM-CSF on the day-14 CFU-granulocyte macrophage (CFU-GM) progenitor compartment. Alternatively, one could suggest that the delayed peak in the neutrophil response is secondary to the induction of lineage-specific factors such as G-CSF, M-CSF, and interleukin-5 (IL-5), which would work in concert with GM-CSF to further amplify and augment the leukocyte response. This is certainly plausible, since GM-CSF has been reported in vitro to induce both G-CSF and M-CSF (Lindemann et al., 1987; Horiguchi et al., 1987). In addition, eosinophils are not noted until after 7 days, perhaps suggesting that some secondary mediator has been brought into play. Which hypothesis is correct remains to be elucidated, but clearly, it would be of interest to know if the circulating levels of G-CSF, M-CSF, or IL-5, respectively, increased during rhGM-CSF administration.

Neutrophilia, following rhGM-CSF, showed a mild left shift: at higher doses (10–20 μg/kg/day of nonglycosylated rhGM-CSF subcutaneously or greater than 120 μg/m^2/day glycosylated (yeast-derived) rhGM-CSF), circulating myelocytes, promyelocytes, and myeloblasts contributed to the cytosis (Morstyn et al., 1988, 1989a; Herrmann et al., 1989a; Lieschke et al., 1989).

Morphological changes in neutrophils following rhGM-CSF have been reported to include toxic granulations (Morstyn et al., 1988, 1989a; Herrmann et al., 1989a; Lieschke et al., 1989), and an increase in leukocyte alkaline phosphatase (Herrmann et al., 1989a; Lieschke et al., 1989), as seen with G-CSF; in addition, cytoplasmic vacuolization (Herrmann et al., 1989a) and hypersegmentation of polymorphonuclear granulocytes (Herrmann et al., 1989a) have been reported.

Neutrophil Function Several investigators have reported preserved in vitro neutrophil function, as measured by phagocytosis and generation of superoxide (Peters et al., 1988; Kaplan et al., 1988). Peters et al. (1988) have reported markedly impaired migration of neutrophils in vivo to a skin abrasion, in patients receiving continuous IV infusions of glycosylated rhGM-CSF. Toner et al. (1989), however, have reported that previously treated ovarian cancer patients, receiving 4-hour infusions of nonglycosylated rhGM-CSF, at doses of 1 to 2 μg/kg/day, did not exhibit impaired migration. However, at higher doses of GM-CSF, migration was also noted to be inhibited with this route of administration and growth factor preparation (Toner and Gabrilove, unpublished observation). The clinical ramifications of this remain to be determined. However, the concern would be that, in patients at risk for, or with, active soft tissue infection, treatment with rhGM-CSF could potentially impair the ability of inflammatory cells to reach the infectious nidus.

Other Cell Lineages A specific increase in eosinophils has been reported after 5 days of rhGM-CSF, administered either as an IV bolus ($\geq$500 μg/m^2: as high as 199.8- ± 20.7-fold) (Herrmann et al., 1989a), continuous infusion ($>$120 μg/m^2/day) (Phillips et al., 1989), or subcutaneous bolus (10–20 μg/kg/day: 33-, 48-, and 71-fold, respectively, by day 10) (Lieschke et al., 1989).

An increase in monocytes has also been noted following the administration of both glycosylated and nonglycosylated GM-CSF, independent of the route of administration (Clark et al., 1988; Steward et al., 1988; Antman et al., 1989; Phillips et al., 1989; Vadhan-Raj et al., 1988a; Devreux et al., 1988; Lindemann et al., 1987). In two studies, monocytes from patients treated with GM-CSF have been reported to express enhanced tumoricidal activity in vitro (Cannistra et al., 1988b; Wing et al., 1988). However, in one other study, no enhanced tumoricidal activity of monocytes was observed (Kleinerman et al., 1988).

During subcutaneous administration of nonglycosylated rhGM-CSF, no consistent effect on hemoglobin, reticulocyte, or platelet counts was noted (Lieschke et al., 1989). Two other studies reported a transient decline in platelets to $<$20% of pretreatment levels after 6 or more days of glycosylated rhGM-CSF and no change in hemoglobin or reticulocyte count (Herrmann et al., 1989a; Clark et al., 1988). Lieschke and colleagues also reported the occurrence of thrombocytopenia possibly secondary to reactivation of idiopathic thrombocytopenia purpura in a patient with a history of the disorder (Bronchud et al., 1988; Lieschke et al., 1989).

Bone Marrow Marrow biopsies obtained from patients receiving glycosylated and nonglycosylated rhGM-CSF have demonstrated an increase in myelopoiesis with an increase in myeloid to erythroid cell ratios (Herrmann et al., 1989a; Lieschke et al., 1989; Antman et al., 1989; Phillips et al., 1989) and a shift toward immaturity with increases, in particular, of promyelocytes and myelocytes (Herrmann et al., 1989a; Lieschke et al., 1989). In patients who develop significant circulating eosinophilia, marrow eosinophilia is also noted (Lieschke et al., 1989).

Bone Marrow and Circulating Progenitors Socinski et al. (1988) were the first to report that PB day-14 CFU-GM and BFU-E per milliliter of blood increased by 18- and 8-fold, respectively, following 6 days of rhGM-CSF stimulation, whereas no significant change in bone marrow progenitors was noted (Socinski et al., 1988). Similar findings have been reported by two other groups utilizing glycosylated preparations of rhGM-CSF (Herrmann et al., 1989a; Cannistra et al., 1988b).

An increase in the percentage of CFU-GM and BFU-E in S phase has been reported in patients receiving 3 and 6 days of glycosylated GM-CSF administered as a continuous IV infusion (Aglietta et al., 1989). In one study, the percentage of bone marrow myeloblasts, promyelocytes, and myelocytes but not erythroblasts in S phase, as measured by 3HTdr autoradiography, was also reported (Aglietta et al., 1989). In addition, these investigators observed an increase in the birth rate of cycling cells from 1.3% to 3.4% per hour and a decrease in (1) the duration of S phase from 14.3 to 9.1 hours and (2) cell cycle time from 86 hours to 26 hours. Finally, the proportion of S-phase bone marrow cells dropped to values lower than pretreatment levels following discontinuation of rhGM-CSF, suggesting a period of relative refractoriness to cell cycle active antineoplastic agents (Aglietta et al., 1989).

Pharmacokinetics Utilizing a radioreceptor assay, a two-compartment model of elimination was reported by Herrmann et al. (1989a), which appeared to be independent of the dose administered. In six patients, clearance of glycosylated rhGM-CSF administered over 30 minutes was found to have an alpha phase of 10 $\pm$ 3 minutes and a beta phase of 85 $\pm$ 35 minutes (Herrmann et al., 1989a).

More extensive pharmacokinetic analysis has been undertaken by Cebon et al. (1988) in patients receiving nonglycosylated GM-CSF. These investigators determined the pharmacokinetics of rhGM-CSF employing both a bone marrow hematopoietic progenitor cell assay and a sensitive (sensitive to 0.02 ng/mL) sandwich enzyme–linked immunosorbent assay (Cebon et al., 1988). Utilizing the latter technique, at the lowest IV and subcutaneous dose levels of 0.3 μg/kg, serum levels of 14 $\pm$ 3 ng/mL and 30 pg/mL, respectively, were measured, with rhGM-CSF being rapidly cleared from the blood within 120 minutes following IV administration, with two apparent phases. Following a 1 μg/kg dose of intravenously administered rhGM-CSF, peak levels of 54 ± 26 ng/mL were achieved with blood levels dropping to less than 5 ng/mL after 60 minutes and to <1 ng/mL by 120 minutes. The same dose administered subcutaneously to two patients resulted in peak levels of 0.75 ± 0.03 and 0.71 ± 0.04 ng/mL 120 minutes after injection. At this dose level, both IV and subcutaneous administrations were associated with at least a twofold increase in WBC by day 10 of treatment. Higher doses of 3 and 10 μg/kg/day subcutaneously, respectively, were associated with earlier initial peaks (within 15 minutes) and prolonged plateau levels of 1 to 3 ng/mL that remained detectable for up to 9 hours.

Overall, a half-life alpha of less than 5 minutes and half-life beta of 50 minutes assuming two phases of elimination from IV administration could be calculated. In contrast, after subcutaneous administration, a rise in rhGM-CSF blood levels occurred within 1 hour, peaked by 2 to 4 hours and fell after 2 to 12 hours. The time during which rhGM-CSF remained detectable was dose-dependent. At the dose level of 10 μg/kg, 0.1 ng/mL levels were detectable for 12 hours: this achievable level is equivalent to sustained levels of 100 units of activity, which is close to the maximal activity required to stimulate both progenitor cell development and granulocyte function (Cebon et al., 1988).

Laboratories

An increase in serum alkaline phosphatase of 1.4-fold was noted in 7 of 16 patients receiving >8 days of subcutaneously administered nonglycosylated GM-CSF (Lieschke et al., 1989). All patients treated for 8 days at 15 and 20 μg/kg/day developed twofold or greater increases of at least two hepatic enzymes, including aspartate aminotransferase levels, with the largest increases being seen in the latter. Increases in lactate dehydrogenase were also observed (Lieschke et al., 1989).

Other Hematopoietic Growth Factors

More recently, studies have been conducted exploring the use of stem-cell growth factors such as IL-1 and IL-3 in an attempt to both enhance stem-cell proliferation, availability, and response to lineage specific factors and to hasten the recovery of hematopoietic cells other than myeloid elements alone. To this end, a study of IL-1 in patients receiving myelosuppressive doses of 5-fluorouracil (5-FU) has recently been undertaken. In this trial, patients with metastatic colorectal cancer have received the following treatment: cycle A: IL-1 alone (.002–.068 μg/kg × 2); cycle B: 5-FU 833 mg/m^2 × 3; cycle C: 5-FU followed by IL-1. Following IL-1 administration, a transient fall in WBC/ANC 5 minutes to 2 hours after IL-1 infusion, followed by a leukocytosis and neutrophilic granulocytosis, is noted in all patients. At the .068-μg/kg dose level, this granulocytosis is associated with an increase in superoxide generation. A transient fall in platelet count within normal range 3 to 4 days after IL-1 administration is also noted followed by a rise in platelet count 4 to 25 days (median, 13) post–IL-1. Effects included metabolic-elevated C-reactive protein and transient hypoglycemia with a mild rebound hyperglycemia. The myeloprotective effects of IL-1 are presently being evaluated.

More recently, human trials of IL-3 have begun in patients with advanced malignancies or bone marrow failure. Ganser et al. (1989a) have treated 14 patients with IL-3 administered for 15 days as a daily subcutaneous injection (60, 125, 250, and 500 μg/m²/day). In 9 available patients, substantial increases in leukocytes, absolute granulocytes as well as reticulocytes, monocyte counts, and platelets have been observed. In 2 patients with thrombocytopenia of 3000/μL and 22,500/μL, respectively, the platelet counts rose to 104,000/μL and 88,000/μL, respectively, with 60 μg/m²/day of IL-3. Side effects have included fever (3), headaches (1), and erythema at injection site (1).

Clinical investigations exploring the use of hematopoietic growth factors such as M-CSF and IL-4 to augment effector-cell function have also been either completed and/or are underway. Recently, Bajorin et al. (1989, 1990) studied the ability of M-CSF to enhance ADCC as well as hematopoiesis in melanoma patients. In this clinical study, the safety, biological effects, and antitumor activity of rhM-CSF were evaluated in 12 patients treated at 10, 30, 50, and 80 μg/kg/day as a continuous IV infusion on days 1 to 7 and 22 to 28. Increases in the percent and absolute PB monocytes were observed at doses ≥30 μg/kg/day. At the 80-μg/kg/day level, the percent PB monocytes (mean + SE) increased from 5.5 ± 0.6 pretreatment to 23.6 ± 2.7 posttreatment, and monocyte counts increased from 356 ± 30/μL to 2063 ± 359/μL. Increases in ADMC were observed in patients treated with 50 and 80 μg/kg/day. The effect of treatment on bone marrow progenitors is ongoing. No partial (PR) or complete (CR) responses were observed. One patient with early tumor progression had delayed regression of skin lesions; tumor biopsy revealed melanophage and $CD8^+$ T lymphocyte infiltration. Thrombocytopenia was mild and dose-related. Changes in cholesterol and lipoproteins were dose-related: at 80 μg/kg, the mean (± SE) reduction from baseline in cholesterol was 27% ± 3.9%, 32% ± 6.5% for low-density lipoprotein (LDL), and 34% ± 5.4% for high-density lipoprotein (HDL). Further dose levels are planned.

Finally, early clinical studies of IL-4 have been designed to either further stimulate lymphocyte activated killer (LAK) cells or to induce other hematopoietic growth factors in vivo to augment myelopoiesis. In one study, 21 patients with advanced cancer have been treated with daily IV bolus for up to 19 days of 20 to 1290 μg/m²/day (Markowitz et al., 1989). Laboratory toxicities included increase in serum alkaline phosphatase, lactate dehydrogenase, gluteunic oxalocitic transaminase, glutamic pyrate transaminase, and creatinine. There were no hematologic changes in PB or bone marrow that could definitely be related to IL-4. There were no dose-related changes in serial immunoglobulin assays, PB mononuclear cell phenotyping, NK-cell activation, or proliferative response of PB lymphocytes (PBL) to IL-2. Monocyte-mediated cytotoxicity was stable or decreased at 80 to 160 μg/m²/day, but significantly enhanced at 320 μg/m²/day.

ADMINISTRATION OF CSF TO PATIENTS RECEIVING MYELOSUPPRESSIVE THERAPY

Recombinant Human G-CSF

Several studies have now been completed that explore the role of rhG-CSF in either abrogating or accelerating the recovery from chemotherapy-induced neutropenia (Bronchud et al., 1988). An initial study explored the efficacy of rhG-CSF in preventing chemotherapy-induced myelosuppression in patients with transitional-cell carcinoma of the urothelium undergoing treatment with methotrexate, doxorubicin, vinblastine, and *cis*-platin (M-VAC) (Gabrilove et al., 1988b). Recombinant human G-CSF was administered in this study, either prior to and/or during their first cycle of combination chemotherapy over a dose range of 1 to 60 μg/kg/day, as a short 30 to 40 minute IV infusion (Gottshall et al., 1987; Natari et al., 1989). Additional patients have also been treated with a dose of 100 μg/kg/day (Jakubowski et al., 1989b). Treatment with rhG-CSF following chemotherapy for the entire study population, including patients treated at the 100-μg/kg/day dose level resulted in (1) significantly fewer days per patient with an ANC of 1000/μL or less, (2) fewer days of antibiotics in the setting of fever and neutropenia, and (3) a significant increase in the percentage of patients qualified to receive planned chemotherapy on day 14 of the treatment cycle. In addition, a significant decrease in the incidence and severity of mucositis was observed (Gabrilove et al., 1988a).

The protocol was subsequently amended to allow some patients to be treated during their second cycle of chemotherapy, and not during their first, or vice versa. These data suggest that the observations made previously are independent of the cycle in which rhG-CSF was administered (Jakubowski and Gabrilove, 1989).

Of note, was the fact that in this study, patients who had received prior pelvic radiation were not protected from neutropenia. In fact, the absolute value of the nadir achieved was when rhG-CSF was administered; however, in all cases, leukocyte counts recovered quickly, so that all such patients were eligible for their additional chemotherapy on schedule (Jakubowski and Gabrilove, 1989; Gabrilove et al., 1988b).

Bronchud et al. (1987) explored the use of the rhG-CSF (1–40 μg/kg/day), administered as a continuous IV infusion, during alternating cycles of combination chemotherapy (daunorubicin [Adriamycin] 50 mg/m^2, ifosfamide 5 gm/m^2 with mesna 9 gm/m^2 on day 1; Etoposide 120 mg/m^2 IV on days 1, 2, 3) for small-cell carcinoma of the lung. In this study, a decrease in neutropenia, fever, and requirement for antibiotics was noted in patients during chemotherapy cycles when they received rhG-CSF, compared to when they did not.

Morstyn et al. (1988, 1989a) initially studied the safety, biological effects, and efficacy of rhG-CSF (1–60 μg/kg/day) administered either intravenously, subcutaneously, or by means of a continuous subcutaneous route prior to, and following, high-dose melphalan. In their studies, a decrease in neutropenia was also observed when rhG-CSF was administered, independent of the route of administration, as compared to when it was not (Morstyn et al., 1989a). In addition, at doses of >30 μg/kg of rhG-CSF, the neutropenia following standard dose melphalan (25 mg/m^2 IV) was completely abrogated (Morstyn et al., 1988).

More recently, these investigators have studied the optimization of timing and duration of rhG-CSF administration in patients receiving melphalan. In this trial, the investigators studied the effect of varying the timing and duration of the postchemotherapy schedules of rhG-CSF. In these studies, rhG-CSF was administered at 10 μg/kg/day by subcutaneous infusion on five schedules including on (1) days 2 to 13, (2) days 2 to 18, (3) days 8 to 13, (4) days 8 to 18, (5) days −8 to −4 and 2 to 13. The major findings were that G-CSF produced a rapid and sustained elevation in neutrophil levels even when it was commenced 8 days after chemotherapy and this was sufficient to abrogate leukopenia (Morstyn et al., 1988).

One additional interesting observation was that the pharmacokinetics of rhG-CSF administered prior to melphalan showed a progressive fall in detectable serum levels despite a sustained rise in neutrophils. This fall was not observed when rhG-CSF was administered after melphalan, suggesting that the level of circulating neutrophilic granulocytes might play a role in the half-life and clearance of the protein (Morstyn et al., 1989a).

Recombinant human G-CSF has been administered to patients receiving more myelosuppressive doses of chemotherapy in the setting of autologous BMT (ABMT). Taylor et al. (1988) examined the ability of 60 μg/kg/day of rhG-CSF, administered as a short 30-minute IV infusion (for 28 days) to decrease the number of days required to achieve an ANC of either 100 cells/μL, 500 cells/μL, or 1000 cells/μL, respectively, in patients with refractory or relapsed Hodgkin's disease undergoing treatment with Cytoxan (1.5 g/m^2/day, days −6 to −3), carmustine (BCNU) (300 mg/m^2, day −6), and VP-16 (125 mg/m^2 q12 hours, days −6 to −4) chemotherapy followed by autologous BMT. In all instances, the number of days required to achieve the desired PB count was significantly decreased as compared to historical controls (Taylor et al., 1988).

Recently Peters et al. (1989) have demonstrated an accelerated recovery from neutropenia in patients treated with rhG-CSF 16 to 64 μg/kg/day infused continuously for 14 days after high-dose cyclophosphamide (5625 mg/m^2), and carmustine (600 mg/m^2), followed 3 days later by autologous bone marrow infusion. Leukocyte counts by day 15 were 6407 ± 1772 cells/μL as compared to 863 ± 645 cells/μL for historical controls. In addition, parameters of neutrophil function were also analyzed, including granulocyte phagocytosis, which was found to be enhanced during rhG-CSF administration, and hydrogen peroxide generation, which remained unchanged. In vivo migration of neutrophils to a sterile inflammatory site was, however, preserved and comparable to patients after hematopoietic recovery but not receiving growth factor. This was in contrast to the significant inhibition of neutrophil migration observed in this same patient population treated with continuous IV infusions of rhGM-CSF (Peters et al., 1989).

Sheridan et al. (1989) studied the use of rhG-CSF after high-dose chemotherapy with busulphan 4 mg/kg/day × 4 days (days −7 to −4) and cyclophosphamide 60 mg/kg/day (days −3 and −2), and ABMT (day 0). In this study, rhG-CSF was administered as a continuous subcutaneous infusion of 20 μg/kg/day beginning on day 1 and reduced progressively when the neutrophil count exceeded 1000 cells/μL. Of 11 patients entered, 9 exceeded neutrophil counts of 500 cells/μL as early as 9 days post-ABMT (range 9–17), with 7 of the 9 reaching this level before day 12, compared to 0 of 17 historical controls (Sheridan et al., 1989). Similar trends in recovery for neutrophil counts to more than 1000 cells/μL were also observed. This enhanced recovery was associated with a decrease in antibiotics and an earlier discharge from the hospital (Sheridan et al., 1989).

Recombinant Human GM-CSF

Several studies exploring the role of rhGM-CSF in ameliorating myelosuppressive toxicity of chemotherapy have also been undertaken.

Antman et al. (1989) treated 16 patients with inoperable or metastatic sarcomas with escalating doses of rhGM-CSF before, and immediately after, a first cycle of Mesna (2500 mg/m^2 days 1–4), doxorubicin (20 mg/m^2, days 1–3), ifosfamide 2500 mg/m^2, days 1–3), and dacarbazine (300 mg/m^2, days 1–3) chemotherapy and compared the myelosuppressive toxicity of this to a second cycle of chemotherapy administered without concomitant growth factor. Neutropenia after cycle 1 was significantly less severe and of shorter duration than after cycle 2. The mean total leukocyte and platelet nadirs were 1.0 and 101 $\times$ 10^9 per liter for cycle 1 as compared to 0.45 and 44 $\times$ 10^9 per liter for cycle 2. The median intervals from day 1 of chemotherapy to neutrophil recovery were 15 and 19 days, respectively, and the duration of neutropenia was 3.5 days as compared to 7.4 days with cycle 2. Despite a decrease in the duration of neutropenia, 2 of 14 patients in the treatment cycle died of sepsis as compared to 0 of the 12 receiving chemotherapy alone, raising the concern that secondary cytokines induced by the administration of rhGM-CSF such as TNF might be synergizing with endogenous endotoxin in the setting of bacterial infection, leading to profound septic shock (Bar et al., 1988).

Morstyn et al. have explored the use of rhGM-CSF in an effort to overcome the myelosuppressive toxicity of patients with small-cell carcinoma of the lung receiving treatment with carboplatin (100 mg/m^2, days 1–3) and VP-16 (120 mg/m^2, days 1–3) every 28 days. Recombinant human GM-CSF was administered as a 15-μg/kg/day dose subcutaneously on either day 4 to 11, day 4 to 18, or day 4 to 25 (Morstyn et al., 1988; Sheridan et al., 1989). The results were compared to historical controls where 31 of 82 patients developed grade IV (modified WHO classification) neutrophil toxicity (Morstyn et al., 1989; Bonnem et al., 1988). In patients receiving rhGM-CSF, only 1 of 11 patients developed a neutrophil count of less than 500 cells/μL.

Mertelsmann et al. (1989) have also investigated the ability of subcutaneously administered glycosylated rhGM-CSF to abrogate hematopoietic toxicity following a variety of chemotherapy regimens for solid tumors. In this study, patients underwent combination chemotherapy, and if significant neutropenia developed, a second cycle of chemotherapy was instituted with concomitant administration of hematopoietic growth factor. Decreases in the degree and duration of neutropenia have been reported, comparable to those studies described previously.

Recombinant human GM-CSF has also been utilized in the setting of BMT (Brandt et al., 1988). The first study to be reported was conducted by Peters et al. in patients with either breast cancer or melanoma treated with combination chemotherapy and ABMT support (Brandt et al., 1988). Groups of three to four patients were treated with 2.0, 4.0, 8.0, 16.0, 32 μg/mg/day or 64 μg/m^2 of glycosylated (CHO-cell derived) rhGM-CSF by continuous IV, beginning 3 hours after bone marrow infusion. Total leukocyte and granulocyte recovery was accelerated in these patients, at all dose levels, as compared to 24 historical controls matched for age, diagnosis, and treatment. No consistent effect on platelet count recovery was noted. Less bacteremia, hepatotoxicity, and nephrotoxicity (perhaps related to the decrease in bacteremia) than previously noted for controls was observed (Brandt et al., 1988).

Nemunaitis et al. (1988) administered escalating doses of glycosylated (yeast-derived) rhGM-CSF, given as a 2-hour IV infusion for 14 days beginning 1 hour following completion of autologous or syngeneic bone marrow infusion to patients with lymphoid malignancies in remission or in relapse. In this study, rhGM-CSF was found to be biologically active at doses of 60 μg/m^2/day, since 5 of 9 patients receiving this dose recovered neutrophil counts to 500 cells/μL or more before day 14, compared to only 1 of 6 patients receiving less than 60 μg/m^2, or 4 of 92 historical controls. A decrease in the number of febrile days was also reduced in patients treated with 60 μg/m^2 or more. In addition, fewer days were required to become platelet transfusion–independent in patients treated with 60 μg/m^2 or more of rhGM-CSF. Two patients treated with 60 μg/m^2 or more had received marrow treated in vitro with pan-B cell antibody plus complement; they both recovered earlier. No enhancement of graft-versus-host (GVH) disease was noted in the small number of patients receiving a syngeneic transplant in combination with rhGM-CSF (Bronchud et al., 1989).

These studies exploring the role of rhG-CSF and rhGM-CSF in ameliorating chemotherapy-induced myelosuppression have suggested that it is possible to reduce the morbidity of chemotherapeutic regimens. From these studies, however, one cannot conclude whether a particular cytoreduction regimen, marrow-purging technique or preparation, or underlying disease affects the responsiveness. Larger, prospective, phase III randomized trials are needed to define more precisely the possible therapeutic advantage offered by these growth factors and to uncover any additional untoward effects (Nemunaitis et al., 1988).

By reducing morbidity and making more tolerable our present antineoplastic regimens, hematopoietic growth factors should certainly render standard cancer treatment more tolerable for patients afflicted with malignant disease. However, an even greater question remains as to whether, by allowing one to administer dose-intensified therapy, these factors will contribute to improved survival. In this regard, Bronchud et al. (1989) have recently explored the use of rhG-CSF to increase the intensity of treatment with doxorubicin in patients with advanced breast and ovarian cancer. High–dose intensity treatment, defined as the amount of cytotoxic drug administered per unit time, is known to improve response rates in patients with advanced breast cancer. In this study, rhG-CSF was given to 17 patients with advanced breast and ovarian cancer in order to increase the intensity and effectiveness of chemotherapy. Treatment with doxorubicin at doses of 75 μg/m^2 (4), 100 μg/m^2 (5), 125 μg/m^2 (6), and 150 μg/m^2 (2) was followed by an infusion of rhG-CSF 5 μg/kg/day for 11 days. In this study, rhG-CSF administration resulted in a return of the ANC to normal, or above normal, levels within 12 to 14 days at all dose levels of doxorubicin used and allowed the administration of up to three cycles of high-dose chemotherapy at 14-day intervals; an ANC of >2500 cells/μL was not reached until days 19 to 21 after 75 μg/m^2 of doxorubicin without rhG-CSF. At doses of 125 μg/m^2 and 150 μg/m^2, all tumors regressed rapidly by days 12 to 14. However, despite the accelerated recovery from neutropenia, marked epithelial toxicity was apparent and became dose-limiting. In this trial, the overall response rate in patients with doxorubicin + rhG-CSF therapy was 80% with a median time to progression of 6 months. Two months after treatment, there was a pronounced improvement of symptoms (by the Rotterdam symptom check list) compared to before treatment.

Logotheliu et al. (1989) recently reported on 19 patients with progressive urothelial tumors failing prior M-VAC (12), cyclophosphamide, daunorubicin, and cisplatin (CISCA) + M-VAC (5), CISCA + CMV (2), treated with escalating M-VAC combination therapy plus rhGM-CSF. Four dosage levels of rhGM-CSF were used, including: (1) 150 μg/m^2 CI × 10 days, 3 patients; (2) 250 μg/m^2 CI × 10 days, 7 patients; (3) 500 μg/m^2 CI × 10, 6 patients; and (4) 500 μg/m^2 SC × 10 days, 3 patients. The mean granulocyte nadir and duration (days <100 granulocyte/μL) for the different levels done are outlined in Table 19-8. In this study, 2 of 15 patients achieved CR, despite prior refractories to lower doses of antineoplastic agents and 6 of 15 exhibited PR (Logotheliu et al., 1989).

Although these two studies are far from definitive, they provide insight into the direction the clinical investigation of these hematopoietic growth factors must take, if the use of these regulators is going to contribute to further progress in the treatment of a variety of cancers. Clearly, additional studies, both phase II and randomized trials, will be required to address these important issues.

TABLE 19-8
GRANULOCYTE RESPONSE FOLLOWING ESCALATING DOSES OF MVAC CHEMOTHERAPY AND VARYING DOSES OF RHGM-CSF

Dose level	Mean granulocyte nadir (cells/μL)	Mean duration (days <1000)*
I IV	600	8.0
II IV	250	8.2
III IV	250	6.5
III SC	80	5.0

*<1000 granulocytes/μL.

NEOPLASTIC DISEASE ASSOCIATED WITH NEUTROPENIA

Neutropenia is also a significant problem directly resulting from a number of hematopoietic malignancies contributing to significant clinical morbidity and mortality.

Hairy-Cell Leukemia

Glaspy et al. (1988) conducted a study to determine whether rhG-CSF was effective in correcting severe neutropenia in patients with hairy-cell leukemia (HCL). Recombinant human G-CSF was administered daily as a subcutaneous injection, beginning at a dose of 1 μg/kg/day. The dose was increased weekly for 2 weeks to 6 μg/kg/day, and treatment continued for 5 to 6 weeks. Four patients were entered; two of these patients had ongoing infection, including (1) conjunctivitis and periorbital skin infections and (2) a perirectal abscess, fever, hypotension, and urinary retention unresponsive to antibiotics and amphotericin. In three of four patients who completed the course of treatment, a significant increase in circulating neutrophil counts associated with an increase in myeloid bone marrow elements was observed. In the two patients with infectious complications, complete resolution of infection occurred with rhG-CSF treatment. One patient had a history of biopsy-proven cutaneous leukocytoclastic vasculitis at the time of her initial presentation. An exacerbation of her dermatological problem, consisting of acute febrile neutrophilic dermatosis (Sweet's syndrome), occurred while receiving rhG-CSF. This most likely resulted from the increase in granulocyte reserves and neutrophil counts stimulated by rhG-CSF administration, giving rise to increased neutrophilic epidermal infiltration (Glaspy et al., 1988).

Myelodysplastic Syndrome

Negrin et al. (1989) conducted a study to determine if rhG-CSF could improve neutropenia associated with myelodysplastic syndrome (MDS). Thirteen patients with MDS (2 with refractory anemia [RA], 8 with refractory anemia with excess blasts in transformation [RAEBIT]) were treated with daily subcutaneous injections of rhG-CSF using an escalating dose, from 0.1 to 3.0 μg/kg/day, for 6–8 weeks. Eleven patients had significant elevations in WBC and ANC. In 5 patients, a greater than twofold increase in reticulocyte count occurred: in 2 of 9 red cell transfusion–dependent patients, this led to a decrease in red cell transfusion requirements. No significant changes in platelet counts were noted during treatment (Negrin et al., 1989). Three patients subsequently received additional treatment for up to 8 weeks, with ANC levels remaining within the normal range. In all cases, treatment has been well tolerated. In vitro suppression of myeloid clonal self-generation was observed with the replating efficiency (PE2) decreasing to 19% of basal levels, posttreatment (Negrin et al., 1989).

Kobayashi et al. (1988) have also treated 5 MDS patients with half-hour IV infusions of rhG-CSF for 6 days and have noted improved neutrophil counts.

Several trials of rhGM-CSF have been conducted in patients with MDS (Vadhan-Raj et al., 1987; Ganser et al., 1989b; Thompson et al., 1989) (Table 19-9). The first study was conducted by Vadhan-Raj et al. (1987). This group of investigators explored the effect of continuously infused glycosylated rhGM-CSF over a dose range of 30 to 500 μg/m^2, given for 14 days in one patient with RA, three patients with refractory anemia with excess blasts (RAEB), and four patients with RAEBIT. Prior therapy for MDS included hormonal and/or vitamin therapy (two patients), daunorubicin/cytosine arabinoside containing regimens (four patients), and ABMT (one patient). Six of the eight patients had >10% blasts in the bone marrow; none of the patients had circulating blasts. In this study, 5- to 20-fold and 5- to 373-fold increases in circulating WBC and ANC were noted. Two of four and two of eight red cell and platelet transfusion–dependent patients, respectively, had significant increases in their red cell and platelet counts; however, one of these patients (with RAEBIT) did not actually have florid RAEBIT at the time of rhGM-CSF treatment, but rather had pancytopenia with a hypoplastic bone marrow 3 months post–cytosine arabinoside and daunorubicin chemotherapy. The augmentation of red cell and platelet count in this patient may or may not be relevant to the actual effect of rhGM-CSF in patients with obvious MDS. In this study, no transformation to acute leukemia was noted. Interestingly, in patients who

TABLE 19-9
CLINICAL TRIALS OF rhGM-CSF IN MYELODYSPLASTIC SYNDROME

Investigators	Source	Dose	Route/ schedule	# Patients	Prior Rx	MDS Subtype
Vadhan-Raj	Glycosylated (yeast)	30–50 μg/m	CI × 14 days	8	2 hormonal/ vitamin 4 Dauna/ Ara-C	1 RA 3 RAEB 3 RAEBIT 1 Hypoplasia after chemo RX*
Ganser	Nonglycosylated	15–50 μg/m	IV bolus/ day 1: 8-hour infusion	11	1 LDAra-C†	3 RA 4 RAEB 2 CMMOL
Thompson	Nonglycosylated	0.3–10 μg/kg/d	Subcutaneous	16	7 hormonal/ vitamin 1 LDAra-C†	7 RA 8 RAEB 1 RAEBIT

*Daunorubicin.
†Low-dose cytosine arabinoside.
‡Not available.

received more than one course of rhGM-CSF, the baseline granulocyte count improved over time with repeated cycles of treatment (Vadhan-Raj et al., 1987).

Ganser et al. (1989b) also conducted a trial (employing the same preparation of glycosylated rhGM-CSF) in patients with MDS, including 3 with RA, 4 with RAEB, and 2 with chronic myelomonocytic leukemia (CMMoL). Recombinant human GM-CSF was administered as an initial bolus on day 1 followed by a daily 8-hour infusion of rhGM-CSF for a total of 8 to 14 days. The treatment schedule included a dose escalation from 15 to 50 $\mu g/m^2$. Previous treatment included only 1 patient treated with low-dose cytosine arabinoside. Results included a 130% to 1800% increase in circulating leukocyte counts in 10 of 11 patients, an increase in monocytes and eosinophils in 7 and 6 patients, respectively, an increase in lymphocytes affecting both helper T and suppressor T cells, but without evidence of activation as measured by the expression of the IL-2 receptor. In all 4 patients with greater than 14% bone marrow blasts, an increase in marrow blasts was observed, and in all 4 patients with circulating blasts pretreatment, an increase in PB blasts was also noted. In addition, 1 patient, initially with no detectable circulating blasts, demonstrated an increase in PB blasts with treatment. No change in circulating red cell, platelet count, or transfusion requirements was observed. Cytogenetic analysis revealed both an increase, as well as a decrease, in the number of abnormal metaphases in 6 patients with chromosomal ab-

TABLE 19-9
(Continued)

% Blasts bone marrow	Blast % blood	Results: decreased RBC TX	Decreased platelets TX	Other
>10% (6)	0/8 with circulating blasts	2/4 (1 who had hypoplasia p RX)	2/8 (1 had hypoplasia p RX)	Increase WBC and ANC
>14% (4)	4/11	No change	No change	Increase WBC and ANC Increase bone marrow and circulating blasts in 1 patient with no prior circulating blasts Increase circulating blasts in 1 patient with prior circulating blasts
≥10% (8)	NA‡	No change	No change	Increase WBC and ANC: Increase monos/eos Transient increase in retics (2); increase in bone marrow blasts (5); decrease in bone marrow blasts (4)

normalities, suggesting both a proliferative, a suppressive, and possibly a differentiating effect on marrow cells with rhGM-CSF treatment (Ganser et al., 1989b).

A third study was conducted by Thompson et al. (1989). These investigators explored the use of daily subcutaneously administered nonglycosylated rhGM-CSF for 10 days to 7 paticnts with RA, 8 patients with RAEB, and 1 patient with RAEBIT. Eight patients had received no prior therapy, 1 patient had received prior low-dose cytosine arabinoside, and 7 patients had previously received only hormonal and/or vitamin therapy. Four dose levels were employed, including: 0.3 μg/kg/day, 1.0 μg/kg/day, 3.0 μg/kg/day, and 10.0 μg/kg/day. Circulating granulocytes increased in a dose-dependent manner. Neutrophil counts decreased to baseline after discontinuation in most patients; however, in 2 patients, the neutrophil count remained elevated over the course of at least 6 months of observation. Increases in monocytes and eosinophils were also noted. Transient increases only in reticulocyte and platelet counts were observed in 2 and 3 patients, respectively. On a percentage basis, 5 of 16 patients had an increase in the percentage of bone marrow blasts, whereas 4 had a slight decrease, and 7 remained unchanged, although the bone marrow cellularity increased (Thompson et al., 1989).

Although these initial results appear promising for select patients, additional studies with longer follow-up will be needed to determine the long-term improvement in morbidity and efficacy of this treatment.

Acute Leukemias

In order to accelerate the hematopoietic reconstitution after chemotherapy in high-risk acute nonlymphatic leukemia (ANLL) and acute lymphatic leukemia (ALL), in 23 patients with relapsed ANLL (8) and ALL (5) or newly diagnosed ANLL (10 patients >65 years of age), Koeniopmann et al. (1989) administered glycosylated rhGM-CSF after chemotherapy with a deescalation in 2- to 4-day steps after neutrophil recovery. The time to achieve a neutrophil count >500 was shorter than historical controls in 16 of 19 patients. Platelets also appeared to recover faster in some patients. Regrowth of leukemic blasts occurred in 1 newly diagnosed and 2 secondary ANLL patients.

At least three studies have been initiated in Europe and the United States to explore the use of either rhGM-CSF or rhG-CSF to promote cell-cycle activation and enhanced leukemic-cell kill with cycle-specific agents such as cytosine arabinoside and/or regulator-induced leukemic-cell maturation. These studies are based on extensive in vitro investigations by several groups (Cannistra et al., 1988b; Tafarri et al., 1988; Bhalla et al., 1988) initially pioneered by McCulloch et al. (Kelleher et al., 1987). These studies demonstrate that one can augment the number of cells as well as leukemic progenitors in S phase by pretreatment in either rhG-CSF, rhGM-CSF, or IL-3 and that, in addition, one can get enhanced cell killing by cytosine arabinoside of both leukemic progenitors and cells of the nonprogenitor compartment with growth factor, as compared to the cell killing with antineoplastic agent alone.

Recently, clinical trials of G-CSF and GM-CSF in ANLL have been initiated. One study explores the proliferative, cycle (S-phase specific)–activating, and cell-maturation effects of rhG-CSF in patients with primary refractory or relapsed ANLL. In this instance, laboratory studies have been designed to also evaluate the utility of in vitro assays to predict clinical outcome (Jakubowski et al., 1989a). The cycle-activating effects and enhanced cell killing with cytosine arabinoside in patients with relapsed ANLL are also under investigation (Cannistra, unpublished). Results of these studies should be forthcoming and revealing. Finally, Buchner and his colleagues (1989) have studied the myeloprotective effects of GM-CSF following reinduction chemotherapy in heavily pretreated patients with relapsed ANLL. In this instance, surprisingly enough, no increase in recurrent leukemia was noted posttreatment and remission was obtained, although the number of patients studied was quite small.

NONNEOPLASTIC DISEASE ASSOCIATED WITH NEUTROPENIA

Several nonneoplastic diseases are characterized by severe neutropenia resulting in significant clinical morbidity. We will discuss each subgroup separately.

Primary Neutropenic Disorders

Primary neutropenic disorders include cyclic neutropenia, congenital neutropenia (Kostmann's syndrome), and adult-acquired "idiopathic" neutropenia. In addition, some of these disorders may, in fact, represent absolute or relative deficiencies of particular hematopoietic growth factors and/or alternations in the relative affinities of their respective receptors. The use of G-CSF in cyclic, congenital, and idiopathic neutropenic disorders is ongoing and appears promising, the initial results of which are summarized.

Cyclic neutropenia is a rare disorder characterized by regular and periodic disappearance of neutrophils. Usually, even at the peak of the cycle, patients are leukopenic. In addition, the typical pattern reveals that all blood counts (in particular, the monocytes) cycle out of phase with each other, but always with the same periodicity. Based on the preclinical observation of Lothrop et al. (1988) in the gray collie cyclic dog, Hammond et al. (1989) conducted a pilot clinical trial of rhG-CSF in which patients were treated with rhG-CSF, 1 to 10 μg/kg intravenously or subcutaneously, for several months to >1 year. Prior to therapy, the patients all had recurrent stomatitis, pharyngitis, lymphadenopathy, and fever at 21-day intervals. The effects of therapy in these patients were (1) to increase the amplitude of the neutrophil cycles, (2) to shorten the cycle length from 21 to 14 days, (3) to shorten the period of neutropenia to about 1 day, and (4) to avoid a fall in count to 0 during the neutropenic period. Clinically, the patients have benefited dramatically by the abbreviated, less severe neutropenic periods (Hammond et al., 1989). With treatment, almost all of the symptoms, including the typical (interestingly enough) mouth ulcers, have virtually been eliminated (Fibbe et al., 1988). In contrast, Fibbe et al. observed no correction of cyclic neutropenia when patients were treated with rhGM-CSF (Bonilla et al., 1989).

Congenital neutropenia or Kostmann's syndrome is a disorder characterized by (1) severe neutropenia with an ANC of <200 cells /μL, (2) maturational arrest of the bone marrow myeloid precursor at the promyelocyte or myelocyte stage, (3) early onset in infancy of severe recurrent bacterial infections, and (4) variable monocytosis and eosinophils and plasma cells in the bone marrow. Bonilla et al. (1989) conducted a phase I/II trial of rhG-CSF administered intravenously and subcutaneously to patients with this disorder. In the first five patients treated, an increase in circulating neutrophil counts to >1000 cells/μL has been observed with varying doses of rhG-CSF. Over a comparable period of observation, this has been associated, in turn, with a decrease in infectious episodes, hospitalizations, and requirements for antibiotics (Bonilla et al., 1989). Similar findings have recently been reported by Welte et al. (1988). In this latter study, patients only developed neutrophilic granulocytosis following rhG-CSF treatment; no augmentation in neutrophil counts was seen in the same patients when rhGM-CSF was administered (Welte et al., 1988).

Idiopathic neutropenia is characterized by progressive neutropenia associated with hypocellular bone marrows, myeloid maturation arrest, recurrent infections, and oral and/or skin ulcerations. Based on preclinical studies in vitro, which demonstrated the efficacy of rhG-CSF in generating either mature neutrophilic granulocytes in bone marrow suspension cultures or neutrophil colonies assays, a pilot study was conducted (Jakubowski et al., 1989a). Two patients were treated with rhG-CSF administered as a daily subcutaneous injection of from 1 to 3 μg/kg/day. Both experienced restoration of their neutrophil counts to within a normal range. This was associated, in turn, with no further infectious episodes and with complete resolution of oral ulcerations in the second. Both of these patients have been maintained on treatment for 8 months to >1 year. No tolerance has developed and no antibody formation has been detected.

Based on the three pilot studies with rhG-CSF in patients with primary neutropenic disorders, a multicenter randomized clinical trial has commenced to further explore the role of this hematopoietic growth factor in the treatment of these rare, but often life-threatening, diseases.

One patient with severe idiopathic agranulocytosis was treated by Antin et al. with glycosylated rhGM-CSF, without any apparent effect (Nissen et al., 1988). Champlin et al. (1989) also attempted to treat two patients with agranulocytosis with rhGM-CSF; however, treatment had to be discontinued in both patients because of dose-related toxicity, before enough time had elapsed to assess clinical response. Recently, Ganser et al. treated four patients with chronic neutropenia. This group of patients included one patient with autoimmune neutropenia, one patient with neutropenia secondary to prior chemotherapy for 3 years for Hodgkin's disease, one patient with asymptomatic neutropenia of unknown cause, and one patient with congenital neutropenia with normocellular bone marrow and normal serum immunoglobulins. Patients were treated with 150 to 1000 μg/m^2 IV (1 patient) or subcutaneously (3 patients) for 12 to 14 consecutive days. All patients demonstrated an initial increase in leukocyte count that was associated with an increase in neutrophilic and eosinophilic granulocytes. All counts returned to baseline upon discontinuation of treatment. One patient with congenital neutropenia demonstrated a much smaller increment in leukocyte count, which was secondary, primarily due to an increase in eosinophils and lymphocytes. Only a minimal increase in neutrophil granulocytes was noted when the patient was challenged again with rhGM-CSF following a 20-day nontreatment interval.

Aplastic Anemia

Four major studies have been conducted exploring the role of different glycosylated rhGM-CSF preparations in the treatment of aplastic anemia (Antin et al., 1988; Champlin et al., 1989; Nissen et al., 1988; Vadhan-Raj et al., 1988a) (Table 19-10). Antin et al. (1988) performed the first phase I/II study of daily rhGM-CSF, 15 to 480 $\mu g/m^2$ administered either as a 1- to 4-hour IV infusion for 14 days. If no toxicity was observed, patients were allowed repeated treatments at progressively higher dose levels than those at which they were entered. Seven red cell transfusion–dependent patients with severe aplastic anemia were studied. Patient characteristics included absolute granulocyte counts of <1000 cells/μL (7 patients); platelet count of <10,000 cells/μL (6); bone marrow cellularity of <10% (6). Prior therapy included antithymocytic globulin (ATG) (4 patients), androgens (3), thymosin (1), prednisone (2), cyclophosphamide + hydroxyurea (1), and no prior treatment (1). Modest increases in granulocyte and monocyte counts, not clearly dose-related, were noted in 13 of 22 and 14 of 22 courses, respectively, with the median time to peak granulocyte count occurring after 4 days (range 1–21). On five occasions, the peak granulocyte count occurred between days 14 and 21, despite the fact that the infusion of rhGM-CSF was stopped on day 7, suggesting that in these patients, the stimulation of early progenitors resulted in improved counts after the growth factor was no longer present. No increase in baseline counts was observed with repeated courses of rhGM-CSF in this patient population. No increases in eosinophils, immature myeloid, or amelioration of red cell or platelet transfusion requirements were noted (Antin et al., 1988).

Nissen et al. (1988) treated four patients with very severe aplastic anemia refractory to ATG. All patients were red cell and platelet transfusion–dependent and had total neutrophil counts of <50 cells/μL. Only one patient had evidence of marrow myelopoiesis. Glycosylated (CHO cell–derived) rhGM-CSF was administered from 4 to 32 μg/kg/day, either as a continuous IV infusion for 14 days (4 patients) or as a subcutaneous twice daily injection (1). In this study, only the one patient with evidence of residual marrow myelopoiesis demonstrated an increase in neutrophil counts that allowed clearance of bilateral pneumonia. No improvement in red cell or platelet transfusions was noted in any patient in this study as well (Nissen et al., 1988).

Vadhan-Raj et al. (1988a) treated eight patients with true moderate (3) to severe (5) aplastic anemia with glycosylated rhGM-CSF over a dose range of 60 to 500 $\mu g/m^2$. In the publication of their clinical trial, two additional patients, one with congenital hypoplastic anemia and one with hypoplasia and pancytopenia following multiple

TABLE 19-10
CLINICAL TRIALS OF GM-CSF IN APLASTIC ANEMIA

Study	GM-CSF Prep	RTE, dose, and schedule	Prior Rx	# Patients	Grade of disease pre-Rx	Mean ANC cells/ μL (range)	Response
Antin	Glycosylated (yeast)	(A) 1-4 h IV infusion × 7 days or (B) 12 h IV infusion × 14 days (15–489 μg/m²)	ATG (4) Androgen (3) Thyrosin (1) Prednisone (2) CTX/HV (1) None (1)	7	Severe	365 (0–925)	(1) Modest increase in granulocytes (2) No change in platelets or RBC transfusion requirements
Nissen	Glycosylated (CHO cell)	(A) CI[1] × 14 days or (B) SC[2] bid (4–32 μg/kg/day)	ATG (4)	4	Severe	<50	(1) 1/4 with increases in granulocytes (2) No change in platelet or red cell transfusion requirements

Vadhan-Raj	Glycosylated (yeast)	(A) CI × 14 days (60–500 μg/m²)	ATG (3) Steroids (7) Androgens (4) Splenectomy (1) No RX (1)	8	Moderate–severe	714 (1560–176)	(1) Increased granulocytes and monocytes (2) Increased bone marrow cellularity (3) No change in platelets or red cell counts or transfusion requirements
Champlin	Glycosylated (CHO cell)	(A) CI × 14–28 days (4–64 μg/kg/day)	ATG (13)	13	Moderate–severe	463 (30–770)	(1) Increased granulocyte counts especially in patients with >300 granulocytes/μL pre-RX (2) Increase bone marrow cellularity

courses of chemotherapy, were included. For the purpose of this review, we have excluded them from the discussion since these two patients possibly represent distinctly different biological entities that might very well respond differently to hematopoietic growth factor administration. Prior therapy for this patient group included ATG (3), steroids (7), androgens (4), splenectomy (1), and no treatment (1). Baselinc neutrophil counts ranged from 1560 to 176 cells/μL with a mean neutrophil count of 714 cells/μL. Recombinant human GM-CSF was administered as a continuous IV infusion daily for 2 weeks. The treatment period was followed by a 2-week rest period and a second cycle of CI treatment. During rhGM-CSF treatment, these investigators reported: an increase in marrow cellularity (8) and myeloid to erythroid cell ratios, and increase in circulating neutrophils (6), eosinophils (8), and monocytes (8). Despite an increase in neutrophil counts, however, four patients (three with a previous history of infectious episodes) had episodes of sepsis while on study. In addition, no changes in red cell or platelet counts were seen (Vadhan-Raj et al., 1988a).

Champlin et al. (1989a) treated 13 patients with refractory aplastic anemia with 4 to 64 μg/kg/day rhGM-CSF administered as a continuous IV infusion for 14 to 28 days. Patients achieving CR or PR were subsequently treated for an additional 2 months. All patients had previously received ATG and had been either primary failures (10) or had experienced transient responses and then relapsed (3). All patients had a marrow cellularity of <20%. The mean neutrophil count was 430 cells/μL (range 30–770 cells/μL) and the mean platelet count 5000 cells/μL (5000–25,000 cells/μL). On treatment, 7 patients had complete normalization of their circulating granulocyte count and 3 patients had an increase to >500 cells/μL. The greatest increments occurred in patients with higher pretreatment granulocyte counts. One patient had no response, and in 1 patient, the granulocyte response was transient. All patients were monocytopenic at study entry; during treatment, 8 of 11 patients had normalization of monocyte counts and 2 achieved PR (>200 cells/μL). Increases in circulating eosinophils were also observed after 2 weeks of rhGM-CSF administration. Circulating erythrocytes, platelets, and their transfusion requirements were unaffected by treatment in all but 1 patient who demonstrated an increase in hemoglobin from 7 to 11 and an increase in platelet count from 20,000 to 45,000 cells/μL, respectively. In addition to an augmentation of circulating blood counts, bone marrow cellularity as well as marrow and PB myeloid progenitors, increased in all responding patients. In all cases, discontinuation of treatment was associated with a return to baseline PB counts and bone marrow cellularity (Champlin et al., 1989). Interestingly, in this study, the investigators noted a significant decrease in serum cholesterol in aplastic patients receiving rhGM-CSF (Nimer et al., 1988).

Acquired Immunodeficiency Syndrome

Acquired immunodeficiency syndrome (AIDS), while primarily due to a deficiency of T4 lymphocytes, is frequently complicated by deficits in neutrophils and monocyte number and function. Therefore, CSF may be useful in AIDS by increasing the number of these host effector cells, but also by enhancing their function. In addition, neutropenia is the major complication of antiviral agents, such as azidothymidine (AZT) and ganciclovir (DHPG), presently used for either the treatment of AIDS or its complications. This toxicity, in turn, limits the dose of medication that can be safely tolerated.

Two major studies have been reported that demonstrate that rhGM-CSF can augment myelopoiesis and improve neutrophil function in patients with AIDS. The first study was conducted by Groopman et al. (1987), who administered a continuous IV infusion of rhGM-CSF to 16 relatively well patients with AIDS and leukopenia, over a dose range of 0.3 to 4.5 μg/kg/day, for 14 days. Treatment resulted in a dramatic augmentation in circulating granulocytes and monocytes without evidence of increased viral production. Baldwin et al. (1988) studied the function of neutrophils produced in 6 of these AIDS patients treated with rhGM-CSF. These investigators found that ADCC and phagocytosis improved with treatment, whereas superoxide generation was more variable.

Mitsuyasu et al. (1988) evaluated the toxicity and clinical, hematologic, and antiviral effects of nonglycosylated rhGM-CSF administered subcutaneously daily for up to 6 months in 15 patients with human immunodeficiency virus (HIV) infection. Cohorts of two to four patients were treated at doses between 0.25 and 8.0 μg/kg/day. All patients were intolerant of AZT or had severe leukopenia precluding its use. The median WBC was 2300 (range, 1300–2800). All patients had a threefold increase in WBC, ANC, and eosinophil counts and a greater than twofold increase in monocytes and lymphocytes within 3 weeks of treatment; however, no change in CD4:CD9 ratio, skin reactivity, hemoglobin, or reticulocyte count was noted. Serum p24 antigen decreased by >50% in two patients, increased by >50% in four, and remained unchanged in seven. No concomitant levels of AZT, to preclude self-administration of this antiviral agent, were obtained in this study. Infections on study included E histolytica + giardia lamblia gastroenteritis (1), hemophilus influenzae bronchitis/pneumonia (2), pneumocystis pneumonia (2), cytomegalovirus septicemia (1), and disseminated mycobacterium avium (1).

Studies have been undertaken to explore the role of rhG-CSF in combination with erythropoietin and AZT in correcting neutropenia and anemia seen in association with AIDS itself, as well as its therapy. In addition to neutropenia, anemia also is not an infrequent complication limiting the dose of antiviral medication that can be administered to these patients. These results appear quite promising, but further data are needed and will be forthcoming to be sure of its ultimate efficacy.

SIDE EFFECTS

The side effects of rhG-CSF and rhGM-CSF in cancer patients in the absence of other chemotherapy and/or BMT are outlined first, respectively, since some observed toxicities may be due to the underlying disease as well as concomitant therapies. Other side effects that thus far have only been observed or reported in particular clinical situations will also be described.

Recombinant Human G-CSF

Treatment with rhG-CSF has been, for the most part, well tolerated. Mild-to-moderate "medullary" bone pain has been the most frequent and significant clinical side effect, observed most commonly when patients are treated with a short IV infusion of rhG-CSF, but also reported following subcutaneous bolus and continuous subcutaneous infusion. The medullary bone pain is most often characterized as a pulsating deep pain or pressure localized primarily in the lower back, pelvis, and/or sternum. In one study, the pain was most problematic in two middle-aged, moderately-to-severely obese post-menopausal women who received 60 and 100 μg/kg/day of rhG-CSF as a short 30- to 40-minute IV infusion (Gabrilove et al., 1988; Jakubowski and Gabrilove, 1989). Both of these patients experienced more diffuse bone pain, which in one patient was only relieved by indomethacin. Other occasional complaints in this setting have included chest tightness, mild headache, and, rarely, flushing.

In one study where rhG-CSF was employed following ABMT, one patient at 64 μg/kg/day developed hypotension. In addition, the occurrence of a maculopapular rash and an increase in serum creatinine were seen at this dose level in general patients (Peters et al., 1988). Historical data for this particular ABMT setting reveal a 30% incidence of elevated creatinine in the transplant setting itself (Peters et al., 1988). In two other transplant studies, the only toxicity observed was medullary bone pain.

In patients with congenital and cyclic neutropenia, splenomegaly has been reported (Bonilla et al., 1989; Welte et al., 1988). Other unusual side effects include a flare in psoriasis in one patient with MDS (Negrin et al., 1988), the recurrence of Sweet's syndrome (cutaneous neutrophilic vasculitis) in a patient with HCL (Glaspy et al., 1988) and cutaneous vasculitis in a patient with congenital neutropenia associated with an increase in ANC to >1000 cells/μL (Welte et al., 1988).

Recombinant Human GM-CSF

A number of side effects have been reported in patients receiving both glycosylated and nonglycosylated rhGM-CSF (Morstyn et al., 1989a, 1989b; Lieschke et al., 1989; Mertelsmann et al., 1989). Fever and bone pain are the most common side effects observed in patients treated with nonglycosylated GM-CSF. Pericarditis was determined to be dose-limiting in 2 of 5 patients treated with 20 to 30 μg/kg/day, whereas this side effect was not observed in 16 patients treated with lower doses (Lieschke et al., 1989). In patients receiving nonglycosylated rhGM-CSF, a peculiar first-dose reaction, including flushing, hypotension, transient hypoxia, and tachycardia, has been described (Morstyn et al., 1989b). After the first dose of rhGM-CSF, subsequent doses do not elicit this response; however, if treatment is discontinued for 10 or more days and rhGM-CSF is reintroduced, the first dose may again produce this reaction (Morstyn et al., 1989b). Morstyn et al. (1989b) have reported that the reaction appears to occur predominantly in patients receiving short infusions and, perhaps more commonly, in patients with pulmonary disease.

The major side effects reported to be associated with glycosylated rhGM-CSF treatment include fever, bone pain, myalgia, and constitutional symptoms of weakness and fatigue (Herrmann et al., 1989a; Rifkin et al., 1988; Clark et al., 1988; Steward et al., 1988; Antman et al., 1989; Phillips et al., 1989; Vadhan-Raj et al., 1988). Fever observed secondary to rhGM-CSF administration can be abrogated by the administration of indomethacin, suggesting that it is possibly mediated by prostaglandins (Peters et al., 1988a). Short IV infusions of glycosylated (yeast-derived) rhGM-CSF have also been associated with dose-limiting epigastric distress, nausea, and vomiting (Herrmann et al., 1989a; Rifkin et al., 1988). In two studies, at higher doses of glycosylated (CHO cell–derived) rhGM-CSF ($\geq$32 μg/kg/day), used either prior to chemotherapy (Rifkin et al., 1988) or following ABMT (Brandt et al., 1988), generalized edema, thrombophlebitis, hypotension, and acute renal failure (1 patient) (Antman et al., 1989; Brandt et al., 1988) have been reported. Comparable side effects with glycosylated yeast-derived rhGM-CSF have not been reported (Nemunaitis et al., 1988); however, comparable doses have not been explored in these identical settings. Treatment with both glycosylated and nonglycosylated rhGM-CSF has, in some studies, also been associated with a transient decline in platelet count, including 2 of 21 in one study and to $<$20% pretreatment values in most patients in another trial (Herrmann et al., 1989a; Lieschke et al., 1989).

Side effects reported to date for IL-1 include fever, chills, phlebitis, hypotension, and abdominal pain. Ganser et al. (1989a, 1989b) have reported an occasional fever and hypotension in patients receiving IL-3. Macrophage-CSF has been relatively well tolerated with essentially no toxicity reported except for mild thrombocytopenia. Reported toxicities of IL-4 have included fever, occasional headache, episodic nasal congestion, and, in one patient, fluid retention.

The clinical ramifications and therapeutic evaluation of hematopoietic growth factors are an ever-expanding area of investigation. A further understanding of the mechanism of action of these factors should provide insight into the pathophysiology and manifestations of many diseases and better delineate how best to employ these regulatory molecules to our therapeutic advantage. Ultimately, combinations of hematopoietic cell factors, alone or in combination with other cytokines, low molecular weight compounds, vitamins, or chemotherapeutic agents used to either accelerate immune reconstitution, boost effector cell function, or promote enhanced differentiation induction of tumor cells should prove useful in the treatment of a number of malignant, infectious, and genetic disorders affecting hematopoiesis.

REFERENCES

Aglietta M, Piacibello W, Sanavio F, et al. Kinetics of human hemopoietic cells after in vivo administration of granulocyte-macrophage colony-stimulating factor. J Clin Invest. 1989; 83:551.

Andreeff M, Welte K. Hematopoietic colony stimulating factors. Semin Oncol. 1989;16:211.

Antin JH, Smith BR, Holmes W, Rosenthal DS. Phase I/II study of recombinant human granulocyte-macrophage colony-stimulating factor in aplastic anemia and myelodysplastic syndrome. Blood. 1988;72:705.

Antman KS, Griffin JD, Elias A, et al. Effect of recombinant human granulocyte-macrophage colony stimulating factor on chemotherapy-induced myelosuppression. New Engl J Med. 1989;319:593.

Arnaout MA, Wang EA, Clark SC, et al. Human recombinant granulocyte-macrophage colony-stimulating factor increases cell-to-cell adhesion and surface expression of adhesion-promoting surface glycoproteins on mature granulocytes. J Clin Invest. 1986;78:597.

Bajorin DF, Jakubowski A, Cody B, et al. Phase I trial of recombinant macrophage colony stimulating factor (rhM-CSF) in patients (PTS) with melanoma (MEL). Blood. 1989;74 (suppl 1):1222.

Bajorin DF, Jakubowski A, Cody B, et al. Recombinant macrophage colony stimulating factor (rhM-CSF): a phase I trial in patients (PTS) with metastatic melanoma. Proc Am Soc Clin Oncol. 1990;9:707.

Baldwin GC, Gasson JC, Quan SG, et al. Granulocyte-macrophage colony-stimulating factor enhances neutrophil function in acquired immunodeficiency syndrome patients. Proc Natl Acad Sci USA. 1988;856:2763.

Bar MH, Aronson FR. Recombinant human GM-CSF in myelosuppression of chemotherapy (continued). New Engl J Med. 1988;320:939.

Begley CG, Nicola NA, Metcalf D. Proliferation of normal human promyelocyte and myelocytes after a single pulse stimulation by purified GM-CSF or G-CSF. Blood. 1988;71:640.

Bevilacqua MP, Pober JS, Majeau GR, et al. Interleukin-1 inducer biosynthesis and cell surface expression of procoagulant activity in human vascular endothelial cells. J Exp Med. 1984; 160:618.

Bhalla K, Berkhofer M, Arlin Z, Grant S, Latzky J, Grahma G. Effect of rhGM-CSF and IL-3 on the metabolism of cytosine arabinoside in normal and leukemic human bone marrow cells. Blood. 1988;72:348.

Bonilla MA, Gillio AP, Ruggeiro M, et al. Effects of recombinant human granulocyte colony stimulating factor on neutropenia in patients with congenital agranulocytosis. New Engl J Med. 1989;320:1574.

Bonnem EM, Morstyn G. Granulocyte-macrophage colony-stimulating factor (GM-CSF) current status and future development. Semin Oncol. 1988;15:46–51.

Brandt SJ, Peters WP, Atwater SK, et al. Effect of recombinant human granulocyte-macrophage colony-stimulating factor on hematopoietic reconstitution after high-dose chemotherapy and autologous bone marrow transplantation. New Engl J Med. 1988;318:869.

Bronchud MH, Potter MR, Morgenstern G, Blasco MJ, Scarffle J. In vitro and in vivo analysis of the effects of recombinant human granulocyte colony-stimulating factor in patients. Br J Cancer. 1988;58:64.

Bronchud MH, Howell A, Crowther D, Hopwood P, Souza L, Dexter TM. The use of granulocyte colony stimulating factor to increase the intensity of treatment with doxorubicin in patients with advanced breast and ovarian cancer. Br J Cancer. 1989;60:121.

Bronchud MH, Scarffe JH, Thatcher N, Crowther D, Dexter TM. Phase I/II study of recombinant human granulocyte colony stimulating factor in patients receiving intensive chemotherapy for small cell lung cancer. Br J Cancer. 1987;56:809.

Buchner T, Hiddemann W, Koenigsmann M, et al. Chemotherapy (CT) followed by recombinant human granulocyte macrophage colony stimulating factor (GM-CSF) for acute leukemias at higher age or after relapse. Proc Soc Clin Oncol. 1989;8:770.

Cannistra SA, Grostrek P, Griffin JD. GM-CSF enhances the cytotoxic effects of cytosine arabinoside in acute myeloblastic leukemia and in myeloid blast crisis phase of chronic myeloid leukemia. Blood. 1988a;72:681.

Cannistra SA, Socinski MA, Groshek P, Elias A, Antman K. Granulocyte-macrophage colony stimulating factor (GM-CSF) enhances monocyte tumoricidal activity. Proc Am Soc Clin Oncol. 1988b;7:645.

Cebon J, Dempsey P, Fox R, et al. Pharmacokinetics of human granulocyte-macrophage colony stimulating factor using a sensitive immunoassay. Blood. 1988;72:1340.

Champlin RE, Nimer SE, Ireland P, Oette DH, Golde DW. Treatment of refractory aplastic anemia with recombinant human granulocyte-macrophage colony-stimulating factor. Blood. 1989;73:694.

Cheng GYM, Kelleher CA, Miyauchi J, et al. Structure and expression of GM-CSF and G-CSF in blast cells from patients with acute myeloblastic leukemia. Blood. 1988;71:204.

Clark J, Longo D, Smith J, et al. Phase I trial of recombinant human granulocyte-macrophage colony stimulating factor (rHuGM-CSF) in cancer patients (Pts) Proc Am Soc Clin Oncol. 1988;7:614.

Correns PG, Wolf BA, Unanue ER, et al. Interleukin-1 is a potent modulator of insulin secretion from isolated rat islets of Langerhans. Diabetes. 1987;36:963.

De France T, Auboy JP, Rousset F, et al. Human recombinant interleukin-4 induces F_C receptors (CD23) on normal human B-lymphocytes. J Exp Med. 1987;165:1459.

Devreux S, Lynch DC, Campos CD, et al. Transient leukopenia induced by granulocyte-macrophage colony stimulating factor. Lancet. 1988;1:667.

Dinarello CA. Biology of interleukin-1. FASEB J. 1988;2:108.

Donahue RE, Wang EA, Stone DK, et al. Stimulation of hematopoiesis in primates by continuous infusion of recombinant human GM-CSF. Nature. 1986;321:872.

Donahue RE, Mitchell S, Metzger M, Rock B, Clark SC. Stimulation of hematopoiesis in primates with human interleukin-3 and granulocyte-macrophage colony stimulating factor. Blood. 1987a;70(suppl 1):388.

Donahue RE, Serhraa J, Norton C, et al. Stimulation of hematopoiesis in primates with human interleukin-3 and granulocyte macrophage colony stimulating factor. Blood. 1987b; 70:388.

Duhrsen U, Villeval J-L, Boyd J, et al. Effects of recombinant human granulocyte colony-stimulating factor on hematopoietic progenitor cells in cancer patients. Blood. 1988;72:2074.

Fernandez-Bohan R, Krammer PH, Diamenstein T, Uhr JW, Vitette ES. B cell stimulatory factor 1 (BSF-1) promotes growth of helper T cell lines. J Exp Med. 1986;164:580.

Fibbe WE, Schaafsman MR, Witteman BJM, Falkenburg JHF, Jones TC, Willemze R. No correction of cyclic neutropenia on treatment with human recombinant GM-CSF. Blood. 1988;72:372.

Fukuoka M, Morit, Taii S, Yasuda K. Interleukin-1 inhibits luteinization of porcine granulosa cells in culture. Endocrinology. 1988;122:367.

Gabrilove JL. Biological effects and clinical applications of human colony stimulating factors. In: Pinedo HM, Longo DL, Chabner BA, eds. Cancer chemotherapy and biological response modifiers annual 10. Amsterdam: Elsevier Science Publishers B.b.; 1988:492.

Gabrilove JL, Welte K, Harris P, et al. Pluripoietin—a second human hematopoietic colony stimulating factor produced by the human bladder carcinoma cell line, 5637. Proc Natl Acad Sci USA. 1986;83:2478.

Gabrilove JL, Jakubowski A, Fain K, et al. A phase I study of granulocyte colony stimulating factor in patients with transitional cell carcinoma of the urothelium. J Clin Invest. 1988a; 82:1554.

Gabrilove JL, Jakubowski A, Scher H, et al. Granulocyte colony stimulating factor reduces neutropenia and associated morbidity of chemotherapy for transitional cell carcinoma of the urothelium. New Engl J Med. 1988b;318:1414.

Ganser A, Lindemann A, Ottman OG, et al. Phase I study of recombinant human interleukin-3 (IL-3). Mol Biother. 1989a;1:68.

Ganser A, Volkers B, Ottman OG, et al. Recombinant human granulocyte-macrophage colony-stimulating factor in patients with myelodysplastic syndromes—a phase I/II trial. Blood. 1989b;73:31.

Gasson JC, Weisbart RH, Kaufman S, et al. Purified human granulocyte macrophage colony stimulating factor: direct action on neutrophils. Science. 1984;226:1339.

Gillio AP, Bonilla MA, Potter GP, et al. Effects of recombinant human granulocyte colony stimulating factor on hematopoietic reconstitution following autologous bone marrow transplantation in primates. Transplant Proc. 1987;7(suppl XIX):153.

Glaspy JA, Baldwin GC, Robertson PA, et al. Therapy for neutropenia in hairy cell leukemia with recombinant human granulocyte colony stimulating factor. Ann Intern Med. 1988; 109:789.

Gottschall PE, Uehara A, Hoffmann ST, Arimura A. Interleukin-1 inhibition follicle stimulating hormone-induced differentiation in rat granulosa cells in vitro. Biochem Biophys Res Commun. 1987;149:502.

Griffin JD. Clinical applications of colony stimulating factors. Oncology. 1988;2:15.

Griffin JD, Young DC, Herrman R, Wiper D, Wagner K, Sabbath KD. Effects of recombinant human GM-CSF on proliferation of clonogenic cells in acute myeloblastic leukemia. Blood. 1986;67:1448.

Griffin JD, Rambaldi A, Vallenga E, Young DC, Ostapovicz D, Cannistra SA. Secretion of interleukin-1 by acute myeloblastic leukemia cells in vitro induces endothelial cells to secrete colony stimulating factors. Blood. 1987;70:1218.

Groopman JE, Mitsuyasu RT, Deleo MJ, et al. Effect of recombinant human granulocyte-macrophage colony-stimulating factor on myelopoiesis in the acquired immunodeficiency syndrome. New Engl J Med. 1987;317:593.

Guilian D, Young DG, Woodward J, et al. Interleukin-1 is an astroglial growth factor in the developing brain. J Neurosci. 1988;8:709.

Hammond WP, Price TH, Souza LM, Dale DC. Treatment of cyclic neutropenia with granulocyte colony stimulating factor. New Engl J Med. 1989;320:1306.

Herrmann F, Schultz G, Lindemann A, et al. Hematopoietic responses in patients with advanced malignancies treated with recombinant human granulocyte-macrophage colony stimulating factor. J Clin Oncol. 1989a;7:159.

Herrmann F, Wieser M, Riedel D, et al. Interleukin-4 (IL-4) is a major inducer of hematopoietic growth factors. Proc Am Assoc Can Res. 1989b;30:268.

Hirano T, Yasukawa K, Harada H, et al. Complementary DNA for a novel human interleukin (BSF-2) that induces B lymphocytes to produce immunoglobulin. Nature. 1986;324:73.

Hoang T, Nara N, Wong G, Clark SC, Minden MD, McCulloch EA. Effects of recombinant GM-CSF on the blast cells of acute myeloblastic leukemia. Blood. 1986;68:313.

Horiguchi J, Warren MK, Kufe D. Expression of the macrophage specific CSF in human monocytes treated with granulocyte-macrophage colony stimulating factor. Blood. 1987; 69:1259.

Howard M, Farraw, Hifiker M, et al. Identification of a T cell–derived B cell growth factor distinct from interleukin-2. J Exp Med. 1982;155:914.

Hu-Li J, Shevach EM, Mizuguchi J, O'Hara U, Mosmann T, Paul WE. B cell stimulatory factor 1 (interleukin-4) is a potent costimulant for normal resting T-lymphocytes. J Exp Med. 1987;165:157.

Ihle JN, Keller J, Henderson L, et al. Procedures for the purification of interleukin-3 to homogeneity. J Immunol. 1982;129:231.

Jakubowski A, Gabrilove JL. RhG-CSF in the treatment of bladder cancer with M-VAC. In: Peters WP, ed. 1989.

Jakubowski A, Andreeff M, Tafuri A, et al. In vivo and in vitro studies of rhG-CSF in acute non-lymphocytic leukemia. Blood. 1989a;74(suppl):1034.

Jakubowski A, Souza LM, Fain K, Clarkson B, Moore MAS, Gabrilove JL. Effects of human granulocyte colony stimulating factor in a patient with idiopathic neutropenia. New Engl J Med. 1989b;320:38.

Kaplan SS, Zdziarski VE, Basford RE, Wing E, Shadduck RK. Effect of in vivo recombinant human granulocyte-macrophage colony stimulating factor on peripheral blood granulocyte function. Clin Res. 1988;36:566.

Kawasaki ES, Ladner MB, Wang AM, et al. Molecular cloning of a complementary DNA encoding human macrophage-specific colony-stimulating factor (CSF-1). Science. 1985; 230:281.

Kelleher C, Miyauchi J, Wong G, Clark S, Minden MD, McCulloch EA. Synergism between recombinant growth factors, GM-CSF and G-CSF, acting on the blast cells of acute myeloblastic leukemia. Blood. 1987;69:1498.

Kishi K, Ihle JN, Urdal DL, Ogawa M. B cell stimulatory factor-1 (BSF-1)/Interleukin-4 (IL-4) is a multi-CSF which acts directly on primitive hemopoietic progenitors. Proc Am Soc Hematol. 1988;72(suppl 1):402.

Kishimoto T. The biology of interleukin-6. Blood. 1989;74:1.

Kleinerman ES, Knowles RD, Lachman LB, Gutterman JU. Effect of recombinant granulocyte/macrophage colony-stimulating factor on human monocyte activity in vitro and following intravenous administration. Cancer Res. 1988;48:2604.

Kobayashi Y, Okabe T, Uzumaki H, Urabe A, Takaku F. Differentiation therapy of myelodysplastic syndrome by granulocyte colony stimulating factor. Clin Res. 1988;36:412.

Koeniopmann M, Buchner TH, Hiddemann W, et al. In vivo hematological effects of human recombinant granulocyte-macrophage colony stimulating factor (GM-CSF) in patients with acute leukemias. Proc Am Soc Oncol. 1989.

Lange B, Valtieri M, Santoli D, et al. Growth factor requirements of childhood acute leukemia: establishment of GM-CSF dependent cell lines. Blood. 1987;70:192.

Leary AG, Yang YC, Clark SC, et al. Recombinant gibbon interleukin-3 supports formation of human multilineage colonies and blast cell colonies in culture: comparison with recombinant human granulocyte-macrophage colony stimulating factor. Blood. 1987;70:1343.

Leary AG, Ikebuchi K, Herai Y, et al. Synergism between IL-6 and IL-3 in supporting proliferation of human hematopoietic stem cells: comparison with IL-1. Blood. 1988;71:1759.

Lieschke GJ, Maher D, Cebon J, et al. Ann Intern Med. 1989;110:357.

Lindemann A, Oster W, Riedel D, Mertelsmann R, Hermann F. GM-CSF induces secretion of monokines by human polymorphonuclear leukocytes. Blood. 1987;70:223.

Logotheliu L, Dexeus F, Sella A, Amatro R, Finn L, Gutterman J. Escalated (ESC) M-VAC (MTX 30 μ/m^2) with recombinant human granulocyte macrophage stimulating factor (rhGM-

CSF) for patients with advanced and chemotherapy refractory urothelium tumors: a Phase I study. Proc Am Soc Clin Oncol. 1989;8:514.

Lopez AF, Williamson J, Gamble JR, et al. Recombinant human granulocyte-macrophage colony-stimulating factor stimulates in vitro mature human neutrophil and eosinophil function, m surface receptor expression and survival. J Clin Invest. 1986;78:1220.

Lothrop CD, Jones JB, Warren DJ, Moore MAS, Souza LM. Correction of cyclic hematopoiesis with recombinant human granulocyte colony stimulating factor. Blood. 1988;72:1324.

Lumpkin MD. The regulation of ACTH secretion by IL-1. Science. 1987;238:452.

Mandrup-Poulsen T, Nesup J, Bendtzen K, et al. Ultrastructural studies of the time-course and cellular specificity of interleukin-1 mediated islet cell toxicity. Acta Pathol Microbiol Immunol Scand. 1987;Sectl. C:95.

Markowitz A, Kleinerman E, Hudson M, et al. Phase I study of recombinant human interleukin-4 (rhuIL-4) in patients with advanced cancer. Blood. 1989;74(suppl 1):540.

Mayer P, Lam C, Obenaus H, Leihe E, Besemer J. Recombinant human GM-CSF induces leukocytosis and activates peripheral blood polymorphonuclear neutrophils in non-human primates. Blood. 1987;70:206.

McNiece IK, McGrath HE, Quesenberry PJ. Granulocyte colony-stimulating factor augments in vitro megakaryocyte colony formation by interleukin-3. Exp Hematol. 1988;16:807.

Mertelsmann R, Lindemann L, Wieser M, et al. Prevention of chemotherapy induced neutropenia and associated morbidity in patients with advanced cancer by subcutaneous recombinant human GM-CSF (rhGM-CSF). Proc Am Assoc Cancer Res. 1989;30:267.

Metcalf D, Begley CG, Johnson GR. Biologic properties in vitro of a recombinant human granulocyte-macrophage colony stimulating factor. Blood. 1986;67:37.

Miller LC, Dinarello CA. Biologic activities of interleukin-1 relevant to rheumatoid diseases. Pathol Immunopathol Res. 1987;6:22.

Mitsuyasu R, Levine J, Miles SA, et al. Effects of long term subcutaneous (SC) administration of recombinant granulocyte macrophage colony stimulating factor in patients with HIV-related leukopenia. Blood. 1988;72:1297.

Miyauchi J, Kelleher CA, Yanf YC, et al. The effects of three recombinant growth factors, IL-3, GM-CSF and G-CSF, on blast cells of acute myeloblastic leukemia maintained in short term suspension culture. Blood. 1987;70:657.

Monsoy RL, Skelly RR, MacVittie TJ, et al. The effect of recombinant GM-CSF on recovery of monkeys transplanted with autologous bone marrow. Blood. 1987a;70:1690.

Monsoy RL, Skelly RR, Davis TA, et al. Effect of interleukin-1 on the recovery of primates after radiation and autologous bone marrow transplantation. Blood. 1987b;70(suppl 1):1103.

Moore MAS, Gabrilove J, Sheridan AP. Therapeutic implications of serum factors inhibiting proliferation and inducing differentiation of myeloid leukemic cells. Blood Cells. 1983; 9:125.

Morstyn G, Souza LM, Keech J, et al. Effect of granulocyte colony stimulating factor on neutropenia induced by cytotoxic chemotherapy. Lancet. 1988;1:667.

Morstyn G, Lieschke GJ, Cebon J, et al. Early clinical trials with colony stimulating factors. Cancer Invest. 1989a.

Morstyn G, Lieschke GJ, Sheridan W, Layton J, Cebon J, Fox RM. Clinical experience with recombinant human granulocyte colony stimulating factor and granulocyte-macrophage colony stimulating factor. Semin Hematol. 1989b;26:9.

Muraguchi A, Kishimoto T, Miki Y, et al. T cell replacing factor (TRF). J Immunol. 1987; 127:412.

Murine B. Cell stimulating factor (interleukin-4) increases expression of the F_C receptor for IgE on mouse B cells. Proc Natl Acad Sci. 1987;84:4606.

Nagata S, Tsuchinya A, Asano S, et al. Molecular cloning and expression of cDNA for human granulocyte colony stimulating factor. Nature. 1986;319:415.

Nara N, Murohashi I, Suzuki T, et al. Effect of recombinant human granulocyte colony stimulating factor (G-CSF) on blast progenitors from acute myeloblastic leukemia patients. Br J Cancer. 1988;56:49.

Natari K, Asano S, Shirafuji N, et al. Serum granulocyte colony stimulating factor levels in healthy volunteers and patients with various disorders as estimated by enzyme immunoassay. Blood. 1989;73:117–121.

Negrin RS, Haeuber DH, Nagler A, et al. Treatment of myelodysplastic syndromes with recombinant granulocyte colony stimulating factor. Ann Intern Med. 1989;110:976.

Nemunaitis J, Singer JW, Buckner D, et al. Use of recombinant human granulocyte-macrophage colony stimulating factor in autologous marrow transplantation. Blood. 1988;72:834.

Neta R, Douches S, Oppenheim JJ. Interleukin-1 is a radioprotector. J Immunol. 1986; 136:2483.

Nienhuis AW, Donahue RE, Karlsson S, et al. Recombinant human granulocyte-macrophage colony stimulating factor (GM-CSF) shortens the period of neutropenia after autologous bone marrow transplantation on primate model. J Clin Invest. 1987;80:573.

Nimer S, Golde D. The 5q abnormality. Blood. 1988;70:1705.

Nimer S, Champlin RE, Golde DW. Serum cholesterol lowering activity of granulocyte macrophage colony stimulating factor. JAMA. 1988;260:3297.

Nissen C, Tichelli A, Gratwohl A, et al. Failure of recombinant human granulocyte-macrophage colony-stimulating factor therapy in aplastic anemia patients with very severe neutropenia. Blood. 1988;72:2045.

Nocile R, Krammer PH, O'Hara J, et al. Increased expression of Ia antigens on resting B cells: an additional role for B-cell growth factor. Proc Natl Acad Sci USA. 1984;81:6149.

Pène J, Rousset F, Brière F, et al. Interleukin-5 enhances interleukin-4 induced IgE production by normal human B cells. Eur J Immunol. 1988;6:929–935.

Peschel C, Paul WE, O'Hara J, Green J. Effects of B-cell stimulatory factor-1 + interleukin-4 on hematopoietic progenitor cells. Blood. 1987;70:254.

Peters WP, Shogan J, Shpall EJ, Jones RB, Kim CS. Recombinant human granulocyte-macrophage colony-stimulating factor produces fever. Lancet. 1988a;1:950.

Peters WP, Stuart A, Affronti ML, et al. Neutrophil migration is defective during recombinant human granulocyte-macrophage colony stimulating factor infusion after autologous bone marrow transplantation in humans. Blood. 1988b;72:1310.

Peters WP, Bar MH, Aronson FR. The effect of recombinant human colony stimulating factors on hematopoietic reconstitutions following autologous bone marrow transplantation. Semin Hematol. 1989a;26:18–23.

Peters WP, Kurtzberg J, Atwater S, et al. Comparative effects of rhG-CSF and rhG-CSF on hematopoietic reconstitution and granulocyte function following high dose chemotherapy and autologous bone marrow transplantation (ABMT). Proc Am Soc Clin Oncol. 1989b;8:691.

Phillips N, Jacob S, Stoller R, Earle M, Przepiorka D, Shadduck RK. Effect of recombinant human granulocyte-macrophage colony stimulating factor on myelopoiesis in patients with refractory metastatic cancer. Blood. 1989;74:26.

Platzer E, Welte K, Gabrilove J, et al. Biological activities of a human pluripotent hematopoietic colony stimulating factor on normal and leukemic cells. J Exp Med. 1985;162:1788.

Platzer E, Oez S, Welte K, et al. Human pluripotent hemopoietic colony stimulating factor: activities on human and murine cells. Immunobiology. 1986;172:185.

Rifkin R, Hersh E, Salmon S. Continuous intravenous (IV) administration of recombinant human granulocyte-macrophage colony-stimulating factor (rGH-CSF) is superior to IV bolus administration: a phase I study. Proc Am Soc Oncol. 1988;7:165.

Roehm NW, Leibson J, Zlotnick A, et al. Interleukin-induced increase in Ia expression by normal mouse B cells. J Exp Med. 1984;160:679.

Sakai K, Hattori T, Matsuoka M, et al. Autocrine stimulating of interleukin 1B in acute myelogenous leukemia cells. J Exp Med. 1987;166:1597.

Scher CJ, Rettenmier CW, Sacca R, et al. The c-*fms* proto-oncogene product is related to the receptor for the mononuclear phagocyte growth factor, CSF-1. Cell. 1985;41:665.

Sheridan W, Morstyn G, Gree M, et al. Phase II study of granulocyte colony stimulating factor (G-CSF) in autologous bone marrow transplantation. Proc Am Soc Clin Oncol. 1989; 8:691.

Shuening FG, Storb R, Goehle S, et al. Effect of recombinant human granulocyte colony stimulating factor on hematopoiesis of normal dogs and on hematopoietic recovery after otherwise lethal total body irradiation. Blood. 1989;in press.

Sideras P, Nowa T, Honjo T. Structure and function of Interleukin 4 and 5. Immunol Rev. 1988;102:189.

Sieff C, Emerson SG, Donahue RE, et al. Human recombinant granulocyte-macrophage colony stimulating factor: a multi-lineage hematopoietin. Science. 1985;230:1171.

Simmers RN, Webber LM, Shannon MF, et al. Localization of the G-CSF gene on chromosome 17 proximal to the breakpoint in the t(15:17) in acute promyelocytic leukemia. Blood. 1987;70:330.

Socinski MA, Elias A, Schnipper L, Cannistra SA, Antman KH, Griffin JD. Granulocyte-macrophage colony stimulating factor expands the circulating haemopoietic progenitor cell compartment in man. Lancet. 1988;1:1194.

Souza LM, Boone TC, Gabrilove J, et al. Recombinant human granulocyte colony stimulating factor: effects on normal and leukemic myeloid cells. Science. 1986;232:61.

Steward WP, Scarffe JH, Austen R, Crowther D, Loyds P. Phase I study of recombinant DNA granulocyte-macrophage colony stimulating factor (rGM-CSF). Proc Am Soc Clin Oncol. 1988;7:614.

Stork JL, Peterson VM, Rundus CH, Robinson WA. Interleukin-1 enhances murine granulopoisis in vivo. Exp. Hematol. 1987;16:163.

Strife A, Lambek C, Wisniewski D, et al. Activities of four purified growth factors on highly enriched human hematopoietic progenitor cells. Blood. 1987;69:1508.

Tafarri A, Hegewisch S, Souza L, Andreeff M. Stimulation of leukemic blast cells in vitro by colony stimulating factors (G-CSF, GM-CSF and IL-3): evidence of recombinant and increased cell killing with cytosine arabinoside. Blood. 1988;72:329.

Taylor K, Spitzer G, Jagannaton S, Dicke K, Souza LM. Phase II study of recombinant human granulocyte colony stimulating factor (rhG-CSF) in Hodgkin's disease after high dose chemotherapy with ABMT. Blood. 1988;72:452.

Thompson JA, Lee DJ, Kidd P, et al. Subcutaneous granulocyte-macrophage colony stimulating factor in patients with myelodysplastic syndrome: toxicity, pharmacokinetics and hematological effects. J Clin Oncol. 1989;7:629.

Toner GC, Jakubowski A, Crown JPL, et al. Colony stimulating factors and neutrophil migration. Ann Intern Med. 1989;110:847.

Vadhan-Raj S, Keating M, Lemaistre A, et al. Effects of recombinant human granulocyte-macrophage colony-stimulating factor in patients with myelodysplastic syndromes. New Engl J Med. 1987;317:1545.

Vadhan-Raj S, Buescher S, Broxmeyer HE, et al. Stimulation of myelopoiesis in patients with aplastic anemia by recombinant human granulocyte-macrophage colony-stimulating factor. New Engl J Med. 1988a;319:1628.

Vadhan-Raj S, Buescher S, Lemaistre A, et al. Stimulation of hematopoiesis in patients with bone marrow failure and in patients with malignancy by recombinant human granulocyte-macrophage colony-stimulating factor. Blood. 1988b;72:134.

Vallenga E, Young DC, Wagner K, Wiper D, Ostapovicz D, Griffin JD. The effects of GM-CSF and G-CSF in promoting growth of clonogenic cells in acute myeloblastic leukemia. Blood. 1987;69:1771.

Warren D, Moore MAS. Interleukin-1 and granulocyte colony stimulating factor synergism: in vivo stimulation of stem cell recovery and hematopoietic regeneration following 5-flourouracil treatment of mice. Proc Natl Acad Sci USA. 1987;84:7134.

Weisbart RH, Golde DW, Clark SC, et al. Human granulocyte-macrophage colony stimulating factor is a neutrophil activator. Nature. 1985;314:361.

Welte K, Platzer E, Lu L, Gabrilove J, Mertelsmann R, Moore MAS. Purification and biological characterization of human pluripotent hematopoietic colony stimulating factor. Proc Natl Acad Sci USA. 1985;82:1526.

Welte K, Bonilla MA, Gillio AP, et al. Recombinant human G-CSF: effects on hematopoiesis in normal and cyclophosphamide treated primates. J Exp Med. 1987a;165:941.

Welte K, Bonilla MA, Gillio AP, et al. In vivo effects of recombinant human G-CSF in therapy induced neutropenias in primates. Exp Hematol. 1987b;15:72.

Welte K, Zeidler C, Reuther A, et al. Correction of neutropenia and associated clinical symptoms with rhG-CSF in children with severe congenital neutropenia. Blood. 1988;72:465.

Westmacott D, Wadsworth J, Bloxham DP. Chemotactic activity of recombinant human interleukin-1. Agents Actions. 1987;21:323.

Wing EJ, Magee DM, Kaplan SS, Shadduck RK. Stimulating of human monocytes by recombinant granulocyte-macrophage colony stimulating factor in patients with metastatic carcinoma. Clin Res. 1988;36:422.

Wong GG, Witek JS, Temple PA, et al. Human GM-CSF: molecular cloning of complementary DNA and purification of the natural and recombinant proteins. Science. 1985;228:810.

Wong GG, Temple PA, Leary AC, et al. Human CSF-1: molecular cloning and expression of 4 kg cDNA encoding the human urinary protein. Science. 1987;235:1504.

Yang Y-C, Ciarletta AB, Temple PA, et al. Human IL-3 (multi-CSF): identification by expression cloning of a novel hematopoietic growth factor related to murine IL-3. Cell. 1986;47:3.

Young DC, Griffin JD. Autocrine secretion of GM-CSF in acute myeloblastic leukemia. Blood. 1986;68:1178.

Young DC, Wagner K, Griffin JD. Constitutive expression of the granulocyte-macrophage colony stimulating factor gene in acute myeloblastic leukemia. J Clin Invest. 1987;79:100.

Yuo A, Kitagawa S, Okabe T, et al. Recombinant human granulocyte colony-stimulating factor repairs the abnormalities of neutrophils in patients with myelodysplastic syndromes and chronic myelogenous leukemia. Blood. 1987;70:404.

Zhang XG, Klin B, Batuille R. Interleukin-6 is a potent myeloma-cell growth factor in patients with aggressive multiple myeloma. Blood. 1989;74:11.

Zsebo KM, Cohen AM, Murdock DC, et al. Recombinant human granulocyte colony stimulating factor: molecular and biological characterization. Immunobiology. 1986;172:175.

CHAPTER **20**

RETINOIDS: PROTOTYPE BIOLOGICAL MODIFIERS OF PREMALIGNANCIES AND CANCERS

James K. Pitcock
Frank L. Meyskens, Jr.

Oncologic interest in the group of compounds known as retinoids (vitamin A and its natural and synthetic derivatives) is primarily based on their ability to prevent the expression of premalignancy and malignancy and to induce differentiation or maturation of malignant cells. Despite an enormous amount of investigative work, these groups of compounds represent a prototype for understanding the structure–function relationships and cellular transformation. Studies of these molecules far exceed those of any other group of chemical or biological maturational agents, and they are used widely as a probe to facilitate an understanding of the biology of normal and transformed cells. The mechanisms for the pleiotropic biological and biochemical effects of retinoids are not yet well understood. In fact, retinoids are pleiotropic in their biochemical and biological effects and provide a rich probe for understanding cellular control processes.

The retinoids represent a group of noncytotoxic compounds that are relatively unexplored at the clinical level and have the potential to dramatically reduce the incidence, morbidity, and mortality of human cancer. Most of the animal and clinical investigations using retinoid compounds have been concerned with tumors of epithelial origin: lung, breast, bladder, prostate, skin, female genital tract, and the upper aerodigestive tract (UADT). This group of malignancies numerically comprises the majority of cancers that affect humans. In this chapter we will address both the chemopreventive potential of retinoids and the possible role of retinoids in the treatment of premalignancies and established human malignancies.

HISTORY

Early vitamin A research was directed to define the role of this nutrient in vision. Night blindness was first described in Egypt around 1500 B.C. Although Hippocrates did not associate blindness with a nutritional deficiency, he empirically established that the eating of beef liver was a treatment for this disorder. During the past century chronic nutritional deficiency (hypovitaminosis A) was recognized as the cause of numerous ophthalmic disorders (Mandel and Cohn, 1980). Ophthalmia Brasiliana, a disease of the eyes, was first described in 1865 in nutritionally deficient slaves. In 1887, endemic night blindness was reported to occur in Russian Orthodox Catholics who fasted during Lent. Of even greater interest was the observation that nursing infants of women who fasted were prone to the spontaneous sloughing of their corneas. During World War I, xerophthalmia (dryness and thickening of the cornea) was related to a decrease in butterfat content in the diet. The importance of ophthalmic diseases is permanently encumbered in the chemical name of vitamin A, retinol, which is derived from the name retina, the photosensitive layer of the eye.

Vitamin A as a discrete compound was first identified in Germany by Stepp (1909). Later in 1913, two groups working independently reported that a fat-soluble substance found in butter, egg yolk, and cod liver oil was capable of reversing in rats a growth deficiency produced by the feeding of a lard-only diet (McCollum and Davis, 1913; Osborne and Mendel, 1913). McCollum, who received most of the credit for this discovery, later named this substance "fat-soluble A" to distinguish it from the essential water soluble substances he called "water-soluble B." Fat-soluble A was subsequently renamed vitamin A in 1920 (Drummond, 1920). Research subsequent to these discoveries identified the chemical structure of vitamin A and its primary biological precursor, β-carotene. Further investigations of vitamin A physiology catalogued the systemic abnormalities associated with hypo- and hypervitaminosis A.

Research into the association between vitamin A and cancer began in 1922 when Mori (1922) reported metaplasia of the respiratory tract and atrophy of the salivary and paraocular glands associated with vitamin A deficiency. In 1925, Wolbach and Howe noted that vitamin A–deficient animals developed epithelia that were similar in appearance to neoplastic tissues (Wolbach and Howe, 1925). Of even greater importance was their finding that dietary vitamin A supplementation rapidly normalized the metaplasia they had observed in the gastrointestinal, respiratory, and urogenital epithelia. In 1926, Fujumaki found that carcinoma developed in the stomachs of rats that were vitamin A deficient (Fujumaki, 1926). Abels et al. (1941) were the first to make an association between human malignancy and vitamin A deficiency.

With the development of organ culture technology, a role for vitamin A in the prevention of cancer emerged. A sentinel study by Lasnitzki (1955) demonstrated that the phenotypic premalignant expression of mouse prostate glands induced by the carcinogenic compound 3-methylcolanthrene was altered toward a more normal appearance with the addition of retinyl acetate. With the development of cell culture technology, Merriman and Bertram (1979) showed that the primary effect of retinoids was on the suppression of the promotion phase of malignant transformation that occurred after initiation of tumor development.

CHEMICAL STRUCTURE

In a general sense, retinoids can be considered to be a group of natural and synthetic compounds that are based on the chemical structure of vitamin A (retinol, all-*trans* retinol). This less than precise definition is required because of differences in the structure of the newer generation of retinoid compounds that have been developed over the past few years. According to the International Union of Pure and Applied Chemistry (IUPAC) (1982), a retinoid is classified as a "diterpenoid derived from a monocyclic parent compound containing five carbon-carbon double bonds and a functional group at the terminus of the acyclic portion." This definition is very limiting and functionally eliminates all of the newer third generation retinoid compounds that are members of the multicyclic retinoidal benzoic acid compounds. Therefore, we prefer to use the definition of Sporn, "a retinoid is a substance that can elicit specific biological responses by binding to and activating a specific receptor or group of receptors" (regardless of structure) (Sporn and Roberts, 1985).

The proband compound of retinoids is vitamin A (retinol or all-*trans* retinol). This 20-carbon compound can be divided into three domains, a cyclic end group, a polyene side chain, and a polar end group (Fig. 20-1) (Frickel, 1984). Alterations in each of these major areas produce retinoid compounds with markedly different biological activities and toxicities. There are now over 2000 retinoid compounds that have been developed and tested for biological activity (Bollwag, 1979, 1983; Loeliger et al., 1980; Cunningham and Ehmann, 1983). The first generation of synthetic retinoid compounds was developed by altering the polar end group and polyene side chain of retinol. This produced the retinyl esters, amides, aldehydes, ethers, amines, and acids. The best known and most widely studied of these compounds is tretinoin (all-*trans*-retinoic acid), which is one of the naturally occurring oxidation products of retinol. A synthetic retinoid formed from all-*trans*-retinoic acid is 13-*cis*-retinoic acid, also known as Accutane (isotretinoin). In addition to its use as an acne medication, 13-*cis*-retinoic acid has been used in many of the initial chemopreventive trials in humans (Moon and Itri, 1984).

The second generation of retinoid compounds was synthesized by altering the cyclic end group, thus forming the aromatic retinoids. The prototype compound in this group is etretinate, which is a drug that has primarily been used in Europe for the treatment of psoriasis and related disorders of keratinization (Peck, 1984). In general it has been considerably less active in preclinical preventive and treatment models of cancer than 13-*cis*-retinoic acid. The third generation of retinoid compounds was developed by the cyclization of the polyene side chain forming the multicyclic retinoidal benzoic-acid derivatives or arotenoids. The arotenoids have the highest level of retinoid activity of all the retinoid compounds known (Gollnick, 1987). Some arotenoid compounds

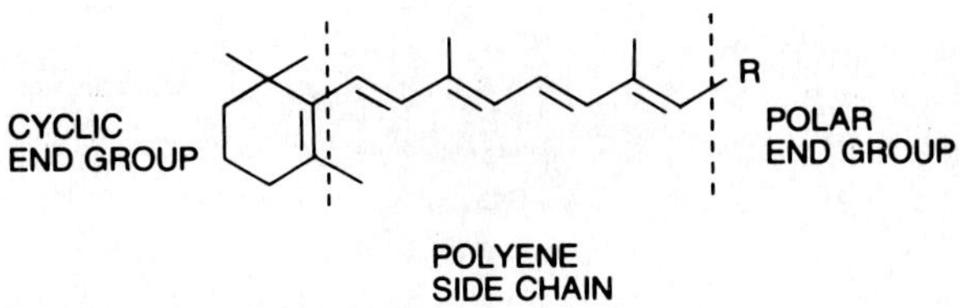

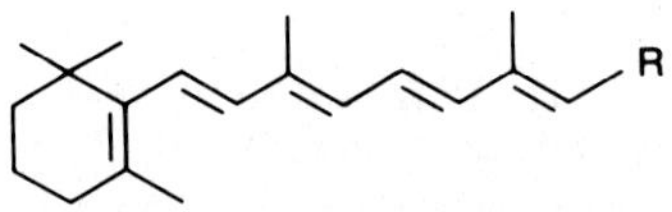

R=CH_2OH=ALL-TRANS-RETINOL
R=COOH=ALL-TRANS-RETINOIC ACID
(Tretinoin)

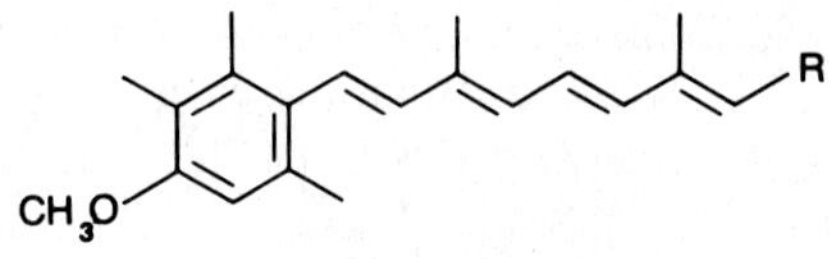

AROMATIC RETINOIDS
R=$COOC_2H_5$=Etretinate
R=$CONHC_2H_5$=Motretinid

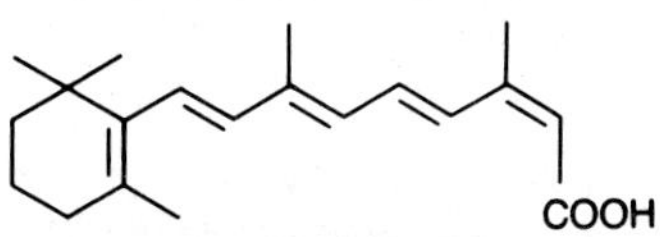

13-CIS-RETINOIC-ACID
(Isotretinoin)

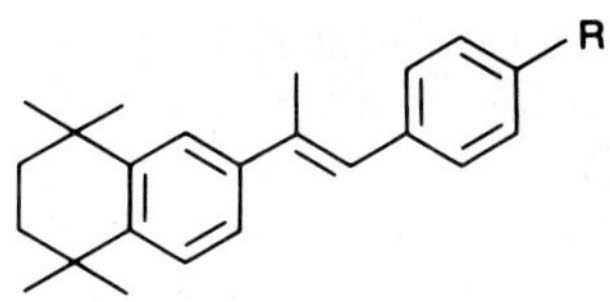

AROTINOIDS
R=$COOC_2H_5$=Arotinoid ethylester
R=COOH=TTNPB

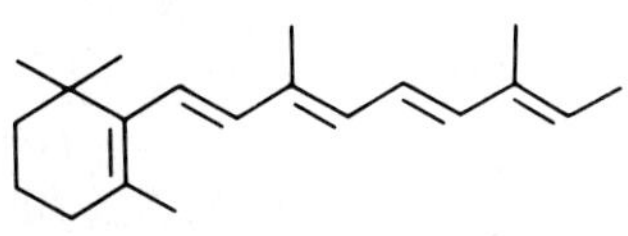

CONH-4-C_6H_4OH
N-(4-hydroxyphenyl) retinamide (4HPR)

FIGURE 20-1
Chemical structures of retinoids. TTNPB = (E)-4-[2-(5,6,7,8-tetrahydro-5,5,8,8-tetramethyl-2-naphthalenyl)-1-propenyl] benzoic acid. (From Lippman et al., 1987.)

(TTNPB, arotenoid acid, Ro13-7410) express over 1000 times the potency of retinol or retinoic acid in biological assays with less systemic toxicity (Vahlquist and Rollman, 1987).

SIDE EFFECTS AND TOXICITY

The clinical picture of acute hypervitaminosis A toxicity has been known for over a century. The syndrome was first identified in Arctic explorers and Eskimos who ate polar bear or seal liver (London). These organs accumulate a very high content of exogenous retinol (5–12 mg retinol/g of liver). Acute human toxicity is seen with the ingestion of 1,000,000 IU of retinol (0.3 μg = 1 IU retinol) in adults and 350,000 IU of retinol in infants (Russell, 1967; Kornell and Vollin, 1975; Windhorst and Nigra, 1982). At this dosage level, central nervous system (CNS) symptoms predominate with signs and symptoms that include severe headache (28%), increased cerebrospinal fluid (CSF) pressure (17%) with exophthalmus, papilledema, and bulging fontanelles in infants (26%), irritability (19%), and dizziness (17%). Nausea, vomiting, fatigue, lethargy, malaise, weakness, and somnolence occur in one third of patients. Acute mucocutaneous side effects of retinol overdosage include chelitis (>90%), dryness and scaling of the skin with palmar-plantar desquamation, pruritus, dry mucous membranes with occasional hemorrhage from the nasal mucosa, pigmentation, and brittle nails. Acute ocular changes include conjunctival inflammation (40%), xerophthalmia, diplopia, and blurred vision. Also seen are gastrointestinal (hepatomegaly [16%], splenomegaly [5%], and portal hypertension with ascites), and musculoskeletal (long-bone pain and edema) side effects.

Laboratory studies of acute retinol toxicity show elevation of serum retinol (25%), serum glutamic-oxaloacetic transaminase (SGOT), serum glutamate pyruvate transaminase (SGPT), alkaline phosphatase, GGT (10%–20%), and erythrocyte sedimentation rate (Pennes et al., 1983). Occasionally, the serum uric acid, calcium, glucose, and coagulation profile can be abnormal (<10%). These laboratory findings may be seen with the ingestion of as little as 50,000 IU of retinol per day in normal patients and at lower levels in patients with underlying hepatic disease or those patients who are concomitantly taking other hepatotoxic drugs (e.g., alcohol, methotrexate).

Chronic low-grade toxicity from hypervitaminosis A may develop over many months to years. The most significant of these toxicities is associated with abnormalities of reproduction (spermatogenesis) and embryological development, serum lipids, the liver, and the skeletal system. Lipid abnormalities include hypertriglyceridemia with a reduction in high-density lipoprotein (HDL) and an elevation of very low density lipoprotein (VLDL) and cholesterol. In addition to gross hepatosplenomegaly, the liver may demonstrate hypertrophy of the fat-storing cells, fibrosis, sclerosis of the central veins, and cirrhosis with subsequent portal hypertension and ascites. Bony abnormalities are primarily seen in children and include periosteal calcifications, retarded growth of long bones, occasional premature closure of the epiphyseal plates, and cranial hyperostosis. In children these retinol-induced changes stop with the cessation of the drug, but the preexisting damage is not reversible. Adults can exhibit some of these bony changes; however, the usual complaint is of bone and joint pain. The minor toxicities associated with chronic retinol overdosage are subtle, nonspecific problems including dry skin and mucous membranes (50%), chelitis (40%), musculoskeletal abnormalities (50%–60%), pruritus (35%), alopecia (40%), visual problems (30%), occipital headache (40%), and occasionally anorexia, weight loss, fatigue, lassitude, and somnolence.

The synthetic retinoids have similar overall toxicities when compared with those of retinol with a notable reduction in the incidence of liver problems and CNS symptoms. However, organ-specific side effects may vary considerably among the different retinoids. The three compounds that have been studied the most are Accutane, tretinoin, and Tegison (Strauss et al., 1984; Edwards et al., 1986; Vahlquist et al., 1985). A side-by-side comparison of the major efficacy and side effects of β-carotene, retinol, 13-*cis*-retinoic acid, and etretinate is shown in Table 20-1.

Isotretinoin, until recently, was the only synthetic retinoid approved for human use in the United States. The most commonly reported side effects of isotretinoin use are mucocutaneous (chelitis [90%], dry mouth or excessive thirst [30%], epistaxis [25%], xerosis-desquamation, especially of the face [30%], pruritus [25%], and, infrequently, erythema, skin fragility, fingertip peeling, pigmentation changes, and hair loss), ocular (conjunctivitis [40%], photosensitivity [5%–10%], dry eyes with contact-lens intolerance, reduced night vision with below normal dark adaptation responses on electroretinogram [6%], and, rarely, corneal opacities), gastrointestinal complaints (20%), musculoskeletal problems (15%), and headache, lethargy, and fatigue (10%) (Weleber et al., 1986). However, serious CNS effects and hepatic damage are rare.

Recently, concern has been expressed over the effect of chronic isotretinoin use on the development of skeletal abnormalities. Patients taking high-dose (2 mg/kg/day) isotretinoin for a year can exhibit X-ray evidence of hyperostosis that with time can become symptomatic if treatment with the drug continues (Pennes et al., 1983). Cunningham and Ehmann (1983) noted an 8% to 28% incidence of vertebral osteophyte formation in patients taking a dose of 2 mg/kg of isotretinoin per day for over 2 years. A prospective trial by Pennes et al. (1983) showed that 75% of patients taking isotretinoin for 1 year at similar doses developed small osteophytes. These findings have not yet been correlated with other dietary factors (e.g., calcium and vitamin D) and have not been reported at lower doses (1 mg/kg/day). At high drug levels (3 mg/kg/day), diffuse idiopathic skeletal hyperostosis has been reported, occurring primarily in patients who are being treated for disorders of keratinization such as refractory ichthyosis (Grupper and Berretti, 1983; Kilcoyne et al., 1984). Laboratory findings in patients on isotretinoin include an elevated erythrocyte sedimentation rate (40%), abnormal hematologic parameters (10%–25%), altered liver profile (10%), elevated blood glucose, elevated triglycerides (25%), elevated VLDL, decreased HDL (15%), increased cholesterol (7%), and a significant increase in the low-density lipoprotein (LDL) cholesterol/HDL cholesterol ratio (Bershad et al., 1985). These changes are reversible upon cessation of the drug.

Etretinate, although used in Europe for many years, has recently been approved for use in the United States for the treatment of refractory psoriasis. Its toxicities are similar to those of isotretinoin with predominance of mucocutaneous side effects that

TABLE 20-1
A COMPARISON OF DIFFERENT RETINOIDS AS ANTICANCER AGENTS

	Efficacy		Side effects			
Compound	**Prevention**	**Treatment**	**Cutaneous**	**Liver**	**Brain**	**Embryo**
Retinol	Modest	No	Low	High	High	Low
Trans-retinoic acid	High	Moderate	High	Low	Low	Moderate
13-*cis*-retinoic acid	High	Moderate	High	Low	Low	High
Etretinate	No	No	High	Low	Low	Very high
β-carotene	High	No	Low	Low	Low	Low

include chelitis (78%), palmar-plantar exfoliation (31%), hair loss (25%), dry mucous membranes (21%), and pruritus (15%) (Ellis and Voorhees, 1987; Ward et al., 1983). A unique side effect of etretinate has been its tendency to increase skin fragility while creating a feeling of stickiness of the skin. Compared to isotretinoin, etretinate produces fewer lipid and skeletal abnormalities; however, it has an increased incidence of hepatotoxicity (8%–40%) (Vahlquist et al., 1985; Gilbert et al., 1986; Schmidt and Foged, 1981; Weiss et al., 1984; Zacharine, 1984).

Both isotretinoin and etretinate are strongly teratogenic, producing an estimated 25-fold increase in the incidence of severe embryopathic changes (Lammer et al., 1985). These changes include spontaneous abortions and a characteristic pattern of malformations involving the craniofacial, cardiac, thymic, and CNS structures. Of the two drugs, etretinate has a greater teratogenic potential because of its long half-life (80–100 days) compared to the relatively short half-life of isotretinoin (12–20 hours). Women of child-bearing potential must be strongly cautioned concerning the potential risks to the fetus during or soon following the use of these drugs, and their use requires mandatory pregnancy testing and birth control counseling prior to the initiation of treatment.

METABOLISM

Humans are totally dependent on exogenous sources of vitamin A and provitamin A for the retinol requirement. Either they ingest a provitamin carotenoid compound such as β-carotene (which is divided to form two retinal molecules within the intestinal mucosal cell) or they ingest preformed retinol from milk (butterfat), eggs, or meat (Wolf, 1984). Physiologically, retinol can be reversibly converted to retinal, which can then be irreversibly converted to retinoic acid. Once in the intestinal mucosal cell, the retinol is esterified with long-chain fatty acids forming retinyl esters. These retinyl esters pass into the lymphatics where they are transported as chylomicrons to the bloodstream and actively absorbed by the liver for storage (DeLuca and Creek, 1986). Mobilization of the retinyl esters from the hepatocytes requires hydrolysis of the free retinol and binding with a 20,000 molecular weight transport protein, retinol binding protein (RBP), produced by the liver. In the blood, retinol is transported as a complex of RBP, transthyretin (formerly known as prealbumin), and thyroxine (Lippman et al., 1987a). The pattern of absorption of retinoic acids from the gut is different than that of retinol. After ingestion or conversion from retinal, retinoic acid is absorbed primarily through the venous portal system and is rapidly metabolized to intermediates before elimination through hepatic and renal paths. This absence of hepatic storage is believed to be the reason that ingestion of retinoic acid rarely results in liver toxicity.

BIOLOGICAL ACTIVITY

Retinol is an essential nutrient for vision, growth, reproduction, and epithelial differentiation and proliferation (Bollag, 1983; Peck, 1984; Moore, 1967; Harris et al., 1973). In the absence of vitamin A, metaplastic changes occur in essentially all epithelial tissues with increased cell division and nucleic acid synthesis (Wolbach and Howe, 1925; Harris et al., 1973). Tissue deficiency of vitamin A also enhances the potency of chemical carcinogens on epithelial tissues (Harris et al., 1973; Nettesheim et al., 1979). Importantly, both the proliferative tendency and anticarcinogen effect are usually reversible with the reintroduction of retinoids into the diet.

Most studies of the biological activity of retinoids have been performed with either the in vitro hamster trachea model or the in vivo mouse skin papilloma model. The tracheal epithelia assay measures the retinoid concentration required to reverse 50% of the keratinization of the trachea during a 10-day culture period. The ED_{50} value is then compared to the ED_{50} obtained from the standardized positive control β-*trans*-retinoic acid to determine the relative effectiveness of the test compound (the lower the concentration of the test compound the more active the retinoid) (Harris et al., 1973; Clamon et al., 1974). The mouse skin papilloma assay determines the ability of a retinoid compound to prevent the formation of papillomas in hairless mice after tumor induction with topical dimethylbenzanthracene (DMBA) and promotion with croton oil. The application or ingestion of retinoids during the promotion phase can prevent or delay the onset of skin tumors (Bollag, 1972, 1974, 1983).

In organ and cell culture models, retinoids have been shown to have an antiproliferative and differentiation-inducing activity on cells from both animal and human tumor lines. Lotan and Nicholson (1977) noted growth inhibition in more than 60% of 31 human tumor cell lines treated with retinoic acid and retinyl acetate. The mechanism by which retinoids are able to affect both replication and differentiation is thought to be different and separate (Koch, 1981; Vitall et al., 1986; Marcelo and Madison, 1984). The differentiating effects of retinoids appear to affect only a specific group of cell types, and this process can be reversible or irreversible, largely dependent on the particular cell type. However, studies using mutant cell lines have not yet identified whether the mechanism of action for differentiation and replication is truly separate or whether the cellular effect is dependent on the specific target cell type (Gallagher et al., 1986; Lotan, 1985; Schindler et al., 1981; Wang and Gudas, 1984).

Retinoic acid and its analogs have, with rare exception, been more active in their effect on both differentiation and replication than retinol, retinyl esters, or retinaldehyde (Bollag, 1979, 1983; Loeliger et al., 1980; Cunningham and Ehmann, 1983; Lotan, 1980; Sporn et al., 1986). Strickland et al. (1983) have shown that the terminal carboxyl group present in retinoic acid is essential for the synthetic retinoids to act as inducers of differentiation in HL-60 and F9 cell lines. In addition, the antiproliferative and differentiating effects of retinoids may produce biphasic responses that vary with concentration. Additionally, the anticarcinogen effect of retinoids occurs largely in the later stages of promotion or against preneoplastic cells.

MECHANISM OF ACTION

At the cellular level, retinoids, in general, block stage II promotion of carcinogens, inhibit proliferation, and induce differentiation or maturation. The exact mechanism via which retinoids affect their action as inducers of differentiation and inhibitors of replication has not been identified despite extensive investigation. It is apparent that the retinoid effect is pleiotropic; several biochemical strategies are used to modulate cellular growth (Table 20-2). The major biochemical mechanisms include direct interaction with the cell membrane and its components, specific binding to intracytoplasmic receptors, specific binding to nuclear receptors, modulation of key enzymes, and repression of oncogene expression. Three major effects occur from retinoid interaction with the cell membrane: (1) direct chemical covalent integration into the membrane via phosphate linkages, (2) direct or indirect (via receptors) interaction with growth factors, and (3) synthesis of new glycoproteins important in membrane function (DeLuca, 1984).

Two major and highly specific intracytoplasmic receptors have been identified, cytoplasmic RBP (cRBP), which binds to native vitamin A, and cytoplasmic retinoic-acid binding protein (cRABP), which binds to retinoids with a free carboxyl group (Chytil and Ong, 1976, 1981; Chytil, 1986). The interaction between retinoids and these receptors has been extensively studied, but the mechanisms involved remain only superficially understood (Wolf, 1984; Sporn et al., 1986; Sherman et al., 1985; Jetten, 1984; Sporn and Roberts, 1984). The current hypothesis is that the holoreceptor interacts with the nuclear membrane to alter transcriptional regulation of genes with differential protein expression and subsequent alterations in the expression of cell phenotype.

Recently, DNA sequences encoding the DNA-binding domain of the steroid/thyroid hormone receptors have been used as hybridization probes to scan the genome for related, but novel, ligand receptors (Slvyser, 1990). Using this strategy, a cDNA was cloned encoding a polypeptide that was a receptor for retinoic acid (Gigueie et al., 1987; Petkowich et al., 1987). Several subtypes of receptors have been identified and their role in limb development formulated (De Jean et al., 1986). The importance of

TABLE 20-2
PLEIOTROPIC EFFECT OF RETINOIDS ON CELLS

Biochemical effects
- Interaction with cellular membranes
  1. Direct chemical covalent integration into the membrane via mannose phosphate linkages
  2. Direct or indirect (via receptors) interaction with growth factors
  3. Synthesis of new glycoproteins important in membrane function
- Binding to intracytoplasmic receptors
- Binding to unclear receptors
- Modulation of key enzymes
- Repression of oncogene expression

Cellular effects
- Blocks stage II promotion in carcinogenesis
- Inhibits proliferation
- Induces differentiation or maturation
- Enhances cellular immunity
- Enhances cell adhesions

these receptors for cancer formation or control is unclear, but they may well have both positive and negative influences on the regulation of proliferation (De Jean et al., 1986; Benbrook et al., 1988). The functional relationship of the classical cRBP and cRABP to these newly described receptors remains to be defined, but it is clear that they are not the same molecule.

Another mechanism may be through the regulation of a number of enzymes including ornithine decarboxylase (ODC). The induction of ODC is a G1 transcriptional event that may be obligatory for cell cycling in both normal and neoplastic cells and that is often correlated with tumor progression (Russell, 1985). Retinoids act to block ODC causing polyamine depletion, which leads to growth inhibition, differentiation, and the accumulation of cells in G1 (Connor et al., 1983; Russell and Haddox, 1981). Russell and Haddox (1981) have shown that unlike difluoromethylornithine (DFMO), which irreversibly binds and inactivates the enzyme, retinoids act by decreasing ODC production. However, the selectivity of ODC expression in determining differentiation and replication effects has not been clearly established (Luk et al., 1982; Jetten and Shirley, 1985).

Recently, we proposed a unifying hypothesis to explain the mechanism of action of retinoids that involves the protein kinase C (PK-C)/phosphoinositol cascade system (Lippman and Meyskens, 1988a; Lippman et al., 1987). Protein kinase C, the phorbol ester receptor, is a $Ca2^{+}$-activated, phospholipid-dependent enzyme, which is a major cell surface signal transduction pathway. The PK-C system therefore plays a critical role in carcinogenesis. The PK-C cascade is activated directly by phorbol esters (TPA) and endogenous ligands and has been implicated in ODC induction, altered oncogene expression, and inhibition of epidermal growth factor (EGF) uptake by phosphorylating the EGF receptor (Nisaizuka, 1986; Jetten and Shirley, 1986; Cope et al., 1986; Verma, 1988; Lippman and Meyskens, 1988b). The studies of Cope et al. (1986) of mouse brain PK-C have shown that unbound retinoid binding proteins (Apo-cRBP and Apo-cRABP) are substrates for PK-C. The Holo- forms, however, inhibit PK-C activity. The regulation of PK-C alters phosphorylation of the RBPs as well as other specific cytosolic and membrane substrates. This mechanism could explain the pleiotropic action of retinoids' anticarcinogenic activity. However, this theory has been challenged by the work of Jetten and Shirley (1986) and others who have demonstrated in rat tracheal epithelial cells that retinoic acid acts to inhibit ODC activity before PK-C activation. Lotan and co-workers (1984, 1987) have also shown that in murine melanoma cells, PK-C does not play a central role in retinoid-induced growth inhibition.

Retinoids also enhance cellular immunity and cell adhesion. The specific effects on immune function are variable and incompletely understood (Russell, 1985; Russell and Haddox, 1981; Connor et al., 1983; Luk et al., 1982). It appears that retinoids have the ability in low and moderate doses to enhance cellular and humoral immunity through a number of mechanisms including potentiation of antibody formation, increase in the tumoricidal and phagocytic activities of macrophages, enhancement of cell-mediated cytotoxicity, interaction with helper T cells to increase production of interleukin-2 (IL-2), which results in killer T-cell proliferation, promotion of delayed cutaneous hypersensitivity, and potentiation of the antitumor effects of the immune enhancer *Mycobacterium bovis* (strain BCG) (Russell and Haddox, 1981; Luk et al., 1982; Jetten and Shirley, 1985, 1986; Lippman and Meyskens, 1988a, 1988b; Nisaizuka, 1986; Cope et al., 1986; Verma, 1988; Lotan, 1986, 1987; Lotan et al., 1984). Despite this degree of retinoid effect with the immune system, the retinoid target cell has yet to be identified.

CLINICAL EFFECTS

Retinoids have been reported to inhibit the growth of many human tumors (review, Lippman et al., 1987b). Retinoids accumulate preferentially in the skin and have been shown to be effective in a number of benign disorders of squamous cell proliferation as well as preneoplastic conditions. A summary of recently published trials of the effect of retinoids on preneoplastic and neoplastic cutaneous lesions is provided in Table 20-3. Actinic keratoses are very common in the Caucasian population, and approximately 5% of these lesions undergo degeneration to nonmelanomatous skin cancer per year.

Both topical and systemic retinoids have been used effectively to treat actinic keratosis and keratoacanthomas, two ultraviolet light–initiated premalignant skin conditions. Substantial response rates in excess of 50% of patients have been documented in a number of trials. Retinoids also appear to be effective in preventing or significantly reducing the development of secondary skin tumors in patients with the nevoid basal cell syndrome, xeroderma pigmentosum, and epidermodysplasia verruciformis.

In the treatment of cutaneous malignancies, retinoids have been effectively used since Bollag and Ott (1975) treated 16 patients with basal cell carcinoma with topical tretinoin (0.1%–0.3%). Fifteen of these patients had a response to treatment (5 complete, 10 partial). Two of the complete responders relapsed within 10 months of treatment. Oral isotretinoin and etretinate have also produced clinical responses. Several reports using isotretinoin have shown a 50% objective response rate in patients with basal cell carcinoma (Meyskens et al., 1982; Peck, 1985). Berretti and Grupper (1983), using oral etretinate (1 mg/kg/day), obtained a similar response rate with relapses occurring more frequently in patients with multiple lesions than in those with an isolated single lesion. As with isotretinoin, maintenance treatment with etretinate was necessary to prevent relapse (Peck, 1987). In recurrent squamous cell carcinoma of the skin, isotretinoin at 1 mg/kg/day has produced prolonged responses in four patients with large, bulky lesions with one patient having a complete response that lasted over 23 months (Lippman and Meyskens, 1987a). The clinical responsiveness of cutaneous squamous cell carcinoma to retinoids has also been demonstrated using etretinate and the arotenoid Ro13-6298 (Abb and Dienhardt, 1980; Kingston et al., 1983).

The dysplastic nevus syndrome is associated with an increased incidence of malignant melanoma. We have reported partial responses of dysplastic nevi with the topical use of tretinoin in three patients (Meyskens et al., 1986). Oral isotretinoin did not produce similar effects, with only one of eight patients responding to treatment (Lippman and Meyskens, 1987b). In malignant melanoma, both topical tretinoin and oral isotretinoin have produced modest partial clinical responses (Meyskens et al., 1982; Levine and Meyskens, 1980). Currently, trials using isotretinoin in combination with interferon-alpha are being conducted to determine if there is synergy between the two agents.

The UADT is a nearly ideal site for the study of chemoprevention (Meyskens, 1985). It is estimated that approximately 43,000 Americans will develop UADT tumors in 1989 and that 93% of these will be squamous cell carcinoma (Silverberg and Lubera, 1989). This incidence of UADT tumors accounts for approximately 6% of all cancers seen in the United States. In other areas of the world, specifically India (30% of all cancers), Pakistan, China, and the rest of Asia, UADT tumors are far more common and comprise a far more significant health risk (Silverberg and Lubera, 1989; Rao and Desai, 1989). As in other areas of the body, the premalignant process is slow and develops from initiated normal appearing mucosa to promoted premalignant mucosa (leukoplakia and erythroplakia) to frank invasive carcinoma. The carcinogen implicated in both progression and promotion of UADT tumors is tobacco. This complete carcinogen is used by patients in a number of ways with the pattern of cancer development related to the method of tobacco use. Smoking cigarettes in combination with the cocarcinogenic effects of alcohol affects the dependent areas of the oral cavity, oropharynx, and supraglottic larynx in addition to the esophagus. Smoking alone appears to most commonly affect the true glottic larynx and lung. Pipe and cigar smoking is associated with an increased incidence of lip, tongue, and oral cavity cancer. The

TABLE 20-3
RETINOIDS IN PREMALIGNANT AND MALIGNANT SKIN CONDITIONS

Retinoid	Evaluable patients	CR%	PR%	CR + PR %	Ref.
Actinic keratoses					
Tretinoin*	93	49	51	100	Belisario, 1972
Tretinoin*	60	40	45	85	Bollag and Ott, 1975
Etretinate	46	76	17	93	Berretti and Grupper, 1983
Etretinate	44	23	61	84	Moriarty et al., 1982
Etretinate	15	93	7	100	Watson, 1986
Etretinate	26	85	12	97	Schumacher and Stuttgen, 1971
Arotenoid	16	0	63	63	Kingston et al., 1983
Keratoacanthoma					
Etretinate	9	67	33	100	Bollag and Ott, 1975; Watson, 1986; Haydey et al., 1980; Verret et al., 1985; Pichler and Fritsch, 1984
Isotretinoin	2	50	50	100	Shaw and White, 1986; Levine et al., 1984
Epidermodysplasia verruciformis					
Etretinate	10	10	60	70	Lutzner et al., 1981; Kanerva et al., 1985; Edelson et al., 1981; Guilhou et al., 1980; Kowalzick and Mensing, 1986
Arotenoid	5	0	80	80	Jablonska et al., 1981

Xeroderma pigmentosum					
Etretinate	1	0	100	100	Berretti and Grupper, 1983
Isotretinoin	5	0	100	100	Moshell, 1989
Basal cell nevoid syndrome					
Isotretinoin	1	0	100	100	Peck, 1985
Etretinate	1	0	100	100	Verret et al., 1985
Basal cell carcinoma					
Tretinoin*/Isotretinoin*	49	33	65	98	Bollag and Ott, 1975; Schumacher and Stuttgen, 1971 Peck et al., 1982; Berretti and Grupper, 1984
Isotretinoin	16	13	56	69	Lippman et al., 1987; Meyskens et al., 1982; Peck, 1985
Etretinate	40	8	35	43	Berretti and Grupper, 1983
Cutaneous squamous cell carcinoma					
Isotretinoin	9	22	56	78	Meyskens et al., 1982; Lippman and Meyskens, 1987a
Etretinate	4	25	25	50	Berretti and Grupper, 1983
Arotenoid (Ro13-6298)	1	0	100	100	Kingston et al., 1983
Retinoid dysplastic nevi					
Tretinoin*	3	0	100	100	Meyskens et al., 1986
Isotretinoin	8	0	13	13	Lippman and Meyskens, 1987b
Melanoma					
Tretinoin*	2	50	50	100	Levine and Meyskens, 1980
Isotretinoin	20	0	15	15	Meyskens et al., 1982

*Topical application of drug.

oral use of tobacco, which has made a dramatic rise in popularity in the past decade in the United States, has long been associated with oral cavity cancer in India (Rao and Desai, 1989). The use of betel quid, which has tobacco, slate lime, and betel nut as its primary components, is the etiologic agent for the high incidence of oral cavity cancer seen in India and Pakistan (Silverberg and Lubera, 1989; Rao and Desai, 1989).

Retinoids alone or in combination with other chemopreventive agents (carotenoids, ascorbic acid, tocopherol, DFMO) have been shown to effectively reverse premalignant mucosal changes associated with tobacco-induced carcinogenesis. Numerous trials using retinoids as chemopreventive agents have been reported, and the results are summarized in Table 20-4. The studies of Stich et al. (1988) and Hong et al. (1986) have demonstrated conclusively that oral leukoplakia is responsive to retinoids with a reduction in the size and improvement in the maturation of the oral lesions. A problem encountered in all these trials has been recurrence of the leukoplakia after drug cessation. It appears that a maintenance phase of treatment will be necessary to sustain a prolonged clinical effect. Drug toxicity, however, makes this phase of treatment less acceptable to patients, and new trials, including our own studies, are trying to identify less toxic agents and/or lowered doses of multiple agents required to maintain clinical effectiveness after induction response.

In the treatment of refractory squamous cell carcinoma of head and neck origin, isotretinoin has been shown to produce clinical responses in 14% of patients, and ongoing trials are being conducted in which retinoids are combined with standard chemotherapeutic agents in an attempt to improve and prolong response rate (Meyskens et al., 1982; Lippman et al., 1988).

Another use of retinoids in UADT is in the treatment of laryngeal papillomatosis. This uncommon disorder is a benign proliferative growth that is found most commonly in children born of mothers with genital condyloma acuminata. This condition has been associated with human papilloma virus subtypes 6 and 11 and can manifest dysplasia and malignant degeneration (Corbitt et al., 1988). Standard treatment for this disorder has been symptomatic with carbon dioxide laser vaporization of the papilloma when they cause respiratory compromise. Medical therapy of this disorder with interferon has provided responses in 50% of patients but with significant toxicity (Brach et al., 1978; Ingimarsson et al., 1979; Haglund et al., 1981; Goepfert et al., 1982). Studies using isotretinoin at 1 to 2 mg/kg/day in six patients produced three complete responders and one partial responder with minimal toxicity (Alberts et al., 1986). Bichler (1983) used etretinate (1 mg/kg/day) to treat 42 patients with laryngeal papilloma who had moderate to severe dysplasia of the papillomas on biopsy. Twenty-eight (67%) of the patients were complete responders and 11 (16%) were partial responders.

In the lung, retinoids have been shown to effectively reverse bronchial squamous metaplasia. The results of recently reported trials are summarized in Table 20-4. Of interest is the finding that cessation of smoking in combination with retinoid therapy produced a higher rate of squamous metaplasia conversion to normal epithelia than the cessation of smoking alone (Misset et al., 1986).

TABLE 20-4
UPPER AERODIGESTIVE TRACT CONDITIONS

Retinoid	Evaluable patients	CR%	PR%	CR + PR %	Ref.
Oral leukoplakia					
Tretinoin*	5	20	80	100	Koch, 1978
Tretinoin	27	0	59	59	Koch, 1978
Tretinoin*†	2	100	0	100	Schofer et al., 1987
Isotretinoin	24	0	88	88	Koch, 1978
Isotretinoin	11	27	73	100	Shah et al., 1983
Isotretinoin	24	8	58	66	Levine and Meyskens, 1980
Isotretinoin*‡	16	50	44	94	Honk et al., 1986
Etretinate	24	0	92	92	Markowska et al., 1987
Etretinate§	24	29	54	83	Koch, 1978
Etretinate	21	24	48	72	Koch, 1981
Etretinate	3	33	67	100	Cordero et al., 1981
Laryngeal papillomatosis					
Isotretinoin	6	50	17	67	Alberts et al., 1986
Etretinate	42	67	26	93	Bichler, 1983
Bronchial metaplasia					
Isotretinoin	19	0	0	0	Saccamanno et al., 1982
Etretinate	30	10	77	87	Mathe et al., 1982
Etretinate	36	11	89	100	Misset et al., 1986
Head and neck squamous carcinoma					
Isotretinoin	38	3	11	14	Meyskens et al., 1982; Lippman et al., 1988

*Topical application of drug.
†Oral hairy leukoplakia in AIDS patients.
‡Vulvar leukoplakia.
§Oral + topical.

Very few trials using retinoids have been reported in the treatment of premalignant gastrointestinal conditions. A study by Wahrendorf et al. (1988) of the incidence of precancerous lesions of the esophagus in China has suggested a decrease in the risk for premalignant changes in the esophagus with an elevation of the serum retinol level. However, Barrett's esophagus, a premalignant condition of the lower esophagus, has not been responsive to retinoid treatment in vivo or in vitro (unpublished data).

Preneoplasias of the cervix have been treated with topical retinoids and premalignant changes successfully reversed (Table 20-5). Based on these favorable responses, a randomized, double-blind, placebo-controlled phase III trial was undertaken to determine whether the natural history of moderate or severe cervical intraepithelial neoplasia can be altered by application of topical *trans*-retinoic acid. However, due to the teratogenic effects of synthetic retinoids, this form of therapy in women of child-bearing age will probably be limited. Due to the complexity of applying daily topical drugs to the cervix, new trials using newer retinoids or carotenoids are in progress (Mathe et al., 1982).

The urinary bladder is another organ system that appears responsive to retinoids. Studies using etretinate (25 mg/day) have demonstrated a response rate of premalignant lesions comparable with the intravesicular instillation of cytotoxic agents (Jacobi and Kurth, 1980; Pavone-Macaluso, 1979; Soloway, 1980). Three recent trials have demonstrated the efficacy of retinoids in the prevention of recurrent superficial bladder carcinoma (Yoshida et al., 1986; Di Silverio et al., 1987; Michalek et al., 1989). Results from the different retinoid urinary bladder trials are summarized in Table 20-5. A new retinoid fenretinide (hydroxyphenylretinamide [HPR], N-[4-hydroxyphenyl] retinamide) may be the most effective retinoid agent in the treatment of premalignant lesions of the urinary bladder and breast. Clinical trials using this compound are underway, with Costa et al. (1989) recently reporting that, based on toxicity studies, 200 mg/day is the recommended dose for clinical trials.

Mammary tumors are not responsive to the standard retinoids that are used in the treatment of cutaneous and UADT lesions. Moon (1989) has shown that the agent of choice using an in vivo mouse model and in vitro human breast model was HPR. A report by Ratko et al. (1989) suggested a combination of HPR and tamoxifen as the most effective combination of chemopreventive agents when used to prevent the development of a second mammary tumor following surgical resection of the first tumor in a mouse model.

Retinoids also produce responses of some hematologic abnormalities (Table 20-6). The myelodysplastic syndromes (MDS) are a heterogeneous group of diseases caused by clonal proliferation of an abnormal stem cell leading to single or multiple cytopenias (Bennet et al., 1982). Since 40% of these patients progress to acute leukemias, MDS is considered to be a preneoplastic or preleukemic state. Previous studies have shown that retinoids with a free terminal carboxyl group had a significant hematopoetic effect. This group included β-all-*trans*-retinoic acid and 13-*cis*-retinoic acid (Tobler et al., 1986). With a reported overall response rate of 38% (26 of 69 patients), isotretinoin

TABLE 20-5
GENITOURINARY TRACT CONDITIONS

	Evaluable patients	CR%	PR%	CR + PR%	Ref.
Cervical dysplasia					
Tretinoin*	18	11	22	33	Cordero et al., 1981
Tretinoin*	36	33	63	97	Surwit et al., 1982
Tretinoin*	20	50	NS	50	Graham et al., 1986
Retinyl acetate	40	NS	NS	NS	Romney et al., 1985
Retinamide†	27	89	7	96	Yoshida et al., 1986
Urinary bladder superficial carcinoma					
Etretinate	5	60	40	100	Shaerer et al., 1982
Isotretinoin	22	NS	NS	NS	Bonney and Prout, 1980
Etretinate	40	0	50	50	Pedersen et al., 1984
Etretinate	15	0	73	73	Alfthan et al., 1983
Etretinate	14	0	29	29	Studer et al., 1984

*Topical application of drug.
†Vaginal suppository.
NS, not stated.

is an active agent in the treatment of this disorder. A report by Garewal et al. (1987) implicated HPR in disease acceleration in MDS. In this report 14 patients were treated; no responses were noted with HPR at a dose of 300 mg/day induction. However, two of the patients with stable sideroblastic anemia showed progression to chronic myelomonocytic leukemia.

In vitro, HL-60 cells respond to retinoic acid, an effect that is enhanced with the addition of a DNA synthesis inhibitor (Ara-C, hydroxyurea) (Ishikura et al., 1985; Nilsson, 1984). In myeloid leukemia, especially acute promyelocytic leukemia (APL), retinoids have produced prolonged complete responses with elevation of the granulocyte count (Nilsson, 1984; Daenen et al., 1986; Fontana et al., 1986; Sampi et al., 1985.) In vitro testing by Kagechika et al. (1988) and Hashimoto et al. (1988) showed a significant responsiveness of HL-60 cells in vitro to arotenoids and have implicated a retinoid specific binding protein in the uptake of retinoids in HL-60 cells.

Mycosis fungoides is a rare cutaneous T-cell lymphoma that has demonstrated remarkable responsiveness to retinoids. In studies totaling 92 patients, 21% of patients had complete responses and 41% had partial responses. Treatment results occurred that had not been achieved by conventional therapy. A new trial involving the combination of Accutane and interferon-II has recently been started to determine whether the complete response rate or duration of remission can be increased. A summary of reported clinical trials is shown in Table 20-5.

TABLE 20-6
HEMATOLOGIC CONDITIONS

	Evaluable patients	CR%	PR%	CR + PR %	Ref.
Myelodysplastic syndrome					
Isotretinoin	15	0	33	33	Gold et al., 1983
Isotretinoin	14	0	21	21	Greenberg et al., 1985
Isotretinoin	18	11	11	22	Besa et al., 1985
Isotretinoin	6	0	67	67	Kerndrup et al., 1986
Isotretinoin	15	7	53	60	Picozzi et al., 1986
Isotretinoin	1	100	0	100	Abrahm et al., 1986
Acute promyelocytic leukemia					
Isotretinoin	6	50	17	67	Nilsson, 1984; Daenen et al., 1986; Fontana et al., 1986; Clark et al., 1987
Etretinate	1	0	0	0	Sampi et al., 1985
Mycosis fungoides					
Isotretinoin	78	14	47	61	Kessler et al., 1987; Molin et al., 1985; Claudy and Rouchouse, 1985; Warrell et al., 1983; Fitzpatrick and Mellete, 1986; Neely et al., 1987
Etretinate	8	50	0	50	Jenkinson and Beare, 1984; Wargon and Downie, 1984; Ippolito and Giacalone, 1982; Souteyrand et al., 1981
Arotenoid (Ro13-6298)	6	67	17	84	Mahrle et al., 1983; Tousignant et al., 1987

FUTURE RESEARCH

A great deal of basic work has been done in an attempt to understand the mechanistic basis of the pleiotropic effects that these agents cause. More needs to be done since a specific appreciation of retinoid structure, cellular or nuclear receptor, and biological effect has not been strongly correlated. For example, nothing close to estrogen–estrogen receptor response relationships has been defined for retinoids. Currently we lack any clue as to why some tumors are retinoid responsive and others are not. Detailing and clarifying this area of retinoid action will be extremely important in maximizing the use of these compounds as anticarcinogen or therapeutic maturational or inhibitory drugs.

The synthetic retinoids appear to produce significantly better responsiveness in the treatment of premalignant and malignant disease than naturally occurring vitamin A. The associated toxicity of retinoid therapy is acceptable for patients with frank malignancy and for the more aggressive premalignant conditions. However, in patients with a small risk of developing a malignancy, toxicity associated with available synthetic retinoids is unacceptable as these agents may need to be used for a lifetime.

Current and future research is also directed toward improving the response of premalignant and malignant diseases to retinoids by combining them with other maturational agents, biological modifiers, or hormonal agents. Retinoids may also have a role in combination with cytotoxic agents, either as a compound with complementary toxicity or as an agent that blocks tumor cells in a portion of the cell cycle in which cells are more susceptible to a particular cytotoxic agent. The actions of retinoids as modifiers of the immune system remain largely unexplored and their interactions with cytokines in influencing immune cells should be of considerable interest. Also of considerable interest to us is the potential for synergistic response of low doses of retinoids with other chemopreventive compounds that have fewer side effects or different mechanisms of action.

ACKNOWLEDGMENT

Supported in part by a grant from the National Cancer Institute (CA 27502).

REFERENCES

Abb J, Dienhardt F. Effects of retinoic acid on the human lymphocyte response to mitogens. Exp Cell Biol. 1980;49:169–179.

Abels JC, Gorham AT, Pack GT, et al. Metabolic studies in patients with cancer of the gastrointestinal tract. I. Plasma vitamin A levels in patients with malignant neoplastic disease, particularly of the gastrointestinal tract. J Clin Invest. 1941;20:749–764.

Abrahm J, Besa EC, Hyzinski M, Finan J, Nowell P. Disappearance of cytogenetic abnormalities and clinical remission during therapy with 13-*cis*-retinoic acid in a patient with myelodysplastic syndrome: inhibition of growth of the patient's malignant monocytoid clone. Blood. 1986;67:1323–1327.

Alberts DS, Coulthard SW, Meyskens FL Jr. Regression of aggressive laryngeal papillomatosis with 13-*cis*-retinoic acid (Accutane). J Biol Response Mod. 1986;5:124–128.

Alfthan O, Tarkkanen J, Grohn P, Heinonen E, Pryhonen S, Saila K. Tigason (etretinate) in prevention of recurrence of superficial bladder tumors. Eur Urol. 1983;9:6–9.

Badwey JA, Robinson JM, Curnette JT, et al. Retinoids stimulate the release of superoxide by neutrophils and change their morphology. J Cell Physiol. 1986;127:223–228.

Belisario JC. Recent advances in topical cytotoxic therapy of skin cancer and precancer. In: Melanoma and skin cancer: Proceedings of the International Cancer Conference. Sydney: McGraw-Hill; 1972;349–365.

Benbrook D, Lernhardt E, Phahl M. A new retinoic acid receptor identified from a hepatocellular carcinoma. Nature. 1988;333:669–672.

Bennet JM, Catovsky D, Daniel MT, et al. The French-American-British (FAB) cooperative group: proposals for the classification of the myelodysplastic syndromes. Br J Haematol. 1982;51:189–199.

Berretti B, Grupper CH. Cutaneous neoplasia and etretinate. In: Spitzy KH, Karrer K, eds. Proceedings of the 13th International Congress of Chemotherapy. Vienna: VH Egermann; 1983;201/24–27.

Berretti B, Grupper CH. Cutaneous neoplasia and etretinate. J Retinoid Ther. 1984;187–194.

Bershad S, Rubinstein A, Paterniti JR, et al. Changes in plasma lipids and lipoproteins during isotretinoin therapy for acne. New Engl J Med. 1985;313:981–985.

Besa EC, Hyzinski M, Nowell PC, Itri LM, Abrahm J. Clinical trials and in-vitro evaluation of 13-*cis*-retinoic acid in myelodysplastic syndrome. Proc Am Soc Clin Oncol. 1985;4:841C (Abstract).

Bichler E. The role of aromatic retinoid in treatment of laryngeal keratinizing disorders and dysplasias. In: Spitzy KH, Karrer K, eds. Proceedings of the 13th International Congress of Chemotherapy. Vienna: VH Egermann; 1983:201–229.

Bollag W. Prophylaxis of chemically induced benign and malignant epithelial tumors by vitamin A acid (retinoic acid). Eur J Cancer. 1972;8:689–693.

Bollag W. Therapeutic effects of an aromatic retinoic acid analog on chemically induced skin papillomas and carcinomas of mice. Eur J Cancer. 1974;10:731–737.

Bollag W. Retinoids and cancer. Cancer Chemother Pharmacol. 1979;3:205–215.

Bollag W. Vitamin A and retinoids: from nutrition to pharmacology in dermatology and oncology. Lancet. 1983;1:860–863.

Bollag W, Ott F. Vitamin A acid in benign and malignant epithelial tumors of the skin. Acta Dermatol Venereol (Stockh). 1975;suppl 74:163–166.

Bonney WW, Prout GR. AUA Monograph, Vol. 1. Baltimore: Williams and Wilkins; 1980:170–171.

Brach BB, Klein RC, Mathews AJ, et al. Papillomatosis of the respiratory tract: upper airway obstruction and carcinoma. Arch Otolaryngol. 1978;91:431–436.

Chytil F. Retinoic acid: biochemistry and metabolism. J Am Acad Dermatol. 1986;15:741–747.

Chytil F, Ong DE. Mediation of retinoic acid induced growth and anti-tumor activity. Nature. 1976;266:49–51.

Chytil F, Ong DE. Cellular vitamin A binding protein. Vitam Horm. 1981;36:1–34.

Clamon GH, Sporn MB, Smith JM, et al. Alpha- and beta-retinyl acetate reverse metaplasias of vitamin A deficiency in hamster trachea in organ culture. Nature. 1974;250:64–66.

Clark RE, Jacobs A, Lush CJ, Smith SA. Effect of 13-cis-retinoic acid on survival of patients with myelodysplastic syndrome. Lancet. 1987;1:763–765.

Claudy AL, Rouchouse B. Treatment of cutaneous T-cell lymphomas with retinoid. In: Saurat JH, ed. Retinoids: new trends in research and therapy. Basel: Karger; 1985:335–340.

Connor MJ, Lowe NJ, Breeding JH, et al. Inhibition of ultraviolet light B carcinogenesis by all-*trans*-retinoic acid regimens that inhibit ornithine decarboxylase induction. Cancer Res. 1983;43:171–174.

Cope FO, Howard BD, Boutwell RK. The in vitro characterization of the inhibition of mouse brain kinase-C by retinoids and their receptors. Experientia. 1986;42:1023–1027.

Corbitt G, Zarod AP, Arrand JR, et al. Human papilloma virus (HPV) genotypes associated with laryngeal papilloma. J Clin Pathol. 1988;41:284–288.

Cordero AA, Allevato MAJ, Barclay CA, et al. Treatment of lichen planus and leukoplakia with the oral retinoid Ro10-9359. In: Orfanos CE, Braun-Falco O, Farber EM, Grupper CL, Polano MK, Schuppli R, eds. Retinoids: advances in basic research and therapy. Berlin: Springer-Verlag; 1981:273–278.

Costa A, Malone W, Perloff M, et al. Tolerability of the synthetic retinoid Fenretinide (HPR). Eur J Cancer Clin Oncol. 1989;25:805–808.

Cunningham WJ, Ehmann CW. Clinical aspects of the retinoids. Semin Dermatol. 1983;2:145–160.

Daenen S, Vellenga E, Van Dobbenburgh OA, Halie MD. Retinoic acid as antileukemic therapy in a patient with acute promyelocytic leukemia and *Aspergillus* pneumonia. Blood. 1986; 67:559–561.

De Jean A, Bougueleret L, Grzeschik KH, Tiollais P. Hepatitis B virus DNA integration in a sequence homologous to v-erb-A and steroid receptor genes in a hepatocellular carcinoma. Nature. 1986;322:70–72.

DeLuca LM. Studies in mammosyl carrier fraction of retinoic acid in epithelial and mesenchymal tissues. J Am Acad Dermatol. 1984;6:611–619.

DeLuca LM, Creek KE. Vitamin A and the liver. In: Popper H, Schaffer F, eds. Progress in liver disease. Vol. XXXV. San Francisco, Ca: Grune and Stratton; 1986:81–98.

Dennert G. Immunostimulation by retinoic acid. In: Nugent J, Clark S, eds. Retinoids, differentiation, and disease. London: Pitman; 1985:117–126.

Dennert G, Crowley C, Koula J, et al. Retinoic acid stimulation of the induction of mouse killer T-cells in allogenic and syngeneic systems. J Natl Cancer Inst. 1979;62:89–92.

Di Silverio F, Concolino G, Tenaglia R, et al. Retinoids in recurrences of superficial bladder tumors. In: Salmon SE, ed. Proceedings of the Fifth International Conference on Adjuvant Therapy of Cancer. Tucson: University of Arizona; 1987:75.

Drummond JC. The nomenclature of the so-called accessory food factors (vitamins). Biochem J. 1920;14:669.

Eccles S. Effects of retinoids on growth and dissemination of malignant tumors: immunological considerations. Biochem Pharmacol. 1985;34:1599–1610.

Eccles JA, Barnett SC, Alexander P. Inhibition of growth and spontaneous metastasis of syngeneic transplantable tumour by an aromatic retinoic acid analog. I. Relationship between tumour immunogenicity and responsiveness. Cancer Immunol Immunother. 1985;29:109–114.

Edelson Y, Berretti B, Grupper C. Treatment of epidermodysplasia verruciformis or multiple verrucae planae by oral aromatic retinoid (Ro10-9359-Tigason). In: Orfanos CE, Braun-Falco O, Farber EM, Grupper CL, Polano MK, Schuppli R, eds. Retinoids: advances in basic research and therapy. Berlin: Springer-Verlag; 1981:401–405.

Edwards L, Alberts DS, Levine N. Clinical toxicity of low dose isotretinoin. Cancer Treat Rep. 1986;70:663–664.

Ellis CN, Voorhees JJ. Etretinate therapy. J Am Acad Dermatol. 1987;16:267–291.

Ermin O, Ashby J, Rhodes J. Inhibition of antibody-dependent cellular cytotoxicity and natural cytotoxicity by retinoic acid. Int Arch Allergy Appl Immunol. 1984;75:2–7.

Fitzpatrick JE, Mellete JR. Treatment of mycosis fungoides with isotretinoin. J Dermatol Surg Oncol. 1986;12:626–629.

Flynn PJ, Miller WJ, Weisdorf DJ, Arthur DC, Brunning R, Branda RF. Retinoic acid treatment of acute promyelocytic leukemia: in vitro and in vivo observations. Blood. 1983;62:1211–1213.

Fontana JA, Rogers JS, Durham JP. The role of 13-*cis*-retinoic acid in the remission induction of a patient with acute promyelocytic leukemia. Cancer. 1986;57:209–217.

Frickel F. Chemistry and physical properties of retinoids. In: Sporn ME, Roberts AB, Goodman DS, eds. Retinoids, Vol. I. Orlando, Fla: Academic Press; 1984:7–145.

Fujumaki Y. Formation of gastric carcinoma in albino rats fed on deficient diets. J Cancer Res. 1926;10:469–477.

Gallagher RE, Chang CS, Schwartz EC. Metabolism of retinoic acid (RA) by wild type (wt) and RA-resistant HL-60 cells: marked effect of serum. Blood. 1986;68(suppl 1):188A (Abstract).

Garewal HS, List A, Meyskens FL, et al. Phase II trial of Fenretinide [N-(4-hydroxyphenyl)retinamide] in myelodysplasia: possible retinoid-induced disease acceleration. Leuk Res. 1987;13:339–343.

Gigueie V, Ong ES, Sequi P, Evans RM. Identification of a receptor for the morphogen retinoic acid. Nature. 1987;330:624–629.

Gilbert M, Ellis CN, Voorhees JJ. Lack of skeletal radiographic changes during short term etretinate therapy for psoriasis. Dermatologica. 1986;172:160–163.

Goepfert H, Sessions RB, Gutterman JU, et al. Leucocyte interferon in patients with juvenile laryngeal papillomatosis. Ann Otol Rhinol Laryngol. 1982;89:472–478.

Gold EJ, Mertelsmann RH, Itri LM, et al. Phase I clinical trial of 13-*cis*-retinoic acid in myelodysplastic syndromes. Cancer Treat Rep. 1983;67:981–986.

Gollnick H. New indications and new retinoids. Dermatologica. 1987;175(Suppl 1):182–195.

Graham V, Surwit EA, Weiner S, Meyskens FL Jr. Phase II trial of beta-all-*trans*-retinoic acid for cervical intraepithelial neoplasia delivered via a collagen sponge and cervical cap. West J Med. 1986;145:192–195.

Greenberg BR, Durie BGM, Barnett TC, Meyskens FL Jr. Phase I-II study of 13-*cis*-retinoic acid in myelodysplastic syndrome. Cancer Treat Rep. 1985;69:1369–1374.

Grupper CH, Berretti B. Cutaneous neoplasia and etretinate. In: Spitzy KH, Karrer K, eds. Proceedings of the 13th International Congress of Chemotherapy. Vienna: VH Egermann; 1983:201/24–27.

Guilhou JJ, Malbos S, Barneon S, et al. Epidermodysplasia verruciformis (2 cases). Immunological study. Ann Dermatol Venereol. 1980;107:611–619.

Haglund S, Lungquist PG, Cantell K, et al. Interferon therapy in juvenile laryngeal papillomatosis. Arch Otolaryngol. 1981;107:327–332, 1981.

Harris CC, Kaufman DG, Sporn MB, et al. Histogenesis of squamous metaplasia and squamous cell carcinoma of the respiratory epithelium in an animal model. Cancer Chemother Rep. 1973;4(Part 3):43–54.

Hashimoto Y, Kagechika H, Kawechi E, et al. Specific uptake of retinoids into promyelocytic leukemia cells HL-60 by retinoid specific binding protein: possibly the true retinoid receptor. Jpn J Cancer Res. 1988;79:473–483.

Haydey RP, Reed ML, Dzubow LM, et al. Treatment of keratoacanthomas with oral 13-*cis*-retinoic acid. New Engl J Med. 1980;303:560–562.

Hemila H, Wikstrom M. Retinoids activate superoxide by polymorphonuclear leucocytes. Scand J Immunol. 1985;21:227–234.

Hong WK, Endicott J, Itri L, et al. 13-*cis*-retinoic acid in the treatment of oral leukoplakia. New Engl J Med. 1986;315:1501–1505.

Ingimarsson S, Cantell K, Strander H. Side effects of long term treatment with human leucocyte interferon. J Infect Dis. 1979;140:560–563.

Ippolito F, Giacalone B. Sur un cas de mycosis fongoide avec manifestations tumorales traité avec Ro10-9359 (Tigason). Ann Dermatol Venerol. 1982;109:65–72.

Ishikura A, Okazaki T, Mochizuki T, et al. Effect of antimetabolites and thymidine blockage on the induction of differentiation at HL-60 cells by retinoic acid or 1-alpha-25-hydroxy vitamin D3. Exp Hematol. 1985;13:981–988.

IUPAC-IUB Joint Commission on Biochemical Nomenclature. Nomenclature of the retinoids. Eur J Biochem. 1982;129:1–5.

Jablonska S, Obalek S, Wolska H, et al. Ro10-9359 in epidermodysplasia verruciformis. Preliminary report. In: Orfanos CE, Braun-Falco O, Farber EM, Grupper CL, Polano MK, Schuppli R, eds. Retinoids: advances in basic research and therapy. Berlin: Springer-Verlag; 1981:401–405.

Jacobi GH, Kurth KH. Studies on the intravesicle action of topically administered G3H-doxyrubicin hydrochloride in men: plasma uptake and tumor penetration. J Urol. 1980;124:34–37.

Jenkinson HA, Beare JM. Mycosis fungoides. Br J Dermatol. 1984;111(Suppl 26):82–84.

Jetten RM. Modulation of cell growth by retinoids and their possible mechanism of action. Fed Proc. 1984;43:134–139.

Jetten AM, Shirley JE. Inhibition of ornithine decarboxylase by retinoic acid and difluoromethyl ornithine in relation to their effects on differentiation and proliferation. Exp Cell Res. 1985;156:221–230.

Jetten AM, Shirley JE. Action of retinoic acid on the diacylglycerol-induced ornithine decarboxylase activity, reduction of EGF binding and protein kinase C activation in rat tracheal epithelial 2C5 cells. Exp Cell Res. 1986;166:519–525.

Kagechika H, Hashimoto Y, Kawechi E, et al. Recent advances in retinoid therapy. Gan To Kagaku Ryoho. 1988;15:2839–2847.

Kanerva LO, Johansson E, Niemi KM, et al. Epidermodysplasia verriciformis. Clinical and light- and electron-microscopic observations during etretinate therapy. Arch Dermatol Res. 1985;278:153–160.

Kerndrup G, Bendix-Hansen K, Pedersen B, Ellegaard J, Hokland P. Primary myelodysplastic syndrome: treatment of 6 patients with 13-*cis*-retinoic acid. Scand J Haematol. 1986;36:128–132.

Kessler JF, Jones SE, Levine N, Lynch PJ, Booth AR, Meyskens FL Jr. Isotretinoin and cutaneous helper T-cell lymphoma (mycosis fungoides). Arch Dermatol. 1987;123:201–204.

Kilcoyne RF, Cope R, Cunninghan W, et al. Isotretinoin therapy is associated with early skeletal radiographic changes. J Am Acad Dermatol. 1984;10:1024–1029.

Kingston T, Gaskell S, Marks R. The effects of a novel potent retinoid (Ro13-6298) in the treatment of multiple solar keratoses and squamous epithelioma. Eur J Cancer. 1983; 19:1201–1205.

Koch HF. Biochemical treatment of precancerous oral lesions: the effectiveness of various analogues of retinoic acid. J Max Fac Surg. 1978;6:59–63.

Koch HF. Effect of retinoids on precancerous lesions of oral mucosa. In: Orfanos CE, Braun-Falco O, Farber EM, Grupper CL, Polano MK, Schuppli R, eds. Retinoids: advances in basic research and therapy. Berlin: Springer-Verlag; 1981:307–312.

Kornell WF, Vollin J. New aspects of the tolerance of retinol in humans. Int J Vitam Nutr Res. 1975;45:312–365.

Kowalzick L, Mensing H. Failure of etretinate in epidermodysplasia verruciformis. Dermatologica. 1986;173:75–78.

Lammer EJ, Chen DT, Hoar RM, et al. Retinoic acid embryopathy. New Engl J Med. 1985;313:837–841.

Lasnitzki I. The influence of A hypervitaminosis on the effect of 20-methylcholanthrene on mouse prostate glands grown in vitro. Br J Cancer. 1955;9:434–441.

Levine N, Meyskens FL Jr. Topical vitamin-A-acid therapy for cutaneous metastatic melanoma. Lancet. 1980;2:224–226.

Levine N, Miller RC, Meyskens FL Jr. Oral isotretinoin therapy: use in a patient with multiple cutaneous squamous cell carcinomas and keratoacanthomas. Arch Dermatol. 1984;120: 1215–1217.

Lippman SM, Meyskens FL Jr. Treatment of advanced squamous cell carcinoma of the skin with isotretinoin. Ann Intern Med. 1987a;107:499–501.

Lippman SM, Meyskens FL. Retinoid therapy of cutaneous neoplasia. Pharmacol Ther. 1987b.

Lippman SM, Meyskens FL. Vitamin A derivatives in the prevention and treatment of human cancer. J Am Coll Nutr. 1988a;7:269–289.

Lippman SM, Meyskens FL. Retinoids as anticancer agents. In: Tryfiates GP, Prasad KN, eds. Proceedings of the First International Symposium on Nutrition, Growth and Cancer. New York, NY: Alan R. Liss; 1988b.

Lippman SM, Kessler JF, Meyskens FL. Retinoids as preventive and therapeutic anticancer agents (Part I). Cancer Treat Rep. 1987a;71:391–405.

Lippman SM, Kessler JF, Meyskens FL. Retinoids as preventive and therapeutic anticancer agents (Part II). Cancer Treat Rep. 1987b;71:493–515.

Lippman SM, Kessler JF, Al-Sarraf M, et al. Treatment of advanced squamous cell carcinoma of the head and neck with isotretinoin: a phase II randomized trial. Invest New Drugs. 1988;6:13–17.

Loeliger P, Bollag W, Mayer H. Arotenoids, a new class of highly active retinoids. Eur J Med Chem Ther. 1980;15:9–15.

London J. Call of the wild.

Lotan R. Effects of vitamin A and its analogs (retinoids) on normal and neoplastic cells. Biochim Biophys Acta. 1980;605:33–91.

Lotan R. Mechanism of inhibition of tumor cell proliferation by retinoids. In: Saurat JH, ed. Retinoids: new trends in research and therapy. Basel: Karger; 1985:97–105.

Lotan R. Immunomodulatory effects of retinoids. J Nutr Growth Cancer. 1986;3:57–65.

Lotan R. Retinoids as biological response modifiers. In: Tryfiates GP, Prasad KN, eds. Proceedings of the First International Symposium on Nutrition, Growth and Cancer. New York, NY: Alan R. Liss; 1987.

Lotan R, Nicholson GC. Inhibitory effects of retinoic acid or retinyl acetate on the growth of untransformed, transformed and tumor cells in vitro. J Natl Cancer Inst. 1977;59:1717–1722.

Lotan R, Dennert G. Stimulatory effects of vitamin A analogs on the induction of cell-mediated cytotoxicity in vivo. Cancer Res. 1979;39:55–58.

Lotan R, Lotan D, Meromski L. Correlation of retinoic acid-enhanced sialytransferase activity and glycosylation of specific cell surface sialyglyco-proteins with growth inhibition in a murine melanoma cell system. Cancer Res. 1984;44:5805–5812.

Luk GK, Civin LI, Weissman RM, et al. Ornithine decarboxylase: essential in proliferation but not differentiation of human promyelocytic leukemia cells. Science. 1982;216:75–77.

Lutzner MA, Blanchet-Bardon C, Puissant A. Oral aromatic etinoid (Ro10-9359) treatment of two patients suffering with the severe form of epidermodysplasia verruciformis. In: Orfanos CE, Braun-Falco O, Farber EM, Grupper CL, Polano MK, Schuppli R, eds. Retinoids: advances in basic research and therapy. Berlin: Springer-Verlag; 1981:407–410.

Mahrle G, Thiele B, Ippen H. Chemotherapie butaner T-cell-lymphocyte mit arotinoid. Dtsch Med Wochenschr. 1983;108:1753–1757.

Mandel HG, Cohn VH. Fat soluble vitamins. In: Gilman AG, Goodman LS, Gilman A, eds. The pharmacologic basis of therapeutics. New York, NY: Macmillan; 1980:1583–1601.

Marcelo CL, Madison KC. Regulation of the expression of epidermal keratinocyte proliferation and differentiation of the vitamin A analogs. Arch Dermatol Res. 1984;276:381–389.

Markowska J, Janik P, Wiese E, et al. Leukoplakia of the vulva locally treated by 13-*cis*-retinoic acid. Neoplasma. 1987;34:33–36.

Mathe G, Guoveia J, Hercend T, et al. Correlation between precancerous bronchial metaplasia and cigarette consumption, the preliminary results of retinoid treatment. Cancer Detect Prev. 1982;5:461–466.

McCollum EV, Davis M. The necessity of certain lipens in the diet during growth. J Biol Chem. 1913;15:167–175.

Merriman RR, Bertram JS. Reversible inhibition by retinoids of 3-methylcholanthrene-induced neoplastic transformation in C3H/10T 1/2 clone 8 cells. Cancer Res. 1979;39:1661–1666.

Meyskens FL. Chemoprevention. In: Wittes RE, ed. Head and neck cancer. New York, NY: John Wiley, 1985:275–283.

Meyskens FL. Clinical trials of retinoids as differentiation inducers. Status of differentiation therapy of cancer. In: Waxman S, Rossi GB, Taraku F, eds. Second Symposia Publications, Vol. 45. New York, NY: Raven Press; 1988:349–359.

Meyskens FL, Surwit MD. Clinical experience with topical tretinoin in the treatment of cervical dysplasia. J Am Acad Dermatol. 1986;15:826–829.

Meyskens FL Jr, Gilmartin E, Alberts DS, et al. Activity of isotretinoin against squamous cell cancers and preneoplastic lesions. Cancer Treat Rep. 1982;66:1315–1319.

Meyskens FL Jr, Edards L, Levine N. Role of topical tretinoin in melanoma and dysplastic nevi. J Am Acad Dermatol. 1986;15:822–825.

Michalek AM, Cummings KM, Phelan J. Vitamin A and tumor recurrence in bladder cancer. Nutr Cancer. 1989;9:143–146.

Misset JL, Mathe G, Santelli G, et al. Regression of bronchial epidermoid metaplasia in heavy smokers with etretinate. Cancer Detect Prev. 1986;9:167–170.

Molin L, Thomsen K, Volden G, Lang E, Wantzin G, Hellbe L. 13-*cis*-retinoic acid in mycosis fungoides: a report from the Scandinavian Mycosis Fungoides Group. In: Saurat JH, ed. Retinoids: new trends in research and therapy. Basel: Karger; 1985:341–344.

Moon RC. Comparative aspects of carotenoids and retinoids as chemopreventive agents for cancer. J Nutr. 1989;119:127–134.

Moon RC, Itri LM. Retinoids and cancer. In: Sporn ME, Roberts AB, Goodman DS, eds. Retinoids, Vol. II. Orlando, Fla: Academic Press; 1984:327–371.

Moore T. Effect of vitamin A deficiency in animals: pharmacology and toxicology of vitamin A. In: Sebrell WH, Harris RS, eds. The vitamins, 2nd ed. New York, NY: Academic Press; 1967:245–294.

Mori S. The changes in the paraocular glands which follow the administration of diets low in fat soluble A with notes of the effect of the same diets on the salivary glands and the mucosa of the larynx and trachea. Johns Hopkins Hosp Bull. 1922;3:357.

Moriarty M, Dunn J, Darragh A, et al. Etretinate in the treatment of actinic keratosis: a double blind crossover study. Lancet. 1982;1:364–365.

Moshell AN. Prevention of skin cancer in xeroderma pigmentosum with oral isotretinoin. Cutis. 1989;43:485–494.

Neely SM, Mehlmauer M, Feinstein DI. The effect of isotretinoin in six patients with cutaneous T-cell lymphoma. Arch Intern Med. 1987;147:529–531.

Nettesheim P, Snyder C, Kim JCS. Vitamin A and the susceptibility of respiratory tract tissues to carcinogenic insult. Environ Health Perspect. 1979;29:89–93.

Nilsson B. Probable in vivo induction of differentiation by retinoic acid of promyelocytes in acute promyelocytic leukaemia. Br J Haematol. 1984;57:365–371.

Nisaizuka Y. Studies and perspectives of protein kinase-C. Science. 1986;233:305–312.

Osborne TB, Mendel LB. The relation of growth to the chemical constituents of the diet. J Biol Chem. 1913;15:311–326.

Pavone-Macaluso M. Intravesicle treatment of superficial (T1) urinary bladder tumours: a review of a 15 year experience. Treatment of superficial bladder tumours. Stockholm: Montedison Lakemedl; 1979:21.

Peck GL. Synthetic retinoids in dermatology. In: Sporn ME, Roberts AB, Goodman DS, eds. Retinoids, Vol. II. Orlando, Fla: Academic Press; 1984:391–411.

Peck GL. Therapy and prevention of skin cancer. In: Saurat JH, ed. Retinoids: new trends in research and therapy. Basel: Karger; 1985:345–354.

Peck GL. Long term retinoid therapy is needed for maintenance of cancer chemopreventive effect. Dermatologica. 1987;175(Suppl 1):138–144.

Peck GL, Gross EG, Butkus D, et al. Chemoprevention of basal cell carcinoma with isotretinoin. J Am Acad Dermatol. 1982;6:815–825.

Pedersen H, Wolf H, Jensen SK, et al. Administration of a retinoid as prophylaxis of recurrent noninvasive bladder tumors. Scand J Urol Nephrol. 1984;18:121–123.

Pennes D, Ellis C, Madison K, et al. Early skeletal hyperostoses secondary to 13-*cis*-retinoic acid for refractory ichthyosis. New Engl J Med. 1983;308:1012–1014.

Petkowich M, Brand NJ, Krust A, Chambon P. A human retinoic acid receptor which belongs to the family of nuclear receptors. Nature. 1987;330:444–450.

Pichler E, Fritsch P. Xeroderma pigmentosum: prevention of tumors with etretinate. Hautarzt. 1984;35:159–161.

Picozzi VJ, Swanson GF, Morgan R, Hecht F, Greenberg PL. 13-*Cis*-retinoic acid treatment for myelodysplastic syndromes. J Clin Oncol. 1986;14:589–595.

Rao RS, Desai PB. Editorial: the challenge of head and neck cancer in India. Head Neck Surg. 1989;11:487–489.

Ratko TA, Detrisal CJ, Dinger NM, et al. Chemopreventive efficacy of combined retinoid and tamoxifen treatment following surgical excision of a primary mammary cancer in female rats. Cancer Res. 1989;49:4772–4776.

Romney SL, Dwyer A, Slagle S, et al. Chemoprevention of cervix cancer: phase I-II: a feasibility study involving the topical vaginal administration of retinyl acetate gel. Gynecol Oncol. 1985;20:109–119.

Russell DH. Ornithine decarboxylase: a key regulatory enzyme in normal and neoplastic growth. Drug Metab Rev. 1985;16:1–88.

Russell DH, Haddox MK. Antiproliferative effects of retinoids related to cell-cycle specific inhibition of ornithine decarboxylase. Ann NY Acad Sci. 1981;359:281–297.

Russell FE. Vitamin A content of polar bear liver. Toxicon. 1967;5:61–62.

Saccomanno G, Moran PG, Schmidt RD, et al. Effects of 13-*cis*-retinoids on premalignant and malignant cells of lung origin. Acta Cytol. 1982;25:78–85.

Sampi K, Honma Y, Hozumi M, Sakurai M. Discrepancy between in-vitro and in-vivo inductions of differentiation by retinoids of human acute promyelocytic leukemia cells in relapse. Leuk Res. 1985;9:1475–1478.

Sankowski A, Janik P, Bogacki-Zatorsica E. Treatment of basal cell carcinoma with 13 *cis*-retinoic acid. Neoplasia. 1984;31:615–618.

Schindler J, Matthaei KI, Sherman MI. Isolation and characterization of murine mutant embryonal carcinoma cells which fail to differentiate in response to retinoic acid. Proc Natl Acad Sci USA. 1981;78:1077–1080.

Schmidt H, Foged E. Some hepatotoxic side effects observed in patients treated with aromatic retinoid (Ro-9359). In: Orfanos CE, Braun-Falco D, Farber ET, et al., eds. Retinoids: advances in basic research and therapy. Berlin: Springer-Verlag; 1981:271.

Schofer H, Ochsendorf FR, Helm EB, et al. Treatment of oral "hairy" leukoplakia in AIDS patients with vitamin A acid (topically) or acyclovir (systemically) [letter]. Dermatologica. 1987;174:150–151.

Schumacher A, Stuttgen G. Vitamin A-saure hyperkeratosen, epithelialia tumoren und akne. Dtsch Med Wochenschr. 1971;40:1547–1551.

Shaerer R, Swiercz P, Mousseau M, Chabert C. Is acid aromatic vitamin A (etretinate or "Tigason") active in low grade malignant bladder carcinoma? Cancer Chemother Pharmacol. 1982;9(Suppl):50.

Shah JP, Strong EW, DeCosse JJ, et al. Effect of retinoids on oral leukoplakia. Am J Surg. 1983;146:466–470.

Shapiro PE, Edelson RL. Effects of retinoids on the immune system. In: Saurat JH, ed. Retinoids: new trends in research and therapy. Basel: Karger; 1985:225–235.

Shaw JC, White CR. Treatment of multiple keratoacanthomas with oral isotretinoin. J Am Acad Dermatol. 1986;15:1079–1082.

Sherman MI, Gubler MC, Barkai U, et al. Role of retinoids in differentiation and growth of embryonal carcinoma cells. In: Nugent J, Clark S, eds. Retinoids, differentiation, and disease. London: Pitman; 1985:42–60.

Sidell N, Rieber P, Golub SH. Immunological aspects of retinoids in humans. I. Analysis of retinoic acid enhancement of thymocyte responses to PHA. Cell Immunol. 1984;87:48–125.

Silverberg E, Lubera JA. Cancer statistics. CA. 1989;39:3–20.

Slvyser M. Steroid/thyroid receptor-like proteins with oncogenic potential: a review. Cancer Res. 1990;50:451–458.

Soloway MS. Rationale for the intensive chemotherapy for superficial bladder cancer. J. Urol. 1980;123:461–466.

Souteyrand P, Thivolet J, Fulton R. Treatment of parapsoriasis en plaques and mycosis fungoides with an oral aromatic retinoid (Ro10-9359). In: Orfanos CE, Braun-Falco O, Farber

EM, Grupper CL, Polano MK, Schuppli R, eds. Retinoids: advances in basic research and therapy. Berlin: Springer-Verlag; 1981:401–405.

Sporn MB, Roberts AB. Role of retinoids in differentiation and carcinogenesis. J Natl Cancer Inst. 1984;73:1381–1387.

Sporn MB, Roberts AB. Introduction: what is a retinoid? In: Nugent J, Clark S, eds. Retinoids, differentiation, and disease. (CIBA Foundation Symposium 113) London: Pitman; 1985:1–5.

Sporn MB, Roberts AB, Roche NS, et al. Mechanism of action of retinoids. J Am Acad Dermatol. 1986;15(Suppl–pt. 2):756–764.

Stankowski A, Janik P, Bogacki-Zatorska E. Treatment of basal cell carcinoma with 13-*cis*-retinoic acid. Neoplasma. 1984;31:615–618.

Stepp W. Versuche uber Futterung mit Lipoidfreir Nahrung. Biochem Z. 1909;22:452–460.

Stich HF. The use of micronuclei in tracing the genotoxic damage in the oral mucosa of tobacco users. In: Hoffman D, Harris CC, eds. Banbury report 23: mechanisms in tobacco carcinogenesis. Cold Spring Harbor, NY: Cold Spring Harbor Laboratory; 1986:99–109.

Stich HF, Hornby AP, Sankaranaraynan R, et al. Response of oral leukoplakias to the administration of vitamin A. Cancer Lett. 1988;40:93–101.

Strauss JS, Rapini RP, Shalita AR, et al. Isotretinoin therapy for acne: results of multicenter dose–response study. J Am Acad Dermatol. 1984;10:490–499.

Strickland S, Breitman TR, Frickel F, et al. Structure–activity relationships of a new series of retinoidal benzoic acid derivatives as measured by induction of differentiation of murine F9 teratocarcinoma cells and human HL-60 promyelocytic leukemia cells. Cancer Res. 1983; 43:5268–5272.

Studer UE, Biedermann C, Chollet D, et al. Prevention of recurrent superficial bladder tumors by oral etretinate: preliminary results of a randomized, double blind multicenter trial in Switzerland. J Urol. 1984;131:47–49.

Surwit EA, Graham V, Droegemueller W, et al. Evaluation of topically applied transretinoid acid in the treatment of cervical intraepithelial lesions. Am J Obstet Gynecol. 1982;143:821–823.

Tachibana K, Sone S, Tsubura E, et al. Stimulatory effects of vitamin A on tumoricidal activity of rat alveolar macrophages. Br J Cancer. 1984;49:343–348.

Tobler A, Dawson MI, Koeffler HP. Retinoids: structure–function relationships in normal and leukemic hematopoesis in vitro. J Clin Invest. 1986;78:303–309.

Tomita Y, Himenko K, Nomoto K, et al. Vitamin A and tumor immunity. Experientia. 1985;41:92–93.

Tousignant J, Raymond GP, Light MJ. Treatment of cutaneous T-cell lymphoma with the arotinoid Ro13-6298. J Am Acad Dermatol. 1987;16:167–171.

Vahlquist A, Rollman D. Clinical pharmacology of three generations of retinoids. Dermatologica. 1987;175(Suppl 1):20–27.

Vahlquist C, Michaelsson G, Vahlquist A, et al. A sequential comparison of etretinate (Tigason) and isotretinoin (Roaccutane) with special regard to their effects on serum lipoproteins. Br J Dermatol. 1985;112:69–76.

Verma AK. Inhibition of protein kinase C-mediated mouse epidermal c-MYC and ornithine decarboxylase gene transcription by retinoic acid. In: Tryfiates GP, Prasad KN, eds. Proceedings of the First International Symposium on Nutrition, Growth and Cancer. New York, NY: Alan R. Liss; 1988.

Verret JL, Schnitzler L, Anevel M, et al. Etretinate and skin cancer prevention. In: Saurat JH, ed. Retinoids: new trends in research and therapy. Basel: Karger; 1985:355–359.

Vitall C, Rakowki I, Raka A. (Abstr.) Number of DNA replication cycles completed by HL-60 cells during differentiation induced by 13-*cis*-retinoic acid (RA). Blood. 1986;68(Suppl 1): 194A.

Wahrendorf J, Muñoz N, Lu JB, et al. Blood, retinol and zinc riboflavin status in relation to precancerous lesions of the esophagus. Finding from a vitamin intervention trial in the Peoples' Republic of China. Cancer Res. 1988;48:2280–2283.

Wang SY, Gudas JJ. Selection and characterizations of F9 teratocarcinoma stem cell mutants with altered responses to retinoic acid. J Biol Chem. 1984;259:5899–5906.

Ward A, Brogen RN, Heel RC, et al. Etretinate: a review of its efficacy in psoriasis and other skin disorders. Drugs. 1983;26:9–43.

Wargon O, Downie D. A case of mycosis fungoides treated with etretinate. Aust J Dermatol. 1984;25:77–79.

Warrell RP Jr, Coonley CJ, Kempin SJ, Myskowski P, Safai B, Itri L. Isotretinoin in cutaneous T-cell lymphoma (letter). Lancet. 1983;2:629.

Watson AB. Preventive effect of etretinate therapy on multiple actinic keratoses. Cancer Detect Prev. 1986;9:161–165.

Weiner SA, Surwit EA, Graham VE, et al. A phase I trial of topically applied *trans*-retinoic acid in cervical dysplasia—clinical efficacy. Invest New Drugs. 1986;4:241–244.

Weiss VC, West DP, Ackerman R, et al. Hepatotoxic reactions in a patient treated with etretinate. Arch Dermatol. 1984;120:104.

Weleber RG, Denman ST, Hanifen JM, et al. Abnormal retinal function associated with isotretinoin therapy for acne. Arch Ophthalmol. 1986;104:831–837.

Windhorst DB, Nigra T. General clinical toxicology of oral retinoids. J Am Acad Dermatol. 1982;6:675–677.

Wolbach SB, Howe PR. Tissue changes following depravation of fat soluble A vitamin. J Exp Med. 1925;42:753–777.

Wolf G. Multiple functions of vitamin A. Physiol Rev. 1984;64:873–937.

Yoshida O, Miyakawa M, Watanabe H, Mishina T, Okajima E. Prophylactic effect of etretinate on the recurrence of superficial bladder tumors—results of a randomized control study. Hinyokika Kiyo. 1986;32:1349–1358.

Zacharine H. Methotrexate and etretinate as concurrent therapy in the treatment of psoriasis. Arch Dermatol. 1984;120:155.

CHAPTER **21**

BONE MARROW TRANSPLANTATION: A FORM OF ADOPTIVE IMMUNOTHERAPY

John R. Wingard

High-dose cytoreductive therapy followed by bone marrow transplantation (BMT) has been found to be effective in the control of malignant lymphohematopoietic diseases in situations where conventional chemotherapy has failed or would be expected to fail based on certain prognostic factors (Clift et al., 1982; Braine et al., 1987; Geller, 1989a; Wingard et al., 1990a; Jones et al., 1990). The initial view of this added beneficial effect of BMT was that the employment of "rescue" bone marrow permitted more intensive cytoreductive treatment with a greater antitumor effect. It soon became apparent with mounting evidence (reviewed by Santos, 1972) that there was an allogeneic antitumor effect independent of the chemoradiotherapy of the preparative regimen. This effect, labeled "adoptive immunotherapy" (Mathe et al., 1965), is, in large measure, accompanied by graft-versus-host (GVH) disease. This chapter will discuss GVH disease after allogeneic and autologous BMT, evidence for a graft-versus-tumor (GVT) effect, the results of efforts to amplify the GVT effect while minimizing GVH disease in the allogeneic BMT setting, and the efforts to create GVH disease in autologous marrow transplantation to augment the antitumor efficacy.

ALLOGENEIC GRAFT-VERSUS-HOST DISEASE

Historically, GVH disease has been a major cause of serious morbidity and death after allogeneic BMT. Graft-versus-host disease and its treatment are accompanied by profound immunodeficiency and immune dysregulation, which places the patient at risk for life-threatening infections and interstitial pneumonitis (Wingard, 1990; Wingard et al., 1988a, 1988b, 1990b). With or without interstitial pneumonitis or infection, GVH disease has accounted for approximately two thirds of the deaths after allogeneic BMT at Johns Hopkins (Santos et al., 1987; Geller et al., 1989a; Wingard et al., 1990a). There have been several reviews of GVH disease after allogeneic BMT (Santos et al., 1985; Sullivan, 1986; Vogelsang et al., 1988; Wagner et al., 1989a).

In view of its major significance in human BMT, it is interesting to note that it was not initially anticipated nor recognized in experimental marrow transplantation. Barnes and Loutit (1955) reported a "secondary" disease manifest by delayed runting and death occurring in 30-day survivors of allogeneic transplants using spleen cells, but not in survivors of syngeneic transplantation. For several years, there were debates as to whether the secondary disease was a delayed host-versus-graft reaction or vice versa. Various syndromes analogous to secondary disease, including runt disease, F1 hybrid disease, parabiosis intoxication, and homologous disease, were noted under differing experimental conditions (reviewed by van Bekkum and de Vries, 1967; Santos, 1983). After extensive experimentation, it was generally agreed that these phenomena represented GVH immune reactions and were mediated by T lymphocytes. The rapidity and severity of disease were dependent on the number of lymphocytes administered along with bone marrow cells, as well as the histocompatibility disparity between host and donor. In the rodent model, early-onset spleen cell–mediated GVH disease appeared to be analogous to the human form of acute GVH disease, while later-onset GVH disease corresponded to the human form of chronic GVH disease.

Billingham (1966–1967) postulated several requirements that must be present for the occurrence of GVH disease: (1) the graft must contain immunologically competent cells; (2) the host must possess important antigens not present in the donor graft cells; and (3) the host must be incapable of mounting an effective immunological reaction against the graft, at least long enough to allow the graft to exert its immunological capabilities (the so-called "security of tenure").

The clinical and pathological characteristics of GVH disease in animals and man have been described (van Bekkum and de Vries, 1967; Slavin and Santos, 1973; Sullivan, 1983). The major target organs in acute GVH disease are the skin, liver, and intestinal tract, although other organs, including bone marrow and thymus, are affected. In chronic GVH disease, the skin and liver are major target organs, but also prominently affected are the lacrimal and salivary glands, oral mucosa and conjunctiva, and the fascia, resulting in a variety of autoimmune and other syndromes, including scleroderma, Sjorgren's syndrome, myasthenia gravis, polymyositis, bronchiolitis obliterans, autoimmune thrombocytopenia, and primary biliary cirrhosis.

Analogous to the findings in animal models of BMT (Korngold and Sprent, 1982), in HLA-identical human marrow transplants, T cells with HLA-restricted cytotoxicity directed at minor histocompatibility antigens have been identified (Goulmy et al., 1984; Reinsmoen et al., 1984) and appear to be the primary mediators of acute GVH disease. In both animals and humans, there may be additional contributors to the pathogenesis of acute GVH disease.

Viral or other infections appear to play a role in the initiation of the GVH response. Germ-free mice, given H-2 incompatible marrow transplants after lethal irradiation, were noted to have a lower incidence of GVH disease than conventionally treated rodents (Jones et al., 1971; Pollard et al., 1976). Moreover, GVH disease has been shown to be mitigated by reduction of the intestinal flora in mice (van Bekkum et al., 1974) and in humans with aplastic anemia by a protective environment (Storb et al., 1983a).

Evidence has been presented that natural killer (NK) cells are mediators of GVH disease in mice (Guillen et al., 1986; Ghayur et al., 1987) and humans (Dokhelar et al., 1981; Muller et al., 1982). Cytotoxic antibody responses (Merritt et al., 1971) have also been described by some as part of the process, but these data are less convincing. There probably are amplication mechanisms participating in the pathogenesis of GVH disease. Thus, activated T lymphocytes may initiate the process, releasing lymphokines, which could secondarily stimulate monocytes, macrophages, or NK cells.

The pathogenesis of chronic GVH disease is less clear. The syndrome is characterized by profound humoral and cellular immune dysregulation with susceptibility for a wide spectrum of opportunistic infectious pathogens. In a rodent model, spleen cells from healthy chimeras react against third-party alloantigens, but not against donor or host cells (Beschorner et al., 1982; Tutschka et al., 1982). In contrast, spleen cells from rats with chronic GVH disease nonspecifically suppress mixed lymphocyte responses with donor and third-party cells. Likewise, in humans, the presence of nonspecific suppressor cells during active chronic GVH disease and the disappearance of nonspecific suppressor cells with resolution of GVH disease have been noted (Tsoi et al., 1979; Witherspoon et al., 1984), apparently by development of specific suppressor cells against the tolerated alloantigens (Tutschka and Bortin, 1981; Tutschka et al., 1981a, 1981b, 1982; Tsoi, 1982). Adoptive transfer of the disease in rodents can be effected by transfer of spleen or marrow cells of rodents with chronic GVH disease to immunosuppressed third-party animals. Hess et al. (1988) were able to show that T lymphocytes recovered from cyclosporine (CsA)-treated rats with chronic GVH disease after allogeneic BMT were cytotoxic to cells bearing class II (Ia) major histocompatibility complex (MHC) determinants (similar or possibly identical to the effector cells that cause syngeneic/autologous GVH disease, see below). This raised the possibility that these effector cells were in fact the previously described nonspecific suppressor cells, but this has not yet been formally proven. Parkman (1986) has also described lymphocyte clones recovered from mice with chronic GVH disease after allogeneic BMT (not treated with CsA) to have autologous Ia-specific blastogenesis, although not demonstrable to be cytotoxic and to express a Thy-1.2^{+},Lyt-2.2-,L3T4^{+} (helper) phenotype. DeClerck et al. (1986) showed that supernatants of these cells can stimulate fibroblasts to secrete collagen, thus offering a possible explanation for the sclerodermatoid features of chronic GVH disease.

The thymus appears to have a central role in the development of transplantation tolerance by deletion of autoreactive lymphocyte clones (MacDonald, 1989) or by participating in the development of suppressor cells specifically suppressing reactivity against host alloantigens (Tutschka and Bortin, 1981). Several observations suggest a role for the thymus in the pathogenesis of chronic GVH disease. Pathological abnormalities of the thymus, impaired T-cell differentiation associated with GVH disease–induced thymic epithelial cell injury, and low levels of serum thymic factor have been consistent observations (Tsoi et al., 1979; Shulman et al., 1980; Seddik et al., 1980; Atkinson et al., 1982).

Injury to the thymus, from acute GVH disease, CsA, or the cytotoxic therapy, may be the initial event in the pathogenesis of chronic GVH disease, preventing lymphocytes from distinguishing self from nonself. Then, as suggested by Parkman (1986), autoreactive cells localize in target tissues and secrete lymphokines, which secondarily stimulate fibroblasts to secrete collagen. This, then, results in sclerosis of various organs damaged by cytotoxic cells during acute GVH disease. The presence of nonspecific suppressor cells can account for the host's inability to mount immune responses to infectious pathogens and the resulting susceptibility to infection.

It is becoming clear that acute and chronic GVH disease are separate entities, with different effector mechanisms. As noted above, Parkman (1986) has shown splenic lymphocytes from mice with chronic GVH disease to proliferate in response to the public epitope of the Ia antigen, whereas lymphocytes from patients with acute GVH disease react specifically to host alloantigens. Similarly, Hess et al. (1988) has shown in a rat model cells specifically cytotoxic to host alloantigens (apparently recognizing private determinants of class I and class II determinants) during acute GVH disease, but later, cells cytotoxic to cells bearing the public specificity of class II (Ia) determinants in chronic GVH disease.

Risk factors for GVH disease have been identified. For acute GVH disease, age, the use of donor buffy coat cells, HLA-nonidentity, lack of some type of immunosuppressive prophylaxis, acute lymphocytic leukemia (ALL) as the underlying disease of the recipient, sex mismatch between donor and recipient, and possibly certain HLA loci have all been implicated as increasing the likelihood for developing acute GVH disease (Storb et al., 1977; Stoch et al., 1983; Storb et al., 1983b; Powles et al., 1984; Bross et al., 1984; Storb and Thomas, 1985). For chronic GVH disease, the greatest risk factor is the prior occurrence of acute GVH disease and in its absence, increasing age and the use of donor buffy coat cells (Storb et al., 1983c).

A test useful for the prediction of acute GVH disease in genotypically HLA-identical allogeneic transplants is the skin explant test (Vogelsang et al., 1985): lymphocytes from both donor and recipient are mixed in vitro for 1 week and, once primed, are then added to skin explant cultures of recipient and donor (as a control); 3 days later, the explants are examined histopathologically for the presence of infiltrating lymphocytes and destructive lesions as an indication of the probability of the occurrence of GVH disease. This test has been found to have a sensitivity and specificity approximating 85%.

Prognosis after the occurrence of acute GVH disease is most dependent on its clinical severity (Glucksberg et al., 1974; Storb et al., 1983a). Multivariate analysis of baseline factors present at the outset of chronic GVH disease indicate that lichenoid cutaneous histology, elevated bilirubin, and the progressive mode of presentation are independent predictors of reduced survival (Wingard et al., 1989).

Methotrexate, cyclophosphamide, and corticosteroids have been traditionally used as GVH disease prophylaxis. In recent years, CsA, either alone or in combination with other immunosuppressive agents, has also been found to be effective (Deeg et al., 1985; Santos et al., 1987). Ex vivo T-cell purging of donor bone marrow has also been shown to effectively reduce GVH disease (Rodt et al., 1981; Slavin et al., 1985; Martin et al., 1985). Once acute GVH disease occurs, the mainstay of therapy is high-dose corticosteroids, which are rapidly tapered over several weeks and discontinued as the GVH disease comes under control. For chronic GVH disease, corticosteroids are also the chief modality of treatment, although given in lower doses and over a prolonged period (Sullivan et al., 1988).

Resolution of acute or chronic GVH disease is dependent on the host eliminating or suppressing the reactive T-cell clones responsible for its pathogenesis. This presumably occurs through either (or both) clonal deletion of the allo- and autoreactive cells, or as mentioned earlier, by the development of alloantigen-specific or (in the case of chronic GVH disease) Ia-specific suppressor cells actively maintaining tolerance.

AUTOLOGOUS GRAFT-VERSUS-HOST DISEASE

From the early days of transplantation, GVHD has been noted to occur sporadically after both syngeneic and autologous BMT in humans (Rappeport et al., 1979; Gluckman et al., 1980; Thein et al., 1981) and in animals (Belanger et al., 1982; Glazier et al., 1983a, 1983b; Hess et al., 1985; reviewed by van Bekkum and de Vries, 1967). In a study of 115 autologous and syngeneic BMT patients, 9 patients developed clinical and histological GVH disease, yielding an incidence of 8% (Hood et al., 1987). These observations were initially controversial because they could not be explained by Billingham's postulates (above), which require histocompatibility differences between donor and host for GVH disease to occur. Syngeneic and autologous GVH disease have been reviewed recently by Santos (1989) and Hess and Fischer (1989).

Glazier et al. (1983a, 1983b) reconstituted lethally irradiated rats with allogeneic, syngeneic, or autologous bone marrow and treated the rats with a short course of CsA. Although it had earlier been noted that delayed GVH disease occurred after CsA withdrawal in the animals reconstituted with allogeneic cells, it was surprising to find a similar occurrence in the animals reconstituted with autologous or syngeneic bone marrow. The studies of Glazier et al. indicated that CsA and irradiation were both necessary ingredients of the transplant procedure, otherwise syngeneic GVH disease did not occur. Further, the thymus had to be in the irradiation field. Sorokin et al. (1986) demonstrated that GVH disease did not occur in thymectomized animals. Autologous GVH disease could be adoptively transferred by T cells (Glazier et al., 1983a), and the transfer could be blocked by treatment of the cells with antithymocyte antibody. The effector cells were subsequently found to be autoreactive $OX8^+$ cytotoxic T cells, which recognize a public determinant of Ia antigens present on syngeneic and allogeneic target cells (Hess et al., 1985), characteristics similar to the effector cells of chronic GVH disease. Additional cellular contributors to the pathogenesis of this phenomenon are cells with a "helper" phenotype, which appear early in the peripheral blood at the onset of the GVH disease; the disease can be adoptively transferred by these cells (Sorokin et al., 1986). Thus, there may be an interaction between these phenotypically distinct lymphocyte subpopulations, through one inducing or amplifying another, and/or both contributing to the end-organ damage (Hess and Fischer, 1989).

In a very different setting, the presence of autoreactive cells can be demonstrated by in vitro manipulation such as in the autologous mixed lymphocyte reaction (Weksler et al., 1981), in which T cells will proliferate in response to autologous non–T cells expressing class II (Ia) MHC antigens. This proliferative response is blocked by anti–Ia antibodies. Thus, it is not surprising that there would be an analogous in vivo situation in syngeneic GVH disease and that self–class II antigens would play an important role.

Initially, syngeneic GVH disease pathologically resembles allogeneic acute GVH disease, but within 2 weeks the histology evolves to resemble chronic GVH disease with prominent fibrosis (Hess et al., 1987; Beschorner et al., 1988a). At onset, the lymphocytes infiltrating target tissues are $CD8^+$ $CD4^-$, but later are predominantly $CD4^+$ (with or without coexpression of $CD8^+$), similar to chronic GVH disease after allogeneic BMT (Beschorner et al., 1982, 1988a; Hess and Fischer, 1989).

Since histocompatibility cannot be the explanation of this phenomenon, it has been suggested that the immune dysregulation that occurs after BMT may play a role in the pathogenesis of syngeneic GVH disease, even after allogeneic BMT (Rappeport et al., 1979; Hess et al., 1988). Indeed, GVH disease in rats after allogeneic BMT and CsA appear to include a syngeneic GVH disease component and can be adoptively transferred to the original donor strain rat (Hess et al., 1988). The effector cells lyse target cells from multiple rat strains and are blocked by monoclonal antibodies against class II MHC antigens, analogous to the properties of the effector cells mediating syngeneic GVH disease (Hess et al., 1985).

Cyclosporine appears to suppress the generation of alloreactive cells while permitting the development of cells that recognize class II antigens and mediate syngeneic GVH disease. The mechanism for this remains unclear. Cyclosporine has profound effects on the thymus with reduction of medullary epithelial cells and reduced class II antigen expression (Glazier et al., 1983a; Beschorner et al., 1988b; Cheney and Sprent, 1985). It has been suggested that T-cell differentiation may be altered in this environment and result in a failure to recognize class II antigens as self or that an autoregulatory cell for self–Ia antigens is inhibited in its development (Hess et al., 1988).

Graft-versus-host disease after syngeneic or autologous BMT is usually mild and has a benign natural history. The most common manifestation is a cutaneous rash, but hepatic or intestinal involvement can also occasionally occur. Often no therapy is necessary, but when treatment is necessary, corticosteroids, in moderately high doses, rapidly tapered and discontinued after several weeks, are effective in controlling the disease.

THE GRAFT-VERSUS-LEUKEMIA EFFECT

Evidence from Animal Models

Mathe et al. (1965) found that nearly all irradiated F1 mice given parental-strain marrow contaminated with L1210 leukemia died. However, 35% of 20-day survivors showed no signs of leukemia, but exhibited histological signs of the secondary syndrome. Similarly, experiments with the AKR spontaneous leukemia demonstrated that transplants conducted in animals aged 6 months (24% of controls at that age had leukemia) using irradiation plus MHC-mismatched donor marrow ended in death in most animals; in most, the cause of death was secondary disease, and only a minority had leukemia. Further, mice inoculated with the Friend leukemia virus were irradiated and given either syngeneic or allogeneic marrow, and then blood from these animals was inoculated into other mice. All of the group given blood from mice transplanted with syngeneic marrow died of leukemia, whereas one third of those given blood from mice treated with allogeneic marrow did not develop leukemia, thus providing evidence for eradication of the leukemia cells in the allogeneic setting.

Bortin et al. (1973) attempted to quantify the magnitude of the "adoptive immunotherapy" of allogeneic BMT. First, AKR mice were lethally irradiated and reconstituted with bone marrow from H-2 matched or mismatched donors with spleen cells from mice bearing BW5147, a lymphoid leukemia, in graded doses. Six days later, mice were sacrificed. Spleen cells were injected into normal AKR secondary hosts that were observed for survival (to determine if any residual leukemia cells had been transferred from the primary hosts). Secondary hosts were more likely to survive if given cells from primary hosts reconstituted with mismatched bone marrow than with H-2 matched bone marrow. Using knowledge of cell generation times and the observed survival time after graded inoculations, it was calculated that a 10^5 reduction of leukemia cells had occurred in the mismatched situation.

Unfortunately, such immunotherapy has been largely ineffective in various animal models where the tumor burden is large (Mathe, 1965; Fefer et al., 1987) and difficult to demonstrate in nonlymphohematopoietic neoplasms (Santos, 1983). On the other hand, it has been suggested that cytoreductive treatment and immunotherapy may be complementary and that immunotherapy might be used as an adjunct to chemotherapy or radiotherapy, once there is minimal residual disease. This has been termed adoptive chemoimmunotherapy.

In most situations, the beneficial antileukemic effect has been offset by the harmful effects of GVH disease, thus negating any improvement in survival. Some investigators have reported findings suggesting that the graft-versus-leukemia (GVL) and the

GVH phenomena could be separated. For example, Bortin et al. (1979) reported immunization of CBA (H-2k) mice by H-2 mismatched allogeneic cells could induce a population of cells that appeared to eliminate AKR leukemia cells when transplanted into lethally irradiated AKR (H-2k) mice along with AKR leukemia; no augmentation of the mild GVH disease was noted, compared to controls.

Greenberg et al. (1981) have presented data suggesting that the phenotype of the predominant T-cell subset that mediates adoptive chemoimmunotherapy in a syngeneic transplant mouse model expresses a noncytologic phenotype, Lyt-1^+2^-, distinctly different from the cell phenotypes that mediate in vitro tumor lysis (Greenberg et al., 1981). In contrast, the cells mediating GVH disease in a minor histoincompatibility mouse model express the cytolytic Lyt-1^+2^+ phenotype (Korngold and Sprent, 1982). Other data suggest that GVH and GVL reactivities are mediated by overlapping cell populations (Truitt et al., 1983).

Evidence from Human Bone Marrow Transplantation

Several lines of evidence suggest the presence of a GVL effect in human BMT. This subject has been reviewed earlier (Gale and Champlin, 1984; Fefer et al., 1987; Butturini et al., 1987; Sullivan et al., 1987). The evidence from pertinent studies is summarized in Table 21-1.

(1) Comparison of Relapse Rates After Allogeneic Versus Syngeneic BMT Weiden et al. (1979); Gale and Champlin (1984); and Fefer et al. (1987) have noted lower relapse rates in recipients of allogeneic BMT than in recipients of syngeneic BMT. For example, the relapse rate in patients transplanted for acute nonlymphocytic leukemia (ANLL) in first remission were 18% and 59%, respectively (Gale and Champlin, 1984).

(2) Comparison of Relapse Rates After Allogeneic BMT With or Without GVH Disease Weiden et al. (1979) noted that in allogeneic BMT recipients transplanted for ANLL or ALL the rate of leukemic relapse was 2.5 times lower in patients with GVH disease than in those without GVH disease. Unfortunately, the antileukemic effect was negated by an increased rate of death from the GVH disease and its sequelae. A subsequent report of patients transplanted for ANLL or ALL (Weiden et al., 1981) sought to determine if the antileukemic effects of acute and chronic GVH disease in 150-day survivors were different. Patients who developed both acute and chronic GVH disease had the lowest relapse rates. The relapse rate was intermediate in those who developed either acute or chronic GVH disease alone and was highest in those without any GVH disease. The effects of chronic GVH disease on relapse rate were additive for those with or without acute GVH disease. Overall survival was best in those with chronic GVH disease alone, intermediate in those with acute plus or minus chronic GVH disease, and poorest in those without any GVH disease. Similar reductions in relapse rates in patients who developed GVH disease have been noted in pa-

TABLE 21-1
EVIDENCE FOR A GRAFT-VERSUS-LEUKEMIA EFFECT FROM REPRESENTATIVE STUDIES EMPLOYING HUMAN BONE MARROW TRANSPLANTATION

Author	Disease	Remission status	GVL effect observed		Factor associated with the GVL effect
			Yes	No	
(1) Comparison of relapse rates after allogeneic versus syngeneic BMT					
Weiden et al. (1979)	ANLL,ALL	CR	Y		Allogeneic, with GVHD
Gale & Champlin (1984)	ANLL	CR1	Y		Allogeneic BMT
Fefer et al. (1987)	ANLL,ALL	CR ≥2,Rel	Y		Allogeneic BMT
Horowitz et al. (1990)	ANLL,ALL,CML	CR1,CP	Y		Allogeneic BMT
(2) Comparison of relapse rates after allogeneic BMT with or without GVHD					
Weiden et al. (1979)	ANLL,ALL	CR	Y		Acute or chronic GVHD
Weiden et al. (1981)	ANLL,ALL	CR	Y		Chronic >acute GVHD
Sanders et al. (1985)	ALL	CR, Rel	Y		Acute and/or chronic
Storb et al. (1986)	CML,ANLL	CP,CR1	Y		Acute GVHD
Weisdorf et al. (1987)	ALL	CR	Y		Acute GVHD

Sullivan et al. (1989b)	ANLL	CR1		N	
	ANLL	CR $\geq$2	Y		Acute GVHD
	ALL	CR $\geq$1	Y		Acute GVHD
	CML	CP		N	
	CML	AP	Y		Acute or chronic GVHD
Geller et al. (1989a)	ANLL	CR and ER	Y		Chronic GVHD
Horowitz et al. (1990)	ANLL,ALL,CML	CR1	Y		Chronic $>$acute GVHD
(3) Influence of type of regimen used for posttransplant GVHD prophylaxis on relapse rates					
Geller et al. (1989a)	ANLL	CR and ER	Y		Non-cyclosporine $>$CsA
Sullivan et al. (1989a)	ANLL,ALL,CML,LY	"poor risk"		N*	
Storb et al. (1989)	ANLL,CML	CR1,CP	Y		CsA $>$combined MTX/CsA
(4) Influence of T-cell purging of marrow graft on relapse rate					
Apperly et al. (1986)	CML	CP	Y		T lymphocytes
Pollard et al. (1986)	CML,ANLL	CP,CR1	Y		T lymphocytes
Goldman et al. (1988)	CML	CP	Y		T lymphocytes
Horowitz et al. (1990)	ANLL,ALL,CML	CR1,CP	Y		T lymphocytes

*Although the incidence of acute GVH disease was affected by the different regimens, the rate of chronic GVH disease was not.

GVL, graft-versus-leukemia; ANLL, acute nonlymphocytic leukemia; ALL, acute lymphocytic leukemia; CR, complete response; GVHD, graft-versus-host disease; BMT, bone marrow transplant; Rel, relapse; CP, chronic phase; CML, chronic myelogenous leukemia; AP, accelerated phase; ER, early relapse; CsA, cyclosporine; MTX, methotrexate.

tients transplanted for ALL (Weisdorf et al., 1987; Sanders et al., 1985) and in patients transplanted for CML and ANLL in first remission (Storb et al., 1986).

From the data using the adoptive chemoimmunotherapy animal models (reviewed above), one might expect the GVL effect to be most noticeable in patients with leukemia in remission, where the minimal residual disease is smallest. Such an effect has been demonstrated (Horowitz et al., 1990). In contrast, a recent report did not find clinical GVH disease to be associated with a GVL effect in patients transplanted for ANLL and ALL in remission or CML in chronic phase, but was evident in patients transplanted for acute leukemia in relapse or CML in accelerated phase (Sullivan et al., 1989a).

(3) Relapse Rates in Patients Using Improved Posttransplant GVH Disease Prophylaxis As more effective regimens for GVH disease prophylaxis have been developed, experience has shown that relapse rates have generally increased as the GVH disease has been better controlled. For example, in patients transplanted for ANLL, Geller et al. (1989a) noted that the use of CsA for GVH disease prophylaxis was associated with a significantly lower death rate from GVH disease and interstitial pneumonia than for patients given some other non–CsA GVH disease prophylaxis. However, there was a higher relapse rate: in patients transplanted in first remission, the increase was nonsignificant (18% vs 6%, $P = .48$), but in patients transplanted in second or subsequent remission or in early relapse, the increase was significant (53% vs 9%, $P = .02$). Acute GVH disease did not significantly affect the risk for relapse, but chronic GVH disease was associated with a lower relapse risk ($P = .06$). Thus, whereas the putative GVL effect may have not been as important in relatively chemotherapy-sensitive disease (as in patients in first remission), it appeared to be more important in patients with more refractory disease (in patients in early relapse or in remission after one or more relapses).

Another study by Storb et al. (1988) did not find an effect of CsA use on relapse (compared to methotrexate as GVH disease prophylaxis). However, this could be explained by the lack of significant reduction in GVH disease associated with the CsA use (Storb et al., 1988). Yet, another study comparing CsA alone versus a combination of a short course of methotrexate with CsA noted a reduction in the frequency and severity of acute GVH disease (but no difference in chronic GVH disease) in patients transplanted for CML or ANLL (Storb et al., 1989). There was no increase in the relapse rate for patients transplanted for CML, but a nonsignificant trend of increased relapses was seen in the group of patients transplanted for ANLL (29% vs 16%, $P = .26$); there were only 17 and 21 ANLL patients in each treatment group, so with larger numbers, this trend might have become significant.

(4) Relapse Rates Observed with Transplants Conducted with Removal of T Lymphocytes from the Marrow Graft Ex vivo T-cell purging of donor marrow by a variety of techniques, including lectins, monoclonal antibodies, corticosteroids, and elutriation, has been used by a number of centers in recent years in an attempt to reduce

GVH disease. Generally, these efforts have succeeded in reducing the frequency and/or severity of GVH disease. Unfortunately, there has been an attendant increase in relapse rates (Apperley et al., 1986; Pollard et al., 1986; Goldman et al., 1988; Horowitz et al., 1990).

(5) Relative Potencies of Various Components of the GVL Effect Data submitted to the International BMT Registry on patients transplanted for ALL or ANLL in first remission or CML in chronic phase have been analyzed to assess the antileukemic effects of GVH disease, to determine the presence of an antileukemic effect in allogeneic BMT in the absence of GVH disease, and to investigate if there is an antileukemic effect altered by T-cell depletion (Horowitz et al., 1990). Patients who developed overt GVH disease had a lower risk for relapse than patients who did not; the risk of relapse decreased progressively as the severity of GVH disease increased, further supporting the antileukemic effect of GVH disease. Syngeneic BMT patients had a relapse rate almost double that of allogeneic BMT patients without GVH disease, suggesting that either subclinical GVH disease had exerted a GVL effect or that there is an allogeneic antileukemic effect independent of GVH disease. The relapse rate in patients given T cell–depleted marrow grafts had a higher relapse rate than patients given non-T cell–purged marrow allogeneic BMT. Among patients given T cell–purged marrow transplants who developed GVH disease, the relapse rate still was higher than allogeneic non-T cell–purged BMT patients with comparable degrees of acute or chronic GVH disease. Patients with T cell–purged marrows who did not develop GVH disease had higher relapse rates than patients without manipulated marrow grafts who also did not experience GVH disease (similarly noted by Goldman et al., 1988). The authors conclude that these data argue for a population of T-cells mediating a GVL effect independent of clinically overt GVH disease. They hypothesize three separate components of the GVL phenomenon associated wtih allogeneic BMT: (1) GVL associated with clinically evident GVH disease; (2) GVL in the absence of overt GVH disease; (3) GVL independent of GVH disease, which can be abrogated by T-cell depletion. Unfortunately, these data do not exclude the possible role of subclinical GVH disease, demonstrable histologically in many patients without overt GVH disease, accounting for some, most, or all of the GVL effect in the absence of clinically overt GVH disease.

(6) Effector Mechanisms for the GVL Phenomenon The nature of the GVL effector cells are poorly understood. They presumably express a T-cell phenotype based on the observations noted above. It remains unclear whether there are GVL effector cells independent of the GVH disease effector cells or whether they are the same. Whether some other cells may mediate part of the GVL effect is yet to be conclusively elucidated. For example, Hercend et al. (1986) found NK cells with in vitro antileukemic activity in a patient following a T-depleted allogeneic transplant. Such observations require further study. The target antigens for GVL effector cells are also poorly understood. They presumably are tumor-associated antigens (TAA), alloantigens, or both.

ATTEMPTS TO EXPLOIT THE GRAFT-VERSUS-LEUKEMIA EFFECT

In the absence of being able to distinguish different populations of human cells mediating the GVL and GVH disease effects, efforts to date to exploit the GVL effect have focused on either amplification of GVH disease after allogeneic BMT or creating GVH disease after autologous BMT.

Sullivan et al. (1989a) studied patients aged 30 or less with acute leukemia in relapse or in late remissions, CML in accelerated phase, or refractory lymphoma; groups in which relapse rates exceeding 60% were expected from previous studies. Patients were randomly assigned to standard-course methotrexate, short-course methotrexate, or standard-course methotrexate plus viable donor buffy-coat cells. The aim was to determine if modification of the GVH disease prophylaxis regimen to promote GVH disease would result in a reduction of the relapse rate. The trial succeeded in the promotion of acute GVH disease, but unfortunately, there was no attendant augmentation of the antileukemic effect seen. Unfortunately, the large number of patients with systemic GVH disease early censored (due to death from complications of the GVH disease) make conclusions less clear, since fewer patients with intense GVH disease lived long enough to discern the antileukemic effect of the more intense GVH disease. Nonetheless, clearly, the lack of antitumor specificity will limit the potential of this approach. Of interest, was the finding that the incidence of chronic GVH disease was equivalent in the three groups despite different rates of acute GVH disease. One could argue that if one were to succeed in promoting chronic GVH disease without exacerbating acute GVH disease, a safer, and perhaps more potent GVL effect might be achieved.

Santos (1989) has reviewed the reasoning behind attempting to create autologous/syngeneic GVH disease as an antitumor therapeutic. In brief, the arguments are (1) the apparent antileukemic effect of GVH disease, especially chronic GVH disease; (2) the presence of autoreactive anti–Ia T cells in chronic GVH disease; (3) the effector cell in syngeneic/autologous GVH disease is an autoreactive cytotoxic T cell directed against Ia antigens; and (4) many acute leukemias and lymphomas express Ia antigens (Foon and Todd, 1986).

Using the animal models demonstrating the capability of CsA to induce syngeneic GVH disease, we have administered CsA to patients undergoing autologous BMT for relapsed lymphoma. We find that most develop mild GVH disease, generally confined to the skin, which can be controlled with either no therapy or short-course corticosteroids (Vogelsang et al., 1989; Jones et al., 1989). Lymphocytes obtained from one of the patients were cytotoxic against the patient's own cells pretransplant and this cytotoxicity was blocked by anti–class II (Dr or Ia) antigens.

Investigations are currently underway to determine whether purposely induced autologous GVH disease has a GVL effect. Such a GVT effect against a rat plasmacytoma cell line (which expresses Ia antigen) has been demonstrated in a syngeneic rat transplant model (Geller et al., 1989b) and it could be blocked by anti–Ia antibody. Moreover, the GVT effect could be augmented by interferon-gamma (IFN-γ) by increasing expression of Ia antigens on tumor cells. The prospective trials underway will ascertain whether induction of autologous GVH disease will have a significant antitumor effect against lymphomas and ANLL.

FUTURE ENDEAVORS

As noted in the discussion above, most studies indicate a correlation between GVH disease and a decreased relapse rate in some leukemias. Furthermore, measures to diminish GVH disease have generally resulted in an increased relapse rate. Finally, there has consistently been observed an increased relapse rate following syngeneic compared to allogeneic transplants. Despite some suggestive animal experiments and clinical observations, there is as yet no conclusive evidence that the GVL effect is mediated by a cell population that does not also contribute to GVH disease. In the future, there will doubtless be much effort to characterize cells that putatively mediate GVL and not GVH disease. The identification of such cells, their preservation in the graft after depletion of unwanted cells or in vitro cultivation, and adoptive transfer to transplant recipients would obviously be of major therapeutic importance. Efforts to engineer a marrow product ex vivo to deplete cell populations that mediated GVH disease, but enriched for NK cells or LAK cells, are directions that will be pursued, and these efforts are likely to resolve the controversy as to whether distinct cell populations mediate these phenomena.

However, such an ideal cell population may not exist and a more fruitful approach for adoptive immunity may be to identify antigens specific for, or enriched on, tumor cells. Large-scale cell-culture techniques are becoming available to generate large numbers of T cells with desired specificities that could be adoptively transferred to transplant recipients. Such cells may need $CD4^+$ helper T cells along with effector T cells to be effective. These transferred cells may be made more effective by genetically engineering them to upgrade their ability to secrete or respond to lymphokines such as interleukin-2 (IL-2).

It is probable that the targeted antigens are not foreign or specific to tumor cells (e.g., the public epitopes of class II MHC antigens recognized by self-reactive cells in syngeneic and chronic GVH disease). If this is the case and a transient reaction is desired, some means must be found to terminate the reaction. This might take the form of treatment with anti-idiotype antibody to the relevant T-cell receptors or the transfusion of specific suppressor cells raised in vitro that would downregulate or terminate the activity of the previously transfused effector cells.

Another posttransplant immunotherapy that will probably find earlier clinical application consists of treatment with antibody specific for TAA (as demonstrated in a rat BMT model of nonlymphocytic leukemia) (Wagner et al., 1989b), or anti-idiotype antibodies directed against clonal lymphoma and ALL cells. The efficacy of such humoral post-BMT treatments might be increased by linkage of the antibody to cellular toxins.

There is an ever-expanding array of cytokines with immunomodulatory properties becoming available for clinical investigation. Some of these factors may permit the augmentation of beneficial, antitumor immune responses following BMT at a time when the tumor burden is minimal. Such an approach may be particularly appealing after autologous BMT. Clinical trials presently underway will ascertain whether the deliberate creation of autologous GVH disease after autologous BMT will have an antitumor effect.

Other cytokines, their receptors, or antibodies to certain cytokines may offer the potential to ameliorate undesirable GVH responses after allogeneic BMT, by interrupting the amplification mechanisms involved in the pathogenesis of GVH disease. If these efforts are successful, use of cytokine cocktails may eventually enhance the immunotherapeutic aspects of BMT and make the procedure safer.

REFERENCES

Apperley JF, Jones L, Hale G, et al. Bone marrow transplantation for patients with chronic myeloid leukaemia: T cell depletion with Campath-1 reduces the incidence of graft-versus-host disease but may increase the risk of leukaemic relapse. Bone Marrow Transplant. 1986;1:53–66.

Atkinson K, Incefy GS, Storb R, et al. Low serum thymic levels in patients with chronic graft-versus-host disease. Blood. 1982;59:1073–1077.

Barnes DWH, Loutit JF. Spleen protection: the cellular hypothesis. In: Bacz ZM, ed. Radiobiology symposium Liege 1954. London: Butterworths; 1955:134–135.

Belanger R, Tutschka PJ, Beschorner WE, Santos GW, Hess AD. Acute graft-versus-host disease in recipients of syngeneic bone marrow. Exp Hematol. 1982;10(suppl):23–32.

Beschorner WE, Tutschka PJ, Santos GW. Chronic graft-versus-host disease in the rat radiation chimera. I. Clinical presentation, hematology, histology, and immunopathology in long-term chimeras. Transplantation. 1982;33:393–399.

Beschorner WE, Shinn CA, Fischer AC, Santos GW, Hess AD. Cyclosporine-induced pseudo-graft-versus-host disease in the early post-cyclosporine period. Transplantation. 1988a; 46(Suppl):112–117.

Beschorner WE, Suresch DL, Shinozawa T, Santos GW, Hess AD. Thymic immunopathology after cyclosporine: effect of irradiation and age on medullary involution and recovery. Transplant Proc. 1988b;20(suppl 3):1072–1978.

Billingham RE. The biology of graft-vs-host reactions. Harvey Lectures. 1966–1967;62:21–78.

Bortin MM, Rimm AA, Saltzstein EC. Graft-versus-leukemia: quantification of adoptive immunotherapy in murine leukemia. Science. 1973;179:811–813.

Bortin MM, Truitt RL, Rimm AA, Bach FH. Graft-versus-host reactivity induced by alloimmunization without augmentation of graft-versus-host reactivity. Nature. 1979;281:490–491.

Braine HG, Santos GW, Kaizer H, et al. Treatment of poor prognosis non-Hodgkin's lymphoma with cyclophosphamide and total body irradiation regimens with autologous bone marrow rescue. Bone Marrow Transplant. 1987;2:7–14.

Bross DS, Tutschka PJ, Farmer ER, et al. Predictive factors for acute graft-versus-host disease in patients transplanted with HLA-identical bone marrow. Blood. 1984;63:1265–1270.

Butturini A, Bortin MM, Gale RP. Graft-versus-leukemia following bone marrow transplantation. Bone Marrow Transplant. 1987;2:233–242.

Cheney RT, Sprent J. Capacity of cyclosporine to induce auto-graft-versus-host disease and impair intrathymic T cell differentiation. Transplant Proc. 1985;17:528–530.

Clift RA, Buckner CD, Thomas ED, et al. Treatment of chronic granulocytic leukaemia in chronic phase by allogeneic marrow transplantation. Lancet. 1982;2:621–623.

DeClerck Y, Draper V, Parkman R. Clonal analysis of murine graft-vs-host disease. II. Leukokines that stimulated fibroblast proliferation and collagen synthesis in graft-vs-host disease. J Immunol. 1986;136:3549–3552.

Deeg HJ, Storb R, Thomas ED, et al. Cyclosporine as prophylaxis for graft-versus-host disease: a randomized study in patients undergoing marrow transplantation for acute nonlymphoblastic leukemia. Blood. 1985;65:1325–1334.

Dokhelar MC, Wiels J, Lipinski M, et al. Natural killer cell activity in human bone marrow recipients. Early reappearance of peripheral natural killer activity in graft-versus-host disease. Transplantation. 1981;31:61–65.

Fefer A, Sullivan KM, Weiden P, et al. Graft versus leukemia effect in man: the relapse rate of syngeneic marrow transplantation. In: Truitt RL, Gale RP, Bortin MM, eds. Cellular immunotherapy of cancer. New York, NY: Alan R. Liss; 1987:401–408.

Foon KA, Todd RF. Immunologic classification of leukemia and lymphoma—review. Blood. 1986;68:1–31.

Gale RP, Champlin RE. How does bone marrow transplantation cure leukaemia? Lancet. 1984;2:28–30.

Geller RB, Saral R, Piantadosi S, et al. Allogeneic bone marrow transplantation following high-dose busulfan and cyclophosphamide in patients with acute nonlymphocytic leukemia. Blood. 1989a;73:2209–2218.

Geller RB, Esa AH, Beschorner WE, Frondoza CG, Santos GW, Hess AD. Successful in vitro graft-versus-tumor effect against an Ia-bearing tumor using cyclosporine-induced syngeneic graft-versus-host disease in the rat. Blood. 1989b;74:1165–1171.

Ghayur T, Seemayer TA, Kong Shaven PAL, Gartner JG, Lapp WS. Graft-vs-host reactions in the beige mice: an investigation of the role of host in donor natural killer cells in the pathogenesis of GVH disease. Transplantation. 1987;44:261–267.

Glazier A, Tutschka PJ, Farmer ER, Santos GW. Graft-versus-host disease in cyclosporine A-treated rats after syngeneic and autologous bone marrow reconstitution. J Exp Med. 1983a;158:1–8.

Glazier A, Tutschka PJ, Farmer ER. Studies on the immunobiology of syngeneic and autologous graft-versus-host disease in cyclosporine-treated rats. Transplant Proc. 1983b;15(suppl 1): 3035–3041.

Gluckman E, Devergie A, Sohier J, Saurat JH. Graft-versus host in recipients of syngeneic bone marrow. Lancet. 1980;1:253–254.

Glucksberg H, Storb R, Fefer A, et al. Clinical manifestations of graft-versus-host disease in human recipients of marrow from HLA-matched sibling donors. Transplantation. 1974; 18:295–304.

Goldman JM, Gale RP, Horowitz MM, et al. Bone marrow transplantation for chronic myelogenous leukemia in chronic phase: increased risk of relapse associated with T-cell depletion. Ann Intern Med. 1988;108:806–814.

Goulmy G, Blokland E, Gratama JW, Zwaan FE, van Rood JJ. Detection of minor histocompatibility antigens by MHC restricted cytotoxic T lymphocytes generated during graft-versus-host disease. Exp Hematol. 1984;12:77.

Greenberg PD, Cheever MA, Fefer A. Eradication of disseminated murine leukemia by chemoimmunotherapy with cyclophosphamide and adoptively transferred immune syngeneic Lyt-1^+2^- lymphocytes. J Exp Med. 1981;154:952–963.

Guillen FJ, Ferrara J, Hancock WW, et al. Acute cutaneous graft-vs-host disease to minor histocompatibility antigens in a murine model. Evidence that large granular lymphocytes are effector cells in the immune response. Lab Invest. 1986;55:35–42.

Hercend T, Takvorian T, Nowill A, et al. Characterization of natural killer cells with antileukemia activity following allogeneic bone marrow transplantation. Blood. 1986;67:722–728.

Hess AD, Fischer AC. Immune mechanisms in cyclosporine-induced syngeneic graft-versus-host disease. Transplantation. 1989;48:895–900.

Hess AD, Horwitz L, Beschorner WE, Santos GW. Development graft-versus-host disease-like syndrome in cyclosporine-treated rats after syngeneic bone marrow transplantation: I. Development of cytotoxic T lymphocytes with apparent polyclonal anti-Ia specificity including autoreactivity. J Exp Med. 1985;161:718–730.

Hess AD, Fischer AC, Vogelsang GB, Beschorner WE, Santos GW. Syngeneic graft-versus-host disease; failure of self/non-self discrimination. In: Baum SW, Santos GW, Takaku F, eds. Experimental hematology today. New York, NY: Springer-Verlag; 1987:12–17.

Hess AD, Vogelsang GB, Silanskis M, Friedman KA, Beschorner WE, Santos GW. Syngeneic graft-versus-host disease after allogeneic bone marrow transplantation and cyclosporine treatment. Transplant Proc. 1988;20(suppl 3):487–492.

Hood AF, Vogelsang GB, Black LP, Farmer ER, Santos GW. Acute graft-versus-host disease: development following autologous and syngeneic bone marrow transplantation. Arch Dermatol. 1987;123:745–750.

Horowitz MM, Gale RP, Sondel PM, et al. Graft-versus-leukemia reactions after bone marrow transplantation. Blood. 1990;75:555–562.

Jones JM, Wilson R, Bealmear PM. Mortality and gross pathology of secondary disease in germ-free mouse radiation chimeras. Radiat Res. 1971;45:577–588.

Jones RJ, Hess AD, Mann RB, et al. Preliminary communication: induction of graft-versus-host disease after autologous bone marrow transplantation. Lancet. 1989;1:754–757.

Jones RJ, Piantadosi S, Mann RB, et al. Bone marrow transplantation for relapsed Hodgkin's disease. J Clin Oncol. 1990;8:527–537.

Korngold R, Sprent J. Features of T cells causing H-2-restricted lethal graft-versus-host disease across minor histocompatibility barriers. J Exp Med. 1982;152:872–883.

MacDonald HR. Mechanisms of immunological tolerance. Science. 1989;246:982.

Martin PJ, Hansen JA, Buckner CD, et al. Effects of in vitro depletion of T cells in HLA-identical allogeneic marrow grafts. Blood. 1985;66:664–672.

Mathe G, Amiel L, Schwarzenberg L, Cattan A, Schneider M. Adoptive immunotherapy of acute leukemia: experimental and clinical results. Cancer Res. 1965;25:1525–1531.

Merritt CB, Mann DL, Rogentine GN. Cytotoxic antibody for epithelial cells in human graft-versus-host disease. Nature. 1971;232:638–639.

Muller C, Schuch K, Pawelec G, Wilms K, Wernet P. Immunohistology of graft-versus-host disease mediated skin lesions and its correlations to a large granular lymphocyte surface phenotype and function. Blut. 1982;44:89–94.

Parkman R. Clonal analysis of murine graft-versus-host disease. I. Phenotypic and functional analysis of T lymphocyte clones. J Immunol. 1986;136:3543–3548.

Pollard CM, Chang CF, Srivastava KK. The role of microflora in development of graft-versus-host disease. Transplant Proc. 1976;8:533–536.

Pollard CM, Powles RL, Millar JL, et al. Leukaemic relapse following Campath I treated bone marrow transplantation for leukaemia. Lancet. 1986;2:1343–1344.

Powles R, Pedrazzini A, Crofts M, Clink H, Millar J, Bhattia G, Perez D. Mismatched family bone marrow transplantation. Semin Hematol. 1984;21:182–187.

Rappeport J, Reinherz E, Mihm M, Lopansri S, Parkman R. Acute graft-versus-host disease in recipients of bone-marrow transplants from identical twin donors. Lancet. 1979;2:717–720.

Reinsmoen NL, Kersey JH, Bach FH. Detection of HLA restricted anti-minor histocompatibility antigens reactive cells from skin GVHD lesions. Hum Immunol. 1984;11:249–257.

Rodt H, Kolb HJ, Netzel B, et al. Munich Cooperative Groups of BMT: effect of anti–T-cell globulin on GVHD in leukemic patients treated with BMT. Transplant Proc. 1981;13:257.

Sanders JE, Flournoy N, Thomas ED, et al. Marrow transplant experience in children with acute lymphoblastic leukemia: an analysis of factors associated with survival, relapse and graft-versus-host disease. Med Pediatr Oncol. 1985;13:165–172.

Santos GW. Application of marrow grafts in human disease: its problems and potential. In: Hanna MG Jr, ed. Contemporary topics in immunobiology, Vol. 1. New York, NY: Plenum Press; 1972:143–177.

Santos GW. History of bone marrow transplantation. Clin Haematol. 1983;12:611–639.

Santos GW. Syngeneic or autologous graft-versus-host disease. Int J Cell Cloning. 1989;7: 92–99.

Santos GW, Hess AD, Vogelsang GB. Graft-versus-host reactions and disease. Immunol Rev. 1985;88:169–192.

Santos GW, Tutschka PJ, Brookmeyer R, et al. Cyclosporine plus methylprednisolone versus cyclophosphamide plus methylprednisolone as prophylaxis for graft-versus-host disease: a randomized double-blind study in patients undergoing allogeneic marrow transplantation. Clin Transplant. 1987;1:21–28.

Seddik M, Seemayer TA, Lapp WS. T cell function defect associated with thymic epithelial cell injury induced by a graft-versus-host reaction. Transplantation. 1980;29:61–66.

Shulman HM, Sullivan KM, Weiden PL, et al. Chronic graft-versus-host syndrome in man. A long-term clinicopathologic study of 20 Seattle patients. Am J Med. 1980;69:204–217.

Slavin RE, Santos GW. The graft-versus-host reaction in man after bone marrow transplantation: Pathology, pathogenesis, clinical features, and implication. Clin Immunol Immunopathol. 1973;1:472–498.

Slavin S, Waldeman H, Or, GC, et al. Prevention of graft-versus-host disease in allogeneic bone marrow transplantation for leukemia by T cell depletion in vitro prior to transplantation. Transplant Proc. 1985;17:465–467.

Sorokin R, Kimura H, Schroder K, Wilson DH, Wilson DB. Cyclosporine-induced autoimmunity. Conditions for expressing disease, requirement for intact thymus, and potency estimates of autoimmune lymphocyte in drug-treated rats. J Exp Med. 1986;164:1615–1625.

Stoch S, Gale RP, Champlin R, Ho W, Falk PM, Feig SA. Partially mismatched marrow transplantation for acute leukemia and aplastic anemia. In: Gale RP, ed. Recent advances in bone marrow transplantation. New York, NY: Alan R. Liss; 1983:785–795.

Storb R, Thomas ED. Graft-versus-host disease in dog and man; the Seattle experience. Immunol Rev. 1985;88:215–238.

Storb R, Prentice RL, Thomas ED. Treatment of aplastic anemia by marrow transplantation from HLA-identical siblings; prognostic factors associated with graft-versus-host disease and survival. J Clin Invest. 1977;59:625–632.

Storb R, Prentice RL, Buckner CD, et al. Graft-versus-host disease and survival in patients with aplastic anemia treated by marrow grafts from HLA-identical siblings. Beneficial effect of a protective environment. New Engl J Med. 1983a;308:302–307.

Storb R, Prentice RL, Hansen JA, Thomas ED. Association between HLA-B antigens and acute graft-versus-host disease. Lancet. 1983b;2:816–819.

Storb R, Prentice RL, Sullivan KM. Predictive factors for chronic graft-versus-host disease in patients with aplastic anemia treated by marrow transplantation from HLA-identical siblings. Ann Intern Med. 1983c;98:461–466.

Storb R, Deeg J, Whitehead J, et al. Methotrexate and cyclosporine compared with cyclosporine alone for prophylaxis of acute graft-versus-host disease after marrow transplantation for leukemia. New Engl J Med. 1986;314:729–735.

Storb R, Deeg HJ, Fisher L, et al. Cyclosporine methotrexate for graft-versus-host disease prevention in patients given marrow grafts for leukemia: long-term follow-up of three controlled trials. Blood. 1988;71:293–298.

Storb R, Deeg HJ, Pepe M, et al. Methotrexate and cyclosporine versus cyclosporine alone for prophylaxis of graft-versus-host disease in patients given HLA-identical marrow grafts for leukemia: long-term follow-up of a controlled trial. Blood. 1989;73:1729–1734.

Sullivan KM. Graft-versus-host disease. In: Blume KG, Petz LD, eds. Clinical bone marrow transplantation. New York, NY: Churchill Livingstone;1983:91–130.

Sullivan KM. Acute and chronic graft-versus-host disease in man. Int J Cell Cloning. 1986; 4:42–93.

Sullivan KM, Fefer A, Witherspoon R, et al. Graft-versus-leukemia in man: relationship of acute and chronic graft-versus-host disease to relapse of acute leukemia following allogeneic bone marrow transplantation. In: Truitt RL, Bortin MM, Gale RP, eds. Cellular immunotherapy of cancer. New York, NY: Alan R. Liss; 1987:391–399.

Sullivan KM, Witherspoon RP, Storb R, et al. Prednisone and azathioprine compared with prednisone and placebo for treatment of chronic graft-versus-host disease: prognostic influence of prolonged thrombocytopenia after allogeneic marrow transplantation. Blood. 1988; 72:546–554.

Sullivan KM, Storb R, Buckner CD, et al. Graft-versus-host disease as adoptive immunotherapy in patients with advanced hematologic neoplasms. New Engl J Med. 1989a;320:828–834.

Sullivan KM, Storb WR, Witherspoon RP, et al. Influence of acute and chronic graft-versus-host disease on relapse and survival after bone marrow transplantation from HLA-identical siblings as treatment of acute and chronic leukemia. Blood. 1989b;73:1720–1728.

Thein SL, Goldman JH, Galton DAG. Acute 'graft-versus-host disease' after autografting for chronic granulocytic leukemia in transformation. Ann Intern Med. 1981;94:210–211.

Truitt RL, Shih CY, LeFever AV, Tempelis LD, Andreani M, Bortin MM. Characterization of alloimmunization-induced T lymphocytes reactive against AKR leukemia in vitro and correlation with graft-vs-leukemia activity in vivo. J Immunol. 1983;131:2050–2058.

Tsoi MS. Immunological mechanisms of graft-versus-host disease in man. Transplantation. 1982;33:459–464.

Tsoi MS, Storb R, Dobbs S, Kopecky KJ, et al. Nonspecific suppressor cells in patients with chronic graft-versus-host disease after marrow grafting. J Immunol. 1979;123:1970–1976.

Tutschka PJ. Graft-versus-host disease: immunobiological aspects. Hematol Blood Transfusion. 1983;28:97–101.

Tutschka PJ, Bortin MM. Graft-versus-host disease. Transplant Proc. 1981;13:1267–1269.

Tutsckha PJ, Hess AD, Beschorner W, Santos GW. Suppressor cells in transplantation tolerance. I. Suppressor cells in the mechanism of tolerance in radiation chimeras. Transplantation. 1981a;32:203–209.

Tutschka PJ, Ki PF, Beschorner WE, Hess AD, Santos GW. Suppressor cells in transplantation tolerance. II. Maturation of suppressor cells in the bone marrow chimera. Transplantation. 1981b;32:321–325.

Tutschka PJ, Teasdall R, Beschorner WE, Santos GW. Chronic graft-versus-host disease in the rat radiation chimera. II. Immunological evaluation in long term chimeras. Transplantation. 1982;34:289–294.

Van Bekkum DW, de Vries JJ. Radiation chimeras. London: Logos; 1967.

Van Bekkum DW, Roodenburg J, Heidt PJ, van der Waaij D. Mitigation of secondary disease of allogeneic mouse radiation chimeras by modification of the intestinal microflora. J Natl Cancer Inst. 1974;52:401–404.

Vogelsang GB, Hess AD, Berkman AW, et al. An in vitro predictive test for graft-versus-host disease in patients with genotypic HLA-identical bone marrow transplants. New Engl J Med. 1985;313:645–650.

Vogelsang GB, Hess AD, Santos GW. Acute graft-versus-host disease: clinical characteristics in the cyclosporine era. Medicine. 1988;67:163–174.

Vogelsang GB, Jones RJ, Hess AD, Geller RB, Schuchter L, Santos GW. Induction of autologous graft-versus-host disease. Transplantation. 1989;21:2997–2998.

Wagner JE Jr, Vogelsang GB, Beschorner WE. Pathogenesis and pathology of graft-versus-host disease. Am J Pediatr Hematol Oncol. 1989a;11:196–212.

Wagner JE Jr, Johnson RJ, Santos, Kim BK, Shin HS. Systemic monoclonal antibody therapy for eliminating minimal residual leukemia in a rat bone marrow model. Blood. 1989b; 73:614–618.

Weiden PL, Flournoy N, Thomas ED. Antileukemic effect of graft-versus-host disease in human recipients of allogeneic marrow grafts. New Engl J Med. 1979;300:1068–1073.

Weiden PL, Sullivan KM, Flournoy N, Storb R, Thomas ED. Antileukemic effect of chronic graft-versus-host disease. Med Intell. 1981;304:1529–1533.

Weisdorf DJ, Nesbit ME, Ramsay KC, et al. Allogeneic bone marrow transplantation for acute lymphoblastic leukemia in remission: prolonged survival associated with acute graft-versus-host disease. J Clin Oncol. 1987;5:1348–1355.

Weksler ME, Moody CE, Kozak RW. The autologous mixed lymphocyte reaction. Adv Immunol. 1981;31:271–312.

Wingard JR. Advances in the management of infectious complications after bone marrow transplantation. Bone Marrow Transplant. 1990;6:371–383.

Wingard JR, Chen DY, Burns WH, et al. Cytomegalovirus infection after autologous bone marrow transplantation with comparison to infection after allogeneic bone marrow transplantation. Blood. 1988a;71:1432–1437.

Wingard JR, Mellits ED, Sostrin MB, et al. Interstitial pneumonitis after allogeneic bone marrow transplantation. Nine-year experience at a single institution. Medicine. 1988b;67:175–186.

Wingard JR, Piantadosi S, Vogelsang GB, et al. Predictors of death from chronic graft-versus-host disease after bone marrow transplantation. Blood. 1989;74:1428–1435.

Wingard JR, Piantadosi S, Santos GW, et al. Allogeneic bone marrow transplantation for patients with high-risk acute lymphoblastic leukemia. J Clin Oncol. 1990a;8:820–830.

Wingard JR, Piantadosi S, Burns WH, et al. Cytomegalovirus infections in patients treated by intensive cytoreductive therapy with marrow transplant. Rev Infect Dis. 1990b;12(suppl 7):793–803.

Witherspoon R, Lum L, Storb R. Immunologic reconstitution after human marrow grafting. Semin Hematol. 1984;21:2–10.

INDEX